Lippincott Professional Guides

Medical terms & abbreviations

Second Edition

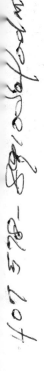

 LIPPINCOTT WILLIAMS & WILKINS
A **Wolters Kluwer** Company

Philadelphia • Baltimore • New York • London
Buenos Aires • Hong Kong • Sydney • Tokyo

Staff

Publisher
Judith A. Schilling McCann, RN, MSN

Editorial Director
David Moreau

Clinical Director
Joan M. Robinson, RN, MSN

Senior Art Director
Arlene Putterman

Clinical Editor
Beverly Ann Tscheschlog, RN, BS

Editor
Juliet McCleery

Copy Editors
Peggy Williams (copy supervisor),
Kimberly Bilotta, Heather Ditch,
Judith Orioli, Patricia Turkington,
Pamela Wingrod

Designers
Mary Ludwicki (art director),
Lynn Foulk

Illustrators
Julie Devito, Dan Fione, Jean Gardner,
John Gist, Francis Grobelny,
Bob Jackson, Bob Jones, BJ Krim,
Bob Neumann, Judy Newhouse

Electronic Production Services
Diane Paluba (manager),
Joyce Rossi Biletz, Richard Eng

Manufacturing
Patricia K. Dorshaw (senior manager),
Beth Janae Orr

Editorial Assistants
Danielle J. Barsky, Beverly Lane,
Linda Ruhf

LPGMT2–D
04 03 02   10 9 8 7 6 5 4 3 2

Library of Congress Cataloging-in-Publication Data

Medical terms & abbreviations. — 2nd ed.
    p. ; cm. — (Lippincott professional guides)
    Rev. ed. of: Medical terms and abbreviations. c1998.
    1. Medicine — 1. Terminology. 2. Medicine —
Abbreviations.
[DNLM: 1. Terminology. 2. Abbreviations. W 15 M489
2002] I. Title: Medical terms and abbreviations. II. Series.
R123 .M396 2002
610'.1'4—dc21
ISBN 1-58255-182-0 (alk. paper)   2001050827

Contents

Contributors   iv

Foreword   v

Medical terms and abbreviations
A through Z   **1**

Appendices   331

Contributors

Gary J. Arnold, MD, FACS
Associate Professor
University of Louisiana
Lafayette

Michelle Green, RHIA, CMA, CTR, MPS
Professor
Alfred (N.Y.) State College

Manuel D. Leal, PA-C, MPAS
Department Head
Naval Medical Clinic
Pearl Harbor, Hawaii

Paul J. Mathews, PhD, RRT, FCCM, FCCP
Associate Professor–Respiratory care
University of Kansas — School of Allied Health
Kansas City

Barbara Maxwell, RNC, MSN, CNS
Nursing Instructor
State University of New York at Ulster
Stone Ridge

Lourdes "Cindy" Santoni-Reddy, MSN, MeD, FAAPM, CPP, CRNP
Faculty/Nurse Practitioner
Frankford Hospital School of Nursing
Philadelphia

Suzanne P. Weaver, RN, RHIT, CPHQ
Director of Nursing
Neshaminy Manor
Warrington, Pa.

Foreword

In our home, we have a dog-eared dictionary that's used almost daily by someone in our family. When my husband is reading Faulkner or when our children are doing homework, it isn't unusual to see someone flip through the dictionary or to hear someone respond, "Look it up."

Medical terms and abbreviations, however, are rarely included in most dictionaries, or, if they are, the definitions are so limited that the meaning is still unclear. A medical dictionary that can fill this gap is essential for students and practitioners in health professions.

Lippincott Professional Guides: Medical Terms & Abbreviations, Second Edition, is a comprehensive storehouse of medical terms and abbreviations, listed in alphabetical order, with clear, concise definitions. The narrative is complemented by diagrams of anatomical features and by charts depicting complex processes, such as lipoprotein synthesis and metabolism.

New features in this second edition highlight information of special importance. Throughout the text, "Clinical tips" assist your understanding of the clinical relevance of a particular term. For example, after the definition for "primary tuberculosis," the clinical tip points out that infants are most susceptible to this disease. The "Alert" logo explains why the pertinent disease or condition is of concern. The "Time line" logo points to a concern that's related to a specific age-group, such as the adolescent patient or the older adult. These added features further enhance your understanding of the clinical relevance and meaning of the medical term.

To further support your learning and retention, the appendices include a listing of medical roots, prefixes, and suffixes along with their meanings. An understanding of these common parts of medical terms enables you to successfully interpret each part of the word and put the parts together to grasp the term's essential meaning. The English-Spanish translator lists the most common anatomic terms, symptoms, and conditions alphabetically in English, next to its corresponding Spanish term. A handy table of metric equivalents rounds out the volume.

Clearly, *Lippincott Professional Guides: Medical Terms & Abbreviations* is a must for health care professionals and students. Packed with a wealth of information yet small and convenient to carry, it serves as a quick, easy-to-use reference at school, in the home, or in the clinical setting.

Cheryl T. Samuels, PhD
Dean, College of Health Sciences
Old Dominion University
Norfolk, Va.

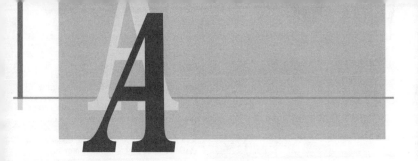

a Symbol for arterial blood.

A Symbol for alveolar gas.

AAB *abbr* American Association of Bioanalysts.

AABB *abbr* American Association of Blood Banks.

AACC *abbr* American Association of Clinical Chemistry.

AACP *abbr* American Associations of Colleges of Pharmacy.

AADS *abbr* American Association of Dental Schools.

AAMA *abbr* American Association of Medical Assistants.

AAMT *abbr* American Association for Music Therapy.

AANNT *abbr* American Association of Nephrology Nurses and Technicians.

AAOHN *abbr* American Association of Occupational Health Nurses.

AAP *abbr* American Association of Pathologists.

AAPA *abbr* American Academy of Physicians' Assistants.

AAPC *abbr* American Association of Professional Coders.

AAPMR *abbr* American Academy of Physical Medicine and Rehabilitation.

AARC *abbr* American Association for Respiratory Care.

AART *abbr* American Association for Respiratory Therapy.

AATA *abbr* **1.** American Art Therapy Association. **2.** American Athletic Trainers Association.

AAV *abbr* adenoassociated virus; adenovirus-associated virus.

abalienation **1.** A state of mental derangement or insanity. **2.** A condition of physical decay.

abandonment of care In law: wrongful failure to continue to provide medical care to a patient (usually by a physician).

abarticular **1.** Describing a site distant from a joint. **2.** Not affecting a joint.

abasia Inability to walk.

abaxial **1.** Describing a position outside the line of axis of the body or of a structure.

2. Pertaining to a location opposite a structure.

abdomen The portion of the trunk between the thorax and the pelvis that contains the major visceral organs: the lower part of the esophagus, the stomach, the intestines, the liver, the spleen, and the pancreas.

abdominal aorta The portion of the descending aorta that lies in the abdomen and conveys blood to body structures below the diaphragm. Its branches are the celiac, superior mesenteric, inferior mesenteric, middle suprarenals, renals, testicular, ovarian, inferior phrenics, lumbars, middle sacral, and common iliacs.

abdominal aponeurosis The point at which the tendons of the oblique and transverse muscles of the abdomen join.

abdominal binder A wide bandage, often elastic, that's placed on the lower portion of the trunk to support the abdomen; for example, a scultetus binder.

abdominal fistula An abnormal, tube-like passage leading from a structure in the abdomen to the surface of the body.

abdominal hernia The protrusion of a loop of bowel through the muscles of the abdominal wall. Also called *ventral hernia.*

abdominal pregnancy An extrauterine pregnancy in the abdominal cavity, usually caused by expulsion of a fertilized ovum from a ruptured fallopian tube.

 ALERT Abdominal pregnancy occurs in about 0.01% of all pregnancies and in about 2% of ectopic pregnancies. It results in fetal death in roughly 90% of cases.

abdominal pulse The pulse in the abdominal aorta.

abdominal reflex A superficial reflex characterized by contraction of the muscles of the abdominal wall when the abdomen is firmly stroked; specifically, the umbilicus moves toward the stimulated area. Absence of this reflex typifies pyramidal tract diseases and disorders.

abdominal surgery Any procedure in which an incision is made into the abdomen.

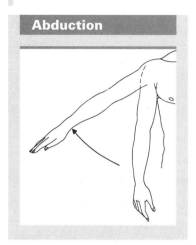

Abduction

abdominoscopy   A diagnostic procedure in which the abdominal cavity is directly examined under magnification by means of a lighted tube inserted through a small incision.

abducens nerve   One of a pair of motor nerves (the sixth cranial nerves) arising from the pons that control movement of the lateral rectus muscle of the eye. Also called **nervus abducens.**

abduct   To move away from the body.

abduction   Movement of an arm or a leg away from the axis of the body.

abduction boots   Casts placed on the lower extremities, connected by a bar at the ankle, which allow hip abduction. They're usually used to promote correct positioning after orthopedic surgery on adductor muscles in the hip or after repair of certain structures of the lower extremities.

abductor   A muscle or other structure that moves an extremity away from the axis of the body.

Abernethy's sarcoma   A cancerous tumor, usually on the trunk, that's composed of fat cells.

aberrant   Deviating from the usual, expected, or normal; may refer to structures in the body or to atypical organisms or individuals in a species.

aberrant conduction   Abnormal pathway of an impulse traveling through the heart's conduction system.

aberrant ductule   A remnant of the tubules of the mesonephros, an excretory structure in the developing male embryo located near the epididymis. A similar structure, the paraoophoron, occurs in the female. Also called *ductulus aberrans.*

aberrant goiter   Enlargement of an ectopic or supernumerary thyroid gland.

abetalipoproteinemia   An inherited disorder of fat metabolism marked by scarcity or absence of serum low-density lipoproteins, the presence of acanthocytes in the blood, and abnormally small amounts of blood cholesterol. The severe form of the disorder may cause retinitis pigmentosa, steatorrhea, voluntary muscle incoordination, and nystagmus.

abiogenesis   A theory of spontaneous generation proposing that living matter can arise from inorganic matter.

abiosis   A condition that's incompatible with life.

abiotrophy   A genetically determined, age-related premature loss of vitality or degeneration of certain cells and tissues.

ablation   The removal or deliberate functional destruction of a body part, such as by amputation or removal of a growth.

abnerval current   An electric current that moves through a muscle fiber in a direction away from the site where the nerve fiber enters.

abnormal behavior   Actions that deviate from the usual and generally acceptable societal norms; typically refers to maladaptive or detrimental actions ranging from inability to cope with a stressful circumstance to serious displays of mental derangement.

abnormal psychology   A branch of psychology devoted to the study of neuroses, psychoses, and other mental and emotional disorders; maladaptive behavior; and normal but poorly understood phenomena, such as dreams, hypnosis, and other altered states of consciousness.

ABO blood groups   The most commonly used system of classifying human blood, based on the presence or absence of certain antigens on the surface of red blood cells. The four blood types are A, B, AB, and O. Both the A and the B antigens are present in type AB blood, whereas neither the A nor the B antigen is present in type O blood. Each blood type has corresponding antibodies, or agglutinins, to the red cell antigens that they lack: those with type A blood have anti-B agglutinin; those with type B blood have anti-A agglutinin; those with type AB blood have neither of the two agglutinins; and those with type O blood have both.

 ALERT Determining blood type is critically important when blood transfusions must be performed.

aborted systole   A premature or weak contraction of the heart that isn't associated with a peripheral pulse.

abortifacient   Any agent or condition that causes abortion.

abortion   The spontaneous or deliberate interruption of a pregnancy before about 20 weeks' gestation, by which time the fetus has developed sufficiently to be expected to survive outside the womb.

abortion-on-demand   A term used to describe a woman's right to request and receive an abortion, provided that the pregnancy is terminated within the time frame specified by law.

abortus fever   An infectious disease caused by *Brucella abortus,* a bacterium that causes abortion in infected cattle. Humans may become infected by drinking the milk or handling the meat of an infected cow, or through contact with the feces of an infected animal. Brucellosis caused by this species is the only form of the disease endemic to North America. Also called *Rio Grande fever.*

abouchement   The junction of a small blood vessel with a large one.

abrachia   The congenital absence of arms.

abrasion   **1.** The removal of superficial layers of skin or mucous tissue by wearing, rubbing, or scraping, either through accidental trauma or for therapeutic purposes (such as in dermabrasion). **2.** The wearing away of a surface, such as the enamel of a tooth, from normal use.

abreaction   A catharsis or emotional release that results when painful, previously repressed memories are brought into consciousness or mentally relived.

abrosia   Abstinence from food; fasting.

abruptio placentae   Premature separation of a normally positioned placenta in a pregnancy of at least 20 weeks' gestation, either before labor or during labor but before delivery. This serious complication of pregnancy, occurring in one of every 200 births and often resulting in hemorrhage, may lead to the death of the mother, the fetus, or both. Also called *ablatio placentae, accidental hemorrhage.*

abscess   A cavity of pus within a circumscribed area of inflammation, resulting from an acute or chronic localized (commonly staphylococcal) infection, or a cavity of pus within solid tissue. Abscesses on or near the surface of skin or mucosal tissue may drain spontaneously, followed by healing; incision of the abscess speeds the healing process. With a deeper abscess, formation of a sinus tract allows pus to drain to the surface.

absence seizure   A seizure marked by a sudden, momentary loss of consciousness, typically accompanied by cessation of voluntary muscle movement and a vacant facial expression. Sometimes this seizure also causes spasms or twitching of the muscles of the head, neck, or arms. Absence seizures can occur many times a day with no warning aura; children and adolescents are most commonly affected. Formerly called *petit mal seizure.*

absent without leave (AWOL)   In psychiatry: a term describing a patient who leaves a psychiatric facility without proper authorization.

absolute alcohol   Ethyl alcohol containing 0.5% water or less by volume. Also called *dehydrated alcohol.*

absolute growth   The total increase in the size of an organism or a part of an organism.

absorb   To take in or assimilate.

absorbable gauze   A gauzelike material derived from oxidized cellulose that can be absorbed by the body. It's placed directly on bleeding tissue for hemostasis.

absorbable gelatin sponge   A local hemostatic agent.

absorbed dose   In radiotherapy: the energy per unit mass absorbed by matter as a result of exposure to ionizing radiation. The absorbed dose is measured in units called *rads* or, in the SI system, *grays;* one rad equals 100 ergs per gram.

absorbent gauze   Gauze used to absorb fluids.

absorption   **1.** The taking in or incorporation of gas, liquid, light, or heat. **2.** In physiology: the passage of any substance across and into cells or tissues. **3.** In radiology: the uptake of radiant energy by the organic or inorganic matter through which it passes.

abstinence   Voluntary avoidance of certain foods, alcoholic beverages, or sexual activities.

abstract   A summary of a scientific article, literary work, or oral presentation.

abstract thinking   Thinking that isn't limited to actual concrete experience; includes engagement in fantasies, idealism, and reasoning about hypothetical possibilities. Abstract thinking is essential to logical problem solving.

> **TIME LINE**   Promoted and enhanced by education, abstract thinking usually develops between ages 11 and 15.

abulia, aboulia   An impairment or loss of the ability to engage in voluntary acts or to make decisions.

abuse   **1.** Behavior toward another that's offensive, harmful, or injurious. **2.** Misuse or particularly excessive use of a substance, service, or equipment; commonly refers to improper use of a drug or similar substance.

abuse of process   In law: a civil action characterized by the allegation that the legal system has been used improperly. A health practitioner might use this action when attempting to countersue a patient.

a.c. *abbr* Latin *ante cibum,* before meals; used in drug prescriptions.

Ac Symbol for actinium.

AC *abbr* alternating current.

academic ladder The system of appointments in a college or university through which a faculty member advances from instructor, to assistant professor, to associate professor and, finally, to professor.

acampsia Stiffening or rigidity of a joint.

acantha A spine or a spurlike projection.

acanthocyte An abnormal red blood cell having numerous spiny projections of cytoplasm, typically present in large numbers in abetalipoproteinemia.

acanthocytosis A condition in which most of an individual's red blood cells are acanthocytes. With abetalipoproteinemia, up to 80% of red cells are acanthocytes. Also called *Bassen-Kornzweig syndrome.*

acanthoma A benign or cancerous tumor composed of epidermal or squamous cells.

acanthosis Abnormal thickening of the cells of the stratum spinosum of the skin, as in eczema and psoriasis.

acanthosis nigricans A skin condition marked by velvety, warty, hyperpigmented growths under the arms, on the neck, in the anogenital area, and in the groin. Usually benign, the condition may be associated with obesity, endocrine disorders, or GI tract cancer.

acardia Congenital absence of the heart. This rare anomaly may be seen in the smaller of conjoined twins who survived by depending on the other's blood supply in utero.

acardius, acardiacus A fetus lacking a heart. Also called *fetus acardiacus.*

acardius acephalus A fetus without a heart who also lacks a head and most of the upper part of the body.

acardius acormus An acardiac fetus in which the head, arms, and legs have failed to develop. Also called *acardius amorphus.*

acariasis Any disease, usually a skin infestation, caused by mites.

acarid A mite; a member of the order Acarina, which also includes ticks. Acarids cause mange in animals and skin diseases in birds. In humans, acarids may directly damage the skin or other tissue, may cause blood loss or loss of other fluids, and may serve as intermediate hosts of disease-causing organisms. An example is the larval form of the trombiculid mite, which acts as a vector for scrub typhus and other rickettsial organisms.

acceleration 1. An increase in the speed of an object or reaction. 2. The rate of increase in speed over a unit of time.

acceleration phase The first period of active labor, as documented on a Friedman curve, in which the rate of dilation of the cervical os increases.

acceptable daily intake (ADI) The maximum amount of any substance that a human being can safely ingest.

acceptance The final stage of death and dying, described by thanatologist Dr. Elisabeth Kübler-Ross, during which the dying person comes to terms with impending death, becomes progressively dissociated from the outside world, and gradually decreases the amount of verbal communication.

acceptor 1. A compound that receives a chemical group from another compound. 2. An individual who receives the blood, organ, or tissue of another individual (donor).

accessory 1. In anatomy: an organ, structure, or tissue that assists other structures in performing a particular function, as the accessory muscles of respiration. 2. A device or piece of equipment that provides or enhances convenience or safety.

 ALERT If the patient displays increased accessory muscle use, immediately look for signs of respiratory distress.

 TIME LINE Because of age-related loss of elasticity in the rib cage, accessory muscle use may be part of the older person's normal breathing pattern.

accessory chromosome An extra chromosome found in wild populations of some species and animals with no apparent influence on the phenotypic effect.

accessory nerve Either of a pair of cranial nerves supplying the muscles of the pharynx, larynx, and soft palate and sternocleidomastoid and trapezius muscles, and which permit speech, swallowing, and certain movements of the head and shoulders. Each nerve is rooted in both the sides of the medulla and in the cervical spine. Also called *eleventh cranial nerve, nervus accessorius, spinal accessory nerve.*

accessory pancreatic duct The double-branched duct at the head of the pancreas; one branch joins the pancreatic duct and the other opens into the duodenum.

accessory phrenic nerve A nerve strand that arises from the fifth cervical nerve and passes downward to join the phrenic nerve at the base of the neck or in the chest.

ACCH *abbr* Association for the Care of Children's Health.

acclimation, acclimatization Physiologic adjustment to a change in climate, such as a different temperature or altitude.

accommodation   **1.** The act or process of adapting to changes in the physiologic or psychological environment to maintain homeostasis. **2.** In ophthalmology: adjustment of the lens of the eye for various distances. **3.** In sociology: the use of compromise, arbitration, or negotiation to resolve conflicts between persons or groups that arise from differences in customs or cultural norms. Also called *adjustment.*

accommodation reflex   The adjustment made by the eyes to focus on near objects, consisting of three actions that change the path of light rays reaching the retina: pupil constriction, ciliary muscle contraction that causes increased rounding of the lens, and convergence of the eyes. Also called *ciliary reflex.*

accomplishment quotient   A numerical device, expressed as a ratio times 100, used to describe an individual's achievement age as compared with mental age.

accouchement   The time or process of childbirth.

accouchement forcé   Rapid delivery of a fetus by means of forcible dilation of the cervix.

 ALERT Because of the danger associated with this procedure, accouchement forcé is no longer used.

accountability   The obligation to accept responsibility for or account for one's actions.

accreditation   The process of recognizing an individual, an institution, or a program as conforming to a certain set of standards, such as the accreditation of a hospital by the Joint Commission on Accreditation of Healthcare Organizations (JCAHO).

accrementition   An increase in the size or amount of tissue through the addition of similar tissue. Examples are cellular division and budding.

accretio cordis   Adhesion of the pericardium to the anatomic structures surrounding the heart.

accretion   **1.** An increase in the size or amount of tissue by the addition of similar tissue; accrementition. **2.** The process of parts gradually growing together. **3.** The accumulation of foreign material, such as plaque on the surface of a tooth or in a cavity.

accretionary growth   An increase in size brought about by the accumulation of new tissue through mitosis or the addition of material similar to the existing material.

acedia   A state of apathy or boredom, manifested as listlessness, lack of demonstrated emotion, and slow mental processes.

acelius   A fetus in which the body cavity is absent.

acentric   **1.** Without a center. **2.** In genetics: a chromosome fragment lacking a centromere.

acephalobrachia   Congenital absence of the head and both arms.

acephalus   A fetus in which the head is absent or improperly developed.

acephaly, acephalia, acephalism   Congenital absence or defective development of the head.

acetabulum, *pl.* **acetabula**   The cup-shaped depression containing the head of the femur, located at the juncture of the ilium, ischium, and pubis.

acetaminophen   An over-the-counter, nonnarcotic medication that relieves pain and reduces fever.

acetate kinase   An enzyme that catalyzes the transfer of a phosphate group from adenosine triphosphate to acetate, resulting in the formation of acetyl phosphate. Also called *acetokinase.*

Acetest   A trademark for a product that tests urine for abnormally high levels of acetone; used by patients with diabetes mellitus and other metabolic disorders.

acetic acid   A clear, colorless, pungent liquid that's the chief acid in vinegar. It's used in the manufacture of such products as plastics, dyes, and insecticides and is found in such health care products as vaginal jellies and antimicrobial remedies for minor external ear infections. Also called *ethanoic acid.*

acetic acid lotion   An astringent.

acetic fermentation   Production of acetic acid or vinegar from a weak solution of ethanol.

acetoacetic acid   One of the three ketone bodies produced during lipid metabolism. It's excreted in trace amounts in the urine of healthy individuals, but accumulates and is excreted in abnormal amounts in patients with metabolic disorders such as diabetes mellitus. It also accumulates during extended fasting or starvation. Also called *acetone carboxylic acid, acetylacetic acid, diacetic acid.*

acetohexamide   An oral drug that stimulates insulin release from the pancreatic beta cells and reduces glucose output by the liver; classified as a sulfonylurea antidiabetic agent.

acetone   A colorless, volatile liquid present in trace amounts in normal urine and in larger amounts in the urine of patients with metabolic disorders, such as diabetics. Acetone has many industrial uses; in health care, commercially prepared acetone is used to clean the skin before injections.

acetylcholine A neurotransmitter released at the autonomic synapses and myoneural junctions, which causes vasodilation, cardiac inhibition, GI peristalsis, and other parasympathetic effects. It's formed by the action of enzymes on choline and is rapidly destroyed by cholinesterase.

acetylcholine chloride A cholinergic drug, classified as an amiotic agent, that causes contraction of the iris, resulting in miosis. It also produces ciliary spasm, deepening of the anterior chamber of the eye, and vasodilation of the conjunctival vessels of the outflow tract.

acetylcoenzyme A (acetyl-CoA) A molecule whose formation is the intermediate step in glucose catabolism, between anaerobic glycolysis and the Krebs (citric acid) cycle.

acetylcysteine An agent that increases the production of liquids in the respiratory tract, thus helping to liquefy and reduce the thickness of mucous secretions. It's classified as an expectorant.

ACh *abbr* acetylcholine.

achalasia Failure of a muscle or, particularly, a muscle sphincter to relax; usually refers to the cardiac sphincter of the stomach.

Achard-Thiers syndrome A hormonal disorder characterized by masculinization such as growth of body hair in a male pattern seen in postmenopausal women with diabetes mellitus.

ache 1. A dull persistent pain of moderate intensity. It may be localized, as in a headache, or generalized, as in the muscle aches typically associated with influenza. 2. To experience dull, persistent pain of moderate intensity.

achievement age A measure of an individual's educational development, using the results of a proficiency test compared with the normal score for individuals of the same chronological age.

achievement motivation A desire to attain a particular goal that's manifested in action directed at reaching that goal.

achievement quotient (AQ) An individual's achievement age divided by chronological age, expressed as a multiple of 100.

achievement test A standardized test designed to measure an individual's level of knowledge or proficiency in a particular field of academic or vocational study.

Achilles tendon reflex Plantar flexion of the foot resulting from contraction in response to a sharp tap on the gastrocnemius muscle at the back of the ankle. Absence of this reflex may occur in patients with diabetes mellitus or peripheral neuropathy. Also called *ankle reflex, calcaneal tendon reflex.*

CLINICAL TIP An abnormally slow return of the foot to the neutral position after the Achilles tendon reflex may indicate hypothyroidism; an abnormally fast return may occur in hyperthyroidism or pyramidal disease.

achlorhydria The absence of hydrochloric acid from the gastric juice.

acholia The absence of bile secretion.

achondroplasia A genetic disorder in which the normal growth of cartilage is disturbed. It results in anchondroplastic dwarfism, characterized by a normal trunk, shortened arms and legs and, commonly, an enlarged head with a protruding forehead, small face, and flattened nose. Also called *chondrodystrophy.*

achondroplastic dwarf An individual whose dwarfism is caused by achondroplasia; the most common type of dwarf.

achromatopsia Total color blindness; the inability to discriminate hues. All colors appear gray, with varying shades of light and dark.

achromocyte A crescent-shaped red blood cell containing less than the normal amount of red pigmentation, probably due to cell rupture and the resulting loss of hemoglobin. Also called *achromatocyte.*

achylia Severe deficiency or absence of gastric juice or other gastric secretions. The term may also refer to deficiency of pancreatic digestive enzymes. Also called *achylosis.*

achylous Describing lack of gastric secretions.

acicular Pointed or needle-shaped; particularly, leaves and crystals having such a shape.

acid A compound that dissociates in solution, releasing hydrogen ions. Acids react with bases to form salts; their chemical properties are essentially opposite to those of bases.

acid-base balance A state in which acid or alkali production is balanced by acid or alkali excretion, resulting in a stable concentration of hydrogen ions in body fluids. Normally, blood pH measures 7.35 to 7.45; if the metabolic processes that maintain acid-base balance are disrupted, the blood may become too acidic (a condition known as acidosis) or too alkaline (a condition called alkalosis).

acid-base metabolism The metabolic processes that maintain acid-base balance in the body.

acid bath Immersion of the body in water containing a mineral acid; used to control excessive perspiration.

acid burn   Tissue damage or destruction resulting from contact with a strongly acidic substance.

acid dust   Accumulation of atmospheric particles that are highly acidic. Acid dust is a common problem in major cities because of hydrocarbons and other pollutants released into the air from such sources as manufacturing plants and automobiles. Acid dust may cause or exacerbate respiratory conditions.

acidemia   Abnormal acidity, or low pH, of the blood.

acid-fast stain   A dye such as carbolfuchsin used to detect certain organisms in tissue or body fluid samples. Acid-fast organisms resist decolorization after being dyed with an acid-fast stain and then washed with acid alcohol. Acid-fast staining is most commonly used to examine sputum for *Mycobacterium tuberculosis,* an acid-fast bacillus.

acid flush   The runoff of highly acidic rain or snow, which may pollute any body of water into which it flows and, in turn, affect the well-being of wildlife and humans who consume or are exposed to the water.

acidify   **1.** To render a substance acid. **2.** To become acid.

acid mist   Mist contaminated with a high concentration of acid or other toxic pollutants. Exposure to acid mist may cause irritation of the mucous membranes, eyes, and respiratory tract as well as other conditions reflecting disturbances of normal body chemistry.

acidophil   **1.** Capable of being stained with acid dyes; usually refers to cells or parts of cells stained for microscopic study. **2.** A bacterium that thrives in an acid medium.

acidophilic adenoma   A pituitary gland tumor containing cells that are stainable with a red acid dye. The condition causes gigantism and acromegaly. Also called *eosinophilic adenoma, growth hormone-producing adenoma.*

acidophilus milk   Milk fermented with *Lactobacillus acidophilus* cultures, used to treat certain GI disorders by altering the intestinal flora.

acidosis   A disturbance of the acid-base balance of the body in which acid accumulates or base is lost. Respiratory acidosis may result from retention of carbon dioxide, as from hypoventilation or pulmonary insufficiency. Metabolic acidosis may occur in patients with such conditions as severe diarrhea, when the body undergoes significant loss of base; or in patients with renal disease, in whom excess amounts of acid may accumulate.

 CLINICAL TIP   The underlying cause of acidosis must be determined and treated to restore acid-base balance.

acid perfusion test   A diagnostic test used to determine if the esophagus is sensitive to acid, which suggests reflux esophagitis. Instillation of a weak solution of hydrochloric acid into the esophagus is alternated with instillation of normal saline solution. A patient with reflux esophagitis experiences symptoms on exposure to the acid and resolution of symptoms on exposure to normal saline solution. Also called *Bernstein test.*

acid phosphatase   An enzyme that synthesizes phosphate especially well in an acid medium.

acid poisoning   Ingestion of a toxic acid agent, such as the compounds commonly found in cleaning products (hydrochloric or sulfuric acid, for example). First-aid measures include dilution of the acid by giving large amounts of water or milk; vomiting can cause further injury and should never be induced.

acid precipitation   Rain or snow with a high acidity due to contamination by atmospheric pollutants from such sources as manufacturing plants and motor vehicles. A pH of 5.6 or less is associated with human health problems, fish kills, and timber destruction. Also called *acid rain, acid snow.*

acid therapy   Treatment with acid-impregnated plaster patches for the removal of warts.

aciduria   Excessive acid in the urine.

Acinetobacter   A genus of bacteria of the family Neisseriaceae that's aerobic, nonmotile, and doesn't produce spores. It contains gram-negative or gram-variable cocci and occurs frequently in clinical specimens. *Acinetobacter* grows on regular media without the addition of serum.

acinic cell adenocarcinoma   A relatively rare, low-grade cancerous adenoma of a racemose gland, particularly the salivary glands. Tumor cells are clear, with a slightly granular cytoplasm and small, dark, eccentric nuclei. Also *called acinar adenocarcinoma, acinous adenocarcinoma.*

acinitis   Inflammation of an acinus or a cluster of acini.

acinus, *pl.* **acini**   **1.** A small, saclike structure. Also called *alveolus.* **2.** The part of the lung consisting of tissue distal to a terminal bronchiole. **3.** Any of the smallest lobules of a gland.

acmesthesia   Sensitivity to a pinprick or the sensation that a sharp point is touching the skin.

acne   An inflammatory skin eruption involving the sebaceous apparatus, which manifests as follicular, papular, and pustular lesions.

acne artificialis A skin eruption resulting from irritation by external substances or from certain ingested drugs (such as iodides or bromides).

acne cachecticorum Acne characterized by large, soft, ulcerative, cystic, purulent, scarred lesions, occurring in patients with debilitating illness.

acne conglobata A severe form of acne characterized by cystic lesions, abscesses, communicating sinuses, and scarring (including keloid scars). It may involve the face, chest, buttocks, lower back, and thighs. Also called *cystic acne.*

acnegenic Producing or exacerbating acne.

acneiform Resembling acne.

acneiform drug eruption A cutaneous reaction to a drug, resembling acne.

acne indurata Acne characterized by deeply seated and extensive papules and pustules, commonly resulting in severe scarring.

acne necrotica miliaris A rare, psychogenic infection characterized by chronic inflammation of the hair follicles, seen chiefly on the head around the hairline.

acne neonatorum A cutaneous condition of newborns characterized by papules and comedones on the face, particularly the nose, forehead, and cheeks.

acne papulosa A form of acne vulgaris in which most of the lesions are papular.

acne vulgaris A form of acne common during puberty and adolescence, characterized by comedones, cysts, papules, and pustules on the face, upper back, and chest. The condition is probably caused at least in part by the effects of hormonal activity on the pilosebaceous apparatus.

ACNM *abbr* American College of Nurse-Midwives.

ACOG *abbr* American College of Obstetricians and Gynecologists.

acoria Hunger that persists even after eating and even if the appetite is small.

acorn-tipped catheter A flexible catheter with an acorn-shaped tip, used especially in urologic diagnostic procedures.

acousma, *pl.* **acousmas, acousmata** Auditory hallucinations marked by indefinite sounds, such as ringing or hissing.

acoustic, acoustical Of or pertaining to sound or hearing.

acoustic microscope A microscope in which very high frequency sound waves are focused on an object, and its image is reconstructed with light waves and stored for display on a monitor. It permits extremely close examination of cells and tissues with little danger of altering the specimen.

acoustic nerve Either of the pair of cranial nerves involved in hearing and in maintaining equilibrium. Each acoustic nerve is composed of the cochlear and vestibular nerves. Also called *eighth cranial nerve.*

acoustic neuroma A benign tumor of the auditory canal arising from the acoustic nerve. It may cause such symptoms as increasing deafness, tinnitus, headache, and dizziness. Also called *acoustic neurilemoma, acoustic neurinoma, acoustic neurofibroma.*

acoustic trauma Sudden hearing loss, either partial or complete, resulting from an accident, such as a severe blow to the head or an explosion, or gradual hearing loss stemming from exposure to loud noise over a prolonged period.

 CLINICAL TIP Hearing loss resulting from acoustic trauma may be temporary or permanent.

ACP *abbr* **1.** American College of Pathologists. **2.** American College of Physicians.

acquired Not inherited or innate, but the result of environmental factors.

acquired immune deficiency syndrome (AIDS) A disorder of the immune system characterized by inability to mount a successful defense against infection, such as by organisms that usually aren't pathogenic (opportunistic infections). The syndrome is caused by infection with the human immunodeficiency virus, which causes a marked depletion in the number of helper T cells. AIDS is currently incurable and fatal. However, recently developed drug treatments and regimens seem to be effective in prolonging the lives of patients with AIDS.

acquired immunity Immunity that isn't inherited or innate but induced, either actively or passively and by natural or artificial means. *Naturally acquired* immunity develops in the fetus as the result of antibodies transmitted from the mother via the placenta or in newborns from antibodies transmitted in early breast milk. Later in life, naturally acquired immunity develops from the production of antibodies in response to exposure to infectious organisms. *Artificially acquired* immunity is produced by vaccination or antiserum injection.

ACR *abbr* American College of Radiology.

acrasia Inability to control oneself.

acrid Having an unpleasant sharp or pungent taste or odor.

acridine A colorless, crystalline compound derived from coal tar and used as the parent compound in the manufacture of many drugs and dyes, including fluorescent yellow dyes and some antiseptic agents.

Acromegalic features

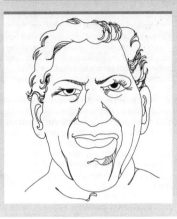
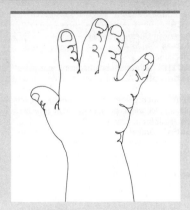

acrocentric   Describing a chromosome with a centromere situated so that one chromatid is significantly longer than the other.

acrochordon   A small, benign outgrowth of skin most commonly seen on the eyelids, on the neck, under the arms, and in the groin. Also called *skin tag.*

acrocyanosis   A circulatory disorder marked by symmetrical cyanosis, blue or red discoloration, and chronic coldness of the hands and, sometimes, the feet. Also called *Raynaud's sign.*

acrodermatitis   An inflammation of the skin of the extremities, particularly of the hands and feet.

acrodermatitis enteropathica   An inherited condition seen in children between 3 weeks and 18 months old marked by defective zinc metabolism that results in oozing, blistering eruptions on the skin and mucous membranes, followed by hair loss, chronic diarrhea, and failure to thrive. Lack of effective treatment may lead to death.

acromegalic eunuchoidism   A disorder occurring in men with advanced acromegaly caused by a chromophil adenoma in the anterior pituitary gland, characterized by genital atrophy and the development of female secondary sex characteristics. With tumor growth, the patient may develop soft skin, a female distribution of fat, impotence, and loss of facial, axillary, and pubic hair. Also called *retrograde infantilism.*

acromegaly, acromegalia   A metabolic disorder occurring in middle-aged persons that results from excessive secretion of somatotropin and is characterized by progressive enlargement of the head, face, hands, and

feet. The condition may be accompanied by organomegaly, diabetes mellitus, or other metabolic disorders.

acromioclavicular articulation   The joint between the acromial end of the clavicle and the medial margin of the acromion of the scapula, having six ligaments.

acromion   The lateral triangular projection of the spine of the scapula that articulates with the clavicle and forms the point of the shoulder. It provides attachment to the deltoid and trapezius muscles. Also called *acromial process.*

acronym   A word formed from the first letter or letters of the words of a name or phrase (for example, PET, an acronym for *Positron-Emission Tomography*).

acropachy   Soft tissue swelling, accompanied by underlying bone changes, where new bone formation occurs.

acroparesthesia   A sensation of prickling, tingling, or numbness in one or more of the extremities resulting from polyneuritis or compression of the nerves in the affected area.

acrophobia   Pathologic fear or dread of high places.

acrosomal reaction   The chemical changes that occur in the anterior portion of the head of a spermatozoon upon contact with an ovum and that result in penetration by the sperm and possible fertilization of the ovum.

acrosome   The caplike structure at the anterior portion of the head of a spermatozoon that releases enzymes upon contact of the spermatozoon with an ovum. Also called *acrosomal cap, anterior head cap.*

acrotic 1. Of or pertaining to the body's surface, particularly the cutaneous glands. 2. Of or pertaining to an extremely weak or absent pulse.

ACS *abbr* 1. American Cancer Society. 2. American Chemical Society.

ACSM *abbr* American College of Sports Medicine.

ACTH *abbr* adrenocorticotropic hormone.

actigraph An instrument that detects and creates a graphic record of changes in the activity of an organism or substance (for example, an electroencephalograph, which records electrical brain activity).

actin One of the two protein components of muscle fibers; actin is active in muscle contraction and cellular movement and helps to maintain the shape of a cell.

actinic Of or pertaining to radiant energy that produces chemical reactions.

actinic dermatitis A sensitivity reaction of the skin resulting from exposure to sunlight or other radiant energy.

actinic keratosis A premalignant, horny growth on portions of the skin that are chronically exposed to the sun or other radiant energy; usually seen in older, light-skinned individuals. Also called *senile keratosis, solar keratosis.*

actinium (Ac) A rare radioactive metallic element found in some uranium ores. Its atomic number is 89; its atomic weight is 227.

Actinomyces A genus of gram-positive anaerobic bacteria. One species, *Actinomyces israelii*, is normally present in the flora of the mouth and throat and may cause disease in humans if it invades the tissue.

actinomycosis A noncontagious infection of the face, mouth, neck, chest, or abdomen with *Actinomyces israelii*. The infection is usually localized but may be systemic; it may manifest as deep, chronic, destructive abscesses or granulomas, with eventual drainage of a thin, granular pus through sinus tracts. Also called *lumpy jaw.*

action current The current generated in a cell membrane of a nerve or muscle by the electrical activity in the tissue. It depolarizes adjacent membrane areas beyond the threshold, thereby triggering repetition of the action potential along the nerve fiber.

action level The level of concentration of a toxic or undesirable substance in a food product that prompts the government to prohibit further sale of that food.

CLINICAL TIP In the United States, the Food and Drug Administration is responsible for monitoring and determining action levels.

action potential The change in electrical potential that occurs across a cell membrane of a nerve, muscle cell, or other excitable tissue when exposed to a stimulus.

activated charcoal Highly absorbent charcoal used to treat individuals who have ingested poisonous substances or with certain types of drug overdoses; it's also used in some cases of severe diarrhea.

activator 1. A substance that converts an inactive substance into an active one. 2. A substance, force, or device that stimulates or accelerates a process or reaction. 3. An agent that stimulates the development of certain embryonic structures during gestation. 4. A device that makes substances radioactive, such as a cyclotron or neutron generator.

active assisted exercise Exercise of a part of the body performed by an individual with the help of a therapist or a device designed for that purpose.

active dental caries Progressive decalcification of the enamel and dentin of a tooth, gradually extending toward the pulp.

active euthanasia A deliberate act, usually the administration of lethal drugs, that results in the death of an individual who's suffering from a terminal illness or who's existing in an irreversible vegetative state. Also called *mercy killing, positive euthanasia.*

active exercise The voluntary, repetitious contraction and relaxation of muscles to improve their strength, tone, and flexibility.

active immunity Acquired immunity caused by the production of antibodies, either following infection or as a result of vaccination.

active movement Movement of muscles at a joint resulting from an individual's voluntary, unassisted effort.

active resistance exercise Exercise of a part of the body against a weight or other resisting force performed by an individual's voluntary, unassisted efforts.

active site The location of catalytic action on the surface of an enzyme.

active transport The movement of substances across a cell membrane as a result of chemical changes that permit the cell to admit larger molecules than would otherwise be able to enter. Certain enzymes provide a chemical "pump" that helps transport substances through the cell membrane. Cells use active transport to absorb glucose and other substances essential to life and health.

activities of daily living (ADLs) The functions an individual usually performs during a typical day, including bathing, dressing, and eating.

ACTP *abbr* adrenocorticotropic polypeptide, a hydrolysate of corticotropin.

actual cautery The use of a heat-generating device rather than chemical means to scar, burn, or cut the skin or other tissue.

acupoints In acupuncture and acupressure, the specific points on the body that are stimulated, either by needles (in acupuncture) or by finger pressure (in acupressure). These points, located along vertical channels called *meridians,* are believed to correspond to specific body organs.

acupressure Application of pressure at certain locations on the body for the purpose of relieving pain or improving the function of some organ or system.

acupuncture A form of traditional Chinese medicine that uses thin needles inserted at designated points on the body (acupoints) to restore health. The needles are believed to work by enhancing the flow of energy *(qi)* in the body; their analgesic effect is thought to involve the release of enkephalin, a neurotransmitter associated with analgesia. Used for many centuries, acupuncture has gained more widespread acceptance among Western clinicians over the last two decades.

acupuncture point One of numerous sites on the skin that lie along a series of lines or channels called *meridians;* stimulation of these points in a carefully prescribed manner may relieve pain or bring about improvement in the function of an organ or system.

acute 1. Beginning suddenly and sharply and having a short course, as describing a disease or symptoms of a disease or condition. 2. Severe or sharp.

acute abdomen Any condition involving the abdomen that requires surgery. Also called *surgical abdomen.*

acute alcoholism Drunkenness caused by excess alcohol ingestion that results in depression of the higher nervous centers, leading to temporary impairment of muscle control, such GI symptoms as nausea and vomiting, and mental disturbance.

acute disease A disease of sudden onset that causes signs and symptoms that are severe and of relatively short duration. An individual with an acute disease either recovers, develops a chronic form of the disease, or dies.

acute epiglottitis, epiglottiditis A severe inflammation of the epiglottis occurring in young children, usually heralded by a sore throat and harsh breath sounds, that may result in respiratory obstruction. It's usually caused by bacterial infection with *Haemophilus influenzae,* although streptococci are sometimes the infecting organisms.

acute glomerulonephritis An inflammatory kidney disease involving the glomeruli and characterized by the sudden onset of facial edema, hematuria, proteinuria, and decreased production of urine. Although not resulting from kidney infection, the condition occurs as a late complication of pharyngitis caused by streptococcal infection (usually beta-hemolytic streptococci).

acute lymphocytic leukemia (ALL) A form of leukemia, most commonly occurring in children, marked by large numbers of immature leukocytes in the blood and blood-forming tissues (including the bone marrow, spleen, liver, and lymph nodes). The disease has a sudden onset and rapid clinical course. Signs and symptoms include fever, pallor, fatigue, loss of appetite, anemia, bleeding, bone pain, spleen enlargement and, because the immune function is disturbed, frequent infection. Also called *acute lymphoblastic leukemia.*

acute myelocytic leukemia (AML) A form of leukemia, usually occurring in adolescents and young adults, marked by the uncontrolled proliferation of myelocytes. Signs and symptoms include frequent infections, anemia, fatigue, enlargement of the spleen, and bone and joint pain. Also called *acute nonlymphocytic leukemia, granulocytic leukemia, acute myelogenous leukemia, myeloid leukemia, splenomedullary leukemia, splenomyelogenous leukemia.*

acute necrotizing gingivitis An inflammation of the gingiva caused by fusiform and spirochetal organisms and characterized by redness, pain, a foul odor, and ulcerated lesions on the gums and in the throat; signs and symptoms also include fever and enlargement of lymph nodes in the neck. Also called *necrotizing ulcerative gingivitis, trench mouth, Vincent's angina, Vincent's infection.*

acute pain Pain that's sharp, severe, and of sudden onset.

acute phase The period in the course of a disease when symptoms are most pronounced.

acute promyelocytic leukemia A form of acute myelogenous leukemia usually occurring in young adults in which more than half the cells are malignant promyelocytes. It's commonly associated with abnormal bleeding secondary to thrombocytopenia, hypofibrinogenemia, and decreased levels of factor V.

acute psychosis The abrupt onset of any of a variety of mental disorders characterized by disorientation and gross distortion of mental activity and emotional responses, an inability to cope effectively with the demands of everyday life, and a diminished capacity to recognize reality or to communicate with and relate to others.

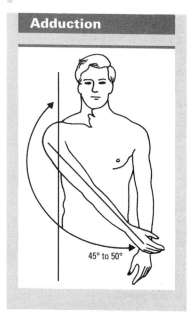

Adduction

45° to 50°

acute pyogenic arthritis   An acute bacterial infection of one or more joints resulting from trauma or a penetrating wound. Typical signs and symptoms include pain, redness, and swelling in the affected joint, muscle spasms, chills, fever, diaphoresis, and leukocytosis.

acute radial nerve palsy   A condition affecting the radial nerve that results in muscle weakness in the forearm. Possible causes include a fracture that compresses or lacerates radial nerve fibers or repeated compression of the nerve by some other means.

acute radiation exposure   Short-term exposure to intense radiant energy, usually as the result of an industrial accident.

ALERT Whole-body exposure to approximately 10,000 rads leads to neurologic and cardiovascular collapse and causes death within 24 hours. A dose between 500 and 1,200 rads destroys the GI mucosa, causes bloody diarrhea, and may be fatal in several days.

acute rheumatic arthritis   Inflammation of the joints due to rheumatic fever.

acute transverse myelitis   An acute inflammation and softening of the spinal cord affecting the function of both sensory and motor nerves. The entire thickness (but not the entire length) of the spinal cord is involved. The condition may arise as a complication of numerous infectious diseases, mul-

tiple sclerosis, or exposure to certain toxins, including carbon monoxide, lead, and arsenic.

ACVD   *abbr* 1. atherosclerotic cardiovascular disease. 2. arteriosclerotic cardiovascular disease.

acyanotic   Not characterized by or accompanied with cyanosis.

acyesis   1. Sterility in a woman. 2. Nonpregnancy.

A/D   *abbr* analog-to-digital.

ADA   *abbr* 1. American Dental Association. 2. American Diabetes Association. 3. American Dietetic Association.

ADAA   *abbr* American Dental Assistants Association.

adactyly, adactylia   Congenital absence of one or more fingers or toes.

Adam's apple   The protrusion at the front of the neck, most prominent in males, formed by the thyroid cartilage of the larynx (*colloquial*). Also called *laryngeal prominence.*

Adams-Stokes syndrome   A syndrome, usually caused by heart block, marked by episodes of slow or absent pulse, dizziness, fainting, Cheyne-Stokes respiration and, sometimes, seizures. Also called *Stokes-Adams syndrome.*

add-a-line set   An I.V. administration set that can deliver intermittent secondary infusions through one or more additional Y-sites.

Addis count   A method used to count the casts and cells in a sedimented 12-hour specimen of urine.

Addison's disease   A life-threatening condition characterized by fatigue, hypotension, loss of appetite and weight, nausea or vomiting, and increased hyperpigmentation of the skin and mucous membranes. It results from partial or complete loss of glucocorticoid, mineralocorticoid, and androgenic function of the adrenal glands owing to tuberculosis, an autoimmune process, or other disease. Also called *addisonism, Addison's syndrome, chronic adrenocortical insufficiency.*

Addison's keloid   A localized area of slightly depressed patches of thickened dermal fibrous tissue, usually appearing as white or pinkish plaques and sometimes surrounded by a purplish or pink halo. Also called *circumscribed scleroderma, localized scleroderma, morphea.*

adduct   To draw a limb toward the median axis of the body.

adduction   Movement of a limb toward the median axis of the body.

adductor   A muscle whose contraction causes adduction.

adductor brevis   One of the five medial femoral muscles, which acts to allow flexion of the leg and to adduct and rotate the thigh toward the median axis of the body.

adductor canal The triangular space in the thigh created by the overlying sartorius muscle that provides passage for the femoral vessels and saphenous nerve. Also called *Hunter's canal.*

adductor longus One of the five medial femoral muscles, which acts to adduct and flex the thigh.

adductor magnus The long, heavy muscle in the medial aspect of the thigh. Its distal portion allows extension and lateral rotation of the thigh; its proximal portion allows medial rotation of the thigh and flexion from the hip.

adenalgia Pain in a gland. Also called *adenodynia.*

adenectomy Surgical removal of a gland.

adenitis Inflammation of a lymph node or gland.

adenoacanthoma A malignant tumor in a gland, consisting mainly of glandular epithelial tissue in which some cells have undergone squamous metaplastic differentiation.

adenoameloblastoma, *pl.* adenoameloblastomas, adenoameloblastomata A benign tumor of the upper jaw that's composed of columnar cells, usually detected on X-ray examination as a lesion surrounding the crown of an impacted tooth.

adeno-associated virus (AAV) A virus that, although unrelated to adenoviruses, can reproduce only in their presence. Its role (if any) in causing disease is unknown.

adenocarcinoma, *pl.* adenocarcinomas, adenocarcinomata A malignant tumor in a gland; it's composed of glandular epithelial cells.

adenocarcinoma in situ Adenocarcinoma confined to a localized site, not having extended into surrounding tissue or metastasized to any distant sites.

adenocele A cystic tumor in a gland.

adenochondroma, *pl.* adenochondromas, adenochondromata A malignant tumor composed of both glandular epithelial cells and cartilaginous cells. Also called *chondroadenoma.*

adenocyst, adenocystoma, *pl.* adenocystomas, adenocystomata A benign, cystic tumor of glandular epithelial tissue. One type is papillary adenocystoma lymphomatosum.

adenocystic carcinoma A slowly progressive malignant tumor of glandular epithelial cells that form cysts. It usually occurs in the breasts, respiratory tract, salivary glands and, sometimes, the vulvar vestibular glands. Also called *adenoid cystic carcinoma, ade-*

nomyoepithelioma, cribriform carcinoma, cylindroma, cylindromatous carcinoma.

adenocyte A secretory cell in a gland.

adenoepithelioma, *pl.* adenoepitheliomas, adenoepitheliomata A malignant tumor composed of both glandular and epithelial elements.

adenofibroma, *pl.* adenofibromas, adenofibromata A benign tumor composed of both connective and glandular tissues. A type of adenofibroma is adenofibroma edematodes.

adenofibroma edematodes An adenofibroma in which there's marked swelling (for example, a nasal polyp).

adenohypophysis The anterior lobe of the pituitary gland, which secretes a number of hormones, including growth hormone, thyrotropin, adrenocorticotropic hormone, melanin-stimulating hormone, follicle-stimulating hormone, luteinizing hormone, prolactin, and beta lipotropin as well as the neurotransmitter endorphin. Also called *anterior pituitary.*

adenoidal speech Abnormal speech with a muted nasal quality, caused by adenoidal hypertrophy.

adenoidectomy Surgical removal of the lymphoid tissues in the nasopharynx (pharyngeal tonsil), usually performed when these tissues are enlarged and cause obstruction or chronic infection.

adenoid hyperplasia Enlargement of the adenoid tissue that results in partial respiratory obstruction, especially in children. The condition commonly occurs in association with enlarged tonsils.

 CLINICAL TIP Adenoid hyperplasia is a frequent cause of recurrent otitis media, sinusitis, and conduction deafness.

adenoleiomyofibroma, *pl.* adenoleiomyofibromas, adenoleiomyofibromata A benign tumor found in the genital tract of women and in the epididymis in men, composed of smooth muscle tissue, connective tissue, and epithelial tissue. Also called *adenomatoid tumor.*

adenolipoma, *pl.* adenolipomas, adenolipomata A tumor composed of both glandular and fatty tissue.

adenolipomatosis A condition marked by multiple adenolipomas, usually on the neck, under the arms, and in the groin.

adenoma, *pl.* adenomas, adenomata A tumor, usually benign, composed of glandular epithelium cells that form glands or glandlike structures. An adenoma may be associated with excess secretion of hormones or other substances from the involved gland.

adenoma sebaceum   A benign tumor of the face, composed mainly of fibrovascular tissue and characterized by small red or yellowish waxy papules. The condition may be associated with tuberous sclerosis.

adenomatosis   Hyperplasia or tumor growth in two or more endocrine glands. The condition usually involves the thyroid, adrenal, or pituitary glands. Also called *multiple endocrine adenomatosis.*

adenomatous goiter   An enlargement of the thyroid gland resulting from an adenoma or numerous colloid nodules within the gland.

adenomyofibroma, *pl.* adenomyofi-bromas, adenomyofibromata   A benign fibrous tumor composed of both glandular and muscular tissue.

adenomyoma, *pl.* adenomyomas, adenomyomata   A benign tumor of muscle tissue (usually smooth muscle), composed of both glandular and muscle tissue and usually occurring in the uterus and uterine ligaments.

adenomyomatosis   A condition marked by the formation of benign nodules resembling adenomyomas, usually affecting the uterus or uterine ligaments.

adenomyosarcoma, *pl.* adenomyosar-comas, adenomyosarcomata   A malignant tumor of the kidneys that occurs in young children, usually under age 5. The tumor is composed of both glandular and striated muscle tissue. Also called *Wilms' tumor.*

adenomyosis   Invasion of the uterine muscular wall by glandular tissue.

adenopathy   Enlargement of a lymph gland.

adenosarcoma, *pl.* adenosarcomas, adenosarcomata   A malignant tumor composed of both glandular epithelial tissue and mesodermal tissue of the same part of the body.

adenosarcorhabdomyoma, *pl.* adenosarcorhabdomyomas, adenosarcorhabdomyomata   A tumor consisting of glandular epithelial, embryonal connective, and striated muscle tissue.

adenosine   A compound formed from the condensation of adenine and D-ribose. It's an important molecular component of deoxyribonucleic acid and ribonucleic acid and of the compounds adenosine monophosphate, adenosine diphosphate, and adenosine triphosphate. Also called *adenine-D-ribose.*

adenosine deaminase   An enzyme that catalyzes the deamination of adenosine to form inosine.

adenosine diphosphate   A nucleotide that's involved in energy metabolism. It's produced by the hydrolysis of adenosine triphosphate.

adenosine hydrolase   An enzyme that catalyzes the conversion of adenosine into adenine and pentose.

adenosine kinase   An enzyme that catalyzes the transfer of a phosphate group from adenosine triphosphate to produce adenosine phosphate.

adenosine monophosphate (AMP)   A nucleotide that's produced by the hydrolysis of adenosine triphosphate.

adenosine phosphate   One of three compounds in which adenosine is attached through its ribose group to one, two, or three phosphoric acid molecules. Kinds of adenosine phosphate, all of which are interconvertible, are adenosine diphosphate, adenosine monophosphate, and adenosine triphosphate.

adenosine triphosphatase (ATPase)   An enzyme that catalyzes the hydrolysis of adenosine triphosphate to adenosine diphosphate and inorganic phosphate. Mitochondrial ATPase has a role in obtaining energy for cellular metabolism; myosin ATPase plays a part in muscle contraction.

adenosine triphosphate (ATP)   A nucleotide found in all cells and required for ribonucleic acid synthesis. It's also involved in energy metabolism and is used to store energy in the form of high-energy phosphate bonds.

adenosis   A general term for a disease in any gland, particularly a lymphatic gland.

adenovirus   Any of the viruses belonging to the Adenoviridae family that cause conjunctivitis, GI infection, and upper respiratory infection in humans.

adenylate kinase   An enzyme found predominantly in skeletal muscle that activates hexokinase to make possible the transfer of phosphate from adenosine diphosphate to fructose or glucose. Also called *myokinase.*

adermia   The congenital absence of skin.

ADH   *abbr* antidiuretic hormone.

ADHA   *abbr* American Dental Hygienists Association.

adhesion   1. The joining of two surfaces or parts. 2. A fibrous band of tissue that holds together anatomic structures that are normally separate. Adhesions usually form in the abdomen, most commonly after surgery or other traumatic tissue injury or an inflammatory disease.

adhesiotomy   The surgical release of adhesions, usually performed when adhesions cause intestinal obstruction.

adhesive absorbent dressing   An absorbent dressing with an adhesive backing.

adhesive pericarditis   An inflammation of the pericardium characterized by adhesions between the two layers of pericardium, between the pericardium and the heart, or between the pericardium and the mediastinum, diaphragm, or chest wall. Adhesive pericarditis may impair normal movements of the heart.

adhesive peritonitis An inflammation of the peritoneum marked by exudation of a fibrinous substance, causing adhesion among intestinal loops or between intestines and other structures.

adhesive pleurisy An inflammation of the pleura marked by exudation of a fibrinous substance, causing adhesion of the visceral and parietal layers of the pleura. Also called *dry pleurisy.*

adhesive skin traction A type of skin traction in which the pull of traction weights is applied with adhesive straps that adhere to the skin over the body structure involved.

CLINICAL TIP Adhesive skin traction is used only when continuous traction is required and skin care for the affected part poses no serious problem.

ADI *abbr* acceptable daily intake.

adiathermancy The state of being unaffected by heat.

adient Tending to move toward, rather than away from, a stimulus.

Adie's syndrome A syndrome involving the pupillary muscle of the eye and characterized by an excessively slow or absent pupillary response to light, impaired accommodation, and slow constriction and relaxation when the focus changes from near to distant. Also called *Adie's pupil.*

adipic Of or relating to adipose, or fatty, tissue.

adipocele A hernia composed of fat or fatty tissue. Also called *lipocele.*

adipofibroma, *pl.* **adipofibromas, adipofibromata** A fibrous tumor that also contains fatty elements; it arises in connective tissue.

adiponecrosis Necrosis of fatty tissue.

adiponecrosis subcutanea neonatorum A dermatologic disease of neonates characterized by patchy areas of hardened subcutaneous fatty tissue and bluish-red discoloration of the overlying skin. Also called *pseudosclerema, subcutaneous fat necrosis.*

adipose Of or pertaining to fat or fatty tissue.

adiposogenital dystrophy A disorder occurring in adolescent boys characterized by obesity, genital hypoplasia, and feminine secondary sex characteristics. The condition results from malfunction of the hypothalamus or an anterior pituitary gland tumor. Also called *adiposogenital syndrome, Fröhlich's syndrome.*

aditus An approach or entrance to a cavity or channel.

ADL *abbr* activity of daily living.

admissible evidence Authentic, relevant, reliable information presented during a trial that may be used to reach a decision.

adnexa, *sing.* **adnexus** Body tissues or structures that lie close to or beside a related structure.

ADP *abbr* adenosine diphosphate.

adrenal cortex The portion of the adrenal gland that produces and secretes steroid hormones. The outer portion of the cortex is a deep yellow; the inner portion, dark red or brown.

adrenal cortical carcinoma A malignant tumor of the adrenal cortex that may result in adrenogenital syndrome or Cushing's syndrome. Such a tumor can arise at any age and may metastasize to the lungs, liver, and other organs.

adrenal crisis An acute, life-threatening insufficiency of adrenocortical hormones resulting from an increased demand for these hormones in a person with excessively low levels (such as from an illness or trauma). Clinical effects may include nausea, vomiting, hypotension, hyperthermia, hyperkalemia, hyponatremia, and hypoglycemia. Also called *acute adrenocortical insufficiency.*

adrenalectomy Complete or partial surgical removal of one or both adrenal glands.

adrenal gland One of the two triangle-shaped, ductless glands situated atop each kidney. The gland secretes cortisol, androgens, and aldosterone (from the adrenal cortex) and the catecholamines epinephrine and norepinephrine (from the adrenal medulla).

adrenalitis Inflammation of the adrenal glands.

adrenalopathy Any disease of the adrenal glands. Also called *adrenopathy.*

adrenal virilism The development of male secondary sex characteristics in a girl, woman, or prepubescent boy due to production of excessive amounts of adrenocortical steroid hormones. Also called *virilization.*

adrenarche 1. The intensified activity of the adrenal cortex that results in menstruation and other signs of puberty. 2. The physiologic changes that result when androgenic hormones or their precursors are secreted by the adrenal cortex.

adrenergic 1. Pertaining to sympathetic nerve fibers of the autonomic nervous system. 2. Of or relating to substances, such as drugs or hormones, that produce adrenergic effects. 3. A drug with adrenergic properties.

adrenergic fibers Sympathetic nerve fibers of the autonomic nervous system (ANS) that use norepinephrine as their neurotransmitter; most postganglionic fibers in the ANS are adrenergic fibers.

adrenergic receptor A site in a muscle or glandular cell that reacts to adrenergic stimulation. Adrenergic receptors are classified as either alpha-adrenergic receptors or beta-adrenergic receptors, according to their response to various activating and blocking agents.

adrenocorticotropic, adrenocorticotrophic Of or pertaining to adrenal cortex stimulation.

adrenocorticotropic hormone, adrenocorticotrophic hormone (ACTH) A hormone secreted by the anterior pituitary gland that stimulates adrenal gland growth as well as the secretion of corticosteroids. Also called corticotropin.

 CLINICAL TIP Exogenous ACTH is used to treat rheumatoid arthritis, acquired hemolytic anemia, severe allergies, multiple sclerosis, and a variety of other diseases and disorders.

adrenogenital syndrome A group of disorders characterized by masculinization in women, feminization in men, or precocious puberty in boys or girls. The condition is caused by abnormal activity of the adrenal cortex, which may be congenital or may be acquired as a result of a malignant tumor or as an adverse effect of a medication that affects adrenocortical function. Also called *congenital adrenal hyperplasia.*

adromia Failure or absence of a nerve that normally innervates a muscle.

adsorb To attract and retain other material on the surface.

ADTA *abbr* American Dance Therapy Association.

adulteration 1. The addition or substitution of a weaker, impure, or inferior agent to any substance. 2. The introduction of a contaminant to a substance, process, or activity.

adult respiratory distress syndrome (ARDS) A syndrome characterized by pulmonary edema, hemorrhage, and acute hypoxemia that can result from a variety of causes, including chest trauma, shock, drug overdose, hemorrhage, aspiration of gastric contents, and near-drowning.

 TIME LINE The older adult may appear to do well following an initial episode of ARDS, but symptoms often reappear within 2 to 3 days.

adult rickets A disease characterized by softening and bending of the bones and accompanied by varying degrees of pain. Also called *osteomalacia.*

advance directives Documents used as guidelines to determine life-sustaining medical care for patients with advanced disease or disability who are no longer able to indicate their own wishes.

advance directive system System implemented by health care institutions (including hospitals, nursing homes, and hospices) to ensure that every patient, on admission, is informed of his right to execute a living will or durable power of attorney for health care decisions.

advanced practice nurse Individual whose education and certification meet criteria established by the state board of nursing; a currently licensed registered nurse with a master's degree or post-basic program certificate in a clinical nursing specialty with national certification, or one with a master's degree in a clinical nursing specialty.

adventitious 1. Acquired or occurring accidentally, as opposed to occurring naturally or through heredity. 2. Occurring sporadically or appearing in a location other than usual.

adventitious bursa A cyst resembling a bursa that forms between two parts as a result of friction or pressure.

adverse drug effect An unintended, harmful reaction to a drug taken in appropriate dosages.

adynamia Lack of physical activity or strength due to muscle disease, cerebellar disease, or psychodynamic weakness. A kind of adynamia is adynamia episodica hereditaria.

adynamia episodica hereditaria An inherited condition marked by muscle weakness and episodes of flaccid paralysis. Also called *hyperkalemic periodic paralysis.*

adynamic fever Temperature elevation accompanied by a feeble pulse, nervous depression, and cool, moist skin. Also called *asthenic fever.*

Aedes A genus of small mosquitoes commonly found in tropical and subtropical climates, several species of which can transmit diseases to humans (for example, dengue and yellow fever).

aerate To charge a substance with air or other gas.

aerobe A microorganism that lives and grows in the presence of oxygen. Types of aerobes are facultative aerobes and obligate aerobes.

aerobic exercise Physical activity that's performed with sufficient exertion to increase the pulse and respiratory rate, with inspired oxygen supplying the required energy.

aerophagy, aerophagia The swallowing of air.

aerosol 1. A fine mist that consists of a liquid or solution with therapeutic, insecticidal, or other properties and is released into the air. **2.** A product packaged under pressure so that its contents are released as a fine mist.

afebrile   Without a fever.

affect   **1.** The mood, feelings, and other emotional reactions to an experience, including the manifestations of those reactions. **2.** To influence or change.

affect memory   The emotional element that accompanies recall of a significant experience.

afferent   Moving toward the center; carrying impulses or substances toward the center. The term usually refers to nerves, but may also refer to arteries, veins, and lymphatics.

affidavit   A sworn statement made in writing and affirmed in the presence of a court officer or notary public.

African trypanosomiasis   A disease occurring in African tropical regions that's caused by the trypanosomal parasitic organisms *Trypanosoma brucei gambiense* or *T. brucei rhodesiense*, transmitted to humans by the bite of tsetse flies. Also called *African sleeping sickness.*

afterbirth   The placenta, membranes, and fluids expelled from the uterus after delivery of a neonate.

afterload   The force opposing ventricular contraction.

afterloading   In radiotherapy: placement of an unloaded applicator or needle within the patient during an operative procedure, followed by loading of the applicator with a radioactive source under controlled conditions.

afterpains   Cramplike contractions of the uterus after childbirth associated with return of the uterus to its normal size.

agamete   A protozoan organism that reproduces asexually by multiple fission.

agamic, agamous   Reproducing in a nonsexual manner; asexual.

agammaglobulinemia   A transient, congenital, or acquired condition in which the gamma fraction of serum globulin is either extremely low or completely absent, causing increased susceptibility to infection. A malignant disease, such as leukemia, myeloma, or lymphoma, usually accompanies the acquired form.

agamogenesis   Reproduction by nonsexual means, as in parthenogenesis. Also called *agamogony.*

agenesia corticalis   Developmental failure of the cortical cells of the embryo's brain, commonly leading to infantile cerebral paralysis and severe mental retardation.

agenesis, agenesia   The congenital absence or incomplete or defective formation of any body part.

agenetic fracture   A spontaneous fracture resulting from imperfect osteogenesis.

agenosomia   The absence or severely defective formation of the sex organs in a fetus, usually associated with intestinal herniation through an incompletely formed abdominal wall.

agglutination   The clumping together of antigen-bearing particles, cells, or bacteria of similar size in a suspension; useful in blood typing and in certain diagnostic procedures relating to the immune system.

agglutination inhibition test   A blood test that identifies unknown circulating soluble antigens. The unknown antigen is mixed with a known agglutinin; if a reaction occurs, the agglutinin can no longer induce aggregation of the cells or particles carrying its corresponding antigen, thus identifying the unknown antigen.

agglutinin   **1.** An antibody that causes clumping, or aggregation, of cells, bacteria, or other organic particles with similar immunologic properties. **2.** Any substance (other than antibody) capable of causing particles to agglutinate.

agglutinin absorption   Removal of an antibody from immune serum through treatment with homologous antigen and centrifugation and separation of the antigen-antibody complex.

agglutinization   The clumping of red blood cells; part of the immune reaction that occurs with Rh incompatibility.

agglutinogen   An antigenic substance that stimulates the production of agglutinin.

aggregate anaphylaxis   An anaphylactic reaction triggered by excess amounts of serum aggregates (such as antigen-antibody complexes), ultimately leading to the release of mediators of immediate hypersensitivity from basophils and mast cells.

aggression   Forceful verbal or physical behavior that arises from anger, hostility, or rage, directed either toward others or toward the self. Aggression is typically associated with destructive actions or tendencies.

aggressive personality   A personality whose behavior is marked by aggression, especially during interactions with others.

aging   The process of growing old, linked to deterioration of body cells, structures, and systems and resulting in decreasing ability to function normally, to replace dead or malfunctioning cells and tissue, and to successfully respond to the environment.

agitated depression   A form of depression associated with hyperactivity (such as restless pacing and obsessive, repetitive actions) rather than the subdued, melancholy affect that's more common in individuals with depression.

agitation   In psychiatry: the condition of psychomotor excitement generated by emotional stress (such as anxiety or fear), manifesting in restless and, commonly, purposeless behavior.

agitographia   Abnormally rapid writing in which words or parts of words are unintentionally omitted.

agitophasia   Abnormally rapid speech in which words or parts of words are produced imperfectly or completely omitted. Also called *agitolalia.*

agnathia, agnathy   The congenital absence of all or part of the lower jaw. The condition is typically accompanied by close approximation of the ears.

agnosia   Partial or complete loss of the ability to recognize objects or persons as a result of organic changes in the brain areas that control the various sensory functions. Agnosia is subdivided into types according to the sensory function involved. Also called *agnosis.*

agonal thrombus   A blood clot that forms in the heart during the process of dying.

agonist   1. In anatomy: any muscle in a state of contraction whose action is opposed by another muscle with which it's paired (called the antagonist). 2. In pharmacology: a drug that has an affinity for and stimulates physiologic activity at cell receptors.

agoraphobia   An intense, irrational fear of being in open spaces or of venturing out from the home or other familiar setting. The anxiety may be generalized to any setting beyond the home or may be specific for certain types of situations and environments, such as open spaces or crowded places.

agranulocyte   A white blood cell that doesn't contain granules in its cytoplasm.

agranulocytosis   An acute disorder in which the number of granulocytes (basophils, eosinophils, and neutrophils) drops to critically low levels. The condition is characterized by infected ulcerous lesions on the mucous membranes and skin; it may develop as an adverse reaction to drug treatment or radiation therapy.

agraphia   Impairment in or loss of the ability to write.

agrypnotic   1. A person who has insomnia. 2. An agent such as a drug that causes wakefulness.

AHA   *abbr* American Hospital Association.
AHH   *abbr* aryl hydrocarbon hydroxylase.
AHIMA   *abbr* American Health Information Management Association.
AI   *abbr* artificial intelligence.

AID   *abbr* artificial insemination donor.
AIDS   *abbr* acquired immunodeficiency syndrome.
AIH   *abbr* artificial insemination husband.
AIHA   *abbr* American Industrial Hygiene Association.

ainhum   A rare condition in which a band of fibrous tissue forms an area of constriction at the base of a toe (usually the fourth or fifth toe), eventually resulting in spontaneous amputation of the toe. Ainhum is most common in tropical climates.

air   The mixture of gases that constitutes the atmosphere of the earth, composed roughly of 78% nitrogen, 21% oxygen, and 1% carbon dioxide, argon, ammonia, nitrites, and organic matter.

air embolism   Sudden obstruction of a blood vessel by air bubbles, usually resulting from introduction of air by a traumatic injury, surgery, or an improperly administered injection.

airplane splint   A splint made from plaster, wire, or leather that holds the arm in abduction at shoulder level and holds the forearm flexed about halfway; used to immobilize a fractured humerus.

air pump   A device that forcibly extracts air from or forces air into a cavity or chamber.

air thermometer   A thermometer in which the expansion of dry air or gas indicates an increase in temperature; used to measure high temperatures. Also called *gas thermometer.*

airway obstruction   The blockage of normal air flow in any part of the respiratory tract, as from a foreign body or from stenosis caused by such conditions as spasm of the bronchi (bronchospasm) or larynx (laryngospasm), chronic obstructive pulmonary disease, or pneumothorax.

akinesia   1. Loss of the ability to move voluntarily. 2. The rest period after systole in the normal heart rhythm. 3. In psychiatry: a neurotic condition characterized by symptoms of paralysis.

akinetic apraxia   Loss of the ability to carry out spontaneous movement.

akinetic mutism   A state in which a person can't make spontaneous movement or sound; commonly caused by a lesion in the upper brain stem.

Al   Symbol for aluminum.

ala, *pl.* **alae**   1. Any structure resembling a wing. 2. The axilla (armpit).

ala auris   The external portion of the ear (pinna).

ala cerebelli   The winglike projection of the central lobule of the cerebellum.

ala cinerea   The wing-shaped area on the floor of the fourth ventricle of the brain.

ala nasi   The winglike flare of the outer wall of each nostril.

alanine aminotransferase (ALT)   One of two enzymes that catalyze a reversible amino group transfer reaction in the Krebs cycle; it's necessary for tissue energy production. ALT is found mainly in the hepatocellular cytoplasm.

ALERT   Falsely elevated ALT levels can follow use of barbiturates, phenothiazines, salicylates, tetracycline, phenytoin, and other drugs that affect the liver.

Al-Anon   An organization based on the 12-step program of Alcoholics Anonymous that provides group support for relatives, friends, and others who live, work, or associate with alcoholics.

ala of the ethmoid   A small, winglike protrusion on each side of the ethmoid bone, each of which articulates with a depression in the frontal bone.

ala of the ilium   The broad, flaring, upper portion of the iliac bone.

ala of the sacrum   The broad, flat, wing-shaped, bony protrusion on either side of the sacrum.

alar cartilage   The curved, winglike greater and lesser cartilages of the nose.

alar ligament   One of the two bands that extend from the tip of the first cervical vertebra to the occipital bone, limiting the extent of head rotation. Also called *check ligament, odontoid ligament.*

alarm reaction   The immediate responses of the body to injury or acute stress, including stimulation of endocrine activity. The alarm reaction constitutes the first phase of the general adaptation syndrome.

alastrim   A mild form of smallpox caused by a less virulent strain of the smallpox virus (*Poxvirus variolae*), characterized by a relatively minor rash and low-grade fever. Also called *Cuban itch, milkpox, variola minor.*

Alateen   An organization based on the 12-step program of Alcoholics Anonymous that provides group support for teenaged children, relatives, or friends of alcoholics.

ala vomeris   A bony protrusion on either side of the upper portion of the vomer, the trapezoid-shaped flat bone in the nasal septum.

alba   *Latin.* White.

albinism   An inherited condition in which defective melanin production causes partial or complete lack of pigmentation in the eyes only or in the eyes, skin, and hair.

Albright's syndrome   An inherited disorder characterized by defective formation of bone, associated with hypoparathyroidism and, in girls, precocious puberty. Also called *Albright-McCune-Sternberg syndrome.*

albumin   A water-soluble protein found in one form or another in the blood, urine, and almost all other animal and plant fluids and tissues.

albumin A   The normal or common type of human serum albumin.

albumin (human)   Serum albumin that has been processed for use as a plasma volume expander.

albuterol   A sympathomimetic drug used in aerosol form as a bronchodilator and in I.V. form as a uterine smooth muscle relaxant to prevent premature labor.

Alcock's canal   The space formed by the obturator fascia and the obturator internus muscle through which the pudendal vessels and nerves pass. Also called *pudendal canal.*

alcohol   1. U.S.P.: a preparation containing at least 92.3% and not more than 93.8% of ethanol (by weight); used as a topical antiseptic and solvent. 2. A clear, colorless, volatile liquid produced by the fermentation of carbohydrates with yeast. 3. A compound analogous to ethanol in constitution that's derived from a hydrocarbon by replacing one or more hydrogen atoms with an equal number of hydroxyl groups. Types of alcohol include rubbing alcohol, sugar alcohol, and unsaturated alcohol.

alcohol bath   A tepid solution of 25% to 50% alcohol in water used as a sponge bath to lower the body temperature of an individual with a fever.

alcoholic fermentation   The chemical conversion of carbohydrates to ethyl alcohol.

alcoholic hallucinosis   Hallucinations (especially auditory) and paranoid delusions resulting from organic brain damage secondary to chronic alcohol abuse; a form of alcoholic psychosis. Also called *acute alcoholic hallucinosis.*

alcoholic-nutritional cerebellar degeneration   Severe incoordination of sudden onset affecting the lower extremities, seen in poorly nourished alcoholics. The condition causes the person to walk (if at all) with an ataxic or wide-based gait.

alcoholic psychosis   One of a group of mental disorders associated with chronic alcohol abuse and characterized by organic brain damage. These disorders include delirium tremens, alcoholic hallucinosis, and Korsakoff's syndrome.

Alcoholics Anonymous (AA)   A nonprofit organization founded by sober alcoholics to help alcoholics achieve and maintain sobriety. Its 12-step plan is designed to promote long-term attitude and behavioral changes, including reliance on a personal experience of a "higher power." The first AA group was started in the United States in 1935. Today, AA is an international organization.

alcoholism   Chronic intake of excess amounts of alcohol, leading to adverse health consequences and impairment of normal social or occupational functioning. An alcoholic person with alcohol tolerance or withdrawal is said to be alcohol dependent. Also called *alcohol abuse.*

alcohol poisoning   Poisoning resulting from ingestion of excessive amounts of ethyl alcohol (grain alcohol, such as in whiskey, gin, and vodka) over a short time, small amounts (8 oz or more) of isopropyl alcohol, or even smaller amounts of methyl alcohol (wood alcohol).

 ALERT Ingestion of as little as 2 oz of methyl alcohol may lead to death.

aldolase   An enzyme of the lyase class found in muscle tissue that catalyzes the step in anaerobic glycolysis in which fructose 1,6-diphosphate breaks down to glyceraldehyde 3-phosphate. Also called *aldehyde-lyase.*

aldosterone   A steroid hormone produced in the adrenal cortex that helps maintain the body's electrolyte balance by regulating serum sodium and potassium balance.

aldosteronism   A disorder marked by the secretion of excess amounts of the hormone aldosterone. Also called *hyperaldosteronism.*

alertness   A state of consciousness in which an individual is oriented to the environment and responsive to auditory, tactile, and visual stimuli.

aleukemic   Leukemia characterized by a normal or below-normal total white blood cell count in the peripheral blood. Also called *subleukemic leukemia.*

aleukia   An extreme reduction in or an absence of white blood cells in the circulating blood.

alexia   A neurologic abnormality characterized by the inability to understand the meaning of printed text, whether as individual words or sentences. Also called *optical alexia, visual aphasia, word blindness.*

algae, *sing.* alga   Any of the genera and species of photosynthetic marine plants, including many varieties of seaweed.

algid malaria   A severe complication of falciparum malaria resulting from vascular collapse and manifested by signs and symptoms of shock and GI distress; may lead to coma and death.

algolagnia   A form of sexual perversion in which inflicting or experiencing pain brings pleasure.

algophobia   An exaggerated fear of experiencing pain or of witnessing pain in others.

alienation   Estrangement or isolation from others or from one's own feelings.

aliphatic acid   An acid of a nonaromatic hydrocarbon that has an open carbon chain.

alkalemia   Abnormal alkalinity, or high pH, of the blood.

alkali   A strongly basic substance that yields hydroxide ions in solution and is able to enter into chemical reactions that yield water-soluble carbonates.

alkali burn   Destruction of tissue caused by exposure to an alkali such as lye. The burned area must be washed with copious amounts of water to remove the chemical, followed by application of vinegar or other mildly acidic substance diluted with water to neutralize any remaining acid.

 ALERT The victim of an alkali burn must be taken immediately to a medical facility, unless tissue damage is only slight and superficial.

alkaline ash   Urine residue with a pH higher than 7.0.

alkaline ash–producing foods   Foods that produce an alkaline urine pH, thereby helping to decrease the incidence of acidic urinary calculi. Foods that result in alkaline ash include fruit (except cranberries, plums, and prunes), vegetables (except corn and lentils), milk, cream, buttermilk, almonds, and olives.

alkaline bath   Immersion in a solution of sodium bicarbonate and water for symptomatic relief of certain skin conditions.

alkaline phosphatase   An enzyme found in the teeth, developing bone, blood plasma, kidneys, and intestines that's involved in bone calcification and the absorption and metabolism of carbohydrates, phospholipids, and other essential compounds.

alkalinize, alkalize   To neutralize an acidic substance or to render a substance chemically base.

alkali poisoning   Poisoning caused by ingestion of a toxic alkaline substance, such as lye and some detergents.

alkalosis   An acid-base imbalance characterized by an excess of base in body fluids (metabolic acidosis) or a loss of hydrogen ions resulting from hyperventilation and excessive loss of carbon dioxide (respiratory alkalosis).

alkylating agent   A substance that promotes alkylation.

alkylation   Substitution of an alkyl group for an active hydrogen atom.

ALL   *abbr* acute lymphocytic leukemia.

allantoidoangiopagous twins   Conjoined twin fetuses of unequal size that are connected by the umbilical cord (allantoic) vessels. Formerly called *omphaloangiogous twins.*

allantois A membrane that develops from the yolk sac and, during the gestation of the human embryo, forms the vessels of the umbilical cord and the chorionic villi.

allele One of the alternative forms of a gene that can occupy a particular locus on a chromosome. Also called *allelomorph.*

allergen A substance capable of inducing a hypersensitive reaction. Common allergens include dust, feathers, animal dander, smoke, certain foods, drugs, and physical agents (such as heat and cold).

allergenic Of or relating to an allergen; causing allergy.

allergic Relating to, caused by, or affected with an allergy.

allergic asthma A form of bronchial asthma in which histamine and other substances that induce airway narrowing are released as part of an allergic process.

allergic bronchopulmonary aspergillosis A bronchial infection, caused by the fungus *Aspergillus fumigatus*, that may occur in asthmatics. Signs and symptoms resemble those of asthma.

allergic conjunctivitis Inflammation and redness of the conjunctiva resulting from exposure to allergens (typically, pollen and atmospheric contaminants such as smoke). The condition commonly affects both eyes and recurs in a seasonal pattern.

allergic coryza Inflammation of the nasal passages caused by exposure to an allergen.

allergic reaction A localized or generalized hypersensitivity response to an allergen to which an individual has developed antibodies. Allergic reactions range in severity from mild cutaneous manifestations to severe systemic symptoms (such as anaphylaxis). Allergic reactions are categorized according to whether they are associated with local or generalized physiologic manifestations and according to the specific immunoglobulin antibodies involved.

allergic rhinitis Acute inflammation of the nasal tissues resulting from exposure to an allergen, characterized by nasal itching, copious nasal secretions, and itching and watering of the eyes.

CLINICAL TIP Allergic rhinitis may be seasonal (as in hay fever) or perennial (as in allergy to dust).

allergic vasculitis An inflammatory condition of the small blood vessels supplying the skin, caused by exposure to an allergen. Signs and symptoms include malaise, itching, and hives or other skin lesions. Also called *allergic angiitis, cutaneous vasculitis.*

allergy A state of hypersensitivity induced by exposure to an intrinsically harmless antigen and resulting in harmful immunologic reactions on reexposure. Allergies are classified as Type I, II, III, or IV hypersensitivity reactions. Types I, II, and III involve different immunoglobulin antibodies and their interaction with antigens. Type IV is associated with contact dermatitis and T cells that react directly with the antigen to cause local inflammation. Some allergies produce immediate or antibody-mediated reactions, whereas others cause delayed or cell-mediated reactions. Immediate allergic reactions involve Types I, II, and III hypersensitivity and the release of certain substances (such as histamine, bradykinin, acetylcholine, gamma globulin G, and leukotaxine) into the circulation. Delayed allergic reactions result from antigens but don't seem to depend on antibodies. Signs and symptoms of allergy vary with the type of hypersensitivity involved. However, common features include bronchial congestion, conjunctivitis, edema, fever, urticaria, and vomiting. Severe allergic reactions, such as anaphylaxis, can lead to shock and death.

allergy testing Any of the various procedures used to determine which allergens trigger allergic reactions in an individual. Skin testing, the most common type of allergy testing, involves intradermal injections of various potential allergens; positive reactions, in the form of a local inflammation, indicate allergic sensitivity and help to guide treatment.

alligator forceps A forceps with long, thin, bent handles, a short clamp, and heavy, interlocking teeth. It's commonly used in orthopedic surgical procedures.

allodiploid, allodiploidic 1. Of or relating to an individual or strain having two genetically distinct sets of chromosomes derived from different ancestral species, as occurs in hybridization. 2. Such an individual or strain.

allodiploidy The state of having two genetically distinct sets of chromosomes originating from different ancestral species.

allometric growth The growth of different organs or parts of the body at different rates.

allometron A quantitative change in bodily form or proportion owing to the evolutionary process.

allometry 1. The growth of a part of an organism, either in relation to the entire organism or to a standard. 2. The measurement and study of such growth.

allopathic medicine System of health care that treats illness with remedies that produce effects opposite those of the disease;

commonly refers to mainstream Western medicine, in contrast with alternative or complementary medicine.

allopathic physician A physician who treats diseases by producing a condition that's antagonistic to or incompatible with the condition produced by the patient's disease. Most practicing physicians in the United States are allopathic.

allopathy A philosophy and system of therapeutics that treats a disease by producing a condition that's antagonistic to or incompatible with the patient's disease.

alloplastic maneuver In psychiatry: a process that promotes adaptation by changing the external environment rather than an individual's beliefs, attitudes, and coping mechanisms.

allopolyploid, allopolyploidic **1.** Of or pertaining to an individual or a strain having more than two genetically distinct sets of chromosomes derived from two or more different ancestral species, as occurs in hybridization. Depending on the number of multiples of haploid sets of chromosomes the individual or strain has, it's referred to as allotriploid, allotetraploid, allopentaploid, allohexaploid, and so on. **2.** Such an individual or strain.

allopolyploidy The state of having more than two genetically distinct sets of chromosomes from two or more ancestral species.

all-or-none law **1.** The observation that the heart muscle, when stimulated, will contract to the fullest extent or not at all. **2.** In nerves and in muscles other than the cardiac muscle, the observation that stimulation of an individual fiber causes an action potential to travel over the entire fiber or not at all.

alopecia Total or partial hair loss resulting from such conditions as normal aging, endocrine or skin disorders, cancer chemotherapy, or drug reactions.

alopecia areata Patchy loss of hair, usually involving the scalp or beard.

alopecia totalis Total loss of the hair on the scalp over a short period of time.

alopecia universalis Total loss of hair from the entire body.

alpha (α) The first letter of the Greek alphabet, often added to the chemical name of a compound to denote that it's a variation, or the first in a series of variations, of the original compound.

alpha-adrenergic receptor One of the postulated sites on effector organs innervated by postganglionic adrenergic fibers of the sympathetic nervous system that responds to norepinephrine and various blocking agents.

alpha-fetoprotein (AFP) An antigen produced in the liver, yolk sac, and GI tract of a human fetus that can be detected in amniotic fluid collected by amniocentesis. Abnormally high or low AFP levels indicate such abnormalities as neural tube defects and Down syndrome.

 CLINICAL TIP In adults, elevated AFP in the blood may be associated with certain malignancies.

alpha hemolysis The presence of a greenish zone around a bacterial colony growing on blood-agar medium, resulting from the partial decomposition of hemoglobin. Alpha hemolysis typifies pneumococci and certain streptococci.

alpha state A condition of tranquil, wakeful relaxation that's devoid of tension, anxiety, and concentration. On an electroencephalogram, this state is indicated by an alpha rhythm.

alpha wave One of the four types of brain waves. As measured by an encephalograph, an alpha wave has a high amplitude or voltage and a frequency of about 10 Hz. Its appearance signifies a wakeful but relaxed state.

ALS *abbr* **1.** Amyotrophic lateral sclerosis. Also called *Lou Gehrig's disease.* **2.** Advanced life support. **3.** Antilymphocyte serum.

altered state of consciousness (ASC) Any state of consciousness that varies from the ordinary condition of mental focus and alertness (including states of deep relaxation, hypnotic trances, and drug-induced states) and is associated with changes in the brainwave patterns signifying normal wakefulness.

alternate generation, alternations of generations A type of reproduction, common among lower plant and animal species, in which successive generations alternate between sexual and asexual reproduction.

alternating current (AC) An electric current that reverses direction at regular, recurrent intervals.

alternating pulse A regular heart rhythm characterized by strong beats alternating with weak ones. It usually indicates serious cardiac disease. Also called *pulsus alternans.*

alternative inheritance The acquisition of all inherited traits from one parent.

alternative medicine A broad spectrum of nontraditional medical and nursing practices and healing arts that are neither widely taught in medical or nursing schools, nor generally used or endorsed by allopathic practitioners. These clinical interventions lack scientific documentation of safety and effectiveness, and usually aren't reimbursable by health care providers.

altitude sickness   A condition caused by relatively low concentrations of atmospheric oxygen (such as encountered during mountain climbing or travel in unpressurized aircraft), characterized by such signs and symptoms as breathlessness, dizziness, and headache.

alum   A chemical compound, either potassium aluminum sulfate or ammonium aluminum sulfate, used as a topical astringent and styptic agent and as an adjuvant in adsorbed toxoids and vaccines.

aluminum (Al)   An abundant, lightweight, silvery metallic element. Its atomic weight is 26.97; its atomic number is 13.

alveolar adenocarcinoma   A type of adenocarcinoma of the lung characterized by columnar or cuboidal epithelial cells that line the alveolar septa and project into alveolar spaces.

alveolar canal   One of the canals of the upper jawbone (maxilla) that serves as a passage for nerves and blood vessels to the upper teeth.

alveolar cell carcinoma   A cancer that begins in a bronchiole, extends along the walls of the alveoli, and forms small masses within the alveoli. Also called *bronchiolar carcinoma*.

alveolar duct   The branch of a bronchiole that leads to the alveolar sacs in the lung.

alveolar soft part sarcoma   A tumor, commonly malignant, that forms in subcutaneous or fibromuscular tissue.

alveolus   **1.** Any small saclike structure. **2.** An air-filled cell in the lung. **3.** The follicle of an alveolar or racemose gland. **4.** One of the honeycomb-like depressions in the stomach wall.

alymphocytosis   The absence of or a significant reduction in circulating lymphocytes, similar to lymphocytopenia but more severe.

Alzheimer's disease   A progressive degenerative brain disease characterized by diffuse atrophy throughout the cerebral cortex, along with senile plaques and neurofibrillary tangles. Affected individuals experience memory loss, confusion, restlessness, disorientation, speech disturbances, and personality and behavioral changes.

TIME LINE   In the elderly, Alzheimer's disease accounts for over 50% of all cases of dementia. The highest prevalence is among those over age 85.

AMA   *abbr* American Medical Association. **1.** Against medical advice; a patient's decision to leave a health care facility against his doctor's advice.

amalgam   A mixture or combination; usually refers to an alloy of mercury and another metal or metals, especially those combinations used in making dental filling materials.

amasesis   Inability to chew food.

amastia   Congenital absence of the breasts in a woman. Also called *amazia*.

amaurosis   Loss of vision, particularly in the absence of an apparent disorder directly involving the eye. The condition usually affects only one eye but sometimes involves both; it may be transient. Causes of amaurosis include brain lesions, poisoning, acute gastritis, or psychogenic conditions (such as hysterical blindness following a severe emotional shock).

amaurosis partialis fugax   Partial blindness of acute onset, accompanied by signs and symptoms resembling those of migraine, such as nausea, vomiting, and dizziness. Vision loss is transient and results from carotid artery insufficiency.

ambient air standard   The maximum tolerable concentration of an air pollutant.

amblyopia   Decreased visual acuity in one eye in the absence of detectable structural or pathologic changes.

ambulatory   **1.** Of or relating to the ability to walk. **2.** Of or relating to a patient who isn't confined to bed because of a medical or surgical condition. **3.** Of or relating to health care provided for individuals not confined to a hospital.

ameba, amoeba   A one-celled, parasitic organism detectable only with a microscope.

amebiasis, amoebiasis   An infectious disease of the intestine or liver caused by *Entamoeba histolytica* or another pathogenic species of ameba, usually acquired by ingesting contaminated food or water.

amelia   The congenital absence of one or more limbs.

amelification   The development of ameloblasts (enamel cells) in the enamel of the teeth.

ameloblast   An epithelial cell that produces and deposits enamel on developing teeth.

ameloblastic fibroma   A benign tumor, arising during tooth formation, in which epithelial and mesenchymal elements of the tooth proliferate but dentin and enamel don't develop.

ameloblastic hemangioma   A benign tumor, consisting of dilated blood vessels, that covers the dental papilla.

ameloblastic sarcoma   A malignant tumor, arising during tooth formation, in which epithelial and mesenchymal elements of the tooth proliferate and dentin and enamel are absent.

ameloblastoma   A rapid-growing tumor of the jaw, usually benign.

Needle position for amniocentesis

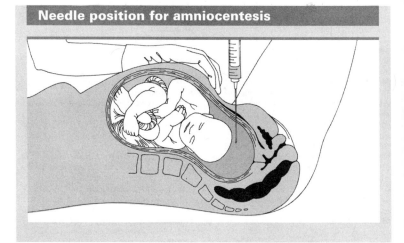

amelodentinal Of or pertaining to the tooth enamel and dentin.

amelogenesis The formation of tooth enamel.

amelogenesis imperfecta An inherited disorder marked by a defect in the amount or structure of the tooth enamel. The condition manifests clinically as a brownish discoloration of the teeth.

amenorrhea The absence or cessation of menstruation.

 CLINICAL TIP Except in preadolescents and in pregnant and postmenopausal women, amenorrhea may reflect dysfunction of the hypothalamus, pituitary gland, ovary, or uterus; congenital absence or surgical removal of both ovaries or the uterus; or an adverse effect of medication.

American Type Culture Collection (ATCC) A nonprofit organization devoted to preserving cultures of cells and microbes and distributing these specimens to academic, scientific, and medical researchers.

americium (Am) An extremely heavy radioactive element created by bombarding plutonium with high-energy neutrons. Its atomic number is 95; its atomic weight is 243.

ametropia An abnormal optical condition in which images of distant objects fail to focus on the retina. Types of ametropia are astigmatism, hyperopia, and myopia.

amine A nitrogen-containing compound derived from ammonia and formed by the replacement of one or more hydrogen atoms.

aminoacetic acid A nonessential amino acid found in many proteins. Also called *glycine, glycocoll.*

amino acids Organic chemical compounds that are the chief components of proteins, either synthesized in the body or derived from dietary sources. All amino acids consist of at least one amino acid group and one acidic carboxyl group.

aminoaciduria The urinary excretion of amino acids, particularly in large amounts. This finding usually indicates a metabolic disorder.

aminobenzoic acid A compound that's part of the vitamin B complex and is typically found in dietary supplements. It's also used as a topical sunscreen. More properly termed p-aminobenzoic acid (PABA).

aminocaproic acid An agent that inhibits plasminogen activator substances, used to prevent or control bleeding.

amitosis Division of a cell and nucleus by simple fission, without mitosis. Also called *direct nuclear division, Remak's nuclear division.*

AML *abbr* acute myelocytic leukemia.

ammonia A pungent, colorless, alkaline gas that's composed of nitrogen and hydrogen and is highly soluble in water.

amnesia Memory loss resulting from such conditions as hysteria, epilepsy, alcoholism, severe psychological trauma, and organic brain disease.

amnesic apraxia, amnestic apraxia Inability to perform a movement on request owing to loss of the ability to recall the request.

amniocentesis   Withdrawal of a sample of amniotic fluid by transabdominal puncture and needle aspiration, usually performed during the fifth month of pregnancy to detect such genetic disorders as Down syndrome, neural tube defects, and Tay-Sachs disease; if the clinician suspects sex-linked genetic defects, the procedure may be done to determine fetal gender.

amniotic fluid   A fluid within the amniotic sac that allows the fetus to move and cushions the fetus's head and umbilical cord during delivery.

amniotic sac   The thin-walled membrane surrounding the fetus and containing amniotic fluid; it eventually lines the chorion. Also called *amnion.*

amorph   A gene that's presumed to exist but has no identifiable effect on the genetic manifestation of a trait. Also called *silent gene.*

amorphic   Of or relating to an amorph.

AMP   *abbr* adenosine monophosphate.

amphetamine   One of a variety of drugs that stimulate the central nervous system. Certain amphetamines are used in the treatment of narcolepsy and attention deficit disorders. Once widely prescribed as appetite suppressants for obese patients, amphetamines commonly were abused and their use for this purpose has decreased markedly. The street name for amphetamines is speed.

 ALERT Long-term amphetamine use may result in dependency, and abuse of drugs in this class is common.

amphigonous inheritance   Acquisition of genetic traits from both parents.

amphikaryon   A diploid nucleus with two haploid chromosome groups.

amphimixis   **1.** The joining of chromatin from the sperm and ovum after fertilization. **2.** In psychoanalysis: the integration of anal and genital eroticism.

amphoric breath sound   A deep, hollow noise heard on percussion or auscultation of the chest, resembling air being blown across the mouth of a bottle. This finding suggests an abnormal bronchial opening or a pneumothorax.

amplification   In genetics: A process by which an increase in genetic material occurs, particularly a proportional increase in the amount of plasmid deoxyribonucleic acid (DNA) over bacterial DNA.

amplitude   **1.** Extent, breadth, or range. **2.** The maximum deviation of a wave from the baseline.

amplitude of accommodation   The range in refractive power between the eye at rest and when completely accommodated.

amplitude of convergence   The difference in the power needed to turn the eyes from their far point to their near point of convergence.

ampule, ampoule, ampul   A small glass or plastic container that can be sealed after it's filled, thus keeping its contents sterile. It typically contains a drug in solution or in powder form to be mixed with an injectable liquid intended for subcutaneous, intramuscular, or I.V. injection.

ampulla, *pl.* ampullae   A saclike swelling or pouch formed in a portion of a duct or canal.

amputation   **1.** Removal of a part of the body, especially a limb or digit, in a surgical procedure. **2.** Traumatic severing of a body part, especially a limb or digit.

amputee   An individual who has sustained the loss of a limb or a part of a limb through trauma or surgery.

AMRT   *abbr* American Society of Radiologic Technologists.

Amsler grid   A grid divided into 5-mm square sections with a dark spot in the center that's used for detecting visual field defects. The patient covers one eye and looks at the spot with the other eye; perception of a blank or distorted section of the grid indicates a visual field defect. Also called *Amsler's chart.*

AMT   *abbr* American Medical Technologists.

amyelinic   Having no myelin sheath.

amyelinic neuroma   A tumor composed only of nonmyelinated nerve fibers.

amylase   An enzyme that causes starches to hydrolyze, or split, into smaller carbohydrate molecules. Alpha-amylases are found chiefly in animals (in saliva and pancreatic juice), whereas beta-amylases occur mainly in plants.

amyloidosis   An abnormal condition in which amyloid, a starchlike, protein-polysaccharide substance, accumulates in tissues and organs, causing functional impairment.

amyotonia   An impairment in or lack of skeletal muscle tone.

amyotrophic lateral sclerosis (ALS) An incurable disease affecting the spinal cord and the medulla and cortex of the brain, characterized by progressive degeneration of motor neurons. Such degeneration leads to weakness and wasting of the muscles, increased reflexes, and severe muscle spasms. Death typically occurs within 2 to 5 years. Also called *Lou Gehrig's disease, Charcot's disease.*

ANA   *abbr* American Nurses Association.

anabolic steroid   Any of a group of synthetic derivatives of testosterone having pronounced anabolic properties; used mainly to promote growth and repair of body tissues or to increase masculinizing effects.

anabolism A constructive metabolic process in which simple substances are converted into more complex compounds.

anacrotic pulse On a sphygmographic tracing: a pulse in which the curve of the primary ascending limb shows a transient drop in amplitude, as in narrowing of the aorta (aortic stenosis).

anadicrotic pulse On a sphygmographic tracing: a pulse in which the curve of the ascending limb shows two transient drops in amplitude. This finding characterizes narrowing of the aorta (aortic stenosis).

anadidymus Conjoined twins that are united in the pelvis and lower extremities but have separate heads and chests.

anadipsia Intense thirst.

anaerobe A microorganism that can live and grow in the absence or near absence of oxygen.

anaerobic 1. Of or relating to the absence of air or oxygen. 2. Pertaining to an anaerobe.

anaerobic exercise Physical activity without a sustained increase in the heart and respiratory rates that causes metabolic acidosis.

anaerobic infection Infection resulting from an anaerobic organism; for example, tetanus and gangrene.

anakatadidymus Conjoined twins that are joined in the middle but are separated in the upper and lower parts of the body.

anal Of or relating to the anus.

anal canal The terminal portion of the large intestine, measuring about 1 1/2" (4 cm) long and situated between the rectal ampulla and the anus.

anal crypt A channel separating the rectal columns.

 CLINICAL TIP When inflamed and swollen, an anal crypt is termed a hemorrhoid.

analeptic Any substance that acts as a central nervous system (CNS) stimulant, particularly a drug or other agent that counteracts CNS depression.

anal fissure An abnormal crack or break in the mucous tissue of the anus.

anal fistula An abnormal passage, usually originating in the rectum, that opens on the skin near the anus.

analgesia The absence of pain in a conscious individual, resulting from therapeutic intervention (such as with medication) or from a functional abnormality of the nervous system.

analgesic 1. Having the ability to relieve pain. 2. A medication that relieves pain.

analog, analogue 1. A feature that superficially resembles another but has evolved in a different way; for example, the wings of a bird and the wings of a fly. 2. In chemistry: a compound that structurally resembles another.

anal reflex Contraction of the external anal sphincter when the skin of the anal region is stroked.

anal stage A stage in psychosexual development, first described by Freud, occurring between ages 1 and 3, when a child is preoccupied with bowel function and the associated body parts and derives most of his or her pleasurable stimulation from attention to these parts.

analysis 1. A process that results in the identification of the components of a substance. 2. The act of breaking up a compound into simpler elements. 3. Psychoanalysis.

anamnesis 1. Recollection of the past. 2. A patient's medical, family, and psychosocial history.

anaphase Third stage of cell division in which chromosomes migrate from the equatorial plate toward the poles; division of the nucleus in meiosis or mitosis.

anaphylactic hypersensitivity reaction An exaggerated systemic reaction of the immune system, usually mediated by immunoglobulin (Ig)E or IgG, that occurs (commonly immediately) in response to exposure to a foreign protein or other agent (such as a drug or other chemical or venom from a bee sting).

 ALERT An anaphylactic hypersensitivity reaction can cause respiratory distress and vascular collapse leading to death.

anaphylactic shock Systemic shock resulting from an anaphylactic hypersensitivity reaction.

anaphylaxis A systemic reaction to a previously encountered antigen.

anaplasia 1. Reversion of a cell to a more primitive form. 2. The loss of structural differentiation of cells, occurring in malignant neoplasms.

anasarca Seepage of fluids into the connective tissue, causing massive, generalized edema. Also called *dropsy.*

anastomosis, pl. anastomoses A surgical procedure in which two blood vessels, ducts, or other tubelike structures are joined to allow the flow of substances between them. Types of anastomoses are end-to-end and side-to-side.

anatomic dead space The area of the respiratory tract in which the exchange of oxygen and carbon dioxide doesn't take place.

anatomic position A body position in which the individual stands erect, facing forward, with arms hanging at the sides, palms forward, and feet slightly apart and pointing forward; used as the position of reference when describing the direction or site of various structures or parts.

anatomic snuffbox A small hollow formed by tendons on the back of the hand near the radial aspect of the wrist, visible when the thumb is abducted and extended.

anatomy 1. The form and structure of an organism. 2. The study, classification, and description of the form and structure of an organism.

anconeus A small muscle at the elbow that extends the forearm and assists in wrist pronation.

ancylostomiasis An intestinal infestation with a species of *Ancylostoma* (hookworm). Also called *hookworm disease.*

Andersen's disease A rare, inborn error of metabolism caused by a defect in the 1,4-alpha-glucan branching enzyme. The condition is associated with liver disorders (hepatosplenomegaly, early cirrhosis, liver failure) and neuromuscular abnormalities. Also called *glycogen storage disease, type IV; familial cirrhosis of the liver; type IV glycogenesis.*

androgen 1. A male sex hormone. 2. Any agent, usually a hormone, that stimulates the activity of male sex organs or increases the development of male sexual characteristics.

androgynous 1. Having both male and female characteristics. 2. Describing a state of phenotypic ambiguity with respect to sexual characteristics.

android pelvis A pelvis with thick, heavy bones, a funnel shape, and a small pubic arch; used to designate a female pelvis possessing characteristics of the male pelvis.

androsterone A weakly androgenic steroid metabolite.

anemia A condition marked by a reduction in the number and volume of red blood cells, the amount of hemoglobin, or the volume of packed red cells. Anemia may reflect decreased hemoglobin or red cell production, increased red cell destruction, or blood loss (or a combination of two or more of these processes).

anencephaly Congenital absence of both cerebral and cerebellar hemispheres and the bones of the cranial vault. The condition isn't compatible with life.

anergy 1. Lack of energy. 2. An immunologic disorder in which exposure to an antigen or a group of antigens fails to produce a normal sensitivity reaction.

aneroid 1. Without fluid. 2. Describing a barometer or sphygmomanometer that doesn't contain mercury.

anesthesia 1. The absence of normal sensation. 2. The inability to feel pain, as produced by an anesthetic substance or by hypnosis or as occurs with damage to nerve tissue.

anesthesia dolorosa Severe pain that arises spontaneously in an area that has been anesthetized.

anesthesiologist A physician who specializes in the administration of anesthesia during surgical procedures and who has special training in resuscitation, intensive respiratory care, and pain control.

anesthesiology A medical-surgical specialty concerned with providing anesthesia, respiratory and cardiovascular support, and pain relief.

anetoderma A skin condition of unknown cause that's characterized by translucent lesions with loose, wrinkled skin.

aneuploid, aneuploidic 1. Of or relating to a chromosome number that isn't an exact multiple of the normal, basic diploid number. 2. An individual or cell with an aneuploid number of chromosomes.

aneurysm A circumscribed, abnormal dilation of the wall of a blood vessel, usually an artery; it may result from congenital weakness or defect in the vessel wall or from other causes, such as atherosclerosis. See illustration on page 28.

TIME LINE Ascending aortic aneurysms, the most common type, are usually seen in hypertensive men under age 60. Descending aortic aneurysms, usually found just below the origin of the subclavian artery, are most common in hypertensive elderly men.

aneurysm needle A needle that has a handle, used to ligate blood vessels.

angina 1. A severe, spasmodic, crushing or constricting pain accompanied by a choking feeling. 2. Angina pectoris.

angina decubitus A condition marked by intermittent attacks of angina pectoris when the individual is lying down.

angina dyspeptica Pain that mimics angina pectoris, resulting from gas accumulation in the stomach.

angina epiglottidea Severe, constricting pain resulting from inflammation of the epiglottis.

angina pectoris Severe chest pain characterized by sensations of spasm, constriction, and a crushing weight, classically radiating from the area over the heart to the left

Types of aneurysms

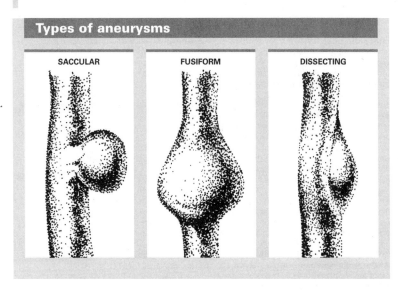

SACCULAR FUSIFORM DISSECTING

shoulder and arm and, possibly, accompanied by a feeling of choking or suffocation. Angina usually results from myocardial oxygen deprivation secondary to atherosclerosis of the coronary arteries.

angioblastic meningioma   A tumor of the blood vessels of the meninges.

angioblastoma, *pl.* angioblastomas, angioblastomata   A benign neoplasm of the brain, consisting of capillary-forming epithelial cells. Also called *hemangioblastoma.*

angiocardiogram   A radiograph of the heart and the vessels of the heart after injection of a radiopaque substance into a blood vessel or a heart chamber.

angioedema   A localized, edematous reaction of the dermis, subcutaneous, or submucosal tissues.

angiofibroma, *pl.* angiofibromas, angiofibromata   A lesion marked by fibrous tissue and blood vessel proliferation, commonly appearing on the face.

angioglioma, *pl.* angiogliomas, angiogliomata   A highly vascular tumor composed of neuroglia.

angiography   Radiographic visualization of blood vessels after injection of radiopaque contrast material, used in diagnosing myocardial infarction and cerebrovascular attack.

angiokeratoma, *pl.* angiokeratomas, angiokeratomata   A superficial tumor of the skin consisting of a cluster of dilated capillaries, warts, and a thickened epidermis; usually found on the feet and legs. Also

called *telangiectasia verrucosa, telangiectatic wart.*

angiokeratoma circumscriptum   A skin disorder, usually occurring in infancy or early childhood, characterized by papules and small nodules that may merge to form plaques. The condition is commonly confined to small patches.

angiokeratoma corporis diffusum   A rare and sometimes fatal inherited disease resulting from deficiency of alpha-galactosidase A, leading to accumulation of ceramide trihexoside in the renal and cardiovascular systems. Also called *Fabry's disease.*

angiolipoma, *pl.* angiolipomas, angiolipomata   A benign tumor consisting of adipose tissue and a large number of blood vessels.

angioma   A swelling or tumor resulting from an abnormal increase in the growth of blood vessels (hemangioma) or lymphatic vessels (lymphangioma).

angioma arteriale racemosum   A vascular neoplasm characterized by the intertwining of small, newly formed blood vessels, later affecting normal blood vessels.

angiomatosis   A condition marked by the development of numerous angiomas.

angiomyoma, *pl.* angiomyomas, angiomyomata   A tumor that arises from the smooth muscle of blood vessels. Also called *angioleiomyoma, vascular leiomyoma.*

angiomyosarcoma, *pl.* angiomyosarcomas, angiomyosarcomata   A malignant tumor composed of elements of angioma, myoma, and sarcoma.

angioneurotic edema   Painless, transient, recurring swelling of the skin, mucous membranes, visceral organs, and brain, sometimes accompanied by joint pain, bleeding into the skin or mucous membranes, or fever.

 CLINICAL TIP Angioneurotic edema may be associated with food or drug allergies, stress, or emotional factors; a hereditary form has also been identified. Also called *angioedema.*

angiosarcoma   A rare, cancerous tumor composed of endothelial and fibroblastic tissue, most commonly seen in the skin or breast tissue.

angiotensin   A family of polypeptides occurring in the blood that's produced by the activity of the enzyme renin on angiotensinogen.

angle   In anatomy and physiology, a figure formed by the joining of two anatomic or physiologic lines, planes, or borders, including those that change when body parts move.

angstrom, Ångström unit (Å)   A unit of measure of length, used for light wavelengths and atomic dimensions, that's equal to 0.1 millimicron, or about the diameter of an atom.

angular movement   A type of motion allowed by joints that either decreases or increases the angle between two adjoining bones.

angular vein   One of a pair of short veins at the front of the eye, arising from the supraorbital and supratrochlear veins and becoming the facial vein.

angulated fracture   A fracture in which the bone sections are displaced and lie at an angle to each other.

anhedonia   Loss of the ability to derive pleasure from experiences that one ordinarily finds pleasurable.

anhidrosis   Absence or abnormally diminished production of sweat as a result of a congenital anomaly or a disease.

anhidrotic   1. Of or relating to anhidrosis. 2. An agent that decreases or prevents sweating.

anicteric hepatitis   A mild form of viral hepatitis characterized by the absence of jaundice.

anion   An ion that carries a negative charge and is attracted to the positively charged anode; the opposite of cation.

anion-exchange resin   A high-molecular weight polymer of simple organic compounds that's capable of exchanging attached anions with other ions in solution.

anion gap   The difference between the concentrations of serum cations and anions, normally 8 to 18 mEq/L.

 CLINICAL TIP The anion gap may be calculated to help evaluate acid-base disorders.

anisocoria   Unequal dilation of the pupils.

anisocytosis   A hematologic condition marked by red blood cells of abnormal and variable size.

anisogamete   A gamete that differs significantly in size or form from the one with which it joins.

anisogamy   The joining of two gametes that differ significantly in size or form.

anisokaryosis   A greater than normal variation in the size of a nucleus of cells of the same type of tissue.

anisometropia   A condition in which the refractive powers of the eyes differ significantly.

anisopoikilocytosis   The presence of red blood cells of varying and abnormal sizes and shapes.

ankle   1. The joint formed by the talus, tibia, and fibula. 2. The bone known as the ankle bone, or talus. 3. The part of the leg where this joint is located.

ankylosing spondylitis   Spinal arthritis that resembles rheumatoid arthritis, sometimes progressing to fusion of the involved vertebrae.

ankylosis   Immobility and consolidation of a joint as a result of disease, injury, or a surgical procedure. Also called *arthrodesis, fusion.*

anlage   A grouping of cells in an embryo from which an organ or structure develops. Also called *primordium.*

ANLL   *abbr* acute nonlymphocytic leukemia.

annular   Having a circular shape; often used to describe a ring-shaped lesion.

annular ligament   A ligament that encircles a bone or other structure.

anomaly   1. A structure, process, or reaction that deviates from what's normal or expected. 2. A congenital defect, such as the absence of a body part or malformation of an organ or structure.

anomia   A type of aphasia characterized by total or partial inability to recall the names of persons or things. Also called *nominal aphasia.*

Anopheles   A genus of mosquito with long, thin appendages. A number of *Anopheles* species serve as vectors for the parasite that causes malaria in humans.

anorchia, anorchism Congenital absence of the testis; may be unilateral or bilateral.

anorectal Of or relating to both the anus and the rectum.

anorexia nervosa An eating disorder, most common among adolescent girls, that's characterized by an aversion to eating, a morbid fear of becoming obese despite significant weight loss, a disturbed body image that results in a feeling of being fat even when extremely thin, and amenorrhea (in females).

anosmia Loss or impairment of the sense of smell as a result of a lesion of the olfactory nerve (essential or true anosmia); mechanical obstruction of the nasal passages (for example, from tissue swelling secondary to an upper respiratory infection); disease in another part of the body (reflex anosmia); or an unidentified cause (functional anosmia). Also called *smell blindness.*

 TIME LINE Anosmia in children usually results from nasal obstruction by a foreign body or enlarged adenoids.

anovulation Suspension or complete cessation of ovulation.

anoxia Absence or near absence of oxygen in inhaled air, body tissues, or arterial blood.

ansa cervicalis A loop of nerves in the cervical plexus, consisting of fibers from the first three cervical nerves.

antagonist 1. In pharmacology: a drug that nullifies the action of another drug. 2. In anatomy: a muscle whose effects counteract the effects of another muscle. 3. In dentistry, a tooth that meets another in the opposite jaw during chewing or clenching of the teeth.

antagonist drug A drug that counteracts the effects of another drug or chemical, such as by receptor-site blockade or neutralization.

anteflexion An acute forward tilt, usually of an organ, especially describing the abnormal forward tilt of the uterus at the junction of the corpus and cervix.

anterior 1. The front of the body or other structure. 2. Describing a part located toward the front of the body or other structure. Also called *ventral.*

anterior atlantoaxial ligament A ligament that joins the atlas and the axis. It's fixed to the ventral surface of the body of the axis and the inferior border of the anterior arch of the atlas.

anterior atlanto-occipital membrane A fibrous layer that extends from the anterior arch of the first cervical vertebra to the occipital bone.

anterior cardiac vein Any of several veins that carry deoxygenated blood to the right atrium of the heart from the ventral portion of the right ventricular myocardium.

anterior longitudinal ligament The wide ligament that extends from the occipital bone and anterior tubercle of the first cervical vertebra to the sacrum. Also called *anterior common ligament.*

anterior mediastinal lymph node A node located along the great vessels of the superior mediastinum and on the anterior part of the diaphragm; it collects lymph from adjacent structures.

anterior nares The external portions of the nasal openings, which permit the inhalation and exhalation of air. Also called *nostrils.*

anterior tibial artery A division of the popliteal artery, arising behind the knee. It divides into six branches, which supply leg and foot muscles.

anterior tibial node A small lymph gland located along the upper portion of the anterior tibial vessels and in front of the interosseous membrane.

anterograde Moving or extending forward.

anterograde amnesia Inability to recall events that occurred after the onset of amnesia or to create new memories.

anterograde memory Inability to recall events of the recent past.

anteroposterior 1. From the front to the back of the body. 2. In radiography: an X-ray taken with the beam passing from the front to the back of the body.

anteversion Leaning forward as a whole, without bending; usually refers to an organ that leans forward, away from the midline.

anthelmintic, anthelminthic Of or describing an agent that destroys or causes the expulsion of intestinal worms, including tapeworms, pinworms, and whipworms.

anthracosis A chronic disease of the lungs caused by the accumulation of carbon from inhaled smoke or coal dust, characterized by the formation of black bronchiolar nodular lesions and symptoms of emphysema. Also called *collier's lung, coal miner's lung.*

anthralin An ingredient in topical ointments that's used to treat psoriasis, ringworm infestations, and other skin conditions.

anthrax A disease of farm animals, usually fatal, that results from *Bacillus anthracis* bacteria. In humans, the anthrax bacillus can cause a serious subcutaneous tissue infection after entering through a break in the skin. Less commonly, humans may develop pulmonary anthrax by inhaling dust containing the bacteria; the pulmonary form, also called *woolsorter's disease,* may be fatal without prompt diagnosis and treatment.

anthropoid pelvis A pelvic type characterized by a long anteroposterior diameter and a narrow transverse diameter, similar in shape to the pelvic bones of apes. A maternal anthropoid pelvis predisposes toward an occipitoposterior position of the fetus.

anthropometric measurements Specific measurements of the human body taken as part of a comprehensive nutritional assessment; include midarm circumference, skinfold thickness, and midarm muscle circumference.

anthropometry An objective, noninvasive method of measuring overall body size, composition, and specific body parts that compares the patient's measurements with established standards. Commonly used anthropometric measurements include height, weight, ideal body weight, body frame size, skinfold thickness, midarm circumference, and midarm muscle circumference.

antiadrenergic **1.** Of or describing blockade of the effects of impulses of the postganglionic sympathetic or adrenergic nerve fibers. **2.** Any agent with antiadrenergic properties.

antiantibody An immunoglobulin that acts as an antibody to another specific antibody.

antibody An immunoglobulin produced in response to exposure to a specific antigen, forming the basis of immunity to invasion by bacteria, viruses, or other antigen-producing agents.

anticholinergic **1.** Of or relating to blockade of the impulses of parasympathetic or other cholinergic nerve fibers. **2.** Any agent with anticholinergic properties.

anticodon In genetics: a sequence of three nucleotides in transfer ribonucleic acid (RNA), complementary to the codon in messenger RNA that specifies the amino acid.

antidiuretic hormone (ADH) A hormone secreted by the hypothalamus that reduces urine production by enhancing water reabsorption by the renal tubules. It's released in response to an increased plasma sodium concentration, a reduction in blood volume, pain, stress, or certain drugs. Also called *vasopressin.*

 CLINICAL TIP ADH may be administered as a pharmacologic agent to cause contraction of smooth-muscle tissue, especially blood vessels.

antidote An agent that blocks or counteracts the effects of a poison.

antidromic conduction Conduction of nerve impulses along an axon in the direction opposite the normal direction. Such impulses are halted at the synapse, permitting conduction in only one direction.

antiembolism hose Elasticized stockings prescribed for some postoperative or bedridden patients to enhance venous blood flow from the lower extremities and thus prevent thromboembolism resulting from pooling of blood in the veins and dilation of veins.

anti-free-flow device A device on an infusion pump that prevents inadvertent bolus infusions if the pump door is accidentally opened.

antigen A substance produced by or introduced into the body that triggers the formation of antibodies that interact specifically with that antigen.

antigen-antibody reaction An immunologic process that causes an antibody to bind with an antigen. The resulting antigen-antibody complexes may induce a variety of results; for instance, they may neutralize the toxic antigen, agglutinize antigens on the surface of microorganisms, or render the antigen more susceptible to ingestion and destruction by phagocytes.

antigenic determinant A site on the surface of an antigen molecule to which an antibody molecule binds. Also called *epitope.*

antigenicity The property of being able to induce a specific immune response. The degree of antigenicity varies with the type and amount of the particular substance, the condition of the host, and the host's sensitivity to the antigen and ability to produce antibodies.

antiglobulin An antibody directed against human globulin (gamma globulin).

antiglobulin test A test that detects nonagglutinating antibodies against red blood cells. Also called *Coombs' test.*

 CLINICAL TIP The direct antiglobulin test is used to detect Rh antibodies in maternal blood and to predict hemolytic disease of the newborn. The indirect antiglobulin test is used in crossmatching blood for type compatibility.

antihemophilic factor (AHF) A blood component essential to normal clotting that's deficient in individuals with classic hemophilia (hemophilia associated with factor VIII deficiency). Also called *factor VIII.*

antihistamine A substance that counteracts or blocks the effects of histamine; used in the treatment of allergies.

antilymphocyte serum (ALS) A serum against lymphocytes; a nonspecific immunosuppressive agent used in humans, usually along with other immunosuppressant drugs or chemicals, to prevent rejection of tissue or organ transplants.

antimitochondrial antibody An antibody that acts against the inner mitochondrial membrane, found in individuals with primary biliary cirrhosis.

antimony A bluish, crystalline metal used in alloys. Its atomic number is 51; its atomic weight is 121.75.

antimony poisoning Poisoning resulting from ingestion, inhalation, or exposure of the skin or mucous membranes to antimony or antimony compounds.

antimorph A mutant gene that antagonizes or inhibits the influence of its allele in the expression of a trait.

antimuscarinic 1. Blocking, counteracting, or reversing postganglionic parasympathetic receptor stimulation. 2. An agent having such an affect.

antimutagen A substance or factor that counteracts or reverses the mutagenic effects of other substances.

antineoplastic 1. Preventing or inhibiting the development of neoplasms or halting the maturation and proliferation of malignant cells. 2. An agent having such an effect.

antioxidants Nutrients, such as vitamin E, that work alone or in a group with other nutrients to destroy disease-causing free radicals.

antipruritic 1. Preventing or relieving itching. 2. A substance or procedure that prevents or relieves itching.

antisense In molecular genetics: a strand of deoxyribonucleic acid containing the same sequence of nucleotides as messenger ribonucleic acid.

antisepsis Prevention of the growth and development of microorganisms by antiseptic means.

antiseptic 1. Preventing decay or putrefaction. 2. A substance that inhibits the growth and development of microorganisms.

antiserum, *pl.* **antisera, antiserums** A serum that contains antibodies against a specific disease, administered to confer passive immunity to that disease. Antiserum is prepared from the blood of animals who have been inoculated with the disease-producing antigens or with antigenic material from the blood of animals and humans who have been exposed to the antigens and who have developed specific antibodies. Also called *immune serum.*

antistreptolysin-O test (ASOT, ASLT) A streptococcal antibody test that measures the relative serum concentrations of the antibody to streptolysin O; used to confirm recent or ongoing infection with beta-hemolytic streptococci.

 CLINICAL TIP Antibiotic or corticosteroid therapy may suppress the streptococcal antibody response and thus alter test results.

antitoxin 1. An antibody against a toxin. 2. A purified antiserum obtained from animals that have been immunized by injections of a toxin or toxoid, given as a passive immunizing agent to neutralize a specific bacterial toxin. Examples include botulism, diphtheria, and tetanus antitoxins.

antivenin An antitoxin whose action is specific against the venom of snakes or insects; used as part of emergency treatment for various snake and insect bites.

antral gastritis The radiographic finding of an abnormal narrowing of the distal portion (antrum) of the stomach; may indicate an ulcer or a tumor.

antrum cardiacum A conical portion of the esophagus situated below the diaphragm. Also called *forestomach.*

anuria The absence of urine formation, usually resulting from a kidney disease or disorder, a decrease in blood pressure below that required to maintain filtration pressure in the kidney, or a mechanical obstruction of urinary flow.

 TIME LINE In elderly patients, anuria is generally a gradual manifestation of underlying pathology. Hospitalized or bedridden elderly patients may be unable to generate the necessary pressure to void, if they remain supine.

anus The external orifice at the lower end of the digestive tract through which feces exit the body.

anxiety An emotional state characterized by fear and dread without a clearly identifiable source, commonly accompanied by a rapid heartbeat, labored breathing, agitation, and tension.

 TIME LINE Anxiety in children usually results from painful physical illness or inadequate oxygenation. Their autonomic signs tend to be more common and dramatic than those of adults. In elderly patients, distractions from the patient's ritual activities may provoke anxiety or agitation.

AOA *abbr* American Osteopathic Association.

aorta The main trunk of the systemic arterial system, having four parts: the ascending aorta, the arch of the aorta, and the two branches of the descending aorta (the thoracic portion and the abdominal portion).

aortic arch syndrome Any of a group of disorders resulting in occlusion of the arteries that arise from the aortic arch. Underlying causes of aortic arch syndrome include atherosclerosis and arterial embolism.

aortic body reflex A reflex normally triggered by a reduction in the blood's oxygen concentration and, to a lesser extent, by a rise in the carbon dioxide and hydrogen ion concentrations that act on chemoreceptors in the wall of the aortic arch. The reflex results in nerve impulses that lead to an increase in respiratory activity.

aortic stenosis An abnormal narrowing of the orifice of the aortic valve, which prevents normal flow of blood from the left ventricle into the aorta. The constriction may result from a congenital malformation or pathologic fusion of the valve cusps.

 ALERT Aortic stenosis causes decreased cardiac output and pulmonary vascular congestion.

aortic valve A valve that guards the opening between the left ventricle and the aorta, preventing the backflow of blood into the left ventricle. It's composed of three half-moon-shaped cusps, which open during systole and close during diastole.

aortitis Inflammation of the aorta, usually occurring in individuals with tertiary syphilis and sometimes associated with rheumatic fever.

aortography Radiographic study of the aorta and its branches after injection of a contrast medium.

AOTA *abbr* American Occupational Therapy Association.

aperture In anatomy: an opening or an orifice in a body structure.

apex, *pl.* apices In anatomy: the extreme end or tip of a body structure, such as the apex of the heart.

apex beat The pulsation of the heart's left ventricle, which may be seen or felt at the fifth intercostal space (about 3 1/4" [9 cm] to the left of midline). It corresponds roughly to the position of the apex of the heart.

 CLINICAL TIP The apex beat is commonly the point of maximal impulse.

Apgar score A numerical evaluation of a neonate's condition in which a rating of 0, 1, or 2 is assigned to each of five criteria: heart rate, respiratory effort, muscle tone, reflex responses, and skin color. The five scores are then combined; a score of 7 to 10 is considered normal, 4 to 7 indicates moderate distress, and 3 or less indicates acute distress. The Apgar score is usually obtained at 1 minute and 5 minutes after birth.

aphagia Difficulty in swallowing. Also called *dysphagia*.

aphagia algera A condition in which an individual refuses to eat or swallow because these acts cause pain.

aphakia, aphacia Absence of the lens of the eye.

aphasia Loss or impairment of the ability to communicate through speech, written language, or signs, resulting from brain disease or trauma.

aphonia Loss of speech resulting from injury, disease (as of the vocal cords, larynx, or other structures involved in speech), or psychological causes (hysterical aphonia).

aphonia clericorum An impairment of speech or difficulty speaking caused by overuse of the voice. Also called *dysphonic clericorum.*

aphonia paralytica Loss of the voice due to paralysis of the vocal cords.

aphonic speech Communication through whispered vocalizations when normal speech sounds can't be produced.

aphtha, *pl.* aphthae A small ulcer.

aphthous fever A highly contagious viral infection of cows and other cloven-hooved animals, characterized by ulcerous lesions (aphthae) around and in the mouth and other mucous tissue. Transmission of the virus to humans, although rare, may occur with exposure to infected animals or their secretions (including contaminated milk). Also called *foot-and-mouth disease.*

aphthous stomatitis A recurring disease of unknown cause marked by the eruption of ulcers on the mucous membranes of the mouth. Also called *canker sore.*

apical dental ligament A ligament, or cord of tissue, that joins the axis to the occipital bone; located near the anterior margin of the foramen magnum.

aplasia 1. The congenital absence of an organ or tissue, or failure of an organ or tissue to develop normally. 2. In hematology: incomplete or defective development of blood cells, or a halt in the normal process of cell regeneration.

aplastic anemia Anemia characterized by significantly reduced formation of red blood cells and hemoglobin, usually accompanied by a reduced number of granular white blood cells and platelets. Aplastic anemia is caused by a bone marrow disorder from a neoplastic disease, or by destruction of bone marrow by toxic chemicals, radiation, or certain medications. Rarely, the disease is idiopathic.

apnea The cessation of spontaneous respiration.

 TIME LINE Premature infants are especially susceptible to periodic apneic episodes because of central nervous system immaturity. In toddlers and older children, the primary cause of apnea is acute

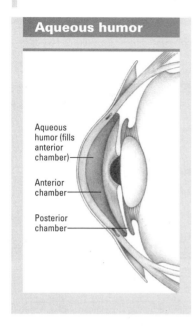

Aqueous humor

Aqueous humor (fills anterior chamber)

Anterior chamber

Posterior chamber

airway obstruction from aspiration of foreign objects.

apocrine gland   One of the numerous glands located under the arms, around the areolae of the breasts, and in the genital and anal areas, whose duct opens into the hair follicle above the sebaceous duct. The action of bacteria on apocrine gland secretions produces the characteristic odor of perspiration.

aponeurosis, *pl.* aponeuroses   A flat, fibrous sheet of connective tissue or an expanded tendon that attaches muscle tissue to bone or other tissue. At some sites, the aponeurosis may also serve as fascia, binding muscles together.

apophysial fracture   A fracture that separates an apophysis, or bony prominence, from the bone.

apophysis   An outgrowth or protuberance, especially one from a bone.

apophysitis   Inflammation of an apophysis, especially in the foot.

apoplexy   1. A sudden neurologic impairment caused by a cerebrovascular accident, characterized by sudden loss of consciousness. 2. A hemorrhage in any organ.

apothecaries' measure   A system of measuring liquids, once commonly used by physicians and pharmacists, that's based on the minim (0.06 ml), fluid dram (60 minims), ounce (8 fluid drams), pint (16 fluid oz), quart (2 pt), and gallon (4 qt).

apothecaries' weight   A system of weighing powders and other solids, once commonly used by physicians and pharmacists, that's based on the grain (65 mg), scruple (20 grains), dram (3 scruples), ounce (8 drams), and pound (12 oz).

appendage   Any part that's attached or appended to a main structure or organ, and which is either vestigial or subordinate in function to the main structure or organ.

appendectomy   Surgical removal of the vermiform appendix.

appendicitis   Inflammation of the vermiform appendix.

> **ALERT** When acute, appendicitis commonly necessitates an appendectomy to prevent perforation of the appendix and subsequent peritonitis.

appendix dyspepsia   Dyspepsia associated with chronic appendicitis. Also called *appendicular dyspepsia.*

applied kinesiology   A method of assessment and evaluation, also known as *muscle testing,* developed by the chiropractic profession in the 1960s that uses the resistance of a patient's muscles to the practitioner's force to assess the relative strength of specific muscles. Particular muscles are associated with specific diseases or organ conditions, so a weak muscle is believed to indicate the cause of the condition.

appropriate-for-gestational-age (AGA) infant   A neonate whose birth weight falls between the 10th and 90th percentiles for gestational age on the Colorado intrauterine growth chart. An AGA infant may be delivered prematurely, at full term, or later than term.

apraxia   The complete or partial inability to perform purposeful movements in the absence of sensory or motor impairment. Sensory or ideational apraxia refers to such impairment caused by loss of perception of the use of an object; motor apraxia refers to inability to make movements or misuse of objects despite correct perception of their intended purpose; amnesic apraxia is the inability to perform a movement on command because of the inability to remember the command.

APTA   *abbr* American Physical Therapy Association.

aptitude   An inherent ability to learn, understand, or perform a certain skill.

aqueous humor   The clear, watery liquid produced by the ciliary processes that fills and circulates in the posterior and anterior chambers of the eye, eventually being reabsorbed into the venous system.

arachnoid   1. Resembling a cobweb or spiderweb. 2. The arachnoid membrane, a delicate, fibrous tissue forming the middle layer of the three tissue layers that cover the brain and spinal cord.

Aran-Duchenne muscular atrophy   A progressive degenerative disease of the motor cells of the spinal cord, usually beginning in the upper extremities and progressing to the lower extremities. Also called *spinal muscular atrophy.*

arbitration   The settlement of a dispute by an impartial person chosen by the disputing parties.

arbitrator   An impartial person appointed to resolve a dispute between parties. The arbitrator listens to the evidence as presented by the parties in an informal hearing, and attempts to arrive at a resolution acceptable to both.

arbovirus   Any of a group comprising approximately 350 identified species of viruses, most of which are borne by arthropods. About 45 species have been identified as being associated with infections in humans.

arcing spring contraceptive diaphragm   A barrier contraceptive device that consists of a latex disk (or diaphragm), having a rim formed from a flexible metal spring. It's available in 10 sizes, in increments of 1/4" (0.5 cm).

ARDS   *abbr* Adult respiratory distress syndrome.

Arenavirus   A genus of viruses of the family Arenaviridae, usually transmitted to man by oral or cutaneous contact with the excreta of wild rodents. Arenaviruses include Bolivian hemorrhagic fever, Lassa fever, and Argentine hemorrhagic fever.

areola, *pl.* areolae   1. A small area or cavity within a tissue. 2. A circular zone of differently pigmented tissue, such as that which surrounds the breast nipples (areola mammae) or a reddened area around a wheal or pustule. 3. In the eye, the part of the iris that surrounds the pupil.

areola mammae   The circular zone of pigmented tissue around the breast nipples. Also called *areola papillaris.*

areolar gland   One of a number of sebaceous glands that protrude from the areolae on a woman's breasts and secrete a lubricating fluid during breast-feeding. Also called *Montgomery's follicles* or *glands.*

areolar tissue   Tissue composed of collagenous and elastic fibers, connective tissue cells, and a semifluid matrix, which forms interstitial tissue, membranes surrounding blood vessels and nerves, and a portion of fascia. Also called *fibroareolar tissue.*

argentaffin cell   A cell containing granules that readily stain with silver, found in the epithelial tissue of the stomach, intestines, and appendix.

argon (Ar)   An odorless, colorless, inert gas. Its atomic number is 18; its atomic weight is 39.9. Argon is found in the atmosphere and in volcanic gases; it's used in argon lasers, electric bulbs, and welding devices.

Argyll Robertson pupil   A pupil that constricts on accommodation but not in reaction to light. Also called *rigid pupil.*

ariboflavinosis   A condition that results from dietary deficiency of riboflavin (vitamin B_2), characterized by magenta tongue, visual disorders, and dry, scaling, cracked lips. Also called *hyporiboflavinosis.*

arm board   A restraining device that helps prevent unnecessary motion that could cause infiltration or inflammation at an I.V. insertion site near a joint, or in the back of the hand.

Arnold-Chiari malformation   A congenital malformation, commonly associated with hydrocephalus and spina bifida, in which the brain stem and lower cerebellum protrude through the foramen magnum into the cervical vertebral canal.

Arnold-Chiari syndrome   Congenital anomaly in which the cerebellum and medulla protrude through the foramen magnum into the spinal canal.

aromatherapy   Therapeutic use of essential plant oils with distinctive scents.

arrested dental caries   Dental caries in which the destruction of the tooth enamel and dentin has ceased.

arrhythmia   A deviation from the normal heart rhythm; an irregular heartbeat.

CLINICAL TIP Types of arrhythmias range from relatively benign (such as occasional mild tachycardia or premature ventricular contractions) to life-threatening (such as ventricular fibrillation).

arsenic (As)   A metallic element that's present in minute traces in all vegetable and animal life. Its atomic number is 33; its atomic weight is 74.9. Arsenic is used in making some dyes and medications; in sufficient quantities it's highly poisonous.

arterial blood gas (ABG)   A term denoting the oxygen and carbon dioxide content of arterial blood, measured to evaluate acid-base balance and to assess and monitor a patient's ventilation and oxygenation status.

arterial circle of the cerebrum   The circular arrangement of arteries at the base of the brain, formed by the anastomosis of the anterior communicating artery, the two anterior cerebral arteries, the two internal carotid arteries, the two posterior communicating arteries, and the two posterior cerebral arteries. Also called *circle of Willis.*

arterial forceps   Self-locking forceps with scissorlike handles, used to grasp and compress an artery.

arterial insufficiency   Inadequate blood flow in the arteries, resulting from such conditions as occlusive atherosclerotic plaques or emboli, aneurysms, vascular disease, arteriovenous fistulas, hypercoagulability states, or heavy tobacco use.

arterial insufficiency of lower extremities   An abnormal condition in which the walls of peripheral arteries become harder, thicker, and less elastic than normal, resulting in reduced circulation, sensation, and function.

arterial pressure   The stress applied by circulating blood against the walls of the arteries, resulting from both cardiac output and systemic vascular resistance.

arterial wall   The enclosure of an artery; made up of three layers, each with a different tissue composition. Types of tissue found in the arterial walls include endothelial tissue, connective tissue, squamous cells, smooth-muscle cells, and elastic tissue.

arteriogram   An X-ray of an artery taken after injection of a contrast medium.

arteriography   A radiologic study that allows visualization of the arteries after injection of a contrast medium.

arteriole   A blood vessel of the smallest branch of the arterial circulation, which communicates with the network of capillaries. Because its muscular wall narrows and widens in response to neurochemical stimulation, the arteriole plays a crucial role in blood pressure regulation and peripheral vascular resistance.

arteriosclerosis   A group of diseases, including atherosclerosis, in which the artery walls become thick and hard and lose their elasticity (commonly called hardening of the arteries).

arteriovenous   Of or relating to both arteries and veins.

arteriovenous angioma of the brain   A congenital anomaly of the vessels of the brain that's characterized by a tangle of coiled arteries and veins, islets of sclerosed brain tissue and, occasionally, cartilaginous cells. Clinical features of this condition include hemorrhage, headache, and focal seizures.

arteriovenous fistula   **1.** An abnormal passage between an artery and vein, usually resulting in an aneurysm. **2.** A surgically created arteriovenous connection that serves as an access site for hemodialysis.

arteritis   Inflammation of one or more arteries, usually associated with a systemic viral or other infectious disease or an autoimmune disease, such as rheumatoid arthritis or systemic lupus erythematosus.

artery   One of the blood vessels in the vast network of vessels that carry oxygenated blood away from the heart and toward the periphery of the body. The wall of an artery consists of an outer coat (tunica adventitia), a middle coat (tunica media), and an inner coat (tunica intima).

arthralgia   Pain in a joint.

arthritis   Inflammation of a joint, or a condition characterized by inflammation of a joint; clinical features include joint pain and swelling.

 ALERT Septic, or infectious, arthritis is a medical emergency that occurs when bacterial invasion of a joint causes inflammation of the synovial lining, effusion and pyogenesis, and destruction of the bone and cartilage.

arthrocentesis   Aspiration of synovial fluid from a joint after needle puncture, performed to obtain a synovial fluid sample for diagnostic evaluation.

arthropathy   Any abnormality or disease affecting a joint.

arthroplasty   Surgical replacement or reconstruction of a joint and repair of tissue, performed to improve joint function and relieve pain (as in osteoarthritis, rheumatoid arthritis, or a congenital deformity).

arthropod   An organism of the phylum Arthropoda, including the Insecta class, Arachnida class (spiders, ticks, mites, and scorpions), and Crustacea class (crabs, shrimps, and lobsters). Many Arthropoda species are medically significant as parasites or disease vectors.

arthroscopy   Endoscopic examination of the interior of a joint, commonly performed to assess pathologic conditions involving the knee. Arthroscopy allows biopsy of cartilage or synovium, aids diagnosis of a torn meniscus, and may permit the removal of loose bodies in the joint space.

articular capsule   A sac of tissue that envelops a joint, composed of an inner synovial membrane and an outer fibrous membrane.

articular disc   The plate of fibrocartilage found in certain joints that attaches to the articular capsule and separates the ends of two bones that don't fit together well.

articular fracture   Fracture of a bone at the joint surface. Also called *joint fracture.*

artifact   Waveforms in an electrocardiogram tracing that don't originate in the heart.

artificial fever An increase in body temperature that has been deliberately induced, as by external heat, for therapeutic purposes.

artificial insemination Placement of semen into the vagina or uterus by means other than sexual intercourse, performed for the purpose of conception.

artificial respiration The forcing of air into and out of the lungs of an individual who has stopped breathing for any reason, commonly performed as an emergency procedure without mechanical equipment. Also called *artificial ventilation.*

aryl hydrocarbon hydroxylase (AHH) An enzyme that transforms carcinogenic chemicals found in tobacco smoke and polluted air into active carcinogens within the lungs.

asbestosis A chronic disease of the lungs characterized by inflammation and leading to fibrotic changes in lung tissue. It results from inhalation of asbestos fibers and is most commonly seen among asbestos miners and workers.

ASC *abbr* American Society of Cytology.

ascariasis A disease caused by infection with parasitic roundworms (nematodes) of the genus *Ascaris*.

Ascaris A genus of large, heavy-bodied roundworms (nematodes), intestinal parasites that are common in vertebrates, including humans.

ascending aorta One of the four main segments of the aorta (the main trunk of the body's arterial circulation). The ascending aorta divides to form the right and left coronary arteries. It measures about 2″ (5 cm) long and has three small aortic sinuses at its origin.

ascending colon The portion of the colon (large intestine) that extends from the cecum to the right hepatic flexure, usually at the umbilical level.

ascites The abnormal accumulation of serous fluid in the peritoneal cavity. Also called *abdominal dropsy.*

ascorbic acid A naturally occurring or synthesized water-soluble vitamin used by the body for the synthesis of collagen and fibrous tissue and the structural integrity of capillary walls. Ascorbic acid is found in citrus fruits, berries, tomatoes, potatoes, and fresh, green, leafy vegetables. Scurvy prevention is among its many therapeutic uses.

asepsis The absence of living, disease-producing organisms. *Medical asepsis* refers to the removal or destruction of disease organisms or infected material. *Surgical asepsis* refers to protection against infection before, during, or after surgery by means of sterile technique.

aseptic fever An abnormal increase in body temperature that isn't associated with infection.

 CLINICAL TIP Aseptic fever is thought to result from the absorption of necrotic tissue after a traumatic injury.

aseptic gauze 1. Any sterile gauze. 2. Sterile gauze that has been prepared and packaged for use during surgery.

aseptic meningitis A nonpurulent, relatively mild form of meningitis (inflammation of the meninges), usually resulting from a virus.

ASET *abbr* American Society of Electroneurodiagnostic Technologists.

asexualization A procedure or process that renders an organism incapable of sexual reproduction, including sterilization by surgical removal of the gonads and other means.

Asherman syndrome A condition characterized by adhesions in the endometrial cavity, commonly associated with amenorrhea and infertility.

ASM *abbr* American Society for Microbiology.

ASMT *abbr* American Society for Medical Technology.

aspartate aminotransferase (AST) One of two enzymes that catalyze the conversion of the nitrogenous portion of an amino acid to an amino acid residue. It's found in various parts of the body, especially the heart, liver, and muscle tissue.

aspartate kinase An enzyme that catalyzes the transfer of a phosphate group from adenosine triphosphate to aspartate, yielding phosphoaspartate.

aspartate transaminase An enzyme that catalyzes the transfer of an amino group from aspartate to alpha-ketoglutarate, yielding glutamate and oxaloacetate. Also called *aspartate aminotransferase.*

aspartic acid A nonessential amino acid found in sugar cane, beet molasses, and the breakdown products of many proteins. It's interconvertible with oxaloacetic acid in the Krebs citric acid cycle. Aspartic acid is also a neurotransmitter in the central nervous system.

aspergillic acid A chemical compound that's produced by the fungus *Aspergillus flavus* and is capable of destroying many gram-negative and gram-positive bacteria.

Aspergillus A genus of fungi whose species are widely distributed in the soil and produce spores that are ubiquitous in the atmosphere. Several species may cause disease in humans, animals, and birds.

asphyxia A condition characterized by impairment or cessation of oxygen and carbon dioxide exchange in the body, resulting in a critically insufficient blood oxygen level and a significantly increased carbon dioxide level. Common causes of asphyxia are choking, drowning, electric shock, poisoning, and inhalation of noxious fumes.

 ALERT Asphyxia leads to loss of consciousness and death if not reversed promptly.

aspirating needle   A hollow needle that's attached to a syringe or suction device and used to withdraw fluid from a body cavity, a body structure, or a cystic mass.

aspiration   **1.** Withdrawal of fluid from a body cavity, structure, or cystic mass using a hollow needle or trocar and cannula. **2.** Accidental inhalation of a fluid or solid into the airway.

aspiration biopsy   Removal of a fluid sample or tissue specimen from a body cavity, structure, or cystic mass for diagnostic purposes.

aspiration biopsy cytology (ABC) Microscopic examination of cells harvested in a fluid sample or a tissue specimen obtained by aspiration.

aspiration pneumonia   Pneumonia caused by accidental inhalation into the bronchi of a liquid (such as vomitus or a beverage) or a solid foreign body (such as a food particle). Aspiration pneumonia is most likely to occur during anesthesia or recovery from anesthesia or as a result of vomiting in an individual who has a decreased level of consciousness.

assault   An attempt or threat by a person to physically injure another person.

ASSE   *abbr* American Society of Safety Engineers.

assisted breech   An obstetric procedure in which a fetus in breech presentation is extracted from the birth canal, either manually or with instruments, after the feet and buttocks have been spontaneously delivered. Also called *breech extraction, partial breech extraction.*

astatine (At)   A highly unstable radioactive element; it's created artificially and may be used to treat hyperthyroidism. Its atomic number is 85; its atomic weight is 210.

astereognosis   Inability to identify objects by touch.

asterixis   Involuntary jerking movements, especially of the hands, which may be induced by having an individual extend the arms, dorsiflex the wrist, and extend the fingers. Asterixis is most commonly seen in patients with metabolic disturbances; it may indicate impending hepatic coma. Also called *flapping tremor, liver flap.*

 ALERT Because asterixis may signal serious metabolic deterioration, quickly evaluate the patient's neurologic status and vital signs.

asteroid body   An eosinophilic inclusion body of irregular star shape, seen in the cytoplasm of giant cells in patients with granulomas (particularly sarcoidosis).

asthma   A respiratory disorder characterized by recurrent attacks of paroxysmal dyspnea, bronchospasm, wheezing on expiration, and coughing. Conditions that may trigger an asthma attack include inhalation of allergens or pollutants, vigorous exercise, emotional stress, and infection.

 ALERT A potentially fatal complication, status asthmaticus arises when impaired gas exchange and heightened airway resistance increase the work of breathing.

 TIME LINE Although this common condition can strike at any age, half of all cases first occur in children under age 10; in this age-group asthma affects twice as many boys as girls.

astigmatism   A refractive abnormality in which unequal curvature of the surfaces of the cornea or lens prevents light rays from focusing at one point on the retina. Astigmatism causes blurred vision and eye discomfort and necessitates corrective lenses to improve acuity.

astringent   **1.** Any substance that causes tissue contraction, controls bleeding, or stops secretions. **2.** Of or pertaining to the effects of such substances.

astroblastoma, *pl.* **astroblastomas, astroblastomata**   A malignant tumor of the brain or spinal cord that's composed of immature astrocytes in a radial arrangement around small blood vessels.

astrocytoma, *pl.* **astrocytomas, astrocytomata**   A tumor of the central nervous system that's composed of astrocytes. It grows slowly and tends to invade surrounding structures.

asymmetrical, asymmetric   Describing a dissimilarity in shape, size, placement (relative to an axis) of corresponding parts of structures on opposite sides of the body that are normally alike.

asynergy   The lack of harmonious function of body structures that normally act harmoniously.

asyntaxia   Lack of the orderly sequence of growth and development in an embryo.

asystole   Absence of a heart beat. Also called *cardiac standstill, cardiac arrest.*

ALERT Asystole rapidly results in death if not reversed, such as with immediate cardiopulmonary resuscitation, cardiac massage, and ventilatory support.

ataxia   Impairment of the ability to coordinate voluntary muscle movement.

ataxic speech   A speech impairment characterized by faulty formation of sounds, resulting from neuromuscular disease.

atelectasis   The collapse of lung tissue or incomplete expansion of a lung, caused by the absence of air in a portion of the lung or in the entire lung.

atelectatic rale   An intermittent crackling sound heard on chest auscultation; usually disappears after the patient takes several deep breaths or coughs.

atheroma, *pl.* atheromas, atheromata   A mass of plaque on the endothelial surface of the walls of arteries, caused by fatty deposits. Atheromas are common in atherosclerosis.

atherosclerosis   A common form of arteriosclerosis in which lipid deposits accumulate in large and medium-sized arteries. These deposits, called atherosclerotic plaques, are associated with calcification and fibrotic changes in the affected arteries.

athetosis   A condition characterized by constant, slow, writhing, involuntary movements of the extremities, especially the hands. Athetosis is most common in certain forms of cerebral palsy and in motor dysfunction secondary to basal ganglionic lesions.

athlete's heart   Enlargement of the heart typically seen in athletes who have undergone long-term endurance training. The physical change in the heart is accompanied by greatly increased functional efficiency, including a slower resting heart rate, an increased rate of recovery after exertion, and more effective delivery of oxygen to the skeletal muscles on exertion.

atlanto-occipital joint   One of a pair of joints at the base of the skull that allows flexion of the neck toward the chest and side-to-side movements of the head.

atlas   The first cervical vertebra, articulating above with the occipital bone and below with the axis and rotating around the tooth-like projection of the second cervical vertebra.

atmosphere   **1.** Air; the envelope of gases (roughly 78% nitrogen, 21% oxygen, and 1% carbon dioxide and other gases) that surrounds the earth. **2.** The gas that surrounds any given body; the gaseous environment of a specific body. **3.** The pressure exerted by the earth's atmosphere at sea level (approximately 760 mm Hg).

atmospheric pressure   The pressure exerted by the weight of the air above it at any point on the earth's surface. Atmospheric pressure varies with altitude, the moisture content of the air, and other factors. The atmospheric pressure at sea level averages 14.7 pounds per square inch. Also called *barometric pressure.*

atom   The smallest part of an element that can exist. An atom consists of a nucleus of protons and neutrons surrounded by moving electrons.

atomic number   The number of protons in the nucleus of an atom of a particular element. The atomic number equals the number of electrons orbiting the nucleus in a neutral atom. Also called *proton number.*

atomic weight   The relative weight of an atom compared with the weight of the standard carbon atom isotope (which has an atomic weight of 12). Also called *relative atomic mass.*

atomizer   A device that releases a liquid into the air in fine droplets; used to deliver medications to or through the nose and throat.

atonia   Lack of normal muscle tone or strength.

atonic   Abnormally relaxed, weak, or flaccid; lacking normal tone.

atonic constipation   Constipation caused by poor muscle tone in the intestine, as in bedridden patients or after prolonged dependence on laxatives.

atopic   Relating to an allergy with a hereditary predisposition that's caused by an allergen associated with immunoglobulin E antibodies (atopic reagin). Examples of atopic allergic reactions are bronchial asthma and chronic hives.

atopic dermatitis   A skin inflammation occurring in individuals with a genetic predisposition to allergies, characterized by intense itching, maculopapular lesions, and excoriation (rash pattern varies with age but usually occurs on the face). See illustration on page 40.

 TIME LINE Almost 10% of childhood cases of atopic dermatitis are caused by allergies to certain foods, especially eggs, peanuts, milk, or wheat.

ATP   *abbr* adenosine triphosphate.

ATPase   *abbr* adenosine triphosphatase.

ATPD   *abbr* ambient temperature, ambient pressure, dry.

ATPS   *abbr* ambient temperature, ambient pressure, saturated (with water vapor).

atresia   Closure or congenital absence of a normal body orifice or tubular structure, such as the external ear canal, vagina, or anus.

atresic teratism   Congenital closure or absence of a body orifice.

atrial failure   A cardiac abnormality in which the atrium doesn't fill adequately, re-

Distribution pattern of atopic dermatitis (ages 2 to 9 months)

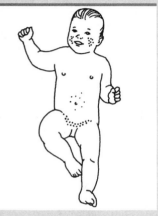

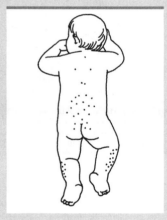

sulting in distention of the associated ventricle.

atrial gallop   An abnormal fourth heart sound heard on auscultation late in diastole, caused by increased resistance to filling of the ventricles. Also called *presystolic gallop, S₄.*

> ⚠ **ALERT** An atrial gallop commonly indicates a serious cardiac problem, such as coronary artery disease or aortic stenosis.

atrial kick   The amount of blood pumped into the ventricles as a result of atrial contraction; contributes approximately 30% of total cardiac output.

atrial myxoma   A soft, gelatinous tumor in the heart, most commonly originating in the left atrium and attached to the septum by a stalk. Clinical effects may include palpitations, nausea, weight loss, fatigue, dyspnea, fever, and sudden loss of consciousness (from obstruction of blood flow through the heart).

atrial septal defect (ASD)   A congenital defect of the heart in which an abnormal passage in the wall between the atria leads to an increased flow of oxygenated blood to the right side of the heart.

atrioventricular (AV) block   Impairment of the normal excitatory impulses between the atria and the ventricles of the heart, usually caused by a block in the atrioventricular node, bundle of His, or bundle branches. The condition may result from such causes as heart disease, acute myocardial infarction, or excessive cardiac glycoside use. It's typically classified as first-, second-, or third-degree AV block.

atrioventricular node   A small area of specialized cardiac muscle cells and fibers in the septal wall of the right atrium that receives impulses from the sinoatrial node and conducts them toward the ventricles.

atrioventricular septum   The membranous structure that separates the atria from the ventricles of the heart.

atrioventricular valve   One of the valves between the atria and ventricles that prevents backflow of blood from the ventricles. The mitral valve is located between the left atrium and left ventricle; the tricuspid valve, between the right atrium and right ventricle.

atrium, *pl.* **atria**   Any chamber or cavity that connects with two or more passageways.

atrium of the heart   One of the two chambers in the upper half of the heart. Deoxygenated blood from the superior vena cava, inferior vena cava, and coronary sinus drains into the right atrium; oxygenated blood from the pulmonary veins drains into the left atrium. During diastole, blood empties from the atria into the ventricles.

atrophic fracture   A spontaneous fracture resulting from atrophy of a bone, as may occur in an elderly person.

atrophic gastritis   A chronic inflammation of the stomach accompanied by wasting of the mucous membranes and breakdown of the peptic glands. The condition sometimes causes pain and is commonly seen in individuals with pernicious anemia or gastric carcinoma or in elderly persons.

attachment **1.** In anatomy: the site at which one structure is affixed to another. **2.** In psychology: an emotional bond between individuals. **3.** In dentistry: a device (such as a partial denture) that's used to affix and stabilize a dental prosthesis.

attention deficit hyperactivity disorder (ADHD) A behavioral disorder characterized by learning disabilities and intrusive, disruptive behavior. The cause is unknown.

 CLINICAL TIP Attention deficit disorder isn't associated with intellectual deficits or neurologic disorders.

Au Symbol for gold.

audiogram A graphic representation of hearing acuity as determined by audiometric and other hearing tests.

audiology A branch of science concerned with hearing, particularly with hearing impairments.

audiometer A device that tests hearing acuity by measuring a patient's perception of tones at various frequencies.

audiometry Evaluation of hearing using an audiometer. Various audiometric tests identify the lowest intensity of sound at which a patient can perceive an auditory stimulus, hear different frequencies, and differentiate speech sounds. Pure tone audiometry evaluates the ability to hear frequencies, usually ranging from 125 to 8,000 hertz, and can determine whether a hearing loss results from a problem in the middle ear, inner ear, or auditory nerve.

auditory ossicles The tiny bones of the middle ear — the incus, malleus, and stapes (commonly called the anvil, hammer, and stirrup) — that vibrate in response to sound waves and form an essential part of the sound conduction system.

Auer body A rod-shaped structure found in the cytoplasm of certain cells, particularly myeloblasts, in individuals with acute myelocytic leukemia. Also called *Auer rod.*

aura, *pl.* **aurae, auras** **1.** A subjective sensation, such as of light or warmth, that immediately precedes the onset of a seizure or an episode of migraine headache. **2.** A field of energy arising from a living being, purportedly seen or perceived by individuals with an acute sensitivity, which has been documented by a technique called Kirlian photography.

ALERT When aura rapidly progresses to the ictal phase of a seizure, quickly evaluate the seizure and be alert for life-threatening complications, such as apnea.

aural **1.** Of or relating to the ears or sense of hearing. **2.** Of or relating to an aura.

aural forceps Forceps with fine, bent tips that are used in surgical procedures involving the ear.

auricle **1.** The shell-like structure of the external ear; the pinna. **2.** A small, cone-shaped pouch that protrudes from the right atrium of the heart.

auricular Of or relating to the auricle of the ear or the atrial auricle.

auricularis anterior The muscle that draws the external portion of the ear (auricle) upward and forward. It's innervated by the temporal branch of the facial nerve.

auricularis posterior The muscle that draws the external portion of the ear (auricle) backward. It's innervated by the posterior auricular branch of the facial nerve.

auricularis superior The muscle that draws the external portion of the ear (auricle) upward. It's innervated by a temporal branch of the facial nerve.

auriculoventriculostomy A surgical procedure in which a polyethylene tube is inserted into the skull and jugular vein to direct excess cerebrospinal fluid away from the brain's ventricles.

 CLINICAL TIP Auriculoventriculostomy is usually performed in newborns with the communicating and obstructive forms of hydrocephalus.

aurothioglucose A gold salt used to reduce inflammation from rheumatoid arthritis.

auscultation The act of listening, either directly or with a stethoscope, for sounds within the body. Usually, the examiner listens for the frequency, intensity, and quality of the sounds made by such organs as the heart, lungs, and intestines or, in a pregnant woman, listens to fetal heart sounds.

Australia antigen Hepatitis B surface antigen (so named because it was first detected in a native of Australia), found in the serum of an individual who has acute or chronic serum hepatitis or who's a carrier for that virus.

autacoid Any of various physiologically active substances that are produced at many sites and act locally as endogenous regulators. Examples include histamine, serotonin, and prostaglandins.

autism A psychiatric disorder characterized by severe withdrawal and an abnormal focus on the self to the extent that communication and interaction with others are extremely limited or nonexistent.

autoantibody An immunoglobulin that's directed against a normal constituent in the host's own tissue.

autoantigen A body constituent that triggers the production of autoantibodies and a resulting autoimmune reaction against host tissues.

autochthonous idea A persistent idea that originates from the unconscious and is perceived by the individual to have been placed into his mind by an outside force.

autodiploid, autodiploidic 1. Of or relating to an individual or a strain having two genetically identical or nearly identical chromosome sets that are derived from the same ancestral species and result from the duplication of the haploid set. 2. An individual or a strain having this property.

autoerythrocyte sensitization syndrome A rare syndrome of recurrent spontaneous bruising and painful, enlarged ecchymoses without trauma. Most common in women, it's thought to represent a type of autosensitization, although some believe that the cause is psychogenic. Also called *painful bruising syndrome.*

autograft The surgical transfer of tissue (commonly skin) from one location of the body to another location in the same individual.

autoimmune disease A disorder resulting from an inappropriate immune response that's directed against the self. Antigens normally found in the internal cells stimulate the development of antibodies; these antibodies can't distinguish antigens of the internal cells from external antigens, and act against the internal cells to cause various reactions.

autoimmunity A condition in which the immune system mounts an attack against the individual's own body tissues. One theory proposes that autoimmunity reflects an inability of the immune system to distinguish between autoantigens and foreign substances, owing to some change in the cellular components of the immune system. Autoimmunity may lead to hypersensitivity and autoimmune disease.

autoinoculation Inoculation with microorganisms from one's own body.

automatic infiltration detector A device that senses a decrease in skin temperature during I.V. fluid infusion, indicating possible infiltration of the fluid. The detector is attached to an I.V. pump and the skin around the insertion site of an I.V. needle. Activation of the device triggers an alarm and halts the infusion.

automaticity The ability of a cardiac cell to initiate an electrical impulse on its own.

automatism 1. The quality of being automatic or of functioning without conscious control. 2. In psychiatry: undirected, aimless behavior that isn't under conscious control,

carried out with no conscious knowledge, as in catatonic schizophrenia and certain other conditions. Also called *automatic behavior.*

autonomic Of or relating to the autonomic nervous system.

autonomic nervous system The division of the nervous system that regulates the activity of cardiac muscle, smooth muscle, and glands. It's subdivided into the sympathetic nervous system, which accelerates the heart rate, narrows blood vessels, and raises blood pressure; and the parasympathetic nervous system, which decreases the heart rate, accelerates intestinal peristalsis and gland activity, and relaxes the sphincters.

autonomic reflex One of the many reflexes associated with the normal activities of the visceral organs, including blood pressure regulation, heart rate, peristalsis, urine production, and glandular secretions.

autonomy The state of being able to function independently of external influences or forces.

autopolyploid, autopolyploidic 1. Of or relating to an individual or a strain whose chromosome complement has more than two complete copies of the genome of a single ancestral species. 2. An individual or strain having this property.

autopolyploidy The state or condition of having more than two complete copies of the genome of a single ancestral species.

autopsy Physical examination of the body and organs of an individual who has died to determine or confirm the cause of death or to study pathologic changes in the body. Also called *postmortem examination* or *necropsy.*

autopsy pathology The study of disease by postmortem examination of the body by a pathologist. The organs and tissues are described by their appearance both at the time of dissection and during microscopic examination of representative tissue samples.

autoserotherapy Treatment consisting of injection with an individual's own serum, used to combat some infectious diseases and skin conditions.

autosite The more normally developed member of conjoined twins upon whom its partner (called the parasite twin) depends for survival and nourishment.

autosomal Of or relating to an autosome or any condition transmitted by an autosome.

autosomal-dominant inheritance An inheritance pattern in which transmission of a dominant gene on an autosome results in manifestation of a particular characteristic. All of the children of a homozygous affected parent are affected, whereas half of the children of a heterozygous affected parent are affected.

autosomal inheritance Inheritance of traits according to the presence or absence of various genes on the autosomes. The pattern may be dominant or recessive and affects males and females with equal frequency.

autosomal-recessive inheritance An inheritance pattern in which the transmission of a recessive gene on an autosome leads to a carrier state if the person is heterozygous for the trait and to the affected state if the person is homozygous for the trait. One-fourth of the offspring of two unaffected heterozygous parents are affected, whereas all of the offspring of two homozygous affected parents are affected. The offspring of a couple in which one parent has the trait and the other doesn't are all carriers who show no effect of the trait.

autosome Any chromosome other than a sex chromosome that occurs as one of a pair in somatic cells and singly in a gamete. Also called *euchromosome.* Autosomes transmit all genetic traits and conditions except those that are sex-linked.

autosplenectomy A progressive disorder of the spleen that's characterized by multiple infarcts leading to fibrosis and dysfunction of the spleen. The condition occurs in sickle cell anemia.

autosuggestion The act of focusing one's concentration on an idea or belief to produce a change in mental or physical functioning.

autotopagnosia Inability to recognize or orient parts of one's own body, resulting from a lesion in the dominant hemisphere of the brain.

autotransfusion The collection and filtration of blood from a patient, then reinfusion of the blood to that same patient.

AV *abbr* atrioventricular, arteriovenous.

avascular 1. Of or relating to a type of tissue (such as some forms of cartilage) that isn't supplied with blood or lymphatic vessels. 2. Of or relating to tissue deprived of sufficient blood flow or lymphatic fluid as a result of trauma, disease, or deliberate interruption of the blood supply (as to control bleeding).

aversion therapy A form of behavior therapy that attempts to modify or arrest certain behaviors by creating a negative response to stimuli that might trigger the undesirable behavior (such as cigarette smoking, excessive alcohol use, or sexual aggression). Techniques used to create and reinforce negative associations include electric shock and drugs to induce nausea. Also called *aversive conditioning.*

aversive stimulus A stimulus, such as electric shock or inducement of nausea, that causes mental or physical discomfort.

avitaminosis A state of vitamin deficiency caused by insufficient dietary intake of one or more vitamins or by failure of the body to absorb and use the available vitamins. Also called *hypovitaminosis.*

AV nicking A retinal vascular abnormality visible on ophthalmologic examination in which an arteriovenous crossing compresses a vein, causing the vein to appear "nicked." The condition may indicate hypertension, arteriosclerosis, or other vascular conditions.

Avogadro's law A law of physics stating that equal volumes of all gases contain equal numbers of molecules at the same pressure and temperature. The law holds true only for ideal gases.

avoidance In psychiatry: physical or psychological behavior that's intended to avoid or provide escape from intrapersonal or interpersonal conflicts, unpleasant feelings, or other negative stimuli.

avoidance-avoidance conflict A situation in which an individual responds to two equally undesirable alternatives by vacillating and behaving indecisively.

avoidance conditioning The act of training an individual or animal to behave in a certain way to prevent exposure to unpleasant stimuli.

avoirdupois weight A system of weighing ordinary commodities in English-speaking countries that's based on the pound (7,000 grains, 256 drams, or 16 oz), with one ounce equaling 28.35 g.

avulsed tooth A tooth that has been dislodged from its socket as the result of a traumatic injury.

avulsion Forcible separation by tearing.

avulsion fracture A fracture occurring when a bone fragment is torn from bone tissue at the attachment site of a strong ligament or tendon.

axial current The portion of the bloodstream located in the center of an artery.

axilla, *pl.* **axillae** The space below the shoulder joint where the upper part of the underside of the arm meets the side of the chest. Also called *armpit.*

axillary artery A vessel that continues from the subclavian artery and subsequently becomes the brachial artery in the arm.

axillary nerve A nerve that arises from the posterior cord of the brachial plexus and supplies the deltoid and teres minor muscles. Also called *circumflex nerve.*

axillary node One of the 20 to 30 lymph glands in the axilla that are situated around the axillary vein. Axillary nodes help to combat infections in the chest, armpit, neck, and arm as well as drain lymph from those areas.

axillary vein   One of a pair of veins that continues from the basilic and brachial veins and becomes the subclavian vein at the outer border of the first rib.

axis, *pl.* **axes**   **1.** In anatomy, an imaginary line that passes vertically through the center of the body or a body part, used to provide a starting point for anatomic angles and other references. **2.** The second cervical vertebra, upon which the atlas (the first cervical vertebra) rotates, permitting turning, extension, and flexion of the head.

axon   The cylinder-shaped process of a neuron that conducts nervous impulses away from the nerve cell body. Also called *axis cylinder.*

axon flare   A spreading area of redness on the skin surrounding the site at which an irritant has been applied or an injury has been sustained. The redness results from dilation of arterioles and capillaries brought about by a response in which a histamine-like substance is released.

axoplasmic flow   The continuous pulsing movement of the cytoplasm between the cell body of a neuron and the axon fiber that supplies substances needed by the axon to maintain activity and repair itself. Any interruption in the axoplasmic flow, such as from disease or trauma, leads to degeneration of the unsupplied areas of the axon.

Ayurvedic medicine   Ancient, traditional Indian system of medicine based on the Hindu philosophy. It shares some fundamental concepts with traditional Chinese medicine: the interconnectedness of body, mind, and spirit; the belief that the cosmos is composed of five basic elements (earth, air, fire, water, and space); and the belief in a human energy field or life force that must be kept in balance to maintain health. Ayurvedic medicine also stresses the importance of a person's metabolic body type, or *dosha,* in determining his health, personality, and susceptibility to disease. See also *doshas.*

azoospermia   The absence of living spermatozoa in the ejaculatory fluid, resulting from testicular dysfunction, blockage of the epididymal tubules, or vasectomy. Azoospermia is associated with infertility but not impotence.

azotemia   The accumulation of excess amounts of nitrogenous bodies, particularly urea, in the blood. Also called *uremia.*

azygospore   A spore created from a gamete that doesn't undergo conjugation.

azygous, azygos   Occurring singly rather than in pairs.

azygous vein   One of the seven thoracic veins. It arises from either the right ascending lumbar vein or the inferior vena cava, passes through the diaphragm at the aortic orifice, travels to the right of the vertebral column to the fourth thoracic vertebra, then rises ventrally over the root of the right lung and terminates in the superior vena cava.

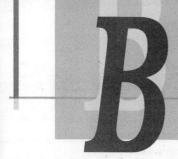

B Symbol for boron.

Ba Symbol for barium.

Babcock's operation Eradication of a varicosed saphenous vein by inserting an acorn-tipped probe and drawing out the vein.

babesiosis An infectious disease caused by protozoa of the genus *Babesia,* transmitted through the bite of ticks of the species *Ixodes dammini.* It occurs in both wild and domestic animals, and may affect humans incidentally.

Babinski's reflex Dorsiflexion of the great toe with hyperextension and fanning of the other toes in response to firm stroking of the lateral aspect of the sole. Also called *Babinski's sign.*

 TIME LINE Babinski's reflex is normal in newborn infants, but may signal a pyramidal tract lesion in children and adults.

Bacillaceae A family of bacteria made up of endospore-forming rods and cocci (most of which are gram-positive and saprophytic), commonly found in soil; some are insect or animal parasites. The family includes the *Bacillus, Clostridium,* and *Desfulfotomaculum.*

bacille Calmette-Guérin (BCG) An organism of the strain *Mycobacterium bovis,* rendered avirulent and used in many countries as a vaccine against tuberculosis (usually administered intradermally).

bacilliform Rod-shaped.

Bacillus A genus of aerobic, gram-positive, spore-producing bacteria of the family Bacillaceae, including 48 species, of which three are pathogenic and the rest saprophytic soil forms.

Bacillus anthracis A species of gram-positive, facultative anaerobes that causes anthrax. Spores of this organism can live for many years in animal products, such as hides and wool, and in soil. Inhaling the spores can lead to a pulmonary form of anthrax.

backcheck valve A device that prevents backflow of secondary I.V. solution into the primary line during drug infusion, often via Y port.

bacteremia The presence of bacteria in the blood.

bacteria, *sing.* **bacterium** A diverse group of unicellular microorganisms that consist of a single cell lacking a distinct nuclear membrane and that multiply by cell division. Bacteria may be classified by shape, Gram stain, and whether or not they require oxygen.

bacterial endocarditis Bacterial infection of the endocardium, the heart valves, or both; may be acute or subacute.

bacterial food poisoning An illness caused by ingesting food contaminated with certain bacteria.

bacterial plaque A soft film comprised of food debris, mucin, and dead epithelial cells, which forms on the surface of the teeth and may cause dental caries and gum infection. Also called *dental plaque.*

bactericidal 1. Destroying bacteria. 2. An agent that destroys bacteria.

bacteriostatic 1. Inhibiting the growth or reproduction of bacteria. 2. An agent that inhibits the growth or reproduction of bacteria.

Bainbridge reflex An increase in the heart rate in response to increased pressure in or increased distention of the large somatic veins or right atrium.

 CLINICAL TIP The Bainbridge reflex may also result from infusion of large amounts of I.V. fluids.

balanced polymorphism A state of equilibrium in which gene frequencies are maintained by the forces of natural selection.

balanced traction A system of balanced suspension that supplements traction, used to treat fractures of the lower extremities or after various procedures affecting the lower parts of the body.

balanced translocation The transfer of segments between nonhomologous chromosomes in such a way that the configuration of the chromosomes changes but the total number of chromosomes remains the same, with each cell or gamete having no more or no less than the normal amount of diploid or haploid genetic material.

45

balanic   Pertaining to the glans penis or the glans clitoridis.

balanitis   Inflammation of the glans penis.

balanopreputial   Pertaining to the glans penis and prepuce.

Balantidium coli   The largest and the only ciliated protozoan species pathogenic to humans, causing balantidiasis.

Balkan frame   A rectangular frame that overhangs and attaches to the bed, used for attachment of splints, changing the position of immobilized limbs, or continuous traction involving weights and pulleys.

ball-and-socket joint   A synovial joint in which the ball-shaped head of an articulating bone fits into a concave socket of another bone. This type of joint permits the widest range of motion.

ballottement   A type of palpation performed to test for a floating object, especially to detect a pregnancy. In late pregnancy, a fetal head that can be ballotted is termed as floating or unengaged.

ball-valve action   The opening and closing of an orifice by the rise and fall of a ball-shaped mass. Objects that may act in this manner include gallstones, renal calculi, and blood clots.

bamboo spine   The rigid spine caused by ankylosing spondylitis. Also called *poker spine.*

band   1. In anatomy: a bundle of fibers that binds one part of the body to another or that encircles a structure. 2. In dentistry: a metal strip that's placed around a tooth to serve as an attachment for orthodontic components.

bandage   A strip or roll of gauze, cloth, or other material that may be placed around a part of the body in various ways to secure a dressing, apply pressure over a compress, or immobilize a part.

bandage shears   Scissors that are used to cut through bandages. Usually, the blade is angled to the shaft of the instrument and the lower blade has a rounded blunt protuberance to allow the shears to be inserted under the bandage without damaging the skin.

band cell   An intermediate leukocyte form between metamyelocytes and adult leukocytes that has a curved or indented nucleus.

banding   Any of several techniques of chromosome staining that allow the appearance of a characteristic pattern of transverse light and dark bands. Banding patterns are identified by the staining technique used, such as C-banding, G-banding, Q-banding, and R-banding. Also called *chromosome banding.*

bank blood   Preserved, anticoagulated donor blood stored under refrigeration (usually for a maximum of 21 days). Bank blood is dated and identified by blood type and, after crossmatching, may be given to a recipient; or any of its components may be extracted and prepared for various purposes.

Bard's sign   Increased oscillations of the eyeball that occur when a patient with organic nystagmus visually follows a target moving from side to side. In patients with congenital nystagmus, such oscillations usually stop during this test.

bargaining agent   A person or group selected by members of a bargaining unit to represent them in negotiations.

bargaining unit   A group of employees who participate in collective bargaining as representatives of all employees.

Barium (Ba)   A pale yellow, metallic element belonging to the alkaline earths group. Its atomic number is 56; its atomic weight is 137.36.

barium enema   Rectal instillation and retention of barium sulfate for radiographic evaluation of obstructions, tumors, and other abnormalities of the lower intestinal tract. Also called *contrast enema.*

barium sulfate   A radiopaque contrast medium used in radiographic diagnostic studies.

Barlow's syndrome   An abnormal heart condition characterized by prolapse of the mitral valve and commonly accompanied by regurgitation. Also called *mitral valve prolapse syndrome.*

barognosis, *pl.* barognoses   The ability to perceive weight, such as when an object is placed in the hand.

baroreceptor   A receptor, or nerve ending, that responds to changes in pressure, specifically a receptor in the wall of the atria, vena cava, aortic arch, or carotid sinus. In response to a pressure change, baroreceptors stimulate mechanisms that permit physiologic adjustment to blood pressure changes through constriction or dilation of blood vessels.

barotrauma   Physical injury caused by increased pressure, such as barotitis media, as may result from the difference between atmospheric and intratympanic pressures.

barrel chest   A large, rounded thorax.

 CLINICAL TIP Barrel chest may indicate pulmonary emphysema. However, it's considered normal in individuals who live in high-altitude areas and thus have an increased vital capacity.

TIME LINE In the elderly, senile kyphosis of the thoracic spine may be mistaken for barrel chest; however,

Barrel chest

NORMAL CHEST

BARREL CHEST

Transverse diameter — Spinal cord — Anteroposterior diameter

Transverse diameter — Spinal cord — Anteroposterior diameter

patients with senile kyphosis lack signs of pulmonary disease.

Barré's pyramidal sign Inability to hold the flexed legs in a vertical position when lying face down; a sign of pyramidal disease.

Barré's sign Slow contraction of the iris, as occurs in mental deterioration.

Barrett's syndrome Peptic ulcer of the lower esophagus that results from the presence of columnar epithelium; sometimes premalignant. The condition is most commonly caused by chronic esophageal irritation secondary to gastric reflux of acidic digestive juices.

Barthel index and scale A functional assessment tool that evaluates an older patient's overall well-being and self-care abilities, based on their capacity to perform 10 self-care activities.

bartholinitis An inflammation of Bartholin's ducts, usually caused by a species

of *Streptococcus* or *Staphylococcus* or a strain of gonococci.

Bartholin's cyst A cyst originating from one of the vestibular glands or from its ducts.

Bartholin's duct The major duct draining the sublingual gland.

Bartholin's gland One of two small, mucus-secreting glands located on either side of the vaginal opening.

Barton's fracture Fracture of the distal end of the radius; it may be accompanied by dorsal dislocation of the carpus on the radius.

Bartter's syndrome A rare condition characterized by hypertrophy and hyperplasia of the juxtaglomerular cells and secondary hyperaldosteronism. It may be hereditary and is sometimes associated with such anomalies as short stature and mental retardation.

basal Pertaining to or located near the base.

basal anesthesia 1. A state of unconsciousness just short of complete surgical anesthesia in which the patient still reacts to noxious stimuli. **2.** Narcosis induced by injection or infusion of potent sedatives, without added narcotics or anesthetic agents.

basal body temperature   Temperature of the body as measured, orally or rectally, in the morning after at least 5 hours of sleep and before the person performs any activities (talking, getting out of bed, moving about, smoking a cigarette, eating, or drinking).

basal bone   **1.** In orthodontics: the relatively fixed osseous structure that limits movement of the teeth in the alveolar or supporting bone if the occlusion is to remain stable. **2.** In prosthodontics: the osseous tissue of the mandible and the maxillae (except for the rami and the processes) that supports dentures.

basal cell   A cell in the basal layer of the epidermis.

basal cell carcinoma   A malignant epithelial tumor of the skin arising from neoplastic differentiation of basal cells, usually occurring as one nodule or several small nodules or plaques with central depressions that erode, crust, and bleed. Basal cell carcinoma is the most common form of skin cancer and usually results from excessive exposure to the sun or X-rays.

basal cell papilloma   A benign neoplasm of the epidermis marked by multiple raised, brown or yellow oval lesions. It usually occurs in middle age. Also called *basal cell acanthoma, seborrheic keratosis.*

basal ganglia   Interconnected islands of gray matter, such as the caudate nucleus, putamen, and pallidium, located deep within the cerebral hemispheres and in the upper brainstem. Also called *basal nuclei.*

basal metabolic rate (BMR)   The rate at which body cells utilize oxygen, or the calculated equivalent heat production by the body in a fasting, resting subject.

 CLINICAL TIP BMR is expressed in calories consumed per hour per square meter of body surface area or per kilogram of body weight.

basal metabolism   The minimal amount of energy expended by the body to maintain essential functions, such as respiration, circulation, temperature, peristalsis, and muscle tone. It's measured by a calorimeter in a waking, resting subject who has fasted for 14 to 18 hours and is in a comfortable, warm environment; it's expressed in calories per hour per square meter of body surface.

basal temperature   The temperature of a healthy individual who has fasted for 14 to 18 hours, measured immediately after at least 8 hours of relaxed sleep.

 CLINICAL TIP Basal body temperature will show a sustained elevation in body temperature post ovulation until just before onset of menses, indicating the approximate time of ovulation.

base   **1.** A chemical compound that combines with acids to form salts; a substance that dissociates to yield hydroxide ions in aqueous solutions. **2.** A molecule or radical that can combine with a proton. **3.** The main ingredient in a compound, especially one used as a medication.

Basedow's goiter   A soft, enlarged thyroid gland that secretes excessive thyroid hormone after iodine administration.

basement membrane   A sheet of fragile, noncellular tissue on which the basal surfaces of epithelial cells rest. Its two layers are the basal lamina and reticular lamina.

base of the heart   The portion of the heart that lies opposite the apex and just below the second rib, forming the upper border of the heart. It consists primarily of the left atrium, part of the right atrium, and the proximal portions of the great vessels.

base of the skull   The floor of the cranium, containing the anterior, middle, and posterior cranial fossae and numerous foramina.

base pair   A pair of complementary nitrogenous bases in a nucleic acid. One of the pair is a purine, the other a pyrimidine. In deoxyribonucleic acid, adenine pairs with thymine and cytosine pairs with guanine.

base ratio   The ratio of molar quantities of the bases in ribonucleic acid and deoxyribonucleic acid.

basic amino acid   An amino acid that carries a positive electric charge in solution. The basic amino acids are arginine, histidine, and lysine.

basilar   Of or describing a base or a basal area.

basilar artery   The artery that's formed by the junction of the right and left vertebral arteries at the base of the skull, divides into the left and right cerebral arteries, and supplies blood to the internal ear and parts of the brain.

basophil   A granulocytic white blood cell whose segmented nucleus contains granules that stain blue when exposed to a basic dye.

basophilic leukemia   A rare acute or chronic malignant neoplasm of the blood-forming tissues in which basophils predominate.

basophilic stippling   The appearance of punctate, basophilic granules in red blood cells, visible microscopically on a Gram-stained smear of blood. Basophilic stippling is typical of lead poisoning.

bathycardia An unusually low position of the heart that isn't associated with disease.
battery The unauthorized touching of a person by another person. For example, a health care professional who treats a patient beyond the patient's consent has committed battery.
Battey bacillus *Mycobacterium intracellulare.*
Battle's sign Discoloration of the skin behind the ear following the fracture of a bone in the lower skull.
Baudelocque's method In obstetrics: a maneuver done to convert a face presentation to a vertex presentation. With the fetal head flexed vaginally, counterpressure is applied to the back of the head abdominally, as the fetus is rotated in the direction of flexion until the vertex is fixed in the pelvis.
Baynton's bandage A spiral adhesive wrap applied to the leg over a dressing, used in the treatment of certain leg ulcers.
B cell A lymphocyte that matures in the bone marrow and is a precursor of the plasma cell. It's primarily responsible for humoral immunity. When stimulated by an antigen, B cells proliferate and differentiate into plasma cells and memory B cells.
BCG *abbr* bacillus Calmette-Guérin.
BCG vaccine A vaccine prepared from bacillus Calmette-Guérin that's given in the United States to immunize individuals at high risk for tuberculosis.

 CLINICAL TIP BCG vaccine is also used as immunotherapy for some cancers because it's thought to stimulate cell-mediated immunity.

B complex vitamins A group of water-soluble substances that are necessary in trace amounts for normal body functioning. They include biotin, choline, cyanocobalamin (vitamin B_{12}), folic acid, inositol, niacin (vitamin B_3), para-aminobenzoic acid, pyridoxine (vitamin B_6), riboflavin (vitamin B_2), and thiamine (vitamin B_1).
Be Symbol for beryllium.
beaded **1.** Of or resembling a string of beads. **2.** Of or describing bacterial colonies that arise along the inoculation line in various stab cultures. **3.** Of or describing stained bacteria that form more deeply stained bead-like granules.
Beckwith's syndrome A hereditary disorder of unknown cause associated with neonatal hyperinsulinism and hypoglycemia. Also called *Beckwith-Wiedemann syndrome.*
Bednar's aphthae Small, yellowish, slightly raised and ulcerated patches normally seen on the posterior portion of the hard palate in newborns.

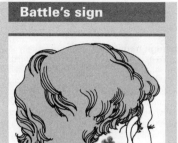

Battle's sign

Behçet's disease A rare, chronic inflammation of unknown cause marked by retinal vasculitis, optic atrophy, ulcerations of the oral and pharyngeal mucous membranes and genitalia, and skin lesions.
Békésy audiometry A technique for evaluating hearing in which the subject presses a signal button while listening to a pure tone of progressively decreasing intensity, and releases the button when the sound no longer is audible.
Bell's palsy Unilateral facial paralysis of sudden onset resulting from trauma to the facial nerve, from compression of the nerve by a tumor, or from an unknown cause.
Bell's phenomenon Upward and outward rolling of the eyeball during an attempt to close the eye; a sign of peripheral facial paralysis.
Bence Jones protein An abnormal plasma or urinary protein occurring almost exclusively in patients with multiple myeloma. The protein is the light chain component of myeloma globulin.
bending fracture A fracture indirectly caused by the bending of a limb.
Benedict's qualitative test A test for urine glucose based on the reduction by glucose of cupric ions to a colored cuprous oxide prebenzodiazepine derivative. If glucose is present, the solution fills with a red, yellow, or green precipitate.
benign Of a tumor: not cancerous and therefore favorable for recovery; however, treatment may eventually be required for health or cosmetic reasons.
benign juvenile melanoma A benign, raised, pinkish papule with a scaly surface,

most commonly seen on the cheek of children ages 9 to 13. Also called *compound melanocytoma, spindle cell nevus, Spitz nevus.*

benign neoplasm   A tumor, usually localized, that has a fibrous capsule, limited growth potential, a regular shape, and well-differentiated cells. Although the tumor may cause harm by pressure, it doesn't invade surrounding tissues or metastasize to distant sites, and it rarely recurs after surgical excision. Types of benign neoplasms include adenoma, fibroma, hemangioma, and lipoma.

benign prostatic hypertrophy   Enlargement of the prostate gland. Although not malignant or inflammatory, the condition is usually progressive and may result in obstruction of the urethra and interference with urine flow, possibly causing frequent urination, nocturia, pain, and urinary tract infections.

 TIME LINE Benign prostatic hypertrophy is common in men by age 50.

benign tumor   A neoplasm that doesn't invade other tissues or metastasize to distant sites. Usually well encapsulated, its cells display less anaplasia than those of a malignant growth.

Bennett's fracture   A fracture of the base of the first metacarpal bone extending into the carpometacarpal joint. It may be associated with dorsal subluxation or dislocation of the first metacarpal.

bent fracture   An incomplete greenstick fracture.

Bergonié-Tribondeau law   In radiotherapy: a principle stating that a cell's sensitivity to radiation varies directly with its reproductive capacity and inversely with the degree of cell differentiation.

beriberi   A disease caused by deficiency of or inability to assimilate thiamine (vitamin B_1). It commonly results from a diet limited to polished white rice and is characterized by polyneuritis, cardiac dysfunction, and edema. The endemic form occurs in eastern and southern Asia.

berkelium (Bk)   An artificial, radioactive, transuranic element produced by bombardment of the isotope of americium. Its atomic number is 97; its atomic weight is 247.

Bernard-Soulier syndrome   A hereditary coagulation disorder characterized by inability of the platelets to aggregate owing to relative lack of an essential glycoprotein in their membranes.

Bernoulli's law   In chemistry: a theorem stating that the velocity of a gas or fluid flowing through a tube is inversely proportional to the pressure exerted by the fluid or gas

against the side of the tube — the greater the velocity, the lower the pressure.

Bernoulli's principle   In physics: a principle stating that at any point in a tube through which a fluid is flowing, the sum of the velocity and the kinetic energy of the fluid flowing is constant. The greater the velocity, the less the lateral pressure on the wall of the tube.

berry aneurysm   A saccular dilation of the wall of a cerebral artery, usually at the junction of the vessels in the circle of Willis.

berylliosis   Poisoning caused by inhalation of fumes, fine dusts, mists, or vapors containing beryllium or beryllium compounds. The condition usually involves the lungs and less often the lymph nodes, liver, skin, and other structures.

 ALERT This disease occurs in two forms: acute nonspecific pneumonitis; and chronic noncaseating granulomatous disease with interstitial fibrosis, which may cause death from respiratory failure and cor pulmonale.

beryllium (Be)   A gray, lightweight metallic element. Its atomic number is 4; its atomic weight is 9.012. Beryllium is toxic and can cause serious lung disease and dermatitis.

beta (ß)   The second letter of the Greek alphabet; it may appear with chemical names as a combining form to differentiate one of two or more isomers or to signify the position of substituted atoms in certain compounds.

beta cells   1. Insulin-producing cells that compose the bulk of the islets of Langerhans. 2. Basophilic cells of the anterior lobe (adenohypophysis) of the pituitary gland.

beta fetoprotein   A protein that's identical to normal liver ferritin, found in the fetal liver and in some adults with liver disease.

beta particle   An electron or a positron emitted from the nucleus of an atom during radioactive (beta) decay.

beta receptor   An adrenergic receptor that responds to epinephrine and blocking agents such as propranolol. Beta receptors occur in two types: $beta_1$ and $beta_2$. Activation of $beta_1$-receptors causes the heart rate and the force of cardiac contraction to increase. Activation of $beta_2$-receptors causes relaxation of the bronchial muscles and vasodilation. Also called *beta-adrenergic receptor.*

betatron   A particle accelerator that produces high-energy electrons by magnetic induction for the production of high-energy X-rays and other research purposes.

beta wave   One of the four types of brain waves recorded by an electroencephalograph, having a frequency of 18 to 30 per second. It typically occurs during periods of intense neurologic activity, principally in the frontal and the central areas of the cerebrum, in an individual who's awake and alert with eyes open.

Bi Symbol for bismuth.

bias 1. A diagonal line. 2. A prejudiced outlook. 3. In statistics: a systematic error resulting from a particular sampling process. 4. In electronics: a voltage applied to an electronic device, as a vacuum tube or a transistor, to establish a reference level for operation.

biceps brachii The long fusiform muscle of the upper arm on the anterior surface of the humerus, arising in two heads from the scapula.

biceps reflex Contraction of the biceps muscle when its tendon is tapped; a normal reflex.

biconcave Concave on both sides.

biconvex Convex on both sides.

bicornate Having two horns or processes.

bicuspid 1. Having two cusps or points. 2. One of the two teeth between the molars and canines of the upper and lower jaw. Also called *premolar tooth.* 3. Pertaining to the bicuspid valve of the heart.

bifid Split into two parts or branches.

bifocal 1. Having two foci. 2. Of a lens: having two areas of different focal lengths — a smaller one for near vision and a larger one for distant vision.

bifurcation 1. Division into two branches. 2. The site where a single structure splits into two.

Bigelow's lithotrite A long-jawed lithotrite, passed through the urethra to crush a calculus (stone) in the bladder.

bigeminal pulse An abnormal pulse in which two beats occur in rapid succession and are followed by an interval during which no pulse is felt.

bigeminy 1. Occurring in pairs. 2. An arrhythmia characterized by two beats in rapid succession followed by a longer interval.

bilabe An instrument used to remove small calculi from the bladder through the urethra.

bilateral Having or occurring on two sides.

bilateral long leg spica cast An orthopedic device that encases and immobilizes the trunk cranially up to the nipple line and both legs caudally as far as the toes. A horizontal crossbar connects the parts of the cast that encase both legs at ankle level.

 CLINICAL TIP A bilateral long leg spica cast is used to promote healing of fractures of the hip, pelvis, femur, or

acetabulum as well as to correct or maintain correction of a hip deformity.

bile A bitter, yellow-green fluid secreted by the liver and stored in the gallbladder. Bile passes from the gallbladder through the common bile duct after an individual has ingested a fatty meal; it emulsifies the fats, preparing them for further digestion and absorption in the small intestine.

bile acid A steroid carboxylic acid of the bile derived from cholesterol. Most bile acids are reabsorbed and returned to the liver by way of the enterohepatic circulation; in the liver, they are reconjugated and excreted again.

bile solubility test A test used to differentiate pneumococcal infection from other streptococcal infection.

biliary Pertaining to bile or to the gallbladder and its ducts, which transport bile.

biliary atresia Congenital absence or underdevelopment of one or more of the biliary structures, resulting in jaundice and liver damage.

biliary cirrhosis Cirrhosis of the liver caused by obstruction or infection of the liver ductules. Signs and symptoms include jaundice, abdominal pain, steatorrhea, and enlargement of the liver and spleen.

biliary colic Pain caused by passage of gallstones through the bile ducts. Also called *gallstone colic, hepatic colic, cholecystalgia.*

biliary duct A duct that conveys bile from the liver to the duodenum.

bilirubin A bile pigment formed by the breakdown of hemoglobin in red blood cells at the end of their normal life span. Water-insoluble, unconjugated bilirubin normally flows through the bloodstream to the liver for conversion to a water-soluble, conjugated form and subsequent excretion into the bile.

biliuria The presence of bile in the urine.

biliverdin A greenish bile pigment formed by hemoglobin breakdown and converted to bilirubin.

Billroth's operation I Surgical removal of the pylorus, with anastomosis of the severed end of the duodenum to the end of the resected stomach.

Billroth's operation II Surgical removal of the pylorus with anastomosis of the resected stomach to the jejunum.

bilobulate, bilobular Having two lobes.

bilocular, biloculate 1. Having two compartments. 2. In biology: divided into or containing two cells.

bimanual Performed with both hands.

bimanual palpation Method of palpation that uses both hands to locate body structures and assess their texture, size, consistency, mobility, and tenderness.

binary fission Direct division of a cell or nucleus into two parts that are approximately equal; a common form of asexual reproduction used by bacteria, protozoa, and other lower life forms.

bind 1. To wrap or bandage in a band. 2. In chemistry: to form a weak, reversible chemical bond, as between toxins and antitoxins.

binder A broad bandage or girdle, especially one that surrounds and supports the abdomen or chest.

binocular 1. Pertaining to both eyes. 2. Describing a microscope, telescope, or field glass having two eyepieces.

binocular fixation A condition in which both eyes are directed at the same object at the same time. It's essential to depth perception.

binocular parallax The apparent difference in the position of an object as seen separately by one eye and then by the other as the head remains stationary. Binocular parallax is a major factor in depth perception. Also called *stereoscopic parallax.*

binocular perception The ability to judge depth or distance by virtue of having two eyes.

binomial 1. A biological species name having two terms. 2. A mathematical expression having two terms that are connected by a plus or minus sign.

bioassay Laboratory determination of the concentration of a substance in a sample or specimen by comparing its effect on an organism, animal, or isolated organ preparation with that of a standard preparation. Also called *biological assay.*

bioavailability The degree to which a drug or other substance becomes available for activity in the target tissue after administration.

biochemistry The chemistry of living organisms and life processes. Also called *biological chemistry, physiologic chemistry.*

bioequivalent Having the same strength and similar bioavailability in the same dosage form as another drug.

biofeedback A technique involving monitoring devices in which an individual receives visual or auditory information about certain physiologic functions, such as blood pressure, muscle tension, and brain wave activity, and then learns to control these functions.

bioflavonoid Any of a group of naturally occurring phenolic compounds required for the maintenance of collagen and of the capillary walls.

 CLINICAL TIP Some researchers believe bioflavonoids may help protect against infection or cancer.

biogenesis, biogeny 1. The theory that living material can arise only from preexisting living matter and not from inanimate matter. 2. The synthesis of chemical compounds or structures in living organisms.

biogenic 1. Produced by the action of a living organism. 2. Necessary for life and the maintenance of health.

biogenic amine One of a large group of organic compounds synthesized by plants and animals, most of which act as neurotransmitters. For instance, norepinephrine plays a role in emotional reactions, memory, sleep, and arousal from sleep.

biological half-life The time required for the body to eliminate one-half of an administered dosage of any substance through regular physiologic processes.

biological response modifiers (BRMs) Agents used in biological therapy that alter the body's response to cancer.

biological safety cabinet (BSC) Specialized work area for preparation of chemotherapeutic drugs.

biology The scientific study of life and living organisms in general. Its branches include biometry, ecology, molecular biology, and paleontology.

biome A major type of ecological community, such as a desert, tropical rain forest, woodland, or tundra, including all of its plants, animals, and microorganisms.

biomechanics The application of mechanical laws to living structures, especially the human body and its locomotor system.

biomedical engineering A group of techniques that applies knowledge of biological processes to solve practical medical problems and to address issues in biomedical research.

bionics The science of applying data about the functioning of biological systems to medical problems. It may involve such devices as artificial pacemakers.

biopsy The removal of tissue from an organ or other part of the body for microscopic examination to aid or confirm diagnosis, gauge the patient's prognosis, or monitor the course of a disease.

biopsychosocial Describing the biological, psychological, and social aspects of life.

biorhythm Any cyclic physiologic event, such as the sleep cycle or the menstrual cycle.

biostatistics The application of statistics to the analysis of biological data, such as births, deaths, diseases, and other factors affecting general health and welfare. Also called *vital statistics.*

biosynthesis The production of biomolecules by a living cell through any one of the thousands of chemical reactions that continually occur within the body. Biosynthesis is the essential feature of anabolism.

biotaxis The selecting and arranging capacities of living cells.

biotechnology Applied biological science. This field involves the development of techniques that apply biological processes to the production of materials for use in medicine and industry.

biotin A water-soluble B complex vitamin. It plays a role in fatty acid metabolism and in the deamination of certain amino acids and promotes the utilization of protein, folic acid, pantothenic acid, and vitamin B_{12}.

biotin deficiency syndrome A syndrome resulting from a deficiency of biotin, marked by dermatitis, hyperesthesia, muscle pain, anorexia, slight anemia, and changes in cardiac activity.

biotransformation The chemical changes that the compounds of the body undergo, as by the activity of enzymes.

Biot's respiration An abnormal breathing pattern characterized by irregular periods of apnea alternating with periods of four or five breaths having the same depth.

 ALERT Biot's respiration indicates meningitis or increased intracranial pressure.

biparietal Pertaining to the two parietal bones or eminences of the skull.

biparietal diameter The distance separating the protuberances of the two parietal bones of the skull.

bipartite Having two parts or divisions.

biped 1. Having two feet. 2. Any animal with two feet.

bipedal 1. Having two feet. 2. Capable of locomotion on two feet.

biphasic Having two phases or stages.

bipolar 1. Having or pertaining to two poles, as in certain electrotherapeutic treatments using two poles. 2. Of a nerve cell: having both an afferent and an efferent process. 3. Pertaining to mood disorders in which both manic and depressive episodes occur.

bismuth (Bi) A pinkish, crystalline, trivalent metallic element with low thermal conductivity. Its atomic number is 83; its atomic weight is 209.

bitegage A device used in prosthetic dentistry to help achieve proper occlusion of the teeth that have roots in the maxilla and the mandible.

bitelock A dental device used to maintain the occlusion rims in the same relation outside the mouth as inside the mouth.

biteplate A removable device that provides the anchorage needed for desired tooth movement. It's used to stimulate eruption of the posterior teeth, to reduce anterior overbite, to correct temporomandibular joint problems, or as a splint in restoring the full mouth.

Bitot's spots Superficial white or gray triangular deposits on the bulbar conjunctiva associated with vitamin A deficiency.

biuret test A method used to detect soluble proteins, such as urea in the serum.

bivalent 1. In genetics: Describing the structure formed by a pair of homologous chromosomes that are joined by synapsis along their length during the early first meiotic prophase of gametogenesis. The structure serves as the basis for the tetrads from which gametes are produced in the two meiotic divisions. 2. In chemistry: Having a valency of two.

bivalve cast An orthopedic cast that immobilizes a part of the body to promote healing of a fractured bone or to correct or maintain the correction of an orthopedic deformity.

Blackfan-Diamond syndrome A congenital hypoplastic anemia that appears during the first 3 months of life, characterized by severe anemia and a very low reticulocyte count with normal numbers of platelets and white blood cells.

blackwater fever A severe complication of malaria characterized by intravascular hemolysis, hemoglobinuria, acute renal failure, and passage of bloody dark red or brown urine. The illness may represent an autoimmune response to malaria.

bladder 1. A saclike organ that acts as a receptacle for secretions. 2. The urinary bladder.

bladder cancer The most common cancer of the urinary tract, marked by a neoplasm or by multiple neoplasms that tend to recur in a more aggressive form.

Blalock-Taussig operation Surgical creation of a shunt as a palliative measure to manage congenital pulmonary stenosis and atrial-septal defects, as in a neonate with tetralogy of Fallot.

blanch 1. To make or become pale or ashen, as from vasoconstriction accompanying anger or fear. 2. To whiten or bleach a surface or substance.

bland diet A diet that's free of irritating or stimulating foods.

CLINICAL TIP A bland diet is commonly prescribed after abdominal surgery or for the treatment of such GI disorders as peptic ulcer, ulcerative colitis, gallbladder disease, diverticulosis, and diverticulitis.

blanket bath The wrapping of a patient in a wet pack and then in blankets.

blast cell An immature cell, such as an erythroblast or a lymphoblast.

blastema, *pl.* blastemas, blastemata A group of cells capable of growth and differentiation that lead to the formation of a new individual, organ, or part.

blastid, blastide The site of nucleus organization in a fertilized ovum.

blastocyst The embryo precursor that follows the morula in human development; a spherical mass of cells with a central, fluid-filled cavity (blastocoele) surrounded by an inner layer of cells (embryoblast) and outer layer of cells (trophoblast). Implantation in the uterine wall typically occurs at this stage.

blastocyte An undifferentiated embryonic cell.

blastoderm The mass of cells produced by cleavage of a fertilized ovum, forming the wall of the blastocyst in mammals during the early stages of embryonic development. Also called *germinal membrane.*

blastogenesis 1. Asexual reproduction. 2. Transmission of inherited characteristics by the germ plasm.

blastogenic 1. Originating in the germ cell. 2. Pertaining to blastogenesis.

blastogeny The germ plasm history of an organism or a species.

blastokinin A globulin secreted by the uterus that may stimulate and regulate implantation of the blastocyst in the uterine wall. Also called *uteroglobulin.*

blastolysis The destruction or splitting up of a germ cell or blastoderm.

blastoma, *pl.* blastomas, blastomata A neoplasm that's composed of embryonic cells derived from the blastema of an organ or tissue.

blastomatosis The occurrence of many neoplasms that derive from embryonic tissue.

blastomere One of a pair of cells produced by cleavage of a fertilized ovum. During the first several days of pregnancy, the two blastomeres divide and subdivide to form the morula.

Blastomyces A genus of imperfect, yeastlike fungus, usually including the species *Blastomyces dermatitidis,* which causes North American blastomycosis.

blastomycosis An infectious disease caused by *Blastomyces dermatitidis,* a fungus that usually affects only the skin but may invade the lungs, kidneys, central nervous system, and bones. The disease is most common in young men living in North America.

 CLINICAL TIP Initial signs and symptoms of pulmonary blastomycosis mimic those of viral upper respiratory tract infection.

blastopore In embryology: the invagination into a blastula that occurs in the process of the blastula becoming a gastrula.

blastulation Transformation of the morula into a blastocyst or blastula by the development of a central cavity (the blastocoele).

bleb Accumulation of fluid under the skin, usually associated with lesions that are smaller than normal blisters.

bleeding time The time required for blood to stop flowing from a tiny wound.

 CLINICAL TIP Bleeding time may be measured by the Duke, Ivy, or Template method. The Template method is the most accurate and widely used. Normal bleeding time is 1 to 3 minutes for the Duke method, 1 to 7 minutes for the Ivy, and 2 to 8 minutes for the Template.

blepharal Of or pertaining to the eyelids.

blepharitis An inflammatory condition of the lash follicles and meibomian glands of the eyelids, characterized by swelling, redness, and crusts of dried mucus on the eyelids.

 CLINICAL TIP Seborrheic blepharitis may be seen in conjunction with seborrhea of the scalp, eyebrows, and ears.

blepharon Eyelid.

blepharoplegia Paralysis of the eyelid.

blepharospasm Spasm of the orbicularis oculi muscle, causing closure of the eyelid.

blind fistula An abnormal passage with only one open end; the opening may be on the body surface or on or within an internal organ or structure.

blind loop A redundant segment of intestine. Bacterial overgrowth may lead to malabsorption, obstruction, and necrosis.

blind spot 1. A normal gap in the visual field occurring when an image is focused on the space in the retina occupied by the optic disk. 2. An abnormal gap in the visual field due to a lesion on the retina or in the optic pathways or to hemorrhage or choroiditis, often perceived as light spots or flashes.

blister A vesicle or bulla.

blocking 1. Preventing the transmission of a nerve impulse by the injection of an anesthetic. 2. Interrupting an intracellular biosynthetic process, as by the injection of actinomycin D. 3. Being unable to remember, or involuntarily interrupting, a train of thought or speech, usually owing to emotional or mental conflict. **4.** Repressing an idea or emotion to keep it from obtruding into the consciousness.

blocking antibody An antibody that fails to cross-link and cause agglutination.

blood agar A culture medium consisting of blood and nutrient agar, used in bacteriology to cultivate certain microorganisms.

blood bank An organizational unit responsible for collecting, processing, and storing blood to be used for transfusion and other purposes. It's usually a subdivision of a laboratory in a hospital and is often charged with the responsibility for all serologic testing.

blood-brain barrier (BBB) An anatomic-physiologic feature of the brain, thought to consist of the walls of capillaries in the central nervous system and surrounding glial membranes.

 CLINICAL TIP The blood-brain barrier slows or helps to prevent the passage of various chemical compounds, radioactive ions, and disease-causing organisms (such as viruses) from the blood into the central nervous system.

blood buffers A system of buffers, composed primarily of dissolved carbon dioxide and bicarbonate ions, that helps to maintain the proper pH level of the blood.

blood cell Any of the formed elements of the blood, including red cells (erythrocytes), white cells (leukocytes), and platelets (thrombocytes). Together, these elements normally constitute about 50% of the total volume of the blood.

blood clot A semisolid, gelatinous mass that results from the clotting process in blood. A blood clot ordinarily consists of red cells, white cells, and platelets enmeshed in an insoluble fibrin network.

blood clotting The conversion of blood from a free-flowing liquid to a semisolid gel. Although blood clotting can occur within the intact blood vessel, the process usually starts with tissue damage and exposure of the blood to air. Within seconds after the vessel wall is injured, platelets aggregate at the site. If calcium, platelets, and tissue factors are present in normal amounts, prothrombin is converted to thrombin. Thrombin then catalyzes the conversion of fibrinogen to insoluble fibrin, and all of the formed elements are immobilized. Also called *blood coagulation.*

blood culture medium A liquid enrichment medium for the growth of bacteria used in the diagnosis of blood infections. It contains a suspension of brain tissue in meat broth with dextrose, peptone, and citrate, and has a pH of 7.4.

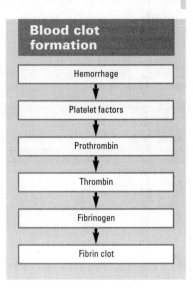

Blood clot formation

Hemorrhage

↓

Platelet factors

↓

Prothrombin

↓

Thrombin

↓

Fibrinogen

↓

Fibrin clot

blood donor An individual who donates blood to a blood bank or directly to another person.

blood fluke A parasitic flatworm of the class Trematoda, genus Schistosoma, including the species *Schistosoma haematobium, S. japonicum,* and *S. mansoni.*

blood gas Gas that's dissolved in the liquid part of the blood. Blood gases include oxygen, carbon dioxide, and nitrogen.

blood gas determination An analysis of the pH of the blood and the concentration and pressure of oxygen, carbon dioxide, and hydrogen ion in the blood. It can be performed rapidly as an emergency procedure to assess acid-base balance and ventilatory status.

blood group The classification of blood based on the presence or absence of genetically determined antigens on the surface of the red cell. More than 14 different grouping systems have been described; their relative importance depends on their clinical significance in transfusion therapy.

blood plasma The liquid portion of the blood, free of its formed elements and particles. Plasma represents approximately 50% of the total volume of blood. It contains glucose, proteins, amino acids, and other nutritive materials, urea and other excretory products as well as hormones, enzymes, vitamins, and minerals.

blood pressure (BP) The pressure exerted by the circulating volume of blood on the walls of the arteries, the veins, and the chambers of the heart. Overall blood pressure is maintained by the complex interaction of the homeostatic mechanisms of the body, moderated by the volume of blood, the lumen of the arteries and arterioles, and the force of the cardiac contraction.

 CLINICAL TIP When routine blood pressure screening reveals elevated pressure, first make sure the cuff size is appropriate for the patient's arm circumference.

blood pump 1. A pump that regulates the flow of blood into a blood vessel during transfusion. 2. A component of a heart-lung machine that pumps the blood through the machine for oxygenation and then through the peripheral circulatory system of the body.

blood substitute A substance used as a replacement for circulating blood or for extending its volume. Plasma, human serum albumin, packed red cells, platelets, leukocytes, and concentrates of clotting factors are commonly administered in place of whole blood transfusions in the treatment of various disorders.

blood transfusion The administration of whole blood or a component, such as packed red cells, to replace blood lost through trauma, surgery, or disease.

blood typing Identification of genetically determined antigens on the surface of the red blood cell, used to determine an individual's blood group.

blood urea nitrogen (BUN) The amount of nitrogenous substance present in the blood as urea.

 CLINICAL TIP BUN is a rough indicator of kidney function.

blood vessel Any tube in the network of tubes that carries blood throughout the body.

blood-warming coil A device made of coiled plastic tubing, used for warming reserve blood before massive transfusions (such as some required by patients with extensive GI bleeding).

blow-out fracture A fracture of the floor of the orbit caused by a blow that suddenly increases the intraocular pressure.

blue baby A neonate born with cyanosis, owing either to a congenital heart lesion, such as transposition of the great vessels or tetralogy of Fallot, or to incomplete expansion of the lungs (congenital atelectasis).

blue nevus A sharply defined, slow-growing nodular tumor, usually benign, blue to black in color. It may be found on the face or upper extremities or, less commonly, on the buttocks or in the sacrococcygeal region.

blunt hook 1. A hook-shaped bar that provides traction between the abdomen and thigh, sometimes used in breech deliveries. 2. A blunt-ended hook used in embryotomy.

blush A brief, diffuse erythema of the face and neck resulting from vascular dilation in response to heat or emotion.

Boas' test 1. A test used to detect hydrochloric acid in the stomach contents. 2. A gastric motility test in which a fasting patient drinks a green-tinted chlorophyll solution; aspiration of the stomach contents 30 minutes later and measurement of the remaining green-tinted water determines how much of the solution has passed through the stomach.

body fluid Fluid contained in the body. Such fluid exists within three compartments — within the blood plasma and lymphatic system (intravascular fluid compartment), within body cells (intracellular fluid compartment), and distributed throughout the loose tissue surrounding the cells (interstitial fluid compartment).

body mechanics The study of the actions and functions of muscles in maintaining posture.

body movement Motion of the body, especially at a joint or joints. Types of body movements include abduction, adduction, extension, flexion, and rotation.

body position The disposition, attitude, or posture of the body. Body positions include anatomic, prone, decubitus, supine, and Trendelenburg's, among others.

body-righting reflex A neuromuscular response that restores the body to an upright position after displacement.

body stalk A precursor of the umbilical cord; a mesodermic bridge between the posterior end of the embryo and the chorion prior to formation of the allantoic stalk.

body temperature The usually constant level of heat that's maintained by heat-producing and heat-dispelling processes.

 CLINICAL TIP Body temperature may vary within a narrow range, depending on the time of day and measurement site.

 TIME LINE Absence of a fever doesn't necessarily mean absence of infection in an elderly person. Many older adults develop subnormal temperatures in response to infection.

boiling point The temperature at which a liquid boils and passes to a gaseous state, equal to the atmospheric pressure.

Bolivian hemorrhagic fever A fever caused by the Machupo virus (an arenavirus), occurring primarily in rural northeastern Bolivia. Humans can contract the disease through contact with the excretions of an infected rodent (usually through contamination of food by rodent urine).

bolus 1. A dose of medication, contrast material, radioactive isotope, or other pharmaceutical preparation given all at once I.V. 2. A round mass of prepared medicinal material or masticated food ready to be swallowed. Also called *alimentary bolus.*

Bombay phenotype A rare phenotype resulting in lack of the H antigen, produced by the interaction of genes in the ABO blood group and a rare recessive gene. The expression of the A, B, and H antigens is suppressed in the cells of individuals with this phenotype.

bone The connective tissue that forms the skeleton of most vertebrates, comprising the 206 bones of the human skeleton. This dense, slightly elastic tissue is composed of organic material (cells and matrix) and inorganic material (mineral components, chiefly calcium phosphate and calcium carbonate).

bone cancer A malignant tumor of the skeleton, usually representing metastasis from cancer elsewhere in the body. Primary bone tumors are relatively rare.

bone marrow The soft tissue that fills bone cavities. *Yellow marrow* is ordinary marrow consisting mainly of fat cells. *Red marrow* is found in developing bone in the sternum, ribs, and vertebral bodies of adults; it's the production site of erythrocytes and granular leukocytes.

booster injection Administration of an antigen, such as a vaccine or toxoid, after administration of the original injection to maintain immunity. Booster injections involve smaller amounts of the antigen than given in the original injection.

Boothby-Lovelace-Bulbulian (BLB) mask A device used to administer oxygen both at high altitudes and in clinical settings. It consists of a mask with a combined inspiratory-expiratory valve and a rebreathing bag.

borborygmus, *pl.* **borborygmi** A rumbling, gurgling, or tinkling noise heard in the abdomen as gas is propelled through the intestines.

Bornholm disease An acute viral disease that usually results from group B coxsackieviruses. It's characterized by sudden pain in the ribs or upper abdomen, and usually affects persons under age 20.

boron (B) A nonmetallic element that occurs as both a crystal and a powder, which serves as the base for boric acid and borax. Its atomic number is 5; its atomic weight is 10.8.

botulism A type of food poisoning, commonly fatal, that results from a neurotoxin produced by the growth of *Clostridium botulinum* in improperly preserved or canned foods.

Bouchard's node A cartilaginous and bony enlargement of the proximal interphalangeal finger joint, as occurs in degenerative joint disease.

bougie A thin, flexible, cylindrical instrument inserted into the urethra or other tubular organ to dilate or examine it.

bounding pulse A pulse that feels full and springy on palpation, resulting from an increase in the thrust of cardiac contraction or a boost in the circulating blood volume.

boutonneuse fever An acute fever caused by *Rickettsia conorii*, transmitted to humans by a tick bite. The disease is heralded by a tache noire (black spot) at the infection site. Fever may last up to 2 weeks, with a papular erythematous rash spreading over the body. Boutonneuse fever occurs mainly in the Mediterranean, Black Sea, and Caspian Sea areas, with a variant form occurring in Africa and India.

bowel training A reflex conditioning technique used to establish regular bowel evacuation in the treatment of fecal incontinence, impaction, and autonomic hyperreflexia.

Bowman's capsule The cup-shaped dilation that forms the beginning of a renal tubule and surrounds the glomerulus. Also called glomerular capsule. See illustration on page 58

Boyle's law In physics: a law stating that the volume of a given mass of gas at a constant temperature is inversely proportional to its pressure. It applies only to an ideal gas.

Br Symbol for bromine.

brace An orthopedic appliance such as a leg brace that's used to support, maintain, or align parts of the body correctly, thereby allowing such functions as standing and walking.

brachial Of or relating to the arm.

brachial artery A continuation of the axillary artery; the major artery of the upper arm.

brachial plexus A network of nerves in the neck that innervate the muscles and skin of the chest, shoulders, and arms. The brachial plexus originates in the last four cervical and the first thoracic spinal nerves and passes under the clavicle and into the axilla.

brachial pulse The pulse of the brachial artery, which can be felt in front of the elbow (antecubital space).

brachioradialis reflex Slight elbow flexion and upper forearm supination when the lower end of the radius is tapped; a deep tendon reflex.

Bowman's capsule of the renal corpuscle

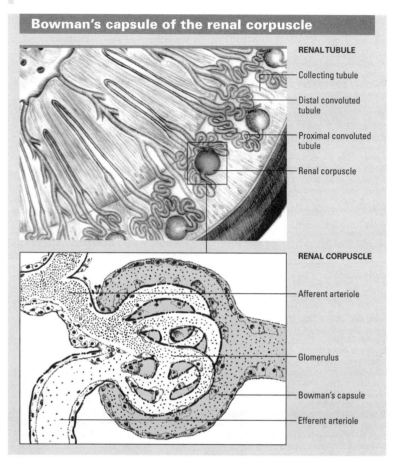

RENAL TUBULE

Collecting tubule

Distal convoluted tubule

Proximal convoluted tubule

Renal corpuscle

RENAL CORPUSCLE

Afferent arteriole

Glomerulus

Bowman's capsule

Efferent arteriole

Bradford frame A rectangular frame made of pipes to which movable straps of canvas are attached. The straps support the patient and keep him immobile while still permitting him to urinate and defecate.
Bradford solid frame A rectangular metal frame covered with canvas that's used for immobilization. The frame supports the patient's entire body, controlling movement by maintaining immobilization, positioning, and alignment. It's sometimes used for young children in traction.
bradycardia A slow but steady heart beat at a rate of less than 60 beats per minute.

 CLINICAL TIP Bradycardia is normal during sleep and in well-conditioned athletes. In other circumstances, it

may indicate an abnormal condition, such as brain tumor, digoxin toxicity, or vagotonus.
bradykinesia Abnormal slowness of physical movement, with sluggish mental responses.
bradykinin Nonpeptide kinin formed from a plasma protein; a powerful vasodilator that increases capillary permeability, constricts smooth muscle, and stimulates pain receptors.
bradypnea Regular but abnormally slow respirations.
brain One of the two components of the central nervous system, encased within the cranium and continuous with the spinal cord. Besides being the seat of intelligence, the brain serves as the main coordinating center for nervous activity, receiving and interpret-

ing nerve impulses sent by sense organs, and then conveying instructions to muscles and other effectors.

brain concussion   Injury to the brain caused by a blow to or violent jarring or shaking of the head, commonly resulting in loss of consciousness.

brain death   Final cessation of activity in the central nervous system, especially as indicated by a flat electroencephalogram for a predetermined length of time. The cessation of all measurable function or activity in every area of the brain, including the brain stem. Compare *death.*

brain electrical activity map (BEAM)   A computer-generated topographic map of the brain that's created by mapping the electrical potentials evoked in the brain by a flash of light.

brain scan   A picture of the brain that uses radioisotope imaging techniques to identify intracranial structures. After injection, the radioisotope circulates to the brain and accumulates in abnormal tissue. Brain scans are used diagnostically to identify intracranial masses, lesions, tumors, and infarcts.

brain stem   The portion of the brain that connects the cerebral hemispheres to the spinal cord, comprised of the medulla oblongata, pons, and mesencephalon. The brain stem houses the corticospinal and the reticulospinal nerve tracts and performs motor, sensory, and reflex functions.

brain stem auditory evoked potential (BAEP)   A test that uses evoked potentials to predict nerve damage in the auditory nerve region during surgery. Electroencephalographic waves from the auditory area are observed as a clicking sound is made; electrical activity typically stops in patients with nerve damage or destruction.

brain tumor   A neoplasm of the brain characterized by uncontrolled and progressive cell multiplication. Brain tumors are usually invasive but don't cross the cerebrospinal axis.

branched tubular gland   A multicellular gland having one excretory duct from two or more tubular secretory branches.

branchial fistula   An abnormal passage leading from the pharynx to the surface of the neck, caused by failure of a branchial cleft to close during fetal development.

Braxton Hicks contraction   Light, painless, irregular uterine tightening during pregnancy, arising during the first trimester and increasing in frequency, duration, and intensity by the third trimester. Also called *false labor.*

 CLINICAL TIP   Strong Braxton Hicks contractions occurring near term may be mistaken for true labor.

breach of contract   Failure to perform all or part of a contracted duty without justification.

breach of duty   The neglect or failure to fulfill in a proper manner the duties of an office, job, or position.

breast   **1.** The anterior portion of the chest **2.** A mammary gland.

breast cancer   A malignant neoplasm of the breast, which may be invasive and metastatic. In premenopausal women, breast cancer may be associated with ovarian hormonal function; in postmenopausal women, with adrenal function.

breast milk jaundice   A form of jaundice affecting breast-fed neonates after the seventh day. Researchers suspect the condition results from increased breast milk levels of the enzyme beta-gluconidase, which may increase intestinal bilirubin absorption and block bilirubin excretion in the newborn. Breast milk jaundice may persist for several weeks or even months. Also called *late-onset jaundice.*

breast self-examination   A procedure in which a woman examines her breasts for lumps, usually performed 7 to 10 days after the first day of the menstrual cycle, when the breasts are smallest and cyclic nodularity is minimal.

breath sound   The sound made as air and carbon dioxide pass in and out of the respiratory system, audible with a stethoscope.

breech birth   A potentially hazardous fetal presentation in which the feet, knees, or buttocks emerge from the birth canal first.

 ALERT   In a breech birth, the danger comes from possible trapping of the fetal head by an incompletely dilated cervix.

breech extraction   The pulling or drawing out of a newborn by the feet or buttocks first, before the trunk is delivered by traction.

breech presentation   A fetal position in which the buttocks or feet present. Types of breech presentation are complete breech, footling breech, frank breech.

broad beta disease   Accumulation in the blood of a lipoprotein having a high concentration of cholesterol and triglycerides. This familial type of hyperlipoproteinemia leads to yellowish nodules (xanthomas) on the elbows and knees, elevated serum cholesterol levels and, to a lesser extent, coronary and peripheral vascular disease. It affects males in their 20s and females in their 30s and 40s.

broad ligament of the uterus A fold of the peritoneum that supports the uterus from either side.

Broca's area A region of the brain that's located on the inferior frontal gyrus and takes part in speech production.

Brodie's abscess A staphylococcal infection of the bone, usually in the metaphyseal region of a long bone, that's characterized by a roughly spherical necrotic cavity surrounded by dense granulation tissue. Brodie's abscess is a form of osteomyelitis.

bromhidrosis The production of axillary (apocrine) sweat with an unpleasant odor.

bromide 1. A negatively charged bromine compound. 2. A bromine salt once widely used to depress the central nervous system, now used only occasionally to treat generalized tonic-clonic seizures.

bromine (Br) A toxic, reddish-brown liquid element of the halogen group that gives off suffocating vapors. Its atomic number is 35; its atomic weight is 79.909.

bronchial breath sound An abnormal sound, audible over the lungs by stethoscope, that signals consolidation caused by pneumonia or compression. Typically, inspiration and expiration produce high-pitched breath sounds of equal duration.

bronchial fremitus A vibration that can be palpated or auscultated as air passes through a bronchus filled with mucus during respiration.

bronchial tree An anatomic structure comprised of the bronchi and its branches. The bronchi divide from the trachea; the bronchial tubes, in turn, branch from the bronchi.

bronchiectasis A chronic condition of the bronchial tree marked by irreversible dilation and destruction of the bronchial walls, resulting in a paroxysmal, mucus-producing cough.

bronchiole A small subdivision of the bronchial tree that extends from the bronchi into the lobes of the lung.

bronchiolitis A lung inflammation that usually begins in the terminal bronchioles, occurring mainly in infants and debilitated persons. Also called *bronchopneumonia.*

CLINICAL TIP Commonly, bronchiolitis results from upper respiratory infection, specific infectious fevers, and other debilitating diseases.

bronchodilator An agent that dilates the smooth muscle of the bronchioles to promote ventilation to the lungs.

bronchogenic carcinoma A malignant new growth of epithelial cells that arises from the bronchial tree, producing such clinical effects as coughing, wheezing, fatigue, chest

tightness, aching joints and, in late stages, sputum, finger clubbing, weight loss, and pleural effusion.

bronchopneumonia Inflammation of the lungs and bronchioles, marked by chills, fever, increased heart and respiratory rates, a cough that produces purulent bloody sputum, severe chest pain, and abdominal distention. The condition typically represents the spread of bacterial infection (such as from *Mycoplasma pneumoniae, Staphylococcus pyogenes,* or *Streptococcus pneumoniae*) from the upper to the lower respiratory tract.

bronchopulmonary Of or pertaining to the lungs and its airways, both bronchial and pulmonary.

bronchoscope A rigid, metal tube or flexible fiberoptic instrument used to examine the tracheobronchial tree, to obtain a specimen for biopsy or culture, and to remove foreign bodies.

bronchoscopy Visual examination of the tracheobronchial tree using a bronchoscope.

bronchospasm A sudden, forceful, involuntary contraction of the smooth muscle of the bronchi, causing narrowing and obstruction of the airway.

bronchus, *pl.* bronchi Any of the larger air passages of the lungs, which convey inhaled air and exhaled waste gases.

Brooke formula A formula used to calculate fluid and electrolyte replacement for burn patients; developed at the Brooke Army Medical Center.

Brown-Séquard syndrome A neurologic disorder caused by damage to one side of the spinal cord above T10 and characterized by paralysis on the affected side, loss of position sense and posture, and loss of pain and temperature sensation on the unaffected side.

brucellosis A generalized infection caused by species of the gram-negative coccobacillus *Brucella;* transmitted to humans by such animals as cattle, swine, goats, deer, and rabbits from ingestion of contaminated milk or milk products or contact with natural reservoirs. The disease occurs mainly in rural areas among individuals who handle animals, such as farm workers, veterinarians, and slaughterhouse workers.

Brudzinski's sign In meningitis, bending the patient's neck usually produces flexion of the knee and hip.

bruit Abnormal sounds heard over peripheral vessels that indicate turbulent blood flow.

 CLINICAL TIP Bruits are most significant when heard over the abdominal aorta; the renal, carotid, femoral, popliteal, and subclavian arteries; and the thyroid gland.

bruxism   The involuntary grinding or clenching of the teeth, usually during sleep. This habit is thought to serve as a mechanism for releasing tension experienced during the waking hours.

bubonic plague   A severe bacterial infection caused by *Yersinia pestis,* transmitted by the bite of infected fleas. The most common form of plague, bubonic plague is characterized by abrupt onset of fever (commonly rising to 106° F [41° C]), followed by painful buboes (inflamed, swollen lymph nodes) in the axilla, groin, or neck; hemorrhagic tendencies; and symmetrical gangrene.

buccal   Of or relating to the inside of the cheek; may also refer to a tooth surface or the gum next to the cheek.

buccinator   The main muscle of the cheek, which compresses the cheek and retracts the angle of the mouth. It's one of the 12 muscles that control the mouth, originating from the maxilla above and the mandible below.

bucket-handle fracture   A fracture in which the semilunar cartilage is torn along the medial side, leaving a loop of cartilage in the intercondylar notch.

Buck's skin traction   Application of a pulling force to the lower extremity, with the hips and knees extended by an apparatus held in place with dressings affixed to the extremity's surface. This orthopedic mechanism may be used unilaterally or bilaterally to treat hip and knee contractures and diseases and to maintain postoperative positioning.

Buck's traction   Exertion of pull on the lower extremity using ropes, weights, and pulleys. It's one of the most common orthopedic mechanisms, used unilaterally or bilaterally to treat contractures and diseases of the hip and knee by immobilizing, positioning, and aligning the lower extremity.

Budd-Chiari syndrome   Obstruction of the hepatic veins by thrombi or fibrous obliteration; more often chronic than acute. The condition leads to enlargement and eventual failure of the liver, ascites, collateral vessel development, and severe portal hypertension.

buffer   A substance or group of substances that prevents changes in the concentration of another substance to minimize pH changes.

bulbourethral gland   One of two small glands next to the prostate that secrete a fluid component of the seminal fluid.

bulbous   Having the form or nature of a bulb.

bulbus   A rounded mass or enlargement.

bulimia, boulimia   An eating disorder characterized by episodes of binge eating that may end in self-induced vomiting, alternating with periods of normal eating or fasting. Depression and awareness that the behavior is abnormal are part of this illness.

bulla, *pl.* bullae   A thin-walled vesicle of the skin or mucous membranes, exceeding 1/4″ (1 cm) in diameter, that contains serous or seropurulent fluid.

bullous myringitis   A viral infection of the middle ear, characterized by fluid-filled or hemorrhagic vesicles on the tympanic membrane and accompanied by sudden severe ear pain.

BUN   *abbr* blood urea nitrogen.

bundle branch block   A cardiac conduction abnormality in which one ventricle is excited before the other owing to a conduction failure in the bundle of His.

bundle of His   A band of fibers arising in the atrioventricular (AV) node of the heart through which cardiac impulses are transmitted to the ventricles. After leaving the AV node, the bundle of His travels through the AV junction and beneath the endocardium of the right ventricle. At the upper end of the muscular part of the interventricular septum, it separates into right and left bundle branches, which descend as Purkinje fibers, into the walls of the right and left ventricle, respectively. Also called *atrioventricular bundle.* See illustration on page 62

Burkitt's lymphoma   A malignant neoplasm that consists of undifferentiated lymphoreticular cells, manifesting as a large osteolytic lesion in the jaw or, in children, an abdominal mass. It may result from the Epstein-Barr virus, a herpesvirus.

burn   Injury to body tissues resulting from exposure to heat, electricity, chemicals (such as caustic or corrosive substances), or gases (such as carbon monoxide gas). The severity of a burn is assessed primarily by evaluating its depth and extent.

 CLINICAL TIP Therapeutic treatment of a burn victim is directed at preventing infection and further loss of soft tissue, cartilage, or bone as well as promoting cosmetic healing and preserving body function.

Burow's solution   A liquid mixture made up of aluminum sulfate, acetic acid, precipitated calcium carbonate, and water; used as a topical astringent, antipyretic, and antiseptic for certain skin disorders.

bursa, *pl.* bursae   A fibrous, saclike cavity containing a viscid fluid, situated between certain tendons and the bones beneath them. The bursae act to prevent friction.

Bundle of His

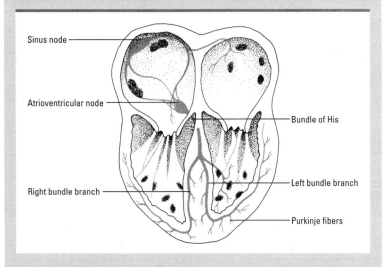

Sinus node

Atrioventricular node

Right bundle branch

Bundle of His

Left bundle branch

Purkinje fibers

bursitis   An inflammation of the bursa, sometimes accompanied by a calcific deposit.

butterfly bandage   A narrow adhesive strip of gauze or other material, with broad, winglike ends that are used to bring together the borders of a superficial injury and close the wound edges as it heals. In some cases, it may be used instead of a suture.

butterfly fracture   A fracture in which the bone is crushed or splintered, forming a pattern resembling a butterfly, with the main fragment abutted by two smaller fragments.

butterfly rash   A scaling eruption of the skin on the nose and adjacent areas of the cheeks, seen in systemic lupus erythematosus, rosacea, and seborrheic dermatitis.

TIME LINE Rare in pediatric patients, a butterfly rash may occur as part of an infectious disease such as erythema infectiousum, or "slapped cheek syndrome."

buttonhole fracture   A fracture in which the bone is perforated by a missile such as a bullet.

bypass   Any of various surgical procedures that redirects the flow of blood or other natural fluids from normal anatomic channels.

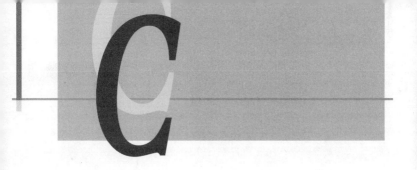

c *abbr* curie. **1.** Symbol for carbon. **2.** Symbol for cervical vertebrae (C1 through C7).

Ca Symbol for calcium.

cachexia A profound state of overall ill health and malnutrition characterized by weakness and emaciation.

Cacophony *pl.* **cacophonies** A discordant or jarring sound or a chaotic mixture of different sounds.

cadaver A dead body or corpse preserved for anatomic study.

cadmium (Cd) A bivalent, bluish-white metal resembling tin. Its atomic number is 48; its atomic weight is 112.40.

café-au-lait spot A pale brown macule.

CLINICAL TIP Café-au-lait spots are an important indicator of neurofibromatosis and other congenital melanotic disorders. The most common cause of café-au-lait spots is neurofibromatosis, also known as von Recklinghausen's disease.

calcaneal spurs Abnormal bony outgrowths on the lower surface of the heel bone that result from chronic pressure on the heel. Such spurs cause pain when walking.

calcaneus The largest tarsal bone, located at the back of the tarsus and generally known as the heel bone. The calcaneus meets proximally with the talus and distally with the cuboid.

calcarine fissure A furrow on the medial surface of the occipital lobe of the brain that separates the cuneus and the lingual gyrus. Also called *calcarine sulcus.*

calciferol A compound with vitamin D activity; a general term for the fat-soluble vitamins crucial for normal bone and tooth formation and for the absorption of calcium and phosphorus from the GI tract.

calcification Hardening of body tissues through the accumulation of calcium salt deposits.

calcitonin A hormone that helps regulate the blood calcium level and inhibit bone resorption. It's produced in the parafollicular cells of the thyroid gland.

calcium (Ca) A metal element; the most abundant mineral in the human body. Calcium is essential for proper functioning of the body, affecting the heart, nerves, muscles, blood coagulation, and formation of teeth and bones. Its atomic number is 20; its atomic weight is 40.

calcium pump A mechanism that transports calcium ions across a cell membrane from an area of low calcium ion concentration to an area of higher concentration.

Calculus *pl.* **calculi** A hardened area within the body, usually found in hollow organs or ducts, that's typically composed of mineral salts. A calculus may result in blockage and inflammation.

Caldwell-Moloy pelvic classification A classification system for identifying the female bony pelvis as android, anthropoid, gynecoid, or platypelloid in structure. See illustration on page 64

CLINICAL TIP Pure pelvic types are unusual. Most women have a combination of two basic types, with the features of one type predominating.

caliber, calibre The diameter of a tube or canal; commonly used in reference to a blood vessel.

californium (Cf) An element of the actinide group that's formed by irradiation of an isotope of curium with helium ions. Its atomic number is 98; californium isotopes have atomic weights from 244 to 245.

calipers A compass with two adjustable, curved legs, used to measure the thickness or diameter of a convex body or solid.

caliper splint A rigid leg appliance consisting of two metal rods extending from a band around the thigh or from a cushioned ring around the lower part of the pelvis. The splint is connected to a metal plate below the arch of the foot.

calix, *pl.* **calices** A cup-shaped organ or cavity such as a renal calix.

callosal fissure A furrow that encircles the convex aspect of the corpus callosum at the bottom of the longitudinal cerebral fissure.

callosomarginal fissure An irregular groove on the medial surface of a cerebral hemisphere, separating the cingulate gyrus

Caldwell-Moloy pelvic classification

GYNECOID

ANDROID

ANTHROPOID

PLATYPELLOID

from the medial frontal gyrus and from the paracentral lobule.

callus An area of skin thickened by repeated exposure to external pressure or friction.

calmodulin A calcium-binding polypeptide protein that's necessary for various biochemical and physiologic processes, including most calcium-sensitive cellular processes.

caloric Of or relating to calories or heat.

calorie The amount of heat needed to raise 1 kg of water 1° C at a specific temperature.

calvaria The skull cap or superior portion of the cranium where the frontal, parietal, and occipital bones meet.

Canadian crutch A device, usually made of wood or metal, that assists a disabled person to stand or walk. Its two uprights extend halfway between the elbow and shoulder; the patient's upper arm leans against a curved upper arm part. Also called *triceps crutch.*

canal of Schlemm A small vein at the angle of the anterior chamber of the eye that drains the aqueous humor and channels it into the bloodstream.

cancer 1. A malignant neoplasm of potentially unlimited growth, expanding locally by invasion and systemically by metastasis. 2. Any malignant neoplastic disease marked by the presence of malignant cells.

Candida A genus of yeastlike fungi that's part of the normal flora of the skin, mouth, intestines, and vagina. Overgrowth of *Candida* can cause infection.

Candida albicans A common, yeastlike fungi normally present in the body. Overgrowth of *C. albicans* can result in candidiasis.

canine tooth Any of the four teeth, two in each jaw, located next to the second incisors. Canine teeth have a long conical crown and the strongest root of all the teeth.

canker An ulcer or sore, especially of the mouth or lips.

cannon wave A tall, abnormal "a" wave seen in tracings of the jugular venous pulse, characteristic of complete heart block and premature ventricular beats. Cannon waves result from contraction of the right atrium after right ventricular contraction has closed the tricuspid valve.

cannula *pl.* **cannulas, cannulae** A flexible tube that's inserted into a duct or cavity. During insertion, it usually contains a stiff, pointed trocar.

Canthus *pl.* **canthi** The angle at either end of the fissure separating the lateral margins of the eyelids. The inner canthus opens into the space containing the lacrimal duct.

Cap. *abbr Latin capiat* 'let him or her take,' used in drug prescriptions.

CAP   In molecular genetics: an abbreviation for catabolic activator protein. CAP aids in the transcription of ribonucleic acid in organisms lacking a true nucleus, such as bacteria.

capillaritis   A progressive pigmentary skin disorder characterized by dilation without inflammation.

capillary   Any of the tiny vessels (roughly 0.008 mm in diameter) that join the arterioles and venules. The walls of the capillary act as semipermeable membranes for the exchange of various substances between the blood and interstitial fluid.

capillary action   The transport of a liquid in a tubular structure, resulting from cohesiveness of the liquid molecules. The more cohesive the molecules, the greater the elevation of the surface of the liquid.

capillary filtration   Movement of fluid and solutes out of the bloodstream, and into the interstitial fluid through capillary wall pores; caused by hydrostatic (fluid) pressure and blood pressure against the capillary walls.

capillary fracture   A thin, hairlike fracture that doesn't result in separation of the bone.

capillary hemangioma   A blood-filled birthmark or benign tumor composed of tightly packed capillaries; the most common type of hemangioma.

capillary reabsorption   The return of water and diffusible solutes to the capillaries that occurs when capillary blood pressure falls below colloid oncotic pressure.

capillus, *pl.* **capilli**   A hair, especially of the scalp.

capitation   A per-member, monthly payment to a provider that covers contracted services and is paid in advance of delivery. Essentially, a provider agrees to provide specified services to enrollees for this fixed payment for a specified term, regardless of how many times each member uses the service.

capitulum, *pl.* **capitula**   A small, rounded eminence on a bone where it articulates with another bone.

capnograph   An instrument that records the proportion of carbon dioxide in expired air and produces a tracing (capnogram). The device is used to help evaluate patients with acute respiratory disorders or who are receiving mechanical ventilation as well as to assess ventilation in anesthetized patients.

capsule   1. A small, hard or soft, soluble structure used to contain a dose of medication. 2. A part of the body that encloses an organ or other body part.

capsulotomy   An incision into a capsule; refers especially to surgical removal of a cataract.

capture   Successful pacing of the heart, represented on the electrocardiogram tracing by a pacemaker spike followed by a P wave or QRS complex.

carbohydrate   Any of a group of organic compounds of carbon, hydrogen, and oxygen (such as sugars, starches, gums, and celluloses). Carbohydrates constitute a major class of animal foods. They are classified according to molecular structure as mono-, di-, tri-, poly-, and heterosaccharides. Most carbohydrates are formed by green plants.

carbohydrate metabolism   The synthesis and breakdown of carbohydrates into galactose, fructose, and glucose through the anabolic and catabolic processes of the body.

carbon (C)   A nonmetallic tetrad element that's found in all living tissue, appearing in nearly pure form in diamond. Its atomic number is 6; its atomic weight is 12.011.

carbon 11   A positron-emitting radioisotope of carbon, produced by a cyclotron. Its atomic mass is 11; its half-life is 20 minutes.

carbon 14   A beta-emitting radioactive isotope of carbon that occurs naturally and is used as a tracer in research on cancer and metabolism. It atomic mass is 14; its half-life is 5,600 years.

carbon cycle   The process by which living organisms extract carbon (in the form of carbon dioxide) from the atmosphere and ultimately return it to the atmosphere. The carbon cycle is one of the major cycles of chemical elements in the environment.

carbon dioxide (CO_2)   A heavy, colorless, odorless gas created by the oxidation of carbon. It's formed in the tissues, carried by the blood (through cell respiration) to the lungs, and is exhaled.

carbon dioxide tension   The partial pressure of carbon dioxide gas in the blood, expressed as $Paco_2$ and measured in millimeters of mercury (mm Hg).

carbon monoxide   A toxic, odorless, colorless gas that's formed by the combustion of carbon or organic fuels having a poor oxygen supply.

 ALERT   Carbon monoxide combines irreversibly with hemoglobin in the blood, causing asphyxiation.

carbuncle   An infection of the skin and subcutaneous tissue, usually caused by *Staphylococcus aureus*, that consists of a cluster of abscesses or boils filled with purulent matter in deep, interconnecting, subcutaneous sinuses.

carcinoembryonic antigen (CEA)   A glycoprotein normally found in the feces and

Cardiac sphincter

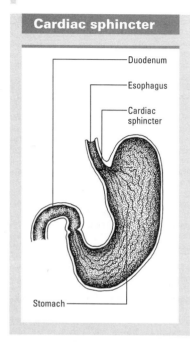

- Duodenum
- Esophagus
- Cardiac sphincter
- Stomach

pancreaticobiliary secretions. It also occurs in the plasma of patients with certain disorders (such as cancer of the breast, colon, lung, pancreas, and stomach), and is used to monitor the response of colorectal cancer to treatment.

carcinogen   A cancer-causing substance.

carcinoid   A small, yellow tumor of the small intestine, appendix, stomach, or colon, originating from argentaffin cells in the mucosa of the GI tract.

carcinoma, *pl.* carcinomas, carcinomata   A malignant growth composed of epithelial cells. It's commonly invasive and metastatic.

carcinoma in situ   A carcinoma that hasn't spread to the basement membrane but shows cytologic features of invasive cancer.

carcinomatosis   Widespread dissemination of carcinoma throughout the body.

cardiac arrhythmia   A deviation from the normal pattern of the heartbeat, involving the rate, regularity, or site of impulse origin or the sequence of activation of the heart chambers.

cardiac asthma   A paroxysmal attack of labored or difficult breathing associated with heart disease such as ventricular failure.

cardiac catheter   A long, fine, tubular instrument used to access the heart through a blood vessel. It permits the measurement of blood pressure and flow rate in the chambers and vessels of the heart and allows identification of abnormal structures.

cardiac catheterization   A diagnostic procedure in which a cardiac catheter is inserted into a large vein (usually of an arm or leg) and then threaded through the vein to the patient's heart.

 CLINICAL TIP Cardiac catheterization allows measurement of blood pressure and flow rate in the heart chambers, collection of blood samples, and recording of films of the ventricles or arteries.

cardiac conduction defect   A fault or failure in the electrical pathways and specialized muscle fibers of the heart that carry impulses leading to contraction of the atria and ventricles.

cardiac cycle   The period from the beginning of one heartbeat to the beginning of the next heartbeat.

cardiac impulse   The palpable movement of the chest that's produced by the beating of the heart.

cardiac monitor   A device that allows continuous observation of cardiac function. It commonly includes electrocardiograph and oscilloscope readings, recording devices, and a record of cardiac function and rhythm.

cardiac murmur   An abnormal sound of finite length made as blood flows through the heart. It may indicate incomplete closure of a heart valve or valvular stenosis.

cardiac muscle   Striated, involuntary muscle of the myocardium, or wall of the heart, containing dark intercalated discs where the cytoplasmic membranes of two cardiac fibers abut. Cardiac muscle moves blood through the heart and into blood vessels. It contracts at a steady rate, regulated by an internal pacemaker.

cardiac output   The volume of blood ejected by the heart per minute (normally ranging from 4 to 8 liters). Cardiac output equals the stroke volume (the difference between end-diastolic volume and end-systolic volume) multiplied by the heart rate.

TIME LINE Cardiac output declines slightly with age. By age 70, cardiac output at rest may have diminished by 30% to 35%.

cardiac plexus   A network of nerves surrounding the base of the heart.

cardiac reserve   The potential capacity of the heart to function beyond its normal level of activity, depending on various physiologic and psychological demands.

cardiac sphincter   A circle of muscle fibers located where the esophagus and stomach meet.

cardiac standstill   Cessation of heart contractions. The condition may result from natural causes, ultimately leading to death, or it may be medically induced for surgical purposes.

cardiac tamponade   Compression of the heart resulting from increased intrapericardial pressure secondary to accumulation of fluid or blood in the pericardial sac (as from cardiac rupture or a penetrating wound).

 ALERT The rapid rise in intrapericardial pressure impairs diastolic filling and leads to such signs and symptoms as neck vein distention, decreased heart sounds, hypotension, tachypnea, weak or absent peripheral pulses (or pulsus paradoxus), and a pericardial friction rub.

cardinal frontal plane   The imaginary plane that separates the body into front and back sections. Also called *vertical plane.*

cardinal horizontal plane   The imaginary plane that separates the body into upper and lower sections.

cardinal ligament   A layer of subserous fascia that travels across the pelvic floor as an extension of the broad ligament.

cardiogenic shock   A condition of low cardiac output that results from heart pump failure, as in acute myocardial infarction, heart failure, or severe cardiomyopathy.

cardiogram   An electronic tracing of the heart's activity. Also *called electrocardiogram (ECG).*

cardiologist   A physician who specializes in the prevention, diagnosis, and treatment of heart disorders.

cardiology   The study of the heart, including its anatomy, normal functions, and diseases and disorders.

cardiomegaly   Hypertrophy or enlargement of the heart. Although usually caused by hypertension, cardiomegaly sometimes is associated with arteriovenous fistula, congenital aortic stenosis, ventricular septal defect, patent ductus arteriosus, or Paget's disease.

cardiomyopathy   Primary noninflammatory disease of the myocardium.

cardiopulmonary bypass   A procedure that diverts blood from the patient's heart and lungs to an external pump oxygenator and then returns it directly to the aorta. It's used in heart surgery to permit repair of the heart.

cardiopulmonary resuscitation (CPR)   An emergency procedure consisting of artificial ventilation and chest compressions, used to force air into the lungs and get blood circulating throughout the body of an individual who has neither a pulse nor a heartbeat.

cardiospasm   A painful, involuntary muscle contraction resulting from failure of the esophagogastric sphincter to relax on swallowing. Also called *achalasia of the esophagus.*

cardiovascular system   The network consisting of the heart, blood vessels, and lymphatics that serves as the body's transport system, bringing oxygen and nutrients to cells, removing metabolic wastes, and carrying hormones from one part of the body to the other. Also called *circulatory system.*

cardioversion   Restoration of a normal sinus heart rhythm by means of a synchronized electric shock delivered to the myocardium through paddles placed on the patient's chest.

carditis   An inflammation of the heart muscle, usually caused by infection.

caries   1. Decay of a tooth or a bone characterized by softening, discoloration, porosity, and destruction of the structure. 2. Dental caries.

carina, *pl.* **carinae**   A ridge-shaped structure, such as the carina of the trachea (a projection from the lowest tracheal cartilage).

carneous   Of or pertaining to flesh.

carnitine   A naturally occurring amino acid found in skeletal muscle and liver, necessary for oxidation of long-chain fatty acids.

carotene, carotin, carrotene, carrotine   A fat-soluble hydrocarbon that's converted into vitamin A by an enzyme in the liver and intestines. Carotene is found in carrots, sweet potatoes, milk fat, egg yolk, and dark green and yellow leafy vegetables.

carotid body   A small neurovascular structure located at the bifurcation of the carotid arteries, which monitors the body's blood oxygen levels and aids respiratory regulation.

carotid body reflex   A normal chemical reflex action occurring in response to a decrease in the blood oxygen concentration and, to a lesser degree, to an increase in carbon dioxide and hydrogen ion concentrations that act on carotid body chemoreceptors. This reflex stimulates nerve impulses that increase respiratory activity.

carotid plexus   Any of the three nerve networks associated with carotid arteries.

carotid pulse   The rhythmic expansion, or pulse, of the carotid artery. It may be palpated in the neck between the larynx and the sternocleidomastoid muscle. See illustration on page 68

carotid sinus   A dilated portion of the internal carotid artery, located near the bifurcation of the common carotid artery. Changes

Location of carotid pulse

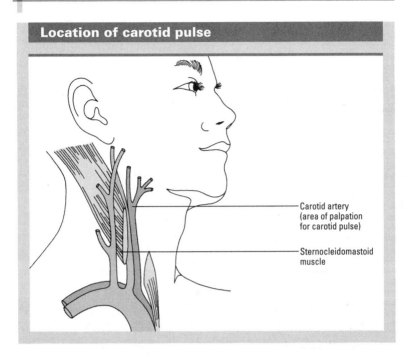

Carotid artery
(area of palpation
for carotid pulse)

Sternocleidomastoid
muscle

in blood pressure stimulate vagal nerve endings in the wall of the carotid sinus.

carotid sinus massage   Manual pressure applied to the carotid sinus to slow the heart rate.

carotid sinus reflex   Slowing of the heart rate in response to stimulation of vagal nerve endings in the carotid sinus.

carotid sinus syndrome   Syncope, or a temporary loss of consciousness, due to over-activity of the carotid sinus reflex from pressure applied to one or both carotid sinuses.

carpal   Of or relating to the carpus, or wrist.

carpal tunnel   A passageway created by the carpal bones and the flexor retinaculum through which the median nerve and the flexor tendons pass.

carpal tunnel syndrome   A painful disorder of the wrist and hand resulting from rapid, repetitive use of the fingers, as when punching the buttons on a keyboard, or from steady, wrist-shaking vibrations, as in working with a chain saw. The repeated trauma causes compression of the median nerve inside the carpal tunnel. Signs and symptoms range from mild numbness and tingling of the hand and wrist to crippling pain in one or both arms, which may be felt in the forearm

or shoulder. The hands may become weak and clumsy, unable to perform simple tasks.

CLINICAL TIP   Treatments for carpal tunnel syndrome include anti-inflammatory medication, resting the hands for several days, wrist splints, wrist massage, and, as a last resort, surgery to remove pressure on the median nerve.

carpopedal spasm   A painful, involuntary contraction of the hand, thumbs, foot, or toes that may accompany tetany.

carpus   The wrist; the joint at which the arm and hand meet, composed of eight bones.

carrier   **1.** A person or an animal who carries and spreads a disease-causing organism to others but doesn't become ill from the disease. **2.** An individual who doesn't express a recessive phenotype but can transmit the recessive gene to offspring.

cartilage   A fibrous connective tissue found in the joints, thorax, and various rigid tubes, such as the larynx, trachea, nose, and ear. In utero, cartilage serves as the temporary skeleton of the embryo, and then as the blueprint for bone development.

cartilaginous joint   A slightly movable joint in which cartilage connects the bony surfaces. The two types of cartilaginous joints are the symphyses (such as the symphysis pubis) and the synchondroses (such as the joints between the ribs and the sternum).

case management   The process by which a designated health care professional, usually a nurse, manages all health-related matters of a patient. Case managers coordinate and ensure continuity of care; match the appropriate intensity of services to the patient's needs; and develop a plan to efficiently and cost-effectively use health care resources to achieve the optimum patient outcome.

caseation   A form of cell death in which the tissue resembles crumbly cheese.

cast   **1.** A rigid dressing that's placed around an extremity or other injured body part to support, immobilize, and protect that part and thus promote healing. Cast materials include plaster of Paris and fiberglass. Some flexible casts use air to cushion and immobilize the injured part. **2.** An impression of an individual's teeth and internal jaw, used in the making of dentures and in other dental procedures. **3.** A particle created from deposits of mineral or other substances on the walls of the renal tubules, bronchioles, or other organs. Casts commonly appear in urine specimens and blood samples. **4.** Strabismus, or deviation of an eye from the normal parallel lines of vision.

castration   Surgical removal of one or both testicles or ovaries, performed most commonly to decrease the production and secretion of hormones thought to stimulate the growth of malignant cells in women with breast cancer and in men with prostate cancer.

CAT   Acronym for computerized axial tomography.

catabasis, pl. catabases   The stage in which a disease declines.

catabiosis   The normal process whereby cells age.

catabolism   The metabolic breakdown of large molecules in living organisms to smaller ones, with the release of energy for use in work, energy storage, or heat production. Respiration is an example of a catabolic series of reactions.

catacrotism   A pulse abnormality marked by a small, extra wave in the descending limb of the pulse tracing.

catalysis   An increase in the rate of a chemical reaction caused by the presence of a material that isn't consumed or affected by the reaction.

catalyst   A substance that affects the rate of a chemical reaction without being consumed or permanently changed.

cataphylaxis   **1.** The movement of leukocytes and antibodies to an infected area. **2.**

The breakdown of the body's natural resistance to infection.

cataplexy   Sudden muscular weakness and hypotonia in response to strong emotions, such as anger, fear, or surprise. Cataplexy is commonly associated with narcolepsy.

cataract   An eye disease in which the lens becomes progressively more opaque, causing vision impairment and blindness.

catarrh   Inflammation of the mucous membranes, especially the air passages of the nose and throat, accompanied by free discharge.

catatonia   A state of pronounced psychomotor disturbance in which the individual remains immobile with extreme muscle rigidity or, less commonly, exhibits uncontrolled excessive movement.

cat-cry syndrome   A rare hereditary, congenital disorder that manifests at birth by a catlike cry and is characterized by an abnormally increased distance between the eyes (hypertelorism), microcephaly, and severe mental deficiency.

catecholamine   Any of a group of compounds having a sympathomimetic action and composed of a catechol molecule and the aliphatic portion of an amine. Some catecholamines are produced by the body and function as key neurologic chemicals. Others are synthesized as drugs for use in the treatment of such disorders as asthma, shock, and heart failure.

catgut   An absorbable sterile strand, prepared from the collagen of mammals, that's used to close injuries or surgical incisions; originally made from the intestines of sheep.

cathartic   An agent that aids evacuation of the bowel by stimulating peristalsis, softening the feces, making the intestinal contents bulkier or more liquid, or lubricating the intestinal wall.

catheter   A hollow, flexible tube that can be introduced into a vessel or body cavity for the purpose of instilling or withdrawing fluids, dilating a body structure, or measuring crucial pressures.

cathode ray   A stream of electrons emitted by the cathode, or negative electrode, in a vacuum tube when it's bombarded by positive ions (as in an oscilloscope). Cathode rays generate X-rays when they strike solids.

cathode ray oscilloscope   An instrument that displays a visual representation of electrical variations on the fluorescent screen of a cathode-ray tube.

cation   An ion with a positive charge that, in solution, is attracted to the negative electrode.

cation-exchange resin Any of various high-molecular-weight, insoluble, organic polymers that exchange their cations for other ions in solution.

cat-scratch fever A disease caused by the scratch or bite of a cat, commonly characterized by a mild fever and inflammation and pustules at the injury site. Within 2 weeks, lymph nodes in the neck, head, groin, or axilla become swollen. The disease is self-limiting and no treatment is needed.

cat's eye amaurosis Blindness in one eye, characterized by a bright reflection from the pupil (as in a cat's eye). The condition represents formation of a white mass in the vitreous humor as a result of inflammation or a malignant lesion.

caudad Away from the head, directed toward the tail or end of the body.

cauda equina The aggregation of spinal roots, resembling the tail of a horse, that descend from the first lumbar vertebrae and occupy the vertebral canal below the cord.

caudal Denoting a position more toward the distal or tail end than some other specified reference point.

caul A piece of the amniotic sac that envelops the fetus's head at birth; sometimes called cowl.

caumesthesia A condition in which a low body temperature is accompanied by a sense of intense heat.

causalgia A burning pain resulting from peripheral nerve damage, typically arising in an extremity and sometimes accompanied by local skin erythema.

cautery A hot instrument or caustic agent that's used to burn or scar tissue.

cavernous hemangioma A large, blood-filled, benign, congenital tumor, which typically appears on the scalp, face, or neck but can also appear in the liver, spleen, pancreas and, sometimes, the brain. It's rarely present at birth.

cavernous rale An abnormal hollow, metallic breath sound resulting from the expansion and contraction of the pulmonary cavity.

cavernous sinus One of two irregularly shaped, bilateral venous spaces located in the head between the sphenoid bone and the dura mater.

cavernous sinus syndrome A condition caused by thrombosis of the cavernous sinus and marked by swelling of the conjunctiva, upper eyelid, and roof of the nose and by paralysis of the third, fourth, and sixth nerves.

cavity 1. A hollow space within the body or one of its organs. 2. Dentistry: a destroyed area of a tooth resulting from dental caries.

CBC *abbr* complete blood count.
CBF *abbr* cerebral blood flow.
CBS *abbr* chronic brain syndrome.
CCRN *abbr* Certified Critical-Care Registered Nurse.
CCU *abbr* coronary care unit.
Cd Symbol for cadmium.
CDC *abbr* Centers for Disease Control and Prevention.
CD4 A cell surface marker onto which the human immunodeficiency virus can bind. The CD4 + T-cell count provides a rough estimate of the state of a patient's immune system.
Ce Symbol for cerium.
CEA *abbr* carcinoembryonic antigen.
ceasmic Relating to or characterized by persistence of an embryonic fissure or abnormal cleavage of parts after birth.

cecostomy The surgical creation of an opening into the cecum, performed to temporarily relieve intestinal obstruction in a patient who's a poor candidate for major surgery.

cecum A cul-de-sac, or blind pouch, that forms the beginning of the large intestine.

celiac Pertaining to the abdomen.

celiac disease A chronic disease in which an individual (usually an adult or young child) can't tolerate foods containing gluten or wheat protein. Signs and symptoms include abdominal distention, vomiting, diarrhea, muscle wasting, and extreme lethargy.

celiac trunk A branch of the abdominal aorta that supplies the stomach, liver, pancreas, spleen, and duodenum.

celiogastrotomy An incision into the stomach that's made through the abdominal wall.

celiotomy A surgical incision into the abdominal cavity.

cell The structural and functional unit of all living organisms. Every cell contains a nucleus, cytoplasm, and organelles enclosed by a cytoplasmic membrane. Cells may exist as independent units of life (as in bacteria and protozoans), or they may cluster into colonies or tissues (as in higher animals and plants).

cella, *pl.* **cellae** An enclosed space or compartment.

cell biology The study of the structures, functions, and living processes of cells.

cell body The part of the cell that contains the nucleus and the surrounding cytoplasm (excluding any projections or processes, which develop as extensions from the cell body).

cell cycle The reproductive and resting phases of every cell, be it normal or malignant.

cell division The process by which a cell separates. Cell division takes place in four stages: prophase, metaphase, anaphase, and telophase.

cell-mediated immune response A delayed type IV hypersensitivity reaction that protects the body against bacterial, viral, and fungal infections and resists transplanted cells and tumor cells. A macrophage processes the antigen, which is then presented to T cells. Some T cells become sensitized and destroy the antigen; others release lymphokines, which activate macrophages that destroy the antigen. Sensitized T cells then travel through the blood and lymphatic systems, providing ongoing surveillance in their quest for specific antigens.

cell membrane The structure that envelops a cell and encloses the cytoplasm.

cell theory The doctrine that cells are the fundamental units of all living substance and that cell activity is the essential process of life.

cellular infiltration The migration and clustering of cells within body tissues.

cellulitis An infection of deep subcutaneous tissue and, sometimes, muscle that's associated with infection of an operative or traumatic wound. Cellulitis is characterized by local heat, pain, redness, and swelling.

cellulose A nondigestible, insoluble polysaccharide carbohydrate that forms the skeleton of most plant structures and plant cells.

cell wall The structure that covers the cell membrane and maintains the shape of some cells, such as certain bacteria and all plant cells.

Celsius (C) Designating a temperature scale in which 0° is the freezing point of water and 100° is the boiling point of water at normal atmospheric pressure.

cement 1. A substance that helps to join two surfaces together to make a solid. 2. Any of a variety of dental bonding materials in which two substances are mixed together and used to fill cavities or to hold bridgework or other dental prostheses in place. 3. A substance used to affix a prosthetic joint to an adjacent bone, such as methyl methacrylate.

cementoma, *pl.* cementomas, cementomata A mass of cementum lying unattached at the apex of a tooth, probably the result of trauma.

cementum The rigid, bonelike connective tissue that protects and supports the roots of the teeth.

centering Technique used before a session of Therapeutic Touch in which the practitioner attempts to become relaxed, calm, and focused on the care that she's going to provide.

Centers for Disease Control and Prevention (CDC) An agency of the U.S. Department of Health and Human Services that provides facilities and services for the investigation, identification, prevention, and control of disease.

centesis A perforation or tapping, as with an aspirator or needle.

centimeter (cm) The metric unit of measurement of length equal to one hundredth of a meter, or 0.3937 inches.

centimeter-gram-second system (CGS, cgs) The international scientific system of measurement in which the unit of length is the centimeter, the unit of mass is the gram, and the unit of time is the second.

central canal of spinal cord The tunnel that runs the entire length of the spinal cord and channels most of the cerebrospinal fluid in the body.

central nervous system (CNS) Collective term for the brain and spinal cord; one of the two main divisions of the nervous system.

central nervous system syndrome (CNS syndrome) A group of neurologic and emotional manifestations ensuing from a massive, whole-body radiation dosage.

central nervous system tumor An abnormal tissue growth in the brain or spinal cord. Although such a tumor may have extensive effects and be invasive locally, it rarely spreads beyond the cerebrospinal axis.

central placenta previa Implantation of the placenta in the lower portion of the uterus, completely covering the internal os of the uterine cervix.

central scotoma A region of blindness or a site of impaired vision involving the macula of the retina.

central sulcus A fissure that divides the frontal and parietal lobes of the brain.

central venous pressure (CVP) monitor An apparatus that measures and records the central venous blood pressure by means of a pressure manometer and an indwelling catheter.

central venous (CV) therapy Treatment in which drugs or fluids are infused directly into a major vein; used when a patient's peripheral veins are inaccessible, in emergencies, or when a patient needs infusion of large volumes of fluid, multiple infusion therapies, or long-term venous access. The catheter tip is inserted in the superior vena cava, inferior vena cava, or right atrium of the heart.

central vision Vision resulting from images falling directly on the macula of the retina.

centrencephalic Of, involving, or relating to the center of the encephalon.

cephalocele The protrusion of a part of the cranial contents through a defect in the skull.

centrifuge A machine that separates lighter portions of a liquid from heavier portions by rotating them in a tube in a horizontal circle.

centriole A cylindrical structure in a cell, typically a component of the centrosome, that plays a part in cell division.

centromere The portion of the chromosome that contains no genes, usually appearing as a constriction when chromosomes contract during cell division.

centrosome The center of the cell (the centrosphere and the two centrioles). It's present in the animal cells and in the cells of some lower plants.

centrosphere The condensed area of cytoplasm surrounding the centrioles in the centrosome of the cell. The centrosphere plays an important role in cell division.

cephalad Toward the head, directed away from the end, or tail.

cephalalgia A pain in the head or headache.

cephalhematoma Limited swelling of a cranial surface from subperiosteal bleeding, commonly seen in newborns as the result of bone trauma.

cephalic presentation A fetal position in which the head of the fetus appears head-first at the uterine cervix.

 CLINICAL TIP Cephalic presentation is seen in about 95% of all births.

cephalometry Scientific measurement of the head, such as by dentists to help determine appropriate orthodontic treatment. Cephalometry uses a combination of linear and angular measurements.

cephalopelvic disproportion (CPD) A condition in which the head of the fetus is too large for the mother's pelvis.

cerclage **1.** Encircling of a part with a loop or a ring, such as encircling an incompetent cervix with suture material to prevent spontaneous abortion. **2.** The binding together of the ends of a fractured bone with a wire loop or a metal band to maintain bone fragments in position until the bone heals. **3.** Application of a taut silicone band around the sclera to restore contact between the retina and the choroid, used in the treatment of a detached retina.

cerebellar artery One of three arteries that supply blood to the cerebellum, medulla, pineal body, and midbrain.

cerebellar cortex The gray matter of the cerebellum that covers the white substance in the medullary core. It consists of an external molecular layer and an internal granule cell layer.

cerebellum, *pl.* cerebellums, cerebella The part of the brain situated behind the brain stem in the posterior cranial fossa, consisting of a middle strip (the vermis) and two lateral cerebellar hemispheres (lobes). The cerebellum plays an important role in coordination, regulation of muscle activity, and maintenance of muscle tone and balance.

cerebral aneurysm A saclike dilation of the wall of a cerebral artery, typically resulting from weakness of the wall.

 ALERT A cerebral, or berry, aneurysm usually occurs in the circle of Willis and is prone to rupture.

cerebral angiography A radiographic procedure in which a radiopaque contrast material is injected into a carotid, subclavian, brachial, or femoral artery to allow visualization of the vascular system of the brain.

cerebral aqueduct The narrow channel between the third and fourth ventricles in the midbrain through which the cerebrospinal fluid travels.

cerebral cortex A thin mantle of gray matter on the surface of each cerebral hemisphere, folded into gyri and separated by fissures. It's responsible for the higher mental functions (memory, thought, intellect, and language) as well as for the control and integration of voluntary movement and the special senses.

cerebral dominance The dominance of one cerebral hemisphere over the other in the integration and control of various functions. The left cerebral hemisphere is dominant in about 90% of the population.

cerebral embolism Occlusion of a cerebral vessel by a blood clot or other material that's carried by the bloodstream, possibly leading to cerebrovascular accident and consequent tissue death distal to the occlusion.

cerebral hemisphere Either of the two halves of the cerebrum. Partly divided by the longitudinal cerebral fissure, the cerebral hemispheres are joined medially at the bottom of the fissure by the corpus callosum.

cerebral hemorrhage Bleeding within the cerebrum. Cerebral hemorrhage is classified by location (subarachnoid, extradural, subdural), the vessel involved (arterial, venous, capillary), and origin (traumatic, degenerative).

cerebral palsy A permanent disorder of motor function resulting from nonprogressive brain damage or a brain lesion.

 TIME LINE Cerebral palsy usually appears before age 3.

Cerebrum

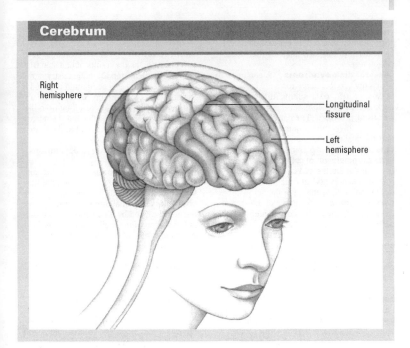

Right hemisphere

Longitudinal fissure

Left hemisphere

cerebrospinal fluid (CSF) The plasma-like fluid contained within the four ventricles of the brain, the subarachnoid space, and the central canal of the spinal cord. CSF is composed of secretions of the ventricles.

cerebrovascular accident (CVA) A condition of sudden onset in which a cerebral blood vessel is occluded by an embolus or cerebrovascular hemorrhage. The resulting ischemia of brain tissue that's normally perfused by the affected vessel may lead to permanent neurologic damage.

cerebrum, *pl.* **cerebrums, cerebra** The largest portion of the brain, located in the uppermost part of the cranium. The longitudinal fissure separates the cerebrum into two hemispheres; the corpus callosum connects the hemispheres at the bottom of the fissure.

cerium (Ce) A gray, metallic, rare-earth element. Its atomic number is 58; its atomic weight is 140.13.

ceroid An insoluble, waxy, golden pigment found in the nervous system and muscles as well as in the cirrhotic livers of some individuals.

ceroma, *pl.* **ceromas, ceromata** An abnormal growth of tissue that has undergone a waxy degeneration.

Certified Nurse-Midwife (CNM) An individual who's educated in both nursing and midwifery and possesses evidence of certification that meets the requirements of the American College of Nurse-Midwives.

cerumen The yellow or brown waxy secretion found in the ear, commonly called earwax. Cerumen is produced by vestigial apocrine sweat glands in the external ear canal.

ceruminosis Excessive accumulation of cerumen in the external auditory canal.

ceruminous gland One of a group of small glands located in the external ear canal that secrete cerumen. Ceruminous glands are thought to be modified sweat glands.

cervical Of or pertaining to the neck or the region of the neck of any organ or structure.

cervical adenitis A condition characterized by enlarged, inflamed, tender lymph nodes of the neck. It may accompany acute throat infections.

cervical canal The canal within the uterine cervix, protruding into the vagina.

cervical cap A barrier contraceptive device consisting of a small rubber cup that's fitted over the uterine cervix to stop spermatozoa from penetrating the cervical canal.

cervical carcinoma A malignant growth of the cervix that tends to infiltrate surrounding tissues. Cervical carcinoma can be detected in the early stage by the Papanicolaou test.

cervical disk syndrome A condition in which the cervical nerve roots are compressed or irritated, resulting in pain in the neck, shoulder, or forearm.

cervical plexus The network of nerves formed by the ventral branches of the upper four cervical nerves.

cervical polyp A common, relatively harmless outgrowth of columnar epithelial tissue in the uterine cervix, typically occurring in the endocervical canal and attached to the wall of the canal by a slender pedicle.

cervical smear A sample of the secretions and superficial cells of the uterine cervix, obtained from the external os using an applicator or endocervical brush.

cervical vertebra One of the upper seven bones of the spinal column that form the neck. Unlike the thoracic and lumbar vertebrae, cervical vertebrae have a foramen in each transverse process.

cervicitis An acute or chronic inflammation of the uterine cervix.

cervicolabial Of, relating to, or located on the labial surface of an anterior tooth.

cervix The narrow lower end of the uterus, connecting to the vagina.

cesarean section Surgical incision through the abdominal and uterine walls to deliver a fetus.

cesium (Cs) A rare alkali metallic element. Its atomic number is 55; its atomic weight is 132.9.

cf *abbr* cardiac failure.

Cf Symbol for californium.

CF *abbr* cystic fibrosis.

C-F test *abbr* complement-fixation test.

CGS, cgs *abbr* centimeter-gram-second (system).

Ch1 Symbol for Christchurch chromosome.

Chaddock's reflex Extension of the great toe and fanning of the other toes elicited by firmly stroking the side of the foot just below the lateral malleolus. A variation of Babinski's reflex, Chaddock's reflex is seen in pyramidal tract disease.

Chadwick's sign Bluish coloration of the vulva and vagina after the sixth week of pregnancy, resulting from local venous congestion. It's an early sign of pregnancy.

chain 1. A line of atoms of the same type in a molecule. 2. A linked grouping of individual bacteria. 3. The functional pattern formed by certain structures. For instance, the ossicles of the middle ear form a chain by moving successively in response to vibration of the tympanic membrane, thus transmitting auditory stimuli.

chain reaction 1. A self-sustaining reaction occurring as the results of one step triggers a subsequent step. 2. In chemistry: a reaction that produces a compound required if the reaction is to continue. 3. In physics: a self-perpetuating reaction resulting from the proliferating fission of nuclei and the release of atomic particles, which lead to more nuclear fissions.

chalasia Incompetence or abnormal relaxation of an opening.

 CLINICAL TIP Chalasia in an opening such as the cardiac sphincter of the stomach results in vomiting.

chalazion A small lump or swelling on the eyelid caused by obstruction and chronic inflammation of the meibomian glands.

chamber A hollow, enclosed space or cavity in an organ, such as the atrial and ventricular chambers of the heart.

Chamberlain's line A line running from the rear of the hard palate to the back of the foramen magnum.

chancre The primary lesion of syphilis, occurring at the entry site of the infection. It initially appears as a papule and then develops into a red, bloodless, painless ulcer with an eroded appearance.

chancroid A highly contagious, sexually transmitted disease caused by infection with *Haemophilus ducreyi*, characterized by an ulcer that appears as a papule on the external genitalia. The ulcer then grows and ulcerates, forming other papules. If the disease goes untreated, the bacillus may cause buboes in the groin.

channel A passageway or groove through which fluid flows.

Charcot-Bouchard aneurysm Dilation of the wall of a small artery in the cerebral cortex.

CLINICAL TIP Some researchers suspect that Charcot-Bouchard aneurysm is the cause of massive cerebral hemorrhage.

Charcot-Leyden crystal A protein crystalline structure found wherever eosinophilic leukocytes are undergoing fragmentation. The crystal, shaped like a narrow double pyramid, appears in the bronchial secretions of patients with bronchial asthma and, sometimes, in the feces of those with intestinal parasites.

Charcot-Marie-Tooth atrophy A progressive hereditary disorder in which the peroneal muscles of the fibula waste away, leading to clubfoot, footdrop, and ataxia.

Charcot's fever   An intermittent fever resulting from impaction of a stone in the liver's common duct and bile duct inflammation. The fever may be accompanied by jaundice and pain in the right upper abdominal quadrant.

charta, *pl.* **chartae**   Paper, especially paper that's medicated or treated with a chemical for a special purpose (for example, litmus paper).

charting by exception (CBE)   Charting system that departs from traditional systems by requiring only documentation of significant or abnormal findings.

chauffeur's fracture   Fracture of the radial styloid, caused by a snapping or twisting injury.

Chaussier's areola   A circular area of indurated tissue surrounding a malignant pustule.

CHC   *abbr* community health center.

cheilitis   Inflammation and cracking of the lips.

cheilosis   A noninflammatory disorder of the lips characterized by chapping and fissures. The condition is caused by a riboflavin deficiency.

cheiralgia   Pain in the hand, particularly arthritic pain.

chelation   A reaction involving a combination with a metal, producing a ring-shaped molecular complex that usually contains a firmly bound and sequestered metal ion.

chelation therapy   A proven treatment for heavy metal poisoning that's also used as an alternative therapy for coronary artery disease and other disorders. Edetic acid (EDTA) is infused into the bloodstream on the theory that it will attach itself to coronary plaque or other harmful substances, and then be excreted in the urine.

chemical action   A chemical change brought about by the combination of natural elements and compounds, yielding a different compound (such as the combination of hydrogen and oxygen to form water).

chemical agent   Any chemical substance, principle, or power capable of producing a physical, chemical, or biological effect in the body by interacting with body substances.

chemical antidote   Any substance that reacts chemically with a poison to yield a harmless compound.

 CLINICAL TIP Few true chemical antidotes exist. Poison treatment usually centers on eliminating the toxic agent before the body absorbs it.

chemical burn   Tissue damage caused by exposure to acids, alkalis, or disinfectants.

chemical equivalence   Of a drug or chemical: possessing the same amount of the same ingredients as another drug or chemical.

chemistry   The scientific study of the elements and the compounds they form. Fields of chemistry include inorganic chemistry and organic chemistry.

chemistry, normal values   The normal quantity of different substances found in the average human body, determined from tests of a large sample of healthy people and expressed in ranges of numbers. Ranges may vary among laboratories.

chemoreceptor   A sensory nerve cell that detects the presence of particular chemicals and transmits this information to sensory nerves. Examples include the carotid body receptors, which send signals that cause the respiratory center in the brain to increase or decrease respiration.

chemoreflex   A reaction initiated by chemoreceptors. For instance, in response to chemical changes in the blood, a chemoreflex of the carotid and aortic bodies leads to an increase or decrease in respiration.

chemosis   Swelling of the conjunctiva of the eye.

chemostat   An apparatus that ensures a constant environment and thus a steady rate of cell division in bacterial populations.

chemotaxis   Movement toward or away from chemical stimulation.

chemotherapy   Treatment of a disease using chemicals that exert a toxic effect on the pathogen or on abnormal cell growth.

cherry angioma   A small, dome-shaped, bright red to purple, vascular tumor of the skin, usually appearing on the torso.

chest pain   A symptom that warrants immediate evaluation. It may reflect a physical problem, such as a disease or disorder of the cardiopulmonary, musculoskeletal, or GI system, or it may have a psychogenic origin.

chest physiotherapy   An array of physical techniques, including postural drainage, chest percussion and vibration, and coughing and deep-breathing maneuvers.

CLINICAL TIP Chest physiotherapy is used to loosen and help eliminate lung secretions, reexpand lung tissue, and promote optimal use of respiratory muscles.

chest tube   A hollow, cylindrical instrument that's inserted into the chest cavity to remove air or fluid.

Cheyne-Stokes respiration   A respiratory pattern marked by alternating periods of apnea and deep, rapid breathing. Typically, the cycle starts with slow, shallow breaths, which slowly increase to abnormal depth and rapidity. Respiration then becomes slow and shallower, ending in a 10- to 20-second apneic episode before the cycle begins again.

TIME LINE Cheyne-Stokes respirations rarely occur in children, except during late heart failure. However, these respirations can occur normally in elderly patients during sleep.

chiasm 1. An X-shaped crossing of two lines or tracts, such as the optic chiasm.
2. In genetics: the sites where pairs of chromatids remain in contact during the prophase of meiosis.

chickenpox A viral disease caused by varicella-zoster virus, a herpesvirus. This acute and highly contagious disease results in pruritic, vesicular skin eruptions that break open and scab over. Although primarily a childhood disease, chickenpox can also affect adults.

chief cell Any of the epithelial cells (columnar or cuboidal) that line the lower portion of the gastric glands. Chief cells secrete pepsin and the extrinsic factor required for vitamin B_{12} absorption and normal development of red blood cells.

chief complaint A patient's description of his most significant or serious symptoms or signs of illness or dysfunction.

chigger The six-legged larva of a mite, which attaches to its host's skin and causes severe itching and dermatitis. Chiggers live in tall grass and weeds.

chilblain Redness and swelling of the skin caused by exposure to cold, damp conditions. Signs of chilblain (such as burning, itching, blistering, and ulceration) may resemble those of a thermal burn.

Chilomastix A genus of flagellate protozoa, such as *Chilomastix mesnili*. This pear-shaped parasite may be found in the intestines of vertebrates (including man); it's considered nonpathogenic.

Chinese medicine, traditional A sophisticated, complex health care system based on the belief that good health depends largely on a person's lifestyle, thoughts, and emotions. It has expanded over the centuries to embrace many theories, methods, and approaches. The cornerstone of traditional Chinese medicine, which evolved from Taoism, Confucianism, and Buddhism, is the concept of *qi*, the vital life force or energy, that flows through the body along channels called meridians.

chip fracture A small fragmental fracture, usually involving a bony process near a joint.

chiropractic A manual healing therapy based on the belief that many medical problems are caused by vertebral misalignment, and can be corrected by manipulating the spine. Chiropractic is the fourth largest health profession in the United States, with more than 50,000 practitioners.

chisel fracture A fracture involving an oblique detachment of a piece of bone from the head of the radius.

Chlamydia A genus of bacteria of the Chlamydiaceae family, occurring as gram-negative organisms, which are common pathogens of animals and cause various diseases in humans.

chloasma Tan or brown pigmentation, especially on the forehead, cheeks, and nose, typically occurring during pregnancy or in individuals using oral contraceptives.

chlorine (Cl) A yellowish-green, gaseous element of the halogen group. Chlorine has a suffocating odor and is used to disinfect, fumigate, and bleach. Its atomic number is 17; its atomic weight is 35.453.

chloroleukemia A green, malignant tumor associated with myelogenous leukemia. Also called *chloroma.*

chlorolymphosarcoma, *pl.* **chlorolymphosarcomas, chlorolymphosarcomata** A greenish tumor arising from myeloid tissue, occurring in patients with myelogenous leukemia.

chlorophyll A green plant pigment that's involved in the photosynthesis of carbohydrates. Chlorophyll absorbs light and converts it to energy.

choana, *pl.* **choanae** Any funnel-shaped cavity or passage.

choanal atresia A congenital abnormality characterized by a bony or membranous blockage of the passage between the nose and pharynx.

cholangiogram An X-ray of the gallbladder and biliary duct system, obtained by injecting a radiopaque material during radiography.

cholangiography Radiographic visualization of the gallbladder and the biliary duct system after injection of radiopaque material.

cholangiohepatoma, *pl.* **cholangiohepatomas, cholangiohepatomata** A carcinoma of the liver composed of a mixture of liver cells and bile duct cells.

cholangitis Inflammation of a bile duct, usually resulting from bacterial infection or from an obstruction of the duct by calculi or a tumor.

cholecystectomy Surgical removal of the gallbladder.

cholecystitis Inflammation of the gallbladder, which may be acute (usually caused by gallstones) or chronic.

cholecystogram   An X-ray picture of the gallbladder obtained after administration of a radiopaque material.

cholecystography   Radiographic study of the gallbladder after administration of a radiopaque material. Cholecystography aids diagnosis of cholecystitis, cholelithiasis, and tumors and helps evaluate a mass in the upper right quadrant of the stomach.

cholecystoduodenostomy   Surgical anastomosis of the gallbladder and duodenum.

cholecystokinin   A polypeptide hormone secreted by the mucosa of the upper intestine and by the hypothalamus. It stimulates contraction of the gallbladder and secretion of pancreatic enzymes.

cholelithiasis   The presence or formation of gallstones in the gallbladder.

cholera   An acute bacterial infection of the small intestine, spread by feces-contaminated water or food. Cholera results from a potent enterotoxin elaborated by *Vibrio cholerae*. The full-blown disease typically causes severe, watery diarrhea; vomiting; muscle cramps; dehydration; shock; and a faint, high-pitched voice.

cholestasis   Stoppage of the flow of bile anywhere in the biliary system.

cholesteatoma   Cystlike mass filled with desquamating debris that frequently includes cholesterol; occurs most commonly in the middle ear and mastoid region.

cholesterase   An enzyme found in blood and body tissues that hydrolyzes cholesterol esters, forming cholesterol and fatty acids.

cholesterol   A fat-soluble, steroid alcohol that's synthesized in the liver and absorbed from the diet. Cholesterol plays an important role in the production of bile acids and steroid hormones. It's found in egg yolk as well as animal fats and oils, and is widely distributed in the body.

cholesterolemia   A condition in which the blood contains excessive amounts of cholesterol.

cholinergic   1. Of or relating to nerve fibers that are stimulated to free acetylcholine at a synapse. 2. An agent that frees acetylcholine.

cholinergic blocking agent   An agent that blocks action of acetylcholine and similar substances, resulting in blocking of cholinergic nerve action.

cholinesterase   An enzyme that catalyzes the hydrolysis of acetylcholine to choline and acetate. It's used in the diagnosis of succinylcholine sensitivity and certain types of insecticide poisoning.

chondriome, chondrioma   All of the mitochondria of a cell, considered as one unit.

chondriomite   One granular mitochondrion or an array of such organelles forming a chain.

chondritis   An inflammatory condition affecting the cartilage.

chondroblastoma, *pl.* **chondroblastomas, chondroblastomata**   A benign tumor that arises from precursors of cartilage cells. It most commonly occurs in the epiphyses of the femur and humerus.

chondrocalcinosis   The presence of calcium salts in peripheral joints. The condition most commonly affects persons over age 50 who suffer from osteoarthritis or diabetes mellitus, and is sometimes accompanied by goutlike symptoms.

chondrodystrophy   Any disorder in which cartilage develops abnormally. Abnormal conversion of cartilage to bone, particularly in the epiphyses of long bones, can cause shortened extremities but a normal trunk.

chondrofibroma, *pl.* **chondrofibromas, chondrofibromata**   An abnormal growth of fibrous tissue containing cartilaginous components.

chondroplasty   The surgical repair of lacerated or displaced cartilage.

chordae tendineae   Tendinous strings that extend from the cusps of the atrioventricular valves to the papillary muscles of the heart, thus preventing valve inversion.

chorditis   1. Inflammation of a vocal cord. 2. Inflammation of a spermatic cord.

chorea   A condition characterized by purposeless, rapid, jerky movements that seem coordinated but are actually involuntary. Examples of such movements include flexing and extending the fingers, raising and lowering the shoulders, and grimacing.

chorion   The outermost extraembryonic membrane, which develops villi about 2 weeks after fertilization, and gives rise to the placenta.

chorionic gonadotropin, human (HCG)   A hormone produced by the placenta that sustains the corpus luteum. Its presence in the urine confirms pregnancy.

> *CLINICAL TIP* An agent derived from HCG in the urine of pregnant women is used to treat infertility, hypogonadism, and nonobstructive cryptorchidism.

chorioretinitis   Inflammation of the choroid and retina of the eye resulting from concussion or parasitic or bacterial infection. The condition causes blurred vision, photophobia, and distorted images.

Choroid plexus

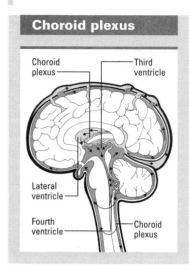

Choroid plexus — Third ventricle

Lateral ventricle

Fourth ventricle — Choroid plexus

chorioretinopathy   A noninflammatory process involving the choroid and retina.

choroid   A thin, pigmented vascular membrane that covers the posterior five-sixths of the eye from the ora serrata to the optic nerve. The choroid supplies blood to the retina and conducts arteries and nerves to the anterior structures.

choroid plexus   Any of the tiny blood vessels that form a network in the pia matter and project into the third, lateral, and fourth ventricles of the brain. See illustration on page 78

choroid vein   A vein of the choroid plexus.

Christchurch chromosome (Ch1)   An acrocentric chromosome of the G group, involving any members of chromosome pairs 21 or 22, in which the short arms are missing or partially deleted. This abnormally small chromosome is associated with chronic lymphocytic leukemia.

chromaffin cell   Any of the special cells that take stain readily with chromium salts. Such cells are found in the adrenal, coccygeal, and carotid glands; the sympathetic nerves; and some organs.

chromatid   One of two identical threadlike strands formed from a chromosome during the early stages of cell division. Each chromosome divides along its length into two chromatids, which later separate completely. The deoxyribonucleic acid (DNA) of the chromosome reproduces itself exactly; thus, each chromatid has the entire amount of DNA and becomes a daughter chromosome with genes identical to those of the original chromosome.

chromatin   The part of the cell nucleus of which eukaryotic chromosomes are composed. The chromatin consists of proteins, deoxyribonucleic acid, and small amounts of ribonucleic acid.

chromatography   Any of several techniques used to separate and analyze mixtures of gases, liquids, or dissolved substances. Chromatography analyzes differences based on pigmentation and on the way in which a particular substance absorbs another substance.

chromesthesia   The association of imaginary color sensations with actual sensations of hearing, smell, or taste.

chromhidrosis   A rare disorder in which the apocrine sweat glands secrete sweat that's yellow, blue, green, or black and that commonly also fluoresces.

chromium (Cr)   A bluish-white, brittle, metallic element. Its atomic number is 24; its atomic weight is 51.9.

chromobacteriosis   A rare systemic infection caused by a gram-negative bacillus, *Chromobacterium violaceum*, which enters the body through a break in the skin.

chromomere   A beadlike granule, one of many that lie along the chromonema of a chromosome during the prophase of cell division.

chromonema, chromoneme, *pl.* **chromonemata**   The coiled thread forming the central part of the chromatid.

chromosomal aberration   An abnormality in the number or structure of a chromosome. It may lead to anomalies of varying severity, including Down syndrome, Turner's syndrome, and Klinefelter's syndrome.

chromosome   A threadlike structure in the cell nucleus that consists of a double strand of deoxyribonucleic acid (DNA) coiled into a helix formation and attached to a protein base. Arranged in a linear pattern along the length of each DNA strand are the genes. Thus, the chromosome transmits genetic information.

chromosome complement   The normal number of chromosomes found in the somatic cell of a given species. In humans, the chromosome complement is 46.

chronic   Persisting over a long time. The term usually describes a disease or disorder that develops slowly and can be managed but not cured.

chronic bronchitis   A persistent respiratory disease marked by increased production of mucus by the glands of the trachea and bronchi. This common disease is characterized by a cough (with expectoration) at least

3 months of the year for more than 2 consecutive years.

chronic carrier An individual who harbors a certain disease for an extended period without showing symptoms and who's capable of transmitting the infection to others.

chronic disease A disease that persists over a long time, usually with symptoms that are less severe than those of the acute form of the same disease.

 CLINICAL TIP Chronic disease may lead to complete or partial disability.

chronic glomerulonephritis An inflammation of the glomerulus of the kidney, characterized by decreased urine production, blood and protein in the urine, and edema. The disease, which may lead to renal failure, may be primary, may follow acute glomerulonephritis, or may occur secondary to a systemic disease.

chronic lymphocytic leukemia (CLL) A progressive, malignant disease of the blood-forming organs, characterized by proliferation of small, long-lived lymphocytes, mainly B cells, in the bone marrow, blood, liver, and lymphoid organs.

chronic myelocytic leukemia (CML) A progressive, malignant disease of the blood-forming organs, characterized by proliferation of granular leukocytes and, commonly, megakaryocytes.

chronic obstructive pulmonary disease (COPD) An abnormal condition marked by reduced inspiratory and expiratory capacity of the lungs. COPD is progressive and irreversible and causes such symptoms as dyspnea on exertion, difficulty inhaling or exhaling deeply and, sometimes, a chronic cough.

chrysotherapy The use of gold salts to treat a disease.

Churg-Strauss syndrome A form of systemic necrotizing vasculitis with lung involvement, characterized by lung granulomatosis, eosinophilia and, usually, severe asthma.

Chvostek's sign A spasm of the facial muscles elicited by light taps on the facial nerve. Seen in patients with hypocalcemia, this spasm is a sign of tetany.

TIME LINE Because Chvostek's sign may be observed in healthy infants, it isn't elicited to detect neonatal tetany. In the elderly patient with Chvostek's sign and hypocalcemia, always consider malabsorption and poor nutritional status.

chyle The milky fluid product of digestion, consisting mainly of lymph and triglyceride fats in an emulsion. Chyle passes through lacteals, fingerlike projections, in the

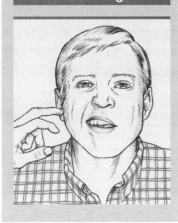
Chvostek's sign

small intestine and then into the lymphatic system for transport to the venous circulation.

chylomicron The largest type of lipoprotein; it transports triglycerides and exogenous cholesterol from the small intestine to the tissues. Chylomicrons are manufactured by the intestinal mucosa and transported by the lacteals and lymphatic system into venous circulation.

chylothorax The presence of effused chyle in the pleural space, most commonly resulting from traumatic injury to the neck or a tumor that invades the thoracic duct.

chyluria The presence of chyle in the urine, causing urine to appear milky.

chyme The creamy, semifluid substance present in the stomach during gastric digestion. It then passes through the pylorus into the duodenum for further digestion.

Ci *abbr* curie.

CI *abbr* **1.** color index. **2.** Colour Index.

CID *abbr* cytomegalic inclusion disease.

cilia, *sing.* cilium **1.** The eyelids or eyelashes. **2.** Tiny, hairlike projections on the surfaces of some cells, which promote metabolism by producing motion or a current in a fluid.

ciliary body The thickened part of the vascular tunic of the eye, joining the choroid with the iris. It's made up of the ciliary crown, ciliary processes and folds, ciliary orbiculus, ciliary muscle, and a basal lamina.

ciliary movement The motion created by the cilia, hairlike processes that project from the epithelium of the respiratory tract and from some microorganisms.

ciliary muscle   A circular band of smooth-muscle fibers attached to the choroid of the eye, which adjusts the eye to view near objects.

ciliary process   Any of about 80 tiny fleshy folds on the posterior surface of the iris, which secrete aqueous humor into the posterior chamber of the eye.

ciliated epithelium   Epithelial tissue bearing cilia, such as portions of the epithelium in the respiratory tract.

cineangiocardiogram   A radiographic image of the heart and great vessels obtained by a combination of X-ray, fluoroscopic, and motion-picture techniques.

cineangiocardiography   The filming of fluoroscopic images of the heart and great vessels using a combination of fluoroscopic, X-ray, and motion-picture techniques.

cineangiogram   A photographic image of blood vessels obtained by filming the action of the vessels as an injected radiopaque medium passes through them.

cineradiography   The filming of fluoroscopic images using a motion-picture camera, especially images of body structures that have been injected with a radiopaque medium.

circadian rhythm   The repetition of certain physiologic phenomena, such as sleeping and eating, every 24 hours.

circinate   Similar to a circle or ring; annular.

circle of Willis   A network at the base of the brain where the internal carotid, anterior cerebral, posterior cerebral, anterior communicating, and posterior communicating arteries interconnect.

circular bandage   A bandage applied in circular turns, commonly used on a limb.

circulation   Movement of an object or substance in a circuitous course, as the movement of blood through the cardiovascular system.

circulation time, normal   The time needed for blood to move from one part of the body to another.

circulatory failure   Inability of the cardiovascular system to supply adequate blood volume to meet the metabolic demands of the body's cells.

circulatory overload   An extremely large volume of fluid that the heart is incapable of pumping through the circulatory system; symptoms include neck vein engorgement, respiratory distress, increased blood pressure, and crackles in the lungs.

circulatory system   The channels through which the nutrient fluids of the body travel.

circumcision   Surgical removal of the penile prepuce (foreskin) or, less commonly, the prepuce of the clitoris.

circumduction   1. Motion of a limb or an eye in a circular pattern. 2. Movement of the head of a bone within its socket, as the hip joint.

cirrhosis   A chronic, degenerative liver disease in which the lobes are covered with fibrous tissue, the liver parenchyma degenerates, and the lobules are infiltrated with fat.

CK   *abbr* creatine kinase.

CK-BB   *abbr* creatine kinase, brain.

CK-MB   *abbr* creatine kinase, muscle.

CK-MM   *abbr* creatine kinase, skeletal muscle.

Cl   Symbol for chlorine.

Clark's rule   A method for calculating the approximate pediatric dosage of a drug using the formula: [weight (in pounds)/150] ×adult dose.

clasp   1. In dentistry: a fitting that attaches over a tooth to hold a partial denture in place. 2. In surgery: a device that holds tissues together, particularly bones.

claudication   An intermittent condition characterized by pain and weakness that worsen during walking until movement is impossible, with symptoms disappearing after rest.

clavicle   A long, horizontal bone shaped like an f, located just above the first rib. It forms the anterior portion of the shoulder girdle on either side. Also *called collar bone.*

clavicular notch   One of the two oval depressions at the superior end of the sternum, located on either side of the sternum and articulating with the clavicle on that side.

cleavage   Mitotic cell division in the fertilized ovum that transforms the single-celled zygote into a multicellular embryo capable of growth and differentiation.

cleavage fracture   A fracture that splits the cartilage and a small piece of bone from the distal portion of the lateral condyle of the humerus.

cleavage plane   1. The region in a fertilized ovum where cleavage occurs; the axis along which cell division takes place. 2. Any area in the body where organs or other structures can be separated with minimum disturbance to surrounding tissue.

cleft   A fissure or elongated opening, particularly one associated with an embryo, such as the facial cleft.

cleft foot   An abnormality characterized by extension of the normal division between the third and fourth toes into the metatarsum of the foot.

cleft palate A congenital defect marked by a fissure in the midline of the palate. The condition occurs when the two sides fail to fuse during embryonic development. The degree of fissure may be partial or complete (through the hard and soft palates into the nasal cavities).

CLINICAL TIP Cleft palate is commonly accompanied by a cleft lip.

click In cardiology: a short, dry, extra heart sound that takes place during systole.

clinical cytogenetics The scientific study of the relationship between chromosomal aberrations and pathologic conditions; a branch of genetics.

clinical diagnosis Determination of a patient's condition or disease from signs, symptoms, and laboratory findings.

clinical genetics A branch of genetics that studies hereditary disorders and examines the possible genetic factors that relate to specific pathologic conditions.

clinical laboratory A laboratory that performs tests on material obtained directly from human patients to aid the diagnosis, prevention, or treatment of diseases and disorders.

clinical nurse specialist (CNS) A registered nurse who holds a master of science degree in nursing (MSN) and who has acquired advanced knowledge and clinical skills in a specific area of nursing and health care.

clinical pathology The laboratory study of disease by a pathologist using techniques appropriate to the specimen being studied, primarily for the purpose of clinical diagnosis.

clinical pathways A clinical tool used by case managers to achieve better quality and cost outcomes by outlining and sequencing the usual and desired care for particular groups of patients. Clinical paths incorporate care requirements from preadmission through postdischarge.

clinical pelvimetry A technique using vaginal palpation of bony landmarks in the pelvis to estimate the size of the birth canal.

clinical practice guidelines A decision-making tool used to help practitioners determine how diseases or disorders can most effectively and appropriately be prevented, diagnosed, treated, and managed clinically. These guidelines include advice and information from recognized clinical experts.

clitoris A small erectile structure located at the anterior angle of the rima pudendi. It's homologous to the corpora cavernosa of the penis.

clonus Involuntary muscular contraction and relaxation in a rapid alternating pattern.

closed amputation The removal of a limb leaving one or two broad flaps of muscular and cutaneous tissue to cover the end of the bone.

closed chain In organic chemistry: a compound in which carbon atoms link together to form a closed ring.

clotting time The length of time required for blood to clot, usually determined by collecting a blood sample and visually examining it for clot formation.

clubbing Enlargement of the soft tissues of distal phalanges, most commonly associated with cyanotic heart disease or advanced chronic pulmonary disease.

TIME LINE In children, clubbing occurs most often in cyanotic congenital heart disease and cystic fibrosis. Arthritic deformities of the fingers or toes may disguise the presence of clubbing.

clubfoot A congenital foot deformity in which the foot is twisted out of shape or position.

cm *abbr* centimeter.

Cm Symbol for curium.

CMAJ *abbr* Canadian Medical Association Journal.

CMHC *abbr* community mental health center.

CML *abbr* chronic myelocytic leukemia.

CMT *abbr* certified medical transcriptionist.

CMV *abbr* cytomegalovirus.

CNM *abbr* certified nurse-midwife.

CNS *abbr* 1. central nervous system. 2. clinical nurse specialist.

Co Symbol for cobalt.

CO_2 Symbol for carbon dioxide.

COA *abbr* Canadian Orthopaedic Association.

coagulation factor One of 12 substances in the blood required for blood clotting. Using standardized numerical nomenclature, the 12 factors are factor I, fibrinogen; factor II, prothrombin; factor III, tissue thromboplastin; factor IV, calcium ions; factor V, labile factor; factor VII, stable factor; factor VIII, antihemophilic globulin; factor IX, plasma thromboplastin component; factor X, Stuart-Prower factor; factor XI, plasma thromboplastin antecedent; factor XII, Hageman factor; factor XIII, fibrin stabilizing factor.

coaptation splint A small splint placed on a fractured limb to prevent overriding of the bone fragments.

 CLINICAL TIP Usually, a longer splint covers the small one to increase the

Coarctation of the aorta

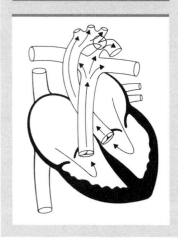

support and provide fixation of the entire limb.

coarctation of the aorta   A congenital heart abnormality characterized by a malformation and localized narrowing of the aorta. Pressure proximal to the defect increases, while pressure distal to the defect decreases. See illustration on page 82

cobalt (Co)   A metallic element used in magnetic alloys and present in vitamin B_1. Its atomic number is 27; its atomic weight is 58.9. Exposure to cobalt powder may cause dermatitis; inhalation of the dust may lead to cobaltosis.

coccidiosis   A parasitic infection caused by the ingestion of oocysts of the protozoa *Isospora belli* or *I. hominis*, occurring in tropical and subtropical regions.

coccygeus   Relating to the coccyx, or tailbone.

coccyx, *pl*. coccyges   The small bone at the base of the spine, named for its resemblance to the bill of the cuckoo. It's formed by three to five rudimentary vertebrae that are joined together and connected to the sacrum by a disk of fibrocartilage.

cochlea   A spirally wound, bony structure of the inner ear, containing apertures for passage of the cochlear division of the acoustic nerve.

codominant inheritance   The genetic transmission of a trait or condition in which both alleles of a pair are dominant and are fully expressed in a heterozygote. For example, the human blood group AB is the result

of two alleles, A and B; both A and B are expressed, and neither is dominant to the other.

codon   A set of three adjacent nucleotides on a single strand of deoxyribonucleic acid or a molecule of messenger ribonucleic acid that directs the incorporation of a specific amino acid in the polypeptide chain during protein synthesis.

coefficient   1. In mathematics: a number of another known factor by which a variable quantity is multiplied. 2. In physics: a measure of a specified property of a specific substance under specified conditions, such as the coefficient of friction of a substance.

coenzyme   An organic nonprotein molecule that combines with an apoenzyme (protein molecule) to form a complete enzyme or holoenzyme.

cognition   Process by which a person becomes aware of objects; includes all aspects of perception, thought, and memory.

coherence   The characteristic of sticking together, such as the molecules within a common substance.

coiled tubular gland   A multicellular gland containing one coiled, tubular secretory portion; for example, a sweat gland.

colation   The process of filtering or straining.

cold agglutinins   Antibodies that could cause red blood cell clumping if cold blood is infused.

cold-sensitive mutation   A change in a gene that leads to a gene that functions only at a high temperature.

colectomy   Surgical removal of part or all of the colon to treat such conditions as colon cancer and severe chronic ulcerative colitis.

colic   Acute abdominal pain caused by torsion, blockage, or smooth-muscle spasm of a hollow or tubular organ, such as an intestine.

colitis   Inflammation of the colon; may refer to an episodic, functional, irritable bowel syndrome or to a chronic, progressive, inflammatory disease of a more serious nature.

collagen   A protein substance consisting of white, glistening, inelastic fibers. It's found in the skin, tendon, bone, cartilage and other connective tissue.

collagen disease   Any one of various conditions characterized by widespread pathologic changes in small blood vessels and connective tissue; examples include scleroderma and lupus erythematosus.

collateral   1. Secondary or accessory. 2. In anatomy: a small side branch, such as an arteriole or venule.

collateral fissure   A longitudinal fissure on the inferior surface of the cerebral hemisphere that separates the fusiform gyrus from the parahippocampal gyrus.

collecting tubule   A channel that passes fluids from secretory cells, such as those in the kidney that funnel urine from the distal convoluted tubules into the renal pelvis.

Colles' fracture   A fracture of the radius at the lower end of the wrist (within 1″ of the wrist joint) in which the bone fragment is displaced posteriorly.

 ALERT Colles' fracture requires reduction with plaster immobilization for 4 to 10 weeks.

colligative   In physical chemistry: of or relating to the number of particles (such as molecules and ions) rather than their size, weight, or chemical makeup.

collimator   A diaphragm or system of diaphragms that limits the direction and dimension of a beam of radiation.

colliquation   The degeneration of body tissue to a liquid, as seen in necrotic tissue.

colliquative   Characterized by excessive discharge of fluid, as seen in suppurating wounds and infected body structures.

colloid   1. A gelatinous substance. 2. A substance consisting of particles that are dispersed throughout another substance (called the dispersion medium). The particles are incapable of passing through a semipermeable membrane.

colloid chemistry   The study of the composition and characteristics of chemical colloids.

colloid goiter   A thyroid disease in which the gland is soft and greatly enlarged and the follicles are distended with colloid.

colloid oncotic pressure (COP)   The osmotic force of albumin in the bloodstream that draws water into the capillaries from interstitial fluids during reabsorption.

colon   The part of the large intestine that extends from the cecum to the rectum, consisting of four segments (ascending, transverse, descending, and sigmoid).

colonoscopy   Examination of the colon using a flexible endoscope to visualize internal body areas or to remove tissue samples or small growths.

colony   In bacteriology: a group of microorganisms in a culture that derives from a single organism or group of organisms. Types of colonies include smooth, rough, and dwarf.

colony counter   An illuminated, transparent plate divided into sections of known area, used to count bacterial colonies that are part of a culture.

colony-stimulating factors (CSFs) Biological response modifiers that regulate hematopoietic growth and differentiation; for example, hematopoietic growth factors (erythropoietin), granulocyte colony stimulating

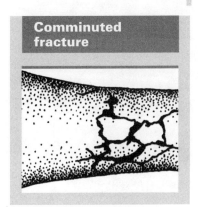

Comminuted fracture

factor, interleukin-3, macrophage colony stimulating factor, and thrombopoietin.

colopexy   Surgical suspension or fixation of the colon.

colpectomy   Excision of the vagina.

colporrhaphy   Suturing of the vagina, such as to restructure the vagina.

Colorado tick fever   An acute, febrile infection caused by an arenavirus and transmitted to man by the bite of a wood tick. It's self-limited and relatively mild.

color blindness   Inability to clearly distinguish color hues.

colorectal cancer   A malignant growth of cells in the large intestine, characterized by a change in bowel habits, black and tarry stools, and the passing of blood.

colorimetry   Measurement of color differences in a fluid or substance.

color vision   Perception of different colors as cones in the retina react to varying wavelengths of light.

colostomy   Surgical creation of an opening between the colon and the surface of the abdomen, used to treat colon cancer or benign obstructive tumors.

colostrum   The highly nutritious fluid secreted by the mammary gland during pregnancy and the first few days postpartum. It contains immunologically active substances and white blood cells, along with water, protein, fat, and carbohydrates.

 CLINICAL TIP Colostrum gradually decreases; at 2 weeks postpartum, it disappears and only mature breast milk remains.

columnar epithelium   Epithelium composed of tall prismatic cells that resemble a column.

column chromatography   A technique for analyzing or separating mixtures of gases, liquids, or dissolved substances based on dif-

Complete breech

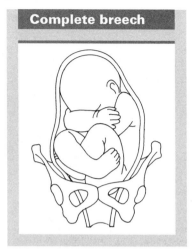

ferences in their absorption affinities for a given absorbent.

coma A state of unconsciousness from which an individual can't be roused, marked by lack of spontaneous eye movements and an absent response to painful stimuli or vocal commands.

commensal An organism that lives on or within another organism and benefits from the relationship while neither benefiting nor harming the host.

comminuted fracture A fracture in which the bone is crushed, creating several fragments.

commissurotomy Surgical division of a connection between corresponding parts of a body structure, performed to enlarge the site.

common bile duct The duct formed by the joining of the cystic duct and hepatic duct.

common hepatic artery An artery that originates in the celiac trunk of the abdominal aorta and carries blood away from the heart to the liver, gallbladder, stomach, pancreas, duodenum, and greater omentum. After passing to the pylorus, it divides into five branches (the gastroduodenal, right gastric, right hepatic, left hepatic, and middle hepatic).

common iliac artery A division of the abdominal aorta that carries blood away from the heart and supplies the pelvis, abdominal wall, and lower limbs. It begins to the left of the fourth lumbar vertebra, passes caudally about 2" (5 cm), and branches into the external and internal iliac arteries.

compatibility For transfusion therapy, typing and crossmatching the donor and recipient blood to minimize the risk of a hemolytic reaction. The most important compatibility tests include ABO blood typing, Rh typing, crossmatching, direct antiglobulin test, and antibody screening test.

compensatory pause Period following a premature ventricular contraction during which the heart regulates itself, allowing the sinoatrial node to resume normal conduction.

complement One of 11 proteins in the blood plasma and tissue fluid that help to defend the body after an immune response; the genes encoding complement form part of the major histocompatibility complex.

CLINICAL TIP Complement is activated after an antibody-antigen reaction, binding to the antibody-antigen complex (complement fixation); it then becomes involved in destroying foreign cells and drawing phagocytes (scavenger cells) to the area.

complement abnormality A condition characterized by a deficiency or malfunction of any of the nine functional components of the enzymatic proteins of blood serum.

complement system Major mediator of inflammatory response; a functionally related system of 20 proteins circulating as inactive molecules pending an inflammatory trigger.

complemental inheritance The expression of a characteristic based on the presence of two independent pairs of nonallelic genes, both of which must be present.

complementary gene Two independent pairs of nonallelic genes, neither of which produces its effect unless the other is present. Also called *reciprocal gene.*

complement-fixation test (C-F test) A test used to determine the presence and extent of antigen-antibody reaction, performed by adding a known antigen or antibody, directed against an unknown antibody or antigen, to serum and incubating the sample. Red blood cells coated with the same known antigen or antibody are added; lack of hemolysis signifies that complement must have been depleted in the original reaction, meaning the unknown antibody or antigen was present in the sample. The unknown antibody or antigen is then assayed.

complete blood count (CBC) Determination of the hematocrit, amount of hemoglobin, and number and proportion of the various white blood cells in a sample of blood.

complete breech A fetal position in which the buttocks are presenting, with the knees folded up to the abdomen. The fetus is in the normal vertex position but upside down.

complete fracture　A fracture in which the bone is broken across its entire width.

complex　**1.** A group of items related in some way, such as in structure or function. **2.** A cluster of signs and symptoms that forms a syndrome.

complex fracture　A closed fracture in which soft tissue around the broken bone is severely injured.

compound fracture　A fracture in which the parts of the broken bone protrude through the skin. Also called *open fracture.*

compound protein　A protein containing a protein molecule and a nonprotein molecule, such as a nucleoprotein or lipoprotein. Also called *conjugated protein.*

compression fracture　A bone fracture caused by compression that collapses the affected bone, such as a vertebral fracture.

compromised host　An animal or a plant that's particularly susceptible to infection as a result of compromised health due to immunosuppressive therapy, an immunologic defect, severe anemia, or disease.

computerized tomography (CT), computerized axial tomography (CAT)　A technique that records detailed internal images of a predetermined plane of body tissue. A device called a tomograph moves an X-ray source in one direction as the film moves in the opposite direction. A scintillation counter measures the emergent X-ray beam; electronic impulses are recorded on a magnetic disk and processed by a computer for display of a cross-section of the body.

concave　Having a surface that curves inward, resembling a hollowed inner segment of a sphere.

concentrate　**1.** To condense, or increase the strength, as of a liquid, by removing inactive ingredients through evaporation or other means. **2.** A drug or other preparation that has been strengthened by the evaporation of its nonactive parts.

conceptus　All products of the fertilized ovum, including its enclosing membranes, from the time of fertilization to birth.

concha　In anatomy: a part or structure of the body that resembles a shell, such as the outer ear.

concussion　A violent shock or jarring, such as from an explosion or a blow.

> **ALERT** Concussion of the brain is characterized by loss of consciousness. Severe concussion may also cause impairment of brain stem functions.

condom　A soft, flexible sheath placed over the penis before sexual intercourse to prevent impregnation and infection.

conduction　The transfer or transmission of heat, energy, nerve impulses, or sound waves from one site to another.

conduction aphasia　A defect in the ability to express oneself despite normal language comprehension.

conductive hearing loss　A form of hearing loss characterized by interference with transmission of sounds through the external and middle ear structures to the sensorineural apparatus of the inner ear.

condyle　A rounded projection at the end of a bone that allows articulation with adjacent bones.

condyloid joint　A synovial joint in which an ovoid head of one bone moves in an elliptical cavity of another.

condyloma, *pl.* condylomata　A wartlike lesion caused by the human papilloma virus, usually occurring on the mucous membrane or skin of the external genitalia or the perianal region. The lesions may cluster to form large masses.

cone　**1.** A solid or hollow structure or body that has a circular base tapering to a point. **2.** A cell in the retina that allows color perception. The human eye contains 6 to 7 million cones. **3.** In radiology: a conical device attached over the portal of the X-ray tube housing that helps to focus the radiation beam on the target tissue.

cone biopsy　Surgical removal of a cone-shaped portion of cervical tissue (including both epithelial and endocervical tissue), usually performed after a positive Papanicolaou test. The tissue specimen is then examined for cancer cells.

cone of light　**1.** A triangular reflection of light seen on the tympanic membrane during an otoscopic examination. **2.** The collection of light rays that enter the pupil and form an image on the retina.

confidentiality　The professional responsibility to keep all privileged information private; confidentiality may be mandated by state or federal statutes and case law.

congenital　Present at or existing from birth.

conjoined twins　Twins who developed from a single ovum and are physically joined at birth, usually at the frontal, transverse, or sagittal plane.

conjugated estrogen　An orally administered drug derived from the sodium salts of estrogen sulfates (principally estrone, equilin, and 17-alpha-dihydroequilin) that approximates the estrogen found in the urine of pregnant mares.

conjunctiva　The mucous membrane that covers the inner surfaces of the eyelids and the anterior portion of the sclera.

conjunctival reflex   A protective response of the eye that causes the eyelids to close when the conjunctiva is touched.

conjunctivitis   Inflammation and redness of the conjunctiva of the eye as a result of infection, allergy, or a chemical reaction.

connecting fibrocartilage   A disk composed of concentric rings of fibrous tissue separated by cartilaginous laminae, found between many joints (particularly those with limited mobility, such as the spinal vertebrae).

connective tissue   Tissue that's derived from the mesoderm and supports and binds together body structures; it includes bone, cartilage, and adipose tissue. Connective tissue is composed of collagenous, reticular, and elastic fibers.

Conn's syndrome   Excessive secretion of aldosterone caused by an adrenocortical adenoma. Also called *primary aldosteronism.*

consensual   Describing the reaction of one body part to stimulation of the homologous or corresponding part; for example, constriction of the pupil of an eye that's covered when the other eye is exposed to light.

consensual reaction to light   Constriction of both pupils when only one pupil has been exposed to light.

consensus sequence   In molecular genetics: a sequence of nucleotides that's common to different genes or genomes.

consent form   A document prepared for the patient's signature that discloses his proposed treatment in general terms and acknowledges his consent to treatment.

conservation of energy   A law of physics stating that within any given closed system, the total amount of energy is constant; energy is neither created nor destroyed, only transformed.

conservation of matter   A law of physics stating that in any chemical reaction, matter can't be created or destroyed and that the universe has a finite amount of matter.

contagious   Transmittable from one individual to another by direct or indirect contact, as a contagious disease.

continuous positive airway pressure (CPAP)   In respiratory therapy: delivery of air at a constant pressure throughout respiration, used to cause inspiration while increasing tidal volume.

continuous positive pressure ventilation   A mechanical ventilation pattern that maintains a positive end-expiratory plateau pressure during expiration.

contraceptive   An agent, such as a medication or device, that prevents or reduces the chance of conception.

contraceptive diaphragm   A thin, rubber dome bonded to a flexible ring and fitted to the uterine cervix. It's inserted into the vagina to prevent conception by creating a mechanical barrier against sperm.

CLINICAL TIP   To be effective, a diaphragm must be used with spermicidal cream or jelly. Additional spermicide must be inserted into the vagina before each act of intercourse and if more than 2 hours have passed between diaphragm insertion and intercourse.

contractility   Ability of a cardiac cell to contract after receiving an electrical impulse.

contracture   Abnormal flexion and fixation of a joint, possibly permanent, which is typically caused by muscle wasting and atrophy or by loss of normal skin elasticity, such as from extensive scar tissue.

contralateral   Occurring on or acting on the opposite side.

contrast medium   A substance introduced into the body to improve radiographic visualization of organs or other body tissues that are otherwise difficult to visualize. Body tissues exposed to the medium absorb more X-rays, providing a contrast with unexposed tissues.

controlled substance   Any substance that's strictly regulated or illegal due to its potential for abuse or addiction. Controlled substances include: cannabis (marijuana), depressants, hallucinogens, narcotics, and stimulants. Compare *prescription drug.*

controlled ventilation   The use of a machine to replace a patient's spontaneous respiration. A respirator, such as an intermittent positive pressure breathing unit, controls breathing.

controller   An electronic device that regulates the flow of I.V. solutions and drugs; used when a precise flow rate is required.

contusion   A bruise; an injury that doesn't break the skin but results in discoloration, swelling, and pain.

convection   Transfer of heat from one part of a fluid to another by movement of the fluid itself.

convex   Having a surface that curves outward, resembling a segment of the external section of a sphere.

convolution   An irregularity caused by the enfolding of a structure upon itself, such as the convolutions on the surface of the cerebral cortex.

convulsion   A sudden, violent involuntary contraction or series of contractions by a group of muscles. Also called *seizure.*

cooling cap   In chemotherapy, a device used to limit superficial blood flow to the scalp during drug administration, thus partially protecting the hair follicles and limiting alopecia.

coordinated reflex A sequential reaction of several muscles in an orderly manner to produce a movement, such as swallowing.

COPD *abbr* chronic obstructive pulmonary disease.

copper (Cu) A malleable, reddish-brown, metallic element. Its atomic number is 29; its atomic weight is 63.54.

coracoid process The strong, curved projection of the superior border of the scapula, to which the pectoralis minor is attached. It overhangs the shoulder joint.

cordectomy Excision of all or part of a cord, such as the spinal cord or a vocal cord.

corditis Inflammation of the spermatic cord, sometimes accompanied by testicular pain, that may result from a urethral infection, groin injury, tumors, hydrocele, or varicocele.

cordopexy A surgical procedure that outwardly displaces the vocal cord, performed to relieve stenosis of the larynx.

coreoplasty Any plastic repair of the pupil.

corium A layer of skin just below the epidermis, consisting of dense vascular connective tissue with blood and lymphatic vessels, nerves and nerve endings, glands, and hair follicles. Also called *dermis.*

corn A horny mass of thickened skin, usually found on the foot. It forms a cone-shaped mass pointing in toward the corium.

cornea The transparent, anterior portion of the eye. It comprises one-sixth of the outermost tunic of the eye, and contains five layers.

corneal abrasion The wearing away of the outer layers of the cornea.

corneal grafting Transplantation of corneal tissue from one human eye to another, performed to remove a perforating ulcer or to improve vision that's marred by corneal scarring.

corneal reflex Closure of the eyelids when the cornea is touched; a protective reaction of the eye.

corneal ulcer A lesion of the cornea.

cornification Thickening of the skin as a result of the accumulation of dead, keratinized epithelial cells.

cornual pregnancy An extrauterine pregnancy that implants in the part of the fallopian tube located within the horn of the uterus.

corona 1. A crown. 2. A structure or projection that's crownlike in shape, such as a bony process.

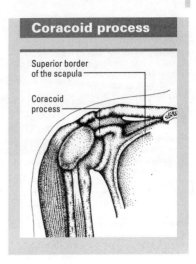

Coracoid process

Superior border of the scapula

Coracoid process

coronal suture The juncture line between the frontal bone and the two parietal bones.

coronary Of or relating to the heart and the arteries that supply it.

coronary artery One of two arteries that branch from the aorta.

coronary artery bypass grafting (CABG) Surgical procedure in which a section of the mammary artery or the saphenous vein is sutured to either side of an obstructed coronary artery.

 CLINICAL TIP CABG improves blood flow to the heart muscle by establishing a shunt to circumvent a blocked coronary artery.

coronary artery disease Any condition that affects the arteries of the heart and causes pathologic effects, such as reduced oxygen flow to the myocardium.

coronary care unit (CCU) A specially-equipped hospital area designed for treatment of patients with sudden, life-threatening cardiac conditions. Cardiopulmonary monitoring, resuscitation techniques, administration of antiarrhythmic drugs, and other appropriate therapeutic measures are provided by personnel specially trained and skilled in the recognition of and immediate response to cardiac emergencies.

coronary heart disease (CHD) A disease of the myocardium in which constriction of the coronary arteries leads to an insufficient myocardial blood supply.

coronary occlusion Blockage of an artery of the heart, typically resulting from atherosclerosis.

coronary thrombosis   Blockage of a coronary artery by a blood clot. It may lead to myocardial infarction and death.

coronary vein   A vein of the heart that channels blood from the capillary beds of the myocardium through the coronary sinus and into the right atrium.

cor pulmonale   A heart condition in which hypertension of the pulmonary circulation leads to enlargement of the right ventricle.

corpus cavernosum clitoridis   One of two columns of erectile tissue embedded in the anterior floor of the vaginal vestibule, which fuse together to form the clitoris.

corpus cavernosum penis   One of two columns of erectile tissue that join together to form the dorsum and the sides of the penis.

corpuscle, corpuscule   1. A small mass or body. 2. A red or white blood cell.

corpus luteum, *pl.* **corpora lutea**   A yellowish, spherical structure on the surface of the ovary that forms after the ovarian follicle releases the ovum. Upon fertilization of the ovum, the corpus luteum grows and remains in place for several months.

Corrigan's pulse   Jerky pulse with full expansion and sudden collapse.

cortex, *pl.* **cortices**   The external layer of an organ or other body structure (as opposed to the internal substance).

cortical blindness   Blindness caused by a lesion in the visual center of the cerebral cortex.

corticospinal tracts   Motor pathways whose fibers come together in the medulla to form the pyramids and whose axons originate from neuron cell bodies in the cerebral cortex. Impulses conducted by these tracts help maintain muscle tone and are essential for voluntary contractions of individual muscles to produce small, discrete movements. Also called *pyramidal tracts.*

corticosteroid   A natural or synthetic hormone associated with the adrenal cortex. Corticosteroids are classified by their primary biological activity as either glucocorticoids (which chiefly affect protein, fat, and carbohydrate metabolism), or mineralocorticoids (which help regulate fluid and electrolyte balance).

Corti's organ   A spiral structure on the basilar membrane in the cochlear duct of the ear that contains special sensory receptors for hearing. Also called *spiral organ of Corti.*

Corynebacterium   A genus of rod-shaped bacilli having many species. *Corynebacterium diphtheriae,* the most common pathogenic species, is the cause of diphtheria.

costochondral   Of or relating to a rib and its cartilage.

costovertebral angle (CVA)   The angle formed on either side of the vertebral column, between the last rib and the lumbar vertebrae.

Cotton's fracture   A fracture that involves the medial, lateral, and posterior malleoli.

coulomb   The SI (Système International d'Unités) unit of electric charge, equal to the charge transferred by a steady current of 1 ampere in 1 second.

Coulomb's law   In physics: a law stating that the force between two electrically charged particles is directly proportional to the product of their charges and inversely proportional to the square of the distance between them.

Coulter counter   A trade name for an electrical instrument that identifies, sorts, and counts formed peripheral blood elements in a blood sample. The device works on the principle that cells are poor conductors of electricity compared with saline solution.

countertraction   Traction that opposes the pull of another traction, used to reduce fractures.

Cowling's rule   A method of calculating the approximate pediatric dosage of a drug; the adult dose is multiplied by the age of the child at his next birthday and divided by 24.

Cowper's gland   Either of two pea-sized glands embedded in the urethral sphincter of the male, posterior to the membranous portion of the urethra. Also called *bulbourethral gland.*

cowpox   A mild, infectious skin disease of milk cows, caused by the vaccinia virus, that can be transmitted to humans from infected cattle. Vesicles, the primary lesions, typically appear on the fingers and may spread to adjacent areas. Other signs and symptoms may include local swelling, lymphangitis, and regional lymphadenitis. Cowpox infection usually confers immunity to smallpox.

coxa valga   A hip deformity marked by an increase in the angle formed by the axis of the head and neck of the femur and the axis of its shaft.

coxa vara   A hip deformity marked by a decrease in the angle formed by the axis of the head and neck of the femur and the axis of its shaft. Also called *coxa adducta, coxa flexa.*

coxitis   Inflammation of the hip joint.

coxsackievirus   Any of a heterogeneous group of enteroviruses causing a disease that resembles poliomyelitis but without paralysis.

CP *abbr* 1. cerebral palsy 2. certified prosthetist.

CPAP *abbr* continuous positive airway pressure.

CPHA *abbr* Canadian Public Health Association.

CPD *abbr* 1. cephalopelvic disproportion. 2. childhood polycystic disease. 3. congenital polycystic disease.

cpm *abbr* cycles per minute.

CPM *abbr* continuous passive motion.

CPPB *abbr* continuous positive pressure breathing.

CPPV *abbr* continuous positive pressure ventilation.

CPR *abbr* cardiopulmonary resuscitation.

CPT *abbr* current procedural terminology.

Cr Symbol for chromium.

CR *abbr* controlled respiration.

cradle cap A form of seborrheic dermatitis of unknown origin. Common among neonates, it's characterized by thick, yellow, greasy scales on the scalp.

ALERT Cradle cap is a potential cause of skin breakdown and infection.

cranioclasis Crushing of the fetal head.

craniorachischisis Congenital fissure of the skull and spinal column.

cranium The skeleton of the head, encasing the brain. It's composed of eight bones — frontal, occipital, sphenoid, and ethmoid bones, and paired temporal and parietal.

cravat bandage A triangular bandage folded lengthwise, used as a circular, spiral, or figure-eight bandage to manage bleeding or to secure a splint in place.

C-reactive protein (CRP) A globulin not normally found in the serum but present in various acute inflammatory conditions and in necrosis.

creatine An end-product of metabolism.

ALERT Greatly elevated serum creatine levels may indicate skeletal muscle disease.

creatine kinase An enzyme found in muscle, brain, and other tissues that triggers the transfer of a phosphate group from adenosine triphosphate to creatine, yielding adenosine diphosphate and phosphocreatine.

creatinine An end-product of creatine metabolism; elevated serum levels may indicate renal disease.

Credé's maneuver 1. A technique used to expel the placenta after birth by forcing the uterus down into the pelvis and squeezing it from all sides toward the birth canal. 2. A similar technique used to expel urine from the bladder.

Credé's treatment Instillation of 1% to 2% silver nitrate solution into each eye of a newborn immediately after birth to prevent ophthalmia neonatorum.

cremasteric reflex Brisk retraction of the testis on the side of the stimulus when the skin of the upper inner aspect of the thigh is stroked.

crenation The development of abnormal notches or leaflike, scalloped edges. A red blood cell exposed to a hypertonic saline solution may acquire crenations from shrinkage.

crepitus 1. Flatulence or noisy discharge of gas from the intestine. 2. A sound resembling the crackling noise made by rubbing hair between the fingers or throwing salt into a fire. 3. The sound made by rubbing the ends of a fractured bone together.

 TIME LINE Children may develop subcutaneous crepitation in the neck from ingestion of corrosive substances that perforate the esophagus.

cretinism A condition caused by congenital absence of thyroid hormone secretion, marked by arrested mental and physical development, bone dystrophy, and reduced basal metabolism. Other signs of cretinism include dwarfism, puffy facial features, dry skin, enlargement of the tongue, umbilical hernia, and muscle incoordination.

cricoid 1. Shaped like a ring. 2. A ring-shaped cartilage attached to the thyroid cartilage by the cricothyroid ligament at the level of the sixth cervical vertebra.

crista A ridge, or projecting structure.

CRNA *abbr* certified registered nurse anesthetist. See *nurse anesthetist.*

Crohn's disease A chronic inflammatory bowel disease of unknown cause, usually involving the terminal ileum, with scarring and thickening of the bowel wall. Signs and symptoms include frequent episodes of diarrhea, severe abdominal pain, nausea, fever, chills, anorexia, and weight loss.

TIME LINE Crohn's disease is most prevalent in adults ages 20 to 40.

cross In genetics: an individual, organism, or strain produced by crossbreeding.

crossbreeding The mating of animals or plants of different varieties, strains, or species; hybridization.

crossed reflex A response on the side of the body opposite the one that has been stimulated.

 CLINICAL TIP The consensual light reflex is an example of a crossed reflex.

crossmatching of blood A procedure used to determine compatibility of a donor's blood with that of a recipient after the specimens have been matched for major blood

Cuboid bone

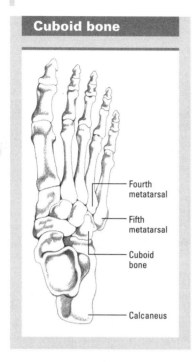

Fourth metatarsal

Fifth metatarsal

Cuboid bone

Calcaneus

type. Donor red blood cells are placed in the serum of the recipient, and vice versa. Then antiglobulin is added to increase reactivity; if hemolysis or agglutination occurs, donor blood and recipient blood are deemed incompatible.

cross-sectional anatomy The study of the relationships among body structures by examining cross sections of the organ or tissue.

cross-sensitivity A patient's hypersensitivity to I.V. drugs that are chemically similar to another drug known to elicit hypersensitivity in that patient.

croup An acute viral infection of the respiratory tract that causes acute upper airway obstruction. It's characterized by stridor, a barking cough, and hoarseness. It primarily affects infants and young children ages 3 months to 3 years and follows an upper respiratory tract infection.

Crouzon's disease A genetic disorder marked by acrocephaly, hypertelorism, exophthalmos, strabismus, and hypoplastic maxilla resulting from premature fusion of the skull bones. Also called **craniofacial dysostosis.**

crown 1. The uppermost part of an organ or structure. 2. An artificial restoration that replaces the entire surface anatomy of the natural crown of a tooth.

CRP *abbr* C-reactive protein.

crude birthrate The number of births per 1,000 persons in a given population during 1 year.

crush syndrome A serious, life-threatening complication of a severe crush injury, marked by hemorrhage, destruction of muscle and bone tissue, and fluid loss leading to hypovolemic shock, hematuria, kidney failure, coma and, possibly, death.

cryocautery 1. Destruction of tissue by applying a substance that causes freezing, such as liquid nitrogen or carbon dioxide. Also called *cautery.* 2. An instrument that destroys tissue by freezing.

cryogen A substance used to induce freezing and thereby destroy diseased tissue without harming adjacent structures.

cryoprecipitate A precipitate produced from cooling, such as antihemophilic factor used to treat hemophilia.

cryptococcosis An infection caused by the fungus *Cryptococcus neoformans,* which may involve the lungs, brain and central nervous system (CNS), skin, or other parts of the body. Acneiform lesions develop with the cutaneous form of the disease; the generalized form typically affects the CNS in immunocompromised patients.

Cryptococcus A genus of yeastlike organisms of the family Cryptococcaceae that reproduces by budding.

Cryptococcus neoformans A species of *Cryptococcus* that causes a potentially fatal fungal infection, cryptococcosis, affecting the lungs, brain, and skin.

cryptodidymus Asymmetrical conjoined twins, with one small, underdeveloped fetus enclosed within the body of the larger twin. Also called *endadelphos.*

cryptorchidism A developmental anomaly marked by failure of one or both of the testicles to descend into the scrotum.

crystal A solid inorganic substance, with a regular polyhedral shape. The atoms, ions, or molecules that form the crystal have a regular, repeating arrangement, called the crystal structure.

crystalline lens The transparent biconvex body of the eye located between the vitreous body and the posterior chamber and enclosed in a capsule. It serves as part of the eye's refracting mechanism.

Cs Symbol for cesium.

CSF *abbr* cerebrospinal fluid.

CSR *abbr* Cheyne-Stokes respiration.

CT *abbr* computerized tomography. Also called *computerized axial tomography.*

Cu Symbol for copper.

cubitus The joint between the arm and forearm; the bend of the arm.

cuboid bone The bone on the lateral side of the foot between the calcaneus and the fourth and fifth metatarsal bones.

cul-de-sac A blind pouch or cecum (such as the conjunctival cul-de-sac), or a tubular cavity closed at one end (such as the diverticulum).

culture procedure In bacteriology: any of several methods for growing colonies of microorganisms for the purpose of identifying a pathogen and determining which antibiotics will successfully combat the infectious organism.

cumulative dose The total dose produced by repeated exposure to radiation.

cuneiform Wedge-shaped.

cupping Component of traditional Chinese medicine in which heated glass cups are placed on the skin to create suction and then removed. This therapy, used primarily to relieve bronchial congestion, is believed to dispel dampness, warm the internal energy force (qi), and reduce swelling.

cupping and vibrating Chest physiotherapy techniques used to help mobilize and eliminate mucus and fluid from the lungs.

CLINICAL TIP To perform percussion (cupping), the practitioner holds the hands in a cupped shape and then percusses each lung segment for 1 to 2 minutes by alternating the hands against the patient in a rhythmic manner. To perform vibration, the practitioner presses the fingers and palms of the hands against the patient's chest wall as the patient exhales slowly through pursed lips. Then the practitioner tenses the arm and shoulder muscles to send fine vibrations through the chest wall.

curet A spoon- or scoop-shaped surgical instrument used to scrape and remove material or tissue from an organ, cavity, or other surface.

curettage The removal of material from the wall of a cavity or other surface, commonly using a curet. It may be done to remove tumors or other abnormal tissue or to obtain tissue for evaluation.

curie (Ci, c) A unit of radioactivity equal to 3.70×10^{10} disintegrations per second.

curium (Cm) A radioactive metallic element with nine known isotopes. Its atomic number is 96; its atomic weight is 247.

Curschmann's spiral One of the coiled mucinous fibrils sometimes found in the sputum of a person with bronchial asthma.

cursor A special character or visual cue on a video display that indicates the position for data entry. The operator uses cursor control keys to maneuver the cursor on the screen.

curvature myopia A form of nearsightedness resulting from an increase in the curvature of the eye's refracting surfaces (especially that of the cornea).

Cushing's syndrome A metabolic disorder caused by chronic, excessive production of adrenocortical hormones or by prolonged high-dose glucocorticoid therapy. It's characterized by such signs and symptoms as hypertension, diabetes mellitus, dusky complexion with purple striae, muscle wasting, weakness, and sudden development of fat around the face, neck, and trunk.

cuspids The four canine teeth, each having one cusp or point.

cutaneous Of or relating to the skin.

cuticle 1. A layer that covers the free surface of an epithelial cell. 2. The narrow band of epidermis that extends from the wall of the nail onto the nail surface. Also called *eponychium.* 3. The sheath of a hair follicle.

cutis laxa A group of connective tissue disorders characterized by abnormally loose, relaxed skin, resulting from decreased elastic tissue formation and an abnormality in elastin formation. The disorders are usually genetic.

CVA *abbr* 1. cerebrovascular accident. 2. costovertebral angle.

cyanocobalamin Vitamin B_{12}; a red, crystalline, water-soluble vitamin required for neural function, normal blood formation, and metabolism of carbohydrates, fats, and proteins.

cyanosis Bluish discoloration of the skin and mucous membranes resulting from an excessive amount of deoxygenated hemoglobin in the blood or a structural defect in the hemoglobin molecule, as in methemoglobin.

cycle-nonspecific drugs In chemotherapy, drugs that act independently of the cell cycle, affecting both reproducing and resting cells. During a single administration of a cycle-nonspecific chemotherapeutic drug, a fixed percentage of both normal and malignant cells die, while the others survive. Slower growing cancers, such as GI and pulmonary tumors, have fewer cells undergoing division at any given moment, and respond best to cycle-nonspecific drugs. Large tumors initially respond better to cycle-nonspecific drugs, but once they shrink, the doctor may switch to a cycle-specific drug.

cycle-specific drugs In chemotherapy, drugs that are only effective during a specific phase of the cell cycle, and are designed to disrupt a specific biochemical process. During administration of cycle-specific chemotherapy, cells in the resting phase survive to eventually reproduce. Faster growing cancers, such as acute leukemias and lymphomas, respond best to cycle-specific chemotherapy. In general, small tumors respond best to drugs that affect DNA synthesis, especially cycle-specific drugs, because they have a higher percentage of actively dividing cells than large tumors.

cyclic adenosine monophosphate (cyclic AMP)   A derivative of adenosine triphosphate, widespread in animal cells, that is an intermediate messenger in many biochemical reactions induced by hormones. It's also involved in immune responses, regulation of gene expression and cell division, and nerve impulse transmission.

cyclic delivery   In parenteral nutrition, delivery of the entire solution overnight; also used to wean a patient from total parenteral nutrition.

cycloplegia   Paralysis of the ciliary muscle or paralysis of accommodation, as induced by certain ophthalmic agents to allow examination of the eye.

cyclothymia   A mood disorder marked by alternation between hypomanic and depressive periods.

cyst   **1.** A closed cavity or sac in or under the skin lined with epithelium, especially one that contains a fluid or semisolid material. **2.** A stage of the life cycle of certain parasites during which they exist within a protective wall.

cystectomy   **1.** Surgical removal of all or part of the urinary bladder, as may be required in treating bladder cancer. **2.** Excision of a cyst.

cysteine   An amino acid found in many proteins in the body, produced by the enzymatic or acid hydrolysis of proteins. A metabolic precursor of cystine, it's sometimes found in the urine.

cystic carcinoma   A malignant growth composed of cysts or cystlike spaces. Such tumors arise in the breast and ovary.

cystic duct   The passage that connects the neck of the gallbladder and the common bile duct, through which bile flows.

cysticercosis   An infection with the larval forms (cysticerci) of the pork tapeworm *Taenia solium.* These forms may invade the intestinal walls and enter such tissues as the brain, muscles, heart, liver, and lung.

cystic fibrosis   An inherited disorder of the exocrine glands that affects multiple organ systems, causing such conditions as chronic pulmonary disease, pancreatic defi-

ciency, sweat gland dysfunction, malabsorption, and liver obstruction.

cystine   An amino acid produced by the metabolism of cysteine, found in many proteins in the body, including keratin and insulin. It also sometimes appears in the urine and in the kidneys as crystals.

cystinuria   Abnormal urinary excretion of the amino acid cystine.

cystitis   An inflammation of the urinary bladder marked by frequent, painful, and urgent urination and by hematuria.

cystometry   Evaluation of the neuromuscular integrity of the bladder by measuring muscle reflex, intravesical pressure and capacity, and reaction to thermal stimulation.

cystoscope   An endoscopic instrument used to examine and treat lesions of the urinary bladder, ureter, and kidney.

cystoscopy   Direct visualization of the urinary tract by inserting a cystoscope in the urethra.

cytochemism   The chemical activity of living cells, specifically their reactions to and affinity for chemical substances.

cytochemistry   The study of the locations, relationships, and interactions of various constituents within a living cell.

cytocide   A substance or other agent that destroys cells.

cytoclesis   A form of energy generated by living tissue; the vital principle of all living tissue. Also called *cytobiotaxis.*

cytogeneticist   One who specializes in cytogenetics.

cytogenetics   The branch of genetics devoted to study of the cellular constituents involved in heredity, primarily the origin, structure, and function of chromosomes.

cytoid body   A small, white spot that appears in degenerated retinal nerve fibers when viewed with an ophthalmoscope. Such bodies are associated with systemic lupus erythematosus.

cytokines   Nonantibody proteins, secreted by inflammatory leukocytes and some nonleukocytic cells, that act as biological response modifiers; for example, interferon, interleukins, tumor necrosis factor, and colony-stimulating factors.

cytological map   A gene map; a graphic representation of the location of genes on a chromosome, obtained by correlating genetic recombination testcrossing results with structural analysis of chromosomes that have undergone deletions, translocations, or other changes.

cytologist   One who specializes in the study of cells, especially one who uses cytological techniques to evaluate neoplasms.

cytology   The study of cells, including their origin, structure, function, and pathology. Types of cytology are aspiration biopsy cytology and exfoliative cytology.

cytomegalic inclusion disease (CID) Any of a group of diseases caused by cytomegalovirus infection, characterized by inclusion bodies in enlarged, infected cells. The classic disease is acquired in utero; however, the disease can be acquired by airborne droplets, by tissue or blood donation, or by sexual contact.

cytomegalovirus (CMV) disease   A viral infection caused by cytomegalovirus (a herpesvirus), marked by malaise, fever, lymphadenopathy, pneumonia, hepatosplenomegaly, and superinfection with various bacteria and fungi.

cytometer   A device used to count and measure the number of cells in a given amount of fluid (typically blood, urine, or cerebrospinal fluid).

cytometry   The counting and measuring of cells (specifically blood cells) and their constituents.

cytoplasm   The entire substance of a cell excluding the nucleus, consisting of the cytosol, an aqueous solution, and the organelles.

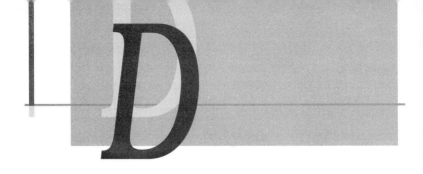

D   Chemical symbol for deuterium.

dacryoadenitis   Inflammation of the lacrimal gland.

dacryocyst   The lacrimal sac, situated at the inner corner of the eye.

dactyl   A digit (a finger or a toe).

daltonism   *Informal.* A genetically transmitted form of color blindness marked by the inability to perceive red.

Dalton's law of partial pressures   In physics: a law stating that the total pressure of a mixture of gases or vapors equals the sum of the partial pressures of its components if they were separated.

damages   The amount of money a court orders the defendant to pay the plaintiff when the case is decided in favor of the plaintiff.

dance reflex   A normal reflex in the neonate to make walking movements by reciprocal flexion and extension of the legs when held upright with the soles lightly touching a hard surface. The reflex is replaced by deliberate movement at about 3 to 4 weeks of age. Also called *stepping reflex.*

D & C   *abbr* dilatation and curettage.

darkfield microscope   A microscope with a central stop in the condenser, allowing scattering of light rays from the observed object and illumination from the side. This promotes easier examination by making the object appear bright against a dark background. The instrument is used primarily to identify the syphilis spirochete.

Darwinian theory   The theory of evolution proposed by Charles Darwin, postulating that evolution results from natural selection of those variants of species best suited to survive in their environment.

db   *abbr* decibel.

DD   *abbr* developmental disability.

DDS   *abbr* Doctor of Dental Surgery.

DDST   *abbr* Denver Developmental Screening Test.

DDT (dichlorodiphenyl-trichloroethane)   A colorless, water-insoluble, chlorinated hydrocarbon used extensively in agriculture during the 1940s and 1950s. The compound concentrates in fatty tissue and may reach dangerous levels in human beings; its use is now restricted.

dead space   A cavity that persists after incomplete closure of a traumatic or surgical wound; this permits accumulation of blood, which may delay healing.

death   **1.** The cessation of life; permanent stoppage of all vital bodily functions. **2.** In law: irreversible cessation of all activity in the brain and the central nervous, cardiovascular, and respiratory systems, as observed and declared by a physician.

debility   Loss or lack of strength; weakness or feebleness.

debride   To remove foreign material and contaminated or devitalized tissue from a wound or a burn so as to prevent infection and to promote healing.

 CLINICAL TIP Debridement of the patient's wound is the first step in wound cleaning.

decalcification   Loss of calcium salts from a bone or tooth, as from such dietary and physiologic conditions as malnutrition and malabsorption.

decay product   In radiology: a stable or radioactive nuclide resulting from the radioactive disintegration of a radionuclide — either directly or from successive transformations in a radioactive series. Also called *daughter product.*

deceleration   Reduction in speed or velocity.

decerebrate positioning   A posture associated with a lesion of the upper brain stem or severe bilateral lesions in the cerebrum; the patient lies with legs extended, head retracted, arms adducted and extended, wrists pronated, and the fingers, ankles, and toes flexed.

 ALERT In decerebrate posturing, remember that your first priority is to ensure a patent airway. Insert an artificial airway, elevate the head of the bed, and turn the patient's head to the side to prevent aspiration. (Don't disrupt spinal alignment if you suspect a spinal cord injury.)

Decerebrate positioning

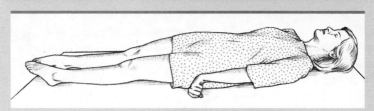

decibel (db) A unit equal to one-tenth of a bel, used to measure the intensity of sound. An increase of 1 bel approximately doubles the perceived loudness.

decidua The endometrium of the pregnant uterus; it envelops the conceptus during gestation and (except for the deepest layer) is shed during the postpartal period.

decidua basalis The decidua of the endometrium in the uterus that lies beneath the implanted ovum.

decidua capsularis The portion of the decidua that lies directly beneath the chorionic vesicle and is attached to the myometrium; it covers the implanted ovum.

decidual endometritis An inflammation or infection of the decidua during pregnancy.

decidua menstrualis The mucosa of the uterus that is shed during menstruation.

decidua vera The portion of the decidua that lines the uterus, except at the attachment site of the chorionic vesicle.

deciduous dentition Eruption of the first of two sets of teeth, usually beginning between ages 6 and 8 months and completed between ages 2 and 3 years.

deciduous teeth The 20 teeth (4 incisors, 2 canines, and 4 molars in each jaw) that erupt during infancy and are usually shed between ages 6 and 13. Deciduous teeth start to develop during gestation as a thickening of the epithelium along the line of the future jaw. Starting at around age 6 months, 1 or more deciduous teeth erupt about every month in the infant until all 20 have appeared.

decompensation **1.** Failure of compensation; inability of the heart to maintain adequate circulation, marked by dyspnea, venous engorgement, and edema. **2.** In psychiatry: failure of defense mechanisms, leading to progressive personality disintegration.

decompression sickness A potentially fatal condition that can affect deep-sea divers and caisson workers who rapidly return to normal pressure environments as well as persons who ascend to high altitudes. The syndrome results from formation of nitrogen bubbles in the tissues when a person moves rapidly from an environment of higher pressure to one of lower pressure. Nitrogen inhaled in air under pressure dissolves in tissue fluids; if ambient pressure decreases too rapidly, nitrogen comes out of solution faster than it can be circulated to the lungs for expiration. Gaseous nitrogen then builds up in the peripheral circulation and joint spaces, compromising tissue oxygenation and causing disorientation, syncope, and severe pain.

decorticate positioning A posture associated with a lesion of the frontal lobes, cerebral peduncles, or internal capsule; the patient lies with arms adducted and flexed, wrists and fingers flexed on the chest, legs stiffly extended and internally rotated, and feet plantar flexed.

TIME LINE Decorticate posturing is an unreliable sign before age 2 because of nervous system immaturity. In children, this posture usually results from head injury. It also occurs in Reye's syndrome. See the illustration on page 96.

decortication Surgical removal of the thick coating over an organ, as in the lung or kidney.

decubitus A horizontal or recumbent position; types of decubitus positions include dorsal decubitus (lying supine), lateral decubitus (lying on the side), and ventral decubitus (lying on the stomach).

decubitus ulcer An inflammation or a sore in the skin over a bony prominence, caused by prolonged pressure on that part with consequent ischemic tissue hypoxia. Also called *bedsore, pressure sore.* Decubitus ulcers most commonly develop on the skin over the shoulder blades, elbows, sacrum, hips, knees, ankles, and heels. They are graded by the anatomic depth of exposed tissue: *Stage 1*—reddened area of intact skin that does not blanch. *Stage 2*—partial-thickness skin loss involving the epidermis, dermis, or both; the ulcer is superficial and appears as a

Decorticate positioning

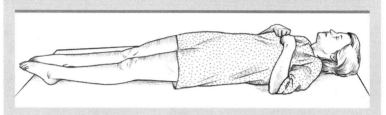

blister, an abrasion, or a shallow crater. *Stage 3*—full-thickness wound penetrating the subcutaneous tissue, which may extend to, but not through, the underlying fascia; the wound resembles a deep crater, and may or may not undermine adjacent tissue. *Stage 4*—ulcer extension through the skin, accompanied by extensive destruction, tissue necrosis, or damage to muscle, bone, or supporting structures.

 CLINICAL TIP Decubitus ulcer prevention is an important aspect of providing health care. Treatment varies with the severity and specific location of the ulcers.

DEd *abbr* Doctor of Education.

deep-breathing and coughing exercises Exercises taught to a patient to maintain respiratory function or improve aeration, particularly after general anesthesia or prolonged inactivity. Deep-breathing exercises require the use of the diaphragm and abdominal muscles in addition to the chest muscles. To perform these exercises, the patient exhales normally, closes the mouth, and inhales deeply through the nose. Then he purses the lips and exhales completely through the mouth, using the abdominal muscles to squeeze all the air out. To perform coughing exercises, the patient takes a slow, deep breath through the nose, exhales through the mouth, and then takes a second breath in the same manner; when inhaling for the third time, he holds his breath and then coughs two or three times to clear the breathing passages.

deep fascia The most extensive of the three kinds of fascia, or fibrous connective tissue, of the body. The deep fasciae form a series of connective sheets and bands that hold the muscles and other structures in place. Comprising a continuous system, they split and merge in a network that is attached to the skeleton.

deep sensation Perception or awareness of pain, pressure, or tension in the deep layers of the skin, muscles, tendons, or joints; sensations travel to the brain by way of the spinal column.

deep tendon reflex (DTR) Involuntary contraction of a muscle after sudden stretching resulting from sharp tapping on the tendon of insertion of the muscle. Types of DTRs include Achilles tendon reflex, biceps reflex, brachioradialis reflex, patellar reflex, triceps reflex. Also called *myotatic reflex, tendon reflex.*

TIME LINE Hyperreflexia may be a normal sign in neonates. After age 6, reflex responses are similar to those of adults. When testing DTRs in children, use distraction techniques to promote reliable results.

deep X-ray therapy Treatment with ionizing radiation from an external source, used for internal neoplastic growths, such as Wilms' tumor, Hodgkin's disease, and other cancers. The dose depends on the patient's condition; the radiosensitivity, size, pathologic grade, and differentiation of the tumor; and the tolerance of normal surrounding tissue for radiation.

defecation Evacuation of fecal material from the digestive tract through the rectum.

defendant The party that is named in a plaintiff's complaint and against whom the plaintiff's allegations are made. The defendant must respond to the allegations. See also *answer* and *litigant.*

deferential artery An artery that distributes blood to the ureter, ductus deferens, testes, and seminal vesicles.

defibrillation The termination of atrial or ventricular fibrillation, usually by electrical countershock to the patient's precordium, either directly or through electrodes placed on the chest wall. This common emergency measure is usually performed by a physician or a specially trained nurse or paramedic.

defibrillator An electronic device that delivers a brief electrical shock to the heart through the chest wall. It is used to restore a normal cardiac rhythm and rate when the heart is fibrillating or has stopped beating.

definitive host   An animal or a plant in which a parasite attains sexual maturity. Human beings are definitive hosts for tapeworms, pinworms, and schistosomes.

deflection   Direction of a waveform, based on the direction of a current.

dehydration   Removal of water from a substance or from body tissues. Dehydration is accompanied by electrolyte imbalances (especially sodium, potassium, and chloride imbalances). Conditions that may induce dehydration include diarrhea, vomiting, prolonged fever, and acidosis. Signs and symptoms of dehydration include poor skin turgor, dry flushed skin, coated tongue, oliguria, irritability, and confusion. The primary goal of therapy is to restore a normal fluid volume and electrolyte balance.

 TIME LINE Dehydration is of special concern in infants and young children, who normally have a precarious electrolyte balance.

delirium tremens (DTs)   An acute, reversible mental syndrome caused by a cessation or decrease in alcohol consumption, typically occurring in long-term alcoholics 2 or 3 days after alcohol withdrawal. The syndrome is marked by a coarse tremor accompanied by sweating, tachycardia, hypertension, delusions, hallucinations, and wild, agitated behavior. Signs and symptoms typically resolve in 3 or 4 days. Also called *alcohol withdrawal delirium.*

delta wave   The slowest of the four types of brain (electroencephalographic) waves, marked by a frequency below 3.5 per second. Delta waves may occur during deep sleep, in infants, and in patients with serious brain disorders.

dementia   An organic mental syndrome marked by general loss of intellectual abilities, with chronic personality disintegration, confusion, disorientation, and stupor. It does not include states of impaired intellectual functioning resulting from delirium or depression.

demulcent   **1.** Any of several mucilaginous or oily substances used to soothe and reduce irritation to abraded or inflamed surfaces. **2.** Soothing, bland.

demyelination   Destruction, loss, or removal of the myelin sheath of a nerve or a nerve fiber.

dendrite   The threadlike process that projects from the cell body of a neuron; it receives impulses and conducts them to the cell body.

dengue, dengue fever   An acute, self-limited arbovirus infection transmitted to man by the bite of infected mosquitos of the *Aedes* genus. The disease occurs in tropical and subtropical regions and usually causes fever, headache, prostration, rash, and severe pain in the head, back, and muscles.

dengue hemorrhagic fever shock syndrome (DHFS)   The most severe stage of hemorrhagic dengue fever (distinguished from classic dengue fever by such hemorrhagic manifestations as thrombocytopenia). Besides having all the signs and symptoms of dengue fever, the patient with DHFS experiences shock with circulatory failure; spontaneous bleeding into the skin, gums, GI tract, and other sites; a weak, thready, or undetectable pulse; and respiratory distress.

dense fibrous tissue   Connective tissue consisting of strong, compact, inelastic bundles of parallel collagenous fibers. Dense fibrous tissue provides structural support. *Organized* (regular) dense fibrous tissue includes the tendons, aponeuroses, and ligaments; *unorganized* (irregular) dense fibrous tissue includes the fascial membranes, dermis, periosteum, and the capsules of organs.

density   The mass of a substance per unit of volume. The greater the mass in a given volume, the greater the density.

density gradient   The continuous variation in the concentration of a solute along the width or height of a confined solution.

dental   Of or pertaining to a tooth or teeth.

dental alveolus   A cavity in the mandible or maxilla in which the roots of the teeth are held by the periodontal ligament.

dental amalgam   An alloy of silver, tin, copper, mercury, and sometimes zinc, used for filling teeth. A soft paste when freshly prepared, it hardens into a solid mass.

dental anesthesia   Any anesthetic drug or procedure used in dental surgery to reduce the ability to feel pain.

dental arch   The curving structure formed by the arrangement of a normal set of teeth. The teeth of the mandible form the inferior dental arch; the teeth of the maxilla form the superior dental arch.

dental assistant   A person who assists a dentist by performing such tasks as chair-side assistance, clerical work, and some radiography and dental laboratory work.

dental caries   A progressive, destructive condition in a tooth that results from the interaction of food with the bacteria that form dental plaque. This material adheres to the surfaces of the teeth, providing the medium for bacterial growth and production of organic acids, which in turn cause breaks in the tooth enamel. Enzymes produced by the bacteria then attack the protein component of the tooth. If left unchecked, this process eventually causes formation of deep cavities and bacterial infection of the pulp chamber and nerves.

 CLINICAL TIP In a debilitated patient, development of dental caries may be worrisome because of the danger that infection of the teeth or gums might spread to the rest of the body.

dental crypt A depression in the alveolar bone occupied by the developing tooth. Also called *tooth crypt.*

dental fistula An abnormal passage leading from the apical periodontal area of a tooth to the surface of the oral mucous membrane; allows discharge of suppurative or inflammatory material.

dental hygienist A person with special training to provide dental services under a dentist's supervision. Tasks typically include dental prophylaxis, radiography, medication application, and dental education.

dental technician A person who makes orthodontic appliances and dental prostheses, such as full dentures, partial dentures, bridgework, and crowns.

dentate fracture A fracture in which sawtooth, or serrated, bone ends fit together like gear teeth.

dentin, dentine The hard material of the tooth surrounding the pulp, consisting of solid organic substratum infiltrated with lime salts. Dentin is softer than enamel but harder and denser than bone.

dentin globule A small, spherical body in the peripheral dentin, created by early calcification of the matrix.

dentinogenesis Formation of the dentin of the teeth. Also called *dentification.*

dentinogenesis imperfecta Hereditary disorder of tooth development resulting in tooth discoloration. Brown, opalescent dentin with an abnormally low mineral content overgrows and obliterates the pulp canal. Typically, the teeth have short roots and wear down rapidly, leaving short, brown stumps.

dentist A person who is skilled and licensed by the state to practice dentistry.

dentistry The profession that deals with the prevention, diagnosis, and treatment of diseases, injuries, and malformations of the teeth, jaws, and oral cavity. Responsibilities include repairing and restoring teeth, replacing missing teeth, and detecting signs of diseases that require a physician's treatment. Besides the general practice of dentistry, eight specialties—endodontics, oral pathology, oral surgery, orthodontics, pedodontics, periodontics, prosthodontics, and public

health dentistry—are recognized. Each specialty requires additional training.

dentition The development and cutting (eruption) of the teeth.

dentoalveolar abscess Formation and accumulation of pus around the base of a tooth, resulting from infection arising secondary to an injury or an infection that causes pulp necrosis. Also called *apical abscess, periapical abscess.*

Denver Articulation Screening Examination (DASE) A language screening test that evaluates speech articulation (pronunciation) and intelligibility in children ages 2¼ to 6 years. The examiner asks a child to repeat certain words, then counts the number of correct pronunciations and evaluates speech intelligibility. Each child's performance may be compared to a standardized norm based on age.

Denver classification A system formerly used to identify and classify human chromosomes according to criteria established at the Denver (1960), London (1963), and Chicago (1966) conferences of cytogeneticists. The system is based on chromosome size and centromere position; chromosomes are arranged in seven groups, designated A to G, in order of decreasing length.

deoxyribonucleic acid, desoxyribonucleic acid (DNA) A nucleic acid found principally in the chromosomes of the cell nucleus that serves as the primary genetic material of most living organisms. By controlling protein synthesis in cells, DNA plays a crucial role in determining hereditary characteristics. The genetic material is coded in two nitrogen-containing bases: a purine and a pyrimidine. These bases form two coiled chains, termed the *double helix,* which are linked together by hydrogen bonds between specific bases. Adenine and guanine are the purines; thymine and cytosine are the pyrimidines.

depilation Removal or extraction of hair by the roots. Mechanical or chemical depilation is temporary; electrolysis, which destroys the hair follicle, is permanent. Also called *epilation.*

depolarization Neutralization of electrical polarity; reversal of the resting potential in excitable cell membranes when stimulated. An example is the reduction of the ion differential of sodium and potassium across the nerve cells at the neuromuscular junction.

deposition A sworn pretrial testimony given by a witness in response to oral or written questions and cross-examination. The deposition is transcribed and may be used for further pretrial investigation. It may also be presented at the trial if the witness can't be present or changes his testimony.

depth perception   The ability to correctly judge depth or the relative distance to different objects in space and to orient one's position in relation to them.

de Quervain's fracture   Fracture of the navicular bone (a tarsal bone of the foot), with dislocation of the lunate bone.

de Quervain's thyroiditis   Inflammatory condition of the thyroid, marked by swelling and tenderness of the thyroid, fever, dysphagia, fatigue, and severe pain in the neck, ears, and jaw. The disorder commonly follows a viral infection of the upper respiratory tract; it tends to remit spontaneously and to recur several times. Also called *subacute granulomatous thyroiditis.*

derived protein   A metabolic product of the protein molecule formed by hydrolysis; types of derived proteins include peptides, peptones, and proteoses.

dermatitis   An acute or chronic inflammatory condition of the skin marked by redness and pain or pruritus. Various skin eruptions occur, which may be unique to a particular allergen, disease, or infection. Types of dermatitis include allergic, atopic, contact, eczematous, exfoliative, occupational, and phototoxic seborrheic.

dermatocellulitis   Inflammation of the skin and underlying connective tissue.

dermatographia   An abnormal skin condition commonly associated with urticaria in which stroking or scratching the skin with a fingernail or a dull instrument causes a raised welt or wheal with a red flare on each side. The skin becomes especially susceptible to irritation.

dermatologist   A physician who specializes in skin diseases and disorders.

dermatology   1. The study of the skin. 2. The medical specialty concerned with diagnosing and treating skin diseases and disorders.

dermatome   1. In embryology: the portion of the segmented mesodermal layer in the developing embryo that originates from the somites and gives rise to the dermal skin layers. 2. In neurology: the area of the skin supplied with afferent (sensory) nerve fibers by a single posterior spinal root. 3. An instrument used to cut thin slices of skin for skin grafts.

dermatomycosis   A superficial fungal infection of the skin or skin appendages caused by a dermatophyte. It typically occurs on moist parts of the body that are protected by clothing, such as the groin or feet.

dermatomyositis   A connective tissue disease marked by pruritic or eczematous

Double helix of DNA

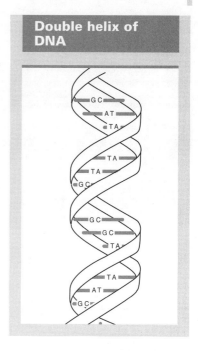

skin inflammation and tenderness and weakness of muscles. Destruction of muscle tissue may be so severe that the patient is unable to walk or perform simple tasks. Common manifestations include weight loss and swelling of the eyelids and face. The cause is unknown, but in about 15% of patients, the condition accompanies an internal malignancy.

dermatophyte   Any of several species of fungi that cause parasitic disease of the skin or skin appendages in humans.

descending aorta   The main portion of the aorta, consisting of the thoracic aorta and abdominal aorta. Continuing from the aortic arch into the trunk of the body, it branches to supply many parts of the body, such as the esophagus, lymph glands, ribs, and stomach.

descending colon   The segment of the colon extending from the end of the transverse colon at the splenic flexure on the left side of the abdomen and coursing downward to the beginning of the sigmoid colon in the pelvic cavity.

developmental anatomy   The study of the differentiation and growth of an organism from a germ cell of each parent to the resulting offspring. Also called *embryology.*

developmental anomaly   A congenital defect caused by imperfect embryonic development.

developmental disability (DD)   A disability with an onset before age 18; examples include cerebral palsy and autism. Most developmental disabilities persist throughout life, although many can be effectively treated.

deviated septum   A deviation in the partition separating the two nasal cavities; the condition is seen in many adults. During normal growth, the nasal septum commonly shifts to the left; a blow to the nose or other trauma may aggravate this deflection. A severe septal deflection may obstruct the nasal passages and lead to infection, sinusitis, headache, shortness of breath, or recurring nosebleeds. Severe septal deviation may be corrected surgically.

deviation from normal   A characteristic quality, symptom, or clinical finding that represents a departure from what is commonly regarded as normal. Examples include an elevated body temperature, an extra digit, and multiple gestation.

dextrocardia   Displacement of the heart to the right side of the thoracic cavity.

dextroposition of the aorta   Displacement of the aorta to the right.

dextrose   A glucose solution that contributes most of the calories in parenteral nutrition solutions and can help maintain nitrogen balance.

diabetes   1. A general term for disorders that are characterized by excessive excretion of urine, such as diabetes mellitus and diabetes insipidus. The excess may result from a deficiency of antidiuretic hormone, as in diabetes insipidus, or from the hyperglycemia that occurs in diabetes mellitus. 2. Diabetes mellitus.

diabetes insipidus   A metabolic disorder marked by extreme polyuria and polydipsia and resulting from deficient secretion or production of antidiuretic hormone (ADH) or inability of the renal tubules to respond to ADH. (Rarely, excessive water intake causes signs and symptoms.) The condition may be acquired (secondary to disease or drug therapy), inherited, idiopathic, or nephrogenic.

diabetes mellitus   A chronic disorder of carbohydrate metabolism characterized by hyperglycemia and glycosuria resulting from inadequate production or utilization of insulin.

diabetic amaurosis   Blindness associated with diabetes mellitus that results from a proliferative, hemorrhagic form of retinopathy marked by capillary microaneurysms and hard or waxy exudates.

diabetic coma   A life-threatening condition occurring in persons with diabetes mellitus, caused by inadequate diabetes treatment, poor compliance with therapy, or stress (as from infection, surgery, or trauma) that increases the body's insulin requirements.

> **ALERT** Warning signs and symptoms of diabetic coma include a dull headache, fatigue, excessive thirst and urination, epigastric pain, nausea, vomiting, parched lips, sunken eyes, and facial flushing.

diabetic ketoacidosis   An acute, life-threatening form of metabolic acidosis that may arise as a complication of uncontrolled diabetes mellitus. Accumulation of ketone bodies leads to urinary loss of water, potassium, ammonium, and sodium, resulting in hypovolemia, electrolyte imbalances, an extremely high blood glucose level and, commonly, coma. Signs and symptoms include flushed, hot, dry skin; confusion; nausea; diaphoresis; restlessness; and fruity breath odor.

diabetic retinopathy   A retinal vascular disorder associated with diabetes mellitus and marked by capillary microaneurysms, hemorrhages, yellow waxy exudates, and cotton-wool patches. The proliferative form of the disorder is characterized by the formation of new retinal vessels and fibrous tissue, vitreous hemorrhage, and retinal detachment.

diabetic xanthoma   An eruption of yellowish orange or yellow papules or plaques on the skin that is associated with uncontrolled diabetes mellitus. The lesions usually disappear when metabolic function is stabilized.

diagnosis-related group   The system of classifying or grouping patients according to medical diagnosis for the purpose of hospital cost reimbursement under Medicare.

diagnostic anesthesia   Induction of analgesia to a depth that allows patient comfort during moderately painful diagnostic procedures of short duration.

diagnostician   A person with expertise in determining the nature of a disease or disorder.

diagnostic radiopharmaceutical   A radioactive chemical or pharmaceutical agent, such as cobalt and radioactive iodine, used as a diagnostic tracer to distinguish normal from abnormal anatomic structures or biochemical or physiologic functions. Most of these agents emit gamma rays to indicate their position within the body.

dialysate   A solution that passes through the membrane in dialysis.

dialysis   1. The process of separating colloids and crystalline substances in solution through diffusion and ultrafiltration. **2.** A procedure that removes certain elements from the blood or lymph by selective diffusion through an external semipermeable membrane or, in the case of peritoneal dialysis, through the peritoneum.

diapedesis   The outward passage of blood corpuscles through the intact walls of blood vessels.

diaphanoscopy   Examination of an internal structure using a diaphanoscope, a device that transilluminates body tissues.

diaphoresis   Perspiration, especially the profuse perspiration associated with an elevated body temperature, physical exertion, heat exposure, and mental or emotional stress.

 ALERT Diaphoresis is an early sign of certain life-threatening disorders such as hypoglycemia, heatstroke, autonomic reflexia, and myocardial infarction or heart failure.

diaphragm   **1.** In anatomy: the musculofibrous partition that separates the abdominal and thoracic cavities. The concave surface of the diaphragm forms the roof of the abdominal cavity; the convex cranial surface forms the floor of the thoracic cavity. During inspiration, the diaphragm moves down and expands the volume of the thoracic cavity; during expiration, it moves up, reducing the volume. **2.** A contraceptive device made of soft plastic material that is placed over the cervix before intercourse to prevent the entrance of spermatozoa.

diaphysis   The shaft, or cylindrical portion, between the epiphyses (ends) of a long bone, consisting of a tube of compact bone enclosing the medullary cavity.

diastole   The phase of the heartbeat occurring between two contractions of the ventricles, during which the heart muscles relax and the ventricles fill with blood from the atria.

 CLINICAL TIP Diastole starts with onset of the second heart sound and ends with the first heart sound.

DIC   *abbr* disseminated intravascular coagulation.

dichotomy   Division or separation into two parts.

diencephalon   The portion of the brain located between the telencephalon and mesencephalon. Forming the central core of the forebrain, it connects the cerebrum with the brain stem. The diencephalon consists of the hypothalamus, thalamus, metathalamus, and epithalamus and includes most of the third ventricle.

dietary fiber   A substance in the diet that is not digested by gastrointestinal enzymes.

The main dietary fiber components are cellulose, lignin, hemicellulose, pectin, and gums.

differentiation   **1.** In embryology: a developmental process marked by changes from simple to more complex forms that is undergone by unspecialized cells or tissues so that they become specialized for a particular physical form, physiologic function, or chemical property. **2.** Progressive diversification leading to complexity. **3.** The distinguishing of one thing from another, as in differential diagnosis.

diffusion   **1.** The process by which molecules or other particles in solution move from an area of greater concentration to an area of lower concentration, resulting in even distribution of the particles in the fluid. **2.** The process of becoming widely scattered.

diffusion of gases   A process essential to respiration in which molecules of a gas move from an area of higher concentration to one of lower concentration.

digestion   The breakdown of ingested food into chemically simpler forms in the gastrointestinal tract. Digestion is achieved through the mechanical and chemical breakdown of food into smaller molecules, aided by glands located inside and outside the bowel.

digestive gland   A structure that secretes agents that help to break down food into the absorbable substances needed for metabolism. Types of digestive glands include the gastric glands, intestinal glands, salivary glands, liver, and pancreas. Important secretions produced by digestive glands include hydrochloric acid, bile, mucus, and various enzymes.

digestive system   The organs, structures, and accessory glands associated with the ingestion, digestion, and absorption of food. Food passes from the mouth to the esophagus, stomach, and intestines. The accessory glands secrete the digestive enzymes needed to break down foods into constituent substances so that they can be absorbed into the bloodstream.

digital   **1.** Of, pertaining to, or performed by a digit (a finger or toe). **2.** Resembling a finger or toe.

digitate wart   A wart with fingerlike projections arising from a pea-shaped base that may appear on the scalp or near the hairline. It is caused by a viral infection of the skin and the adjacent mucous membrane.

 CLINICAL TIP Digitate warts may spontaneously disappear or they may warrant treatment, such as electrodesiccation, cryotherapy, and curettage.

dihybrid   In genetics: an individual, organism, or strain that is heterozygous for two pairs of genes, is the offspring of parents differing in two specific gene pairs, or is heterozygous for two specific traits or gene loci under consideration.

dihybrid cross In genetics: the mating of two individuals, organisms, or strains with different gene pairs that determine two specific traits or in which two particular characteristics are being followed.

dilatation 1. A normal physiologic increase in the diameter of a body opening or tubular structure, such as a blood vessel or the pupil of the eye. 2. An artificial increase in the diameter of such an opening by instrumentation (as with use of a dilator to open the uterine cervix) or by medication (as with administration of cycloplegic eyedrops to open the pupil wide for retinal examination). 3. The diameter of the cervical opening in labor, expressed in centimeters or finger-breadths.

dilatation and curettage (D & C) Dilatation of the uterine cervix and scraping of the endometrium, performed to diagnose uterine disease, to treat heavy or prolonged vaginal bleeding, to remove the products of conception (such as retained placental fragments), to remove tumors, or to find the cause of infertility.

dilatator pupillae An involuntary muscle innervated by nerve fibers from the sympathetic system that contracts the iris of the eye and induces pupil dilation. Radiating fibers in this muscle converge from the circumference of the iris toward the center, blending with fibers of the sphincter pupillae near the margin of the pupil.

diluent A liquid used to reconstitute I.V. drugs that are supplied in powder form, including normal saline solution, sterile water for injection, and dextrose 5 % in water.

dimpling Puckering or depression of breast skin, possibly caused by an underlying growth. Also called *retraction.*

diphtheria An acute infectious disease caused by the bacterium *Corynebacterium diphtheriae,* usually confined to the upper respiratory tract. It is marked by the development of a false membrane attached to the underlying tissue of the throat, which bleeds if forcibly removed.

diplegia Bilateral paralysis; paralysis affecting like parts on opposite sides of the body or both sides of any part of the body.

diplococcus, *pl.* diplococci 1. A coccus that predominantly occurs in pairs. 2. An organism of the genus *Diplococcus.*

diploë The loose osseous tissue situated between the two tables of the cranial bones.

diploid Describing an individual, an organism, a strain, or a cell having two full sets

of homologous chromosomes, as normally found in the somatic cells and the primordial germ cells before maturation. The normal diploid number in humans is 46. Symbol: 2n.

diplopagus Conjoined twins of roughly equal development, although one or more internal organs may be shared.

diplopia Perception of two images of a single object, caused by defective function of the extraocular muscles or a disorder of the nerves innervating these muscles. Also called *amblyopia, binocular polyopia, double vision.*

TIME LINE Strabismus, which can be congenital or acquired at any age, produces diplopia; however, in young children, the brain rapidly compensates for double vision by suppressing one image, so diplopia is a rare complaint.

direct calorimetry Measurement of the amount of heat that is directly produced through an oxidation reaction.

direct lead 1. A conductor connected to an electrocardiograph in which the exploring electrode is placed directly on the surface of the exposed heart. 2. *Informal.* An electrocardiographic tracing produced by a direct lead.

direct reaction to light Brisk constriction of a pupil in response to a light shined directly onto its retina, resulting from stimulation of parasympathetic nerves.

disciform keratitis Corneal inflammation marked by formation of disklike opacities. The condition commonly follows an attack of dendritic keratitis and is thought to represent an immunologic response to an ocular herpes simplex infection.

discoid lupus erythematosus (DLE) A chronic form of cutaneous lupus erythematosus marked by scale-covered red macules that extend into follicles. Lesions typically have a butterfly distribution and cover the cheeks and bridge of the nose.

disengagement An obstetric manipulation in which the presenting part of the fetus is liberated from the maternal pelvis.

disinfection The act of killing pathogenic organisms or of rendering them inert.

displaced fracture A fracture in which two ends of the fractured bone are separated from each other. The ends may pierce surrounding skin, as in an open fracture, or may be contained within the skin, as in a closed fracture.

dissect To cut apart or separate tissues using a scalpel, probe, or scissors.

dissecting aneurysm A localized dilatation of an artery (most commonly the aorta) marked by longitudinal splitting of the arterial wall and a tear in the intima, which establishes communication with the lumen.

Mechanisms of DIC

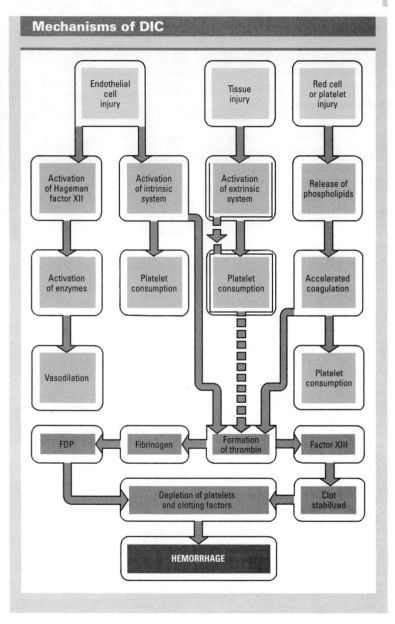

Rupture of a dissecting aneurysm may be fatal within 1 hour. Also called *aortic dissection.*

disseminated intravascular coagulation (DIC) A life-threatening disorder of excessive clot formation caused by overstimulation of the body's clotting and anticlotting processes in response to disease or injury. The overstimulation results in excess thrombin, followed by fibrinolysis with excess fibrin formation and fibrin degradation products (FDP); activation of fibrin-stabilizing factor (factor XIII); consumption of platelet and clotting factors; and eventual hypocoagulability and hemorrhage.

dissociative anesthesia   An anesthetic procedure marked by analgesia and amnesia without loss of respiratory function or pharyngeal and laryngeal reflexes. It is sometimes used during brief, superficial operative or diagnostic procedures, especially in patients who are sensitive to general or local anesthetics or who may not be safely anesthetized with inhalant gases for other reasons.

distal   1. Farthest away. 2. Away from the point of origin, the midline, or a central part of the body.

distal convoluted tubule   A convoluted portion of the renal tubule located distal to the loop of Henle.

distal phalanx   A small distal bone in the third row of phalanges of the hand or foot.

disuse phenomena   Physical and psychological changes caused by lack of use of a body part or body system. Usually degenerative, disuse phenomena are associated with confinement and immobility.

diuresis   Increased urine formation and excretion. Diuresis may result from ingestion of coffee, tea, certain foods, and diuretic drugs; it is pronounced in such conditions as diabetes mellitus and diabetes insipidus.

diuretic   1. Tending to increase the formation and excretion of urine. 2. An agent that promotes the formation and excretion of urine.

divalent cations   An electrolyte that carries two positively charged ions, such as Ca^{++}. In I.V. therapy: a solution containing divalent cations has a higher incidence of incompatibility.

diverticulitis   Inflammation of one or more diverticula, or saclike herniations, in the muscular layer of the colon. Colonic diverticula may undergo perforation with abscess formation; repeated inflammation may cause narrowing of the lumen of the colon, with subsequent obstruction.

diverticulosis   The presence of saclike herniations through the muscular layer of the colon without accompanying inflammation. Most patients with this condition have few signs or symptoms except for occasional rectal bleeding.

TIME LINE About 50% of older adults develop diverticulosis. In elderly patients, a rare complication of diverticulosis (without diverticulitis) is hemorrhage from colonic diverticula. Such hemorrhage is usually mild to moderate and easily controlled but may occasionally be massive and life-threatening.

diverticulum, *pl.* **diverticula**   A pouchlike herniation through a defect in the muscular wall of a tubular organ. The most common site of diverticula formation is the colon; other sites include the stomach and small intestine.

dizygotic   Describing twins from two fertilized ova, as dizygotic (fraternal) twins.

dizygotic twins   Two offspring developed from two separate ova released from the ovary simultaneously and fertilized at the same time. They may be of the same or opposite sex, differ both physically and in genetic composition, and have two separate and distinct placentas and membranes. Also called *dichorial, false, fraternal,* or *heterologous twins.*

dizziness   A sensation of unsteadiness, faintness, or inability to maintain normal balance, sometimes associated with giddiness, mental confusion, nausea, and weakness.

ALERT Dizziness is often confused with vertigo, which is the sensation of revolving in space or of one's surroundings revolving. However, unlike dizziness, vertigo is often accompanied by nausea, vomiting, nystagmus, staggering gait, and tinnitus or hearing loss.

CLINICAL TIP A patient who complains of dizziness should be carefully lowered to a safe position on a bed, a chair, or the floor to reduce the risk of injury from falling.

DLE   *abbr* discoid lupus erythematosus.

DM   *abbr* diabetes mellitus.

DMD   *abbr* Doctor of Dental Medicine.

DNA   *abbr* deoxyribonucleic acid.

DNA chimera   In molecular genetics: a recombinant molecule of deoxyribonucleic acid (DNA) consisting of segments derived from more than one source.

DNA ligase   An enzyme that synthesizes a bond between adjoining nucleotides and thus can repair breaks in a strand of deoxyribonucleic acid (DNA). Under some circumstances, the enzyme can join together loose ends of DNA strands or repair breaks in ribonucleic acid. DNA ligases are used in genetic engineering to insert foreign DNA into cloning vectors.

DNA polymerase   In molecular genetics: an enzyme that catalyzes the elongation of a new deoxyribonucleic acid (DNA) strand during DNA replication, with single-stranded DNA serving as the template.

DNR   *abbr* do not resuscitate.

DNSc *abbr* Doctor of Nursing Science.

DO *abbr* Doctor of Osteopathy.

DOA *abbr* dead on arrival.

Dobie's globule A minute stainable body in the middle of the transparent disk of a muscle fiber.

doll's eye reflex A normal response in newborns in which the eyes remain stationary as the head is rotated laterally.

 CLINICAL TIP Doll's eye reflex disappears as ocular fixation develops. However, it may occur in an adult with a severely reduced level of consciousness.

 TIME LINE Normally, the doll's eye reflex is not present for the first 10 days after birth, and it may be irregular until age 2. After that, this sign reliably indicates brain stem dysfunction.

dominance In genetics: a principle stating that not all genes governing a given trait possess the same vigor. Two genes that produce a different effect at a given locus compete for expression; the dominant gene is the one that manifests, masking the effect of the other gene, which is recessive.

dominant gene A gene that is phenotypically expressed whether or not its allele is the same or different.

Donovan bodies Facultatively anaerobic, encapsulated gram-negative rods of the species *Calymmatobacterium granulomatis,* typically present as intracellular organisms in the cytoplasm of large mononuclear phagocytes obtained from the lesions of granuloma inguinale. They may be visible under the microscope in a Wright-stained smear of infected tissue.

Doppler effect The apparent change in the observed frequency of a sound wave or light wave as a result of relative motion between the source and the observer. The frequency increases as the two move toward each other and decreases as they move apart (as the rising pitch of the whistle of an approaching train and the falling pitch of the whistle of a departing train).

dorsal Of or pertaining to the back or posterior.

dorsiflexion Flexion or bending toward the extensor aspect of a limb, as in the upward bending of the hand on the wrist or the foot on the ankle.

dorsiflexor A muscle that causes backward flexion of a body part.

dorsiflexor gait An abnormal style of walking marked by footdrop during the entire gait cycle, with excessive knee and hip flexion to permit clearance of the involved extremity during the swing phase. Inability of the dorsiflexor to decelerate the body weight as the heel strikes the ground causes the sole of the affected foot to slap against the ground during heelstrike. Dorsiflexor gait results from weakness of the dorsiflexors of the ankle.

dosage The regimen that determines the size, frequency, and number of doses of a therapeutic agent to be administered to a patient.

dose The quantity of a drug or other substance to be administered at one time.

dose rate In radiotherapy: the amount of radiation delivered per unit of time.

dose ratemeter In radiotherapy: an instrument that measures the dose rate of radiation.

dose threshold In radiotherapy: the minimum amount of absorbed radiation required to produce a detectable degree of some effect.

dose to skin In radiotherapy: the amount of absorbed radiation at the center of the skin's irradiation field. It equals the sum of the dose in the air and the scatter from body parts.

dosimeter A device used to detect and measure exposure to ionizing radiation. Commonly, a pencil-sized ionization chamber with a self-reading electrometer monitors exposure.

double innervation Innervation of a structure by two kinds of nerve fibers, such as the sympathetic and parasympathetic divisions of the autonomic nervous system. Operating at cross purposes, the fibers of the two divisions achieve a balance and maintain homeostasis. Doubly innervated structures include the pelvic viscera, bronchioles, heart, eyes, and digestive system.

Down syndrome A chromosomal disorder marked by varying degrees of mental retardation and multiple defects caused by the presence of an extra chromosome 21 in the G group or translocation of chromosome 14 or 15 in the D group and chromosomes 21 or 23. Down syndrome occurs in approximately 1 in 600 to 650 live births and is associated with advanced maternal age. Also called *trisomy 21.*

DPT vaccine *abbr* diphtheria and tetanus toxoids and pertussis vaccine.

DQ *abbr* developmental quotient.

drainage Removal of fluids or discharge from a body cavity, wound, or other source. Various methods are used to accomplish drainage. In *closed drainage*, tubing and other apparatus removes fluid from the body using an airtight circuit to guard against entry of environmental contaminants into the wound or cavity. In *open drainage,* a cavity is drained through an open-ended tube into a receptacle. In *postural drainage,* gravity aids fluid removal as the patient is positioned to permit the outflow of discharge, as through the trachea to drain fluid from the lungs. In *suction drainage,* a pump or other device is used to aid fluid extraction. In *tidal drainage,* a body area is alternately flooded and then emptied with the aid of gravity; this technique may be used to treat a urinary bladder disorder.

drainage tube A heavy-gauge catheter used to remove air or fluid from a body cavity or wound. The tube may simply allow flow by gravity into a receptacle, or it may be connected to a suction device.

dram A unit of weight equivalent to an apothecaries' measure of 60 grains or $1/8$ oz and to an avoirdupois system of measure of $1/16$ oz or 27.34 grains.

drape A sheet of fabric or paper used to cover all or a part of a patient's body during a physical examination or treatment.

dream state A state of altered consciousness lasting for several minutes in which the person does not recognize the environment and reacts in an uncharacteristic manner. The state is associated with epilepsy and certain neuroses.

dressing A clean or sterile material used to cover and protect a wound or diseased tissue. Kinds of dressings include absorbent, antiseptic, occlusive, pressure, and wet dressings.

CLINICAL TIP A dressing is applied to absorb secretions, protect against trauma, administer medications, or stop bleeding.

dressing forceps Forceps with scissor-like handles, used to grasp drainage tubes, remove lint, or extract fragments of necrotic tissue when dressing wounds.

Dressler's syndrome A disorder that may arise several days after an acute myocardial infarction and is marked by fever, pericarditis, pleurisy, pleural effusions, and joint pain. It occurs as an immunologic response to a damaged myocardium and pericardium. A similar syndrome may follow cardiac surgery. Also called *postmyocardial infarction syndrome.*

drug 1. Any chemical substance administered to aid the diagnosis, treatment, or prevention of a disease, disorder, or other abnormal condition, to relieve pain or to manage a pathologic condition. Also called *medicine.* 2. *Informal.* A narcotic substance.

drug abuse Use of a drug for a nontherapeutic purpose, especially one for which it was not prescribed or intended. Commonly abused substances include alcohol, amphetamines, and barbiturates. Drug abuse may lead to organ damage, addiction, and disturbed behavior.

drug action The interaction between a drug and cellular constituents; the means by which a drug exerts a desired effect. Drugs are usually classified by their actions; for example, antibacterial agents, which are prescribed to treat infection, act by killing bacteria or suppressing their growth or reproduction.

drug addiction A state marked by an overwhelming desire to continue to take a drug to which one has become habituated through repeated use to obtain a particular effect—usually an alteration of mental activity, attitude, or outlook. Common addictive drugs are barbiturates, ethanol, and morphine and other narcotics, especially heroin.

drug allergy Hypersensitivity induced by exposure to a particular drug, manifested by reactions ranging from a mild rash to anaphylactic shock, depending on the person, allergen, and dose. Agents that commonly cause allergic responses include aspirin, contrast media containing iodine, aspirin, phenylbutazone, cephalosporins, penicillin, and other antibiotics.

drug dependence A state marked by a compulsion to take a drug in order to experience its psychological effects or a state of physiologic reliance on a drug brought about by habituation, abuse, or addiction.

drug-drug interaction An alteration of the effect of a drug when given concomitantly with another drug. The effect may be an increase or decrease in the action of either substance, or it may be an adverse effect not normally associated with either drug. The particular interaction may result from a change in the drug absorption rate or the quantity of the drug absorbed in the body, chemical-physical incompatibility between the two drugs, a change in the binding ability of either drug, or a change in the ability of receptor sites and cell membranes to bind either drug.

Drug Enforcement Administration (DEA) A federal agency that enforces regulations pertaining to the import or export of narcotic drugs and certain other substances or the traffic of these substances across state lines.

drug eruption A skin rash or lesion resulting from ingestion, parenteral administration, or local application of a drug. Also called *drug rash.*

drug fever A fever induced by administration of a medication that results from an immunologic reaction mediated by drug-induced antibodies, the drug's pharmacologic or thermoregulatory action, or a local complication of parenteral administration. The fever usually appears 7 to 10 days after drug therapy begins and subsides within 2 days of drug discontinuance.

dry catarrh   A dry cough accompanied by little or no expectoration occurring in severe coughing spells. It is associated with asthma and emphysema in older people.

dry dressing   Dry gauze or absorbent cotton containing no medication, applied directly to an incision or a wound to absorb secretions or to prevent contamination or trauma.

dry rale   An abnormal chest sound with a whistling, squeaking, or musical quality produced by passage of air through a constricted bronchial tube, as in asthma and bronchitis.

dry tooth socket   An inflammatory condition of a tooth socket (alveolus) that sometimes follows tooth extraction and results from disintegration or loss of the blood clot that normally forms over the bone after extraction. Exposure of bone tissue to the environment can lead to infection. The condition is usually painful.

DSM   *abbr* Diagnostic and Statistical Manual of Mental Disorders.

DSN   *abbr* Doctor of Science in Nursing.

DSR   *abbr* dynamic spatial reconstructor.

DTR   *abbr* deep tendon reflex.

DTs   *abbr* delirium tremens.

DUB   1. A genetically determined human blood factor associated with immunity to certain diseases such as sickle cell anemia. 2. A strain of mice used in medical experiments. 3. *abbr* dysfunctional uterine bleeding.

Duchenne's disease   A term denoting three different neurologic conditions: spinal muscular atrophy, bulbar paralysis, and tabes dorsalis. The term is also strongly associated with pseudohypertrophic muscular dystrophy, the most common form of muscular dystrophy.

duct   A passage with well-defined walls, especially a tubular structure through which material is secreted or excreted.

duct carcinoma   A neoplasm arising from the epithelium of a duct, especially in the breast or pancreas.

ductless gland   A gland without an excretory duct, such as an endocrine gland, which secretes hormones into the blood or lymph.

ductule   A tiny duct.

ductus epididymis   The duct, or tube, into which the coiled ends of the efferent ductules of the testis empty.

dumping syndrome   A condition of nausea, weakness, profuse sweating, and dizziness occurring in patients who have had a subtotal gastrectomy. Signs and symptoms arise soon after eating, when the contents of the stomach empty too rapidly into the duodenum. Also called *postgastrectomy syndrome.*

 CLINICAL TIP Eating small, frequent, high-protein, high-calorie meals may help prevent discomfort and ensure adequate nutrition.

Dunlop's skin traction   An orthopedic device that helps immobilize the upper limb in the treatment of contracture and supracondylar fracture of the elbow. The device uses a system of traction weights, pulleys, and ropes and is usually applied unilaterally. It may be applied as adhesive or nonadhesive skin traction.

duodenal   Of or pertaining to the duodenum.

duodenal ulcer   A peptic ulcer in the duodenum.

duodenectomy   Partial or total excision of the duodenum.

duodenoscopy   Examination of the duodenum using a fiberoptic endoscope.

duodenum   The first or proximal portion of the small intestine, which takes an almost circular course from the pyloric valve of the stomach so that it terminates near its starting point. Measuring about 25 cm (10") long, it is divided into superior, descending, horizontal, and ascending portions. The duodenum plays a key role in digestion.

Dupuytren's contracture   A progressive, painless thickening, shortening, and fibrosis of the subcutaneous tissue of the palm, producing a flexion deformity of a finger. The fourth and fifth fingers are most commonly affected.

dura mater   The outermost, toughest, and most fibrous of the three membranes that surround the brain and spinal cord.

durable power of attorney   A legal instrument that authorizes another person to act as the agent or attorney, an "attorney-in-fact," if the principal person becomes incompetent. This power is revoked when the principal person dies.

Duverney's fracture   Fracture of the ilium just below the anterior superior spine.

dwarfism   1. Underdevelopment of the body. 2. The state of being a dwarf.

dyad   In genetics: one of the paired homologous chromosomes that result from the halving of a tetrad in the first meiotic division.

dyadic interpersonal communication Communication in which two people interact face-to-face as senders and receivers, as in a conversation.

dynamometer   A device used to measure the force of muscular contraction, as a

Dysphagia

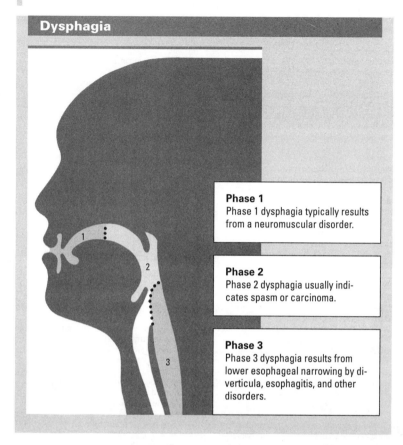

Phase 1
Phase 1 dysphagia typically results from a neuromuscular disorder.

Phase 2
Phase 2 dysphagia usually indicates spasm or carcinoma.

Phase 3
Phase 3 dysphagia results from lower esophageal narrowing by diverticula, esophagitis, and other disorders.

squeeze dynamometer, which measures the force of the hand when squeezing the device.
dysarthria Poor speech articulation resulting from a disturbance in muscular control of speech, usually produced by damage to a central or peripheral motor nerve.

ALERT If the patient displays dysarthria, ask him about associated difficulty swallowing. Next, determine respiratory rate and depth, measure vital capacity, and assess blood pressure and heart rate. Usually, shortness of breath, slightly increased blood pressure, and tachycardia are early signs of respiratory muscle weakness.
dyscrasia Synonymous with disease, usually refers to an imbalance of component elements.
dysentery An inflammation of the intestine, especially the colon, marked by frequent and bloody stools, abdominal pain, and

tenesmus. Causes include chemical irritants, bacteria, protozoa, and parasites.
dysfunctional uterine bleeding (DUB)
Uterine bleeding in the absence of a recognizable organic cause, usually owing to an endocrine imbalance rather than a pathologic condition.
dysgenesis, dysgenesia **1.** Defective or abnormal development of an organ or part, primarily during embryonic development. **2.** Loss or impairment of the ability to procreate.
dysgenics The study of conditions or situations that are genetically detrimental to a race or species.
dyshidrosis Abnormal sweating. Types of dyshidrosis are hyperhidrosis, miliaria, pompholyx.
dyskinesia Impairment or distortion of voluntary movement.

dyslexia   An inability to read, write, or spell words that results from a variety of pathological conditions. A person with the condition commonly reverses letters and words and cannot adequately distinguish the letter sequences in written words.

dysmelia   An abnormal congenital condition marked by missing or shortened extremities and caused by abnormal embryonic development.

dysmenorrhea   Painful menstruation. Primary dysmenorrhea results from factors intrinsic to the uterus and the menstruation process; it occurs at least occasionally in nearly all women.

dyspareunia   A condition in women in which sexual intercourse is difficult or painful. The cause may be an abnormal genital condition, a dysfunctional psychophysiologic reaction to sexual union, incomplete sexual arousal, or forcible coition.

dyspepsia   Gastric discomfort, such as fullness, heartburn, bloating, and nausea, that occurs after eating. Dyspepsia may signal an underlying intestinal disorder, such as peptic ulcer or gallbladder disease.

dysphagia   Difficulty swallowing, commonly resulting from obstructive or motor disorders of the esophagus. Obstructive disorders, such as an esophageal tumor or lower esophageal ring, interfere with the ability to swallow solids; motor disturbances such as achalasia impair swallowing of solids and liquids.

ALERT   If a patient suddenly complains of dysphasia and displays signs of respiratory distress, such as dyspnea and stridor, suspect an airway obstruction. Quickly perform abdominal thrusts; then administer oxygen by mask or nasal cannula; or assist with endotracheal intubation.

dysphasia   Impairment of speech involving lack of coordination and failure to arrange words in their proper order, usually resulting from injury to the speech area in the cerebral cortex. Dysphasia may follow a cerebrovascular accident or a brain tumor.

dysphonia   Difficulty speaking; any impairment of the voice.

dysphoria   Sadness; anguish; depression.

dyspnea   Shortness of breath, difficulty breathing, or labored breathing resulting from certain heart conditions, anxiety, or strenuous exercise.

TIME LINE   Normally, an infant's respirations are abdominal, gradually changing to costal by age 7. Suspect dyspnea in an infant breathing costally, in an older child breathing abdominally, or in any child using accessory muscles to breathe.

dyspraxia   Partial loss of the ability to perform coordinated movements, with no associated defect in motor or sensory functions.

dysreflexia   An abnormal motor response to stimuli.

dystocia   Abnormal or difficult labor caused by a disturbance in uterine expulsive powers, obstruction or contraction of the birth passage, or abnormal size, shape, or position of the fetus.

dysuria   Painful or difficult urination, usually caused by a bacterial infection or an obstruction in the urinary tract.

CLINICAL TIP   Dysuria may occur in such conditions as cystitis, urethritis, prostatitis, urinary tract tumors, and some gynecologic disorders.

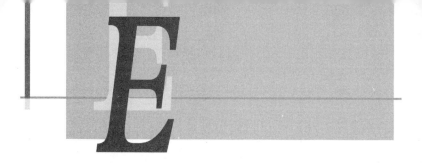

ear The sense organ for hearing, specialized for detecting sound and assisting with maintaining equilibrium. It consists of the internal, middle, and external ear.

earache Pain in the ear, as from a disease of the ear or an infection or other disorder of the nose, oral cavity, larynx, or temporomandibular joint. The pain may be perceived as dull, sharp, or burning and may be intermittent or constant.

Ebola virus disease An acute, fatal hemorrhagic fever caused by the Ebola virus, occurring in the Sudan and adjacent parts of northwestern Zaire. The virus passes from person to person by direct contact with infected blood, body secretions, or organs; nosocomial and community-acquired transmission can occur. Ebola disease typically begins with flulike symptoms; as the virus spreads through the body, capillaries rupture and a maculopapular eruption appears. The patient may also display melena, hematemesis, epistaxis, and bleeding gums. In the final disease stages, the skin blisters and sloughs off, blood seeps from all body orifices, and the patient begins vomiting his liquefied internal organs. Also called *Ebola hemorrhagic fever.*

EBV *abbr* Epstein-Barr virus.

ecchymosis, *pl.* **ecchymoses** Bluish or purplish discoloration of the skin or mucous membrane secondary to extravasation of blood into the subcutaneous tissues, resulting from fragility of the vessel walls or injury to the underlying blood vessels.

eccrine Describing a sweat gland that secretes onto the skin surface through a duct.

eccrine gland One of two types of sweat glands in the dermal layer of the skin. Eccrine glands promote cooling through evaporation of their secretion — a clear substance with a faint odor that contains water, sodium chloride, and traces of albumin, urea, and other compounds.

ECF *abbr* extracellular fluid.

ECG *abbr* 1. electrocardiogram. 2. Electrocardiograph or echocardiogram.

echo *Informal.* Echoradiography or echocardiogram.

echocardiography A diagnostic technique that studies the structure and motion of the heart by the echocardiogram obtained from beams of ultrasonic waves directed through the chest wall. The waves are then recorded on a strip chart.

echoencephalogram A recording produced by an echoencephalograph.

echoencephalography A diagnostic technique used to study structures within the brain, especially to evaluate for ventricular dilatation and a major shift of midline structures owing to an expanding lesion.

echoradiography An ultrasonographic diagnostic procedure used to visualize internal structures of the body.

eclampsia The most serious form of toxemia of pregnancy, marked by such signs and symptoms as hypertension, proteinuria, edema, generalized tonic-clonic seizures, and coma.

ECT *abbr* electroconvulsive therapy.

ecthyma A form of impetigo characterized by large pustules, crusts, and ulcerations surrounded by erythema and usually caused by group A beta-hemolytic streptococcal infection at the site of minor trauma. The most common site of ecthyma is the skin of the legs.

ectoderm The outermost of the three primary germ layers of the embryo.

ectodermal dysplasia A hereditary condition marked by abnormal development of the sweat glands, with poorly functioning sweat glands, sparse hair follicles, missing or abnormal fingernails or toenails, and skin rash.

ectopic 1. Of an organ or object: located in an unusual place, away from the normal position, as in ectopic pregnancy. 2. Of an event: occurring at the wrong time, as a premature heartbeat.

ectopic pregnancy Implantation of the fertilized ovum outside the uterine cavity. Types of ectopic pregnancy are abdominal pregnancy, interstitial pregnancy, tubal pregnancy.

ectrodactyly, ectrodactylia Congenital absence of part or all of one or more of the fingers or toes.

ectrogeny Congenital defect or absence of an organ or part of the body.

ectropion Eversion (turning outward) of an edge or margin, most commonly of the eyelid (which exposes the conjunctival membrane lining the eyelid and part of the eyeball). Causes include paralysis of the facial nerve and, in older persons, loss of elasticity of eyelid tissues.

ectropion uveae Eversion or outward turning of the margin of the pupil. The condition is commonly congenital, although it is sometimes associated with diabetes.

eczema Superficial dermatitis arising as a reaction to any of a wide range of endogenous and exogenous agents. In the early stage, eczema may be pruritic, erythematous, papulovesicular, edematous, and exudative. Later, it becomes crusted, scaly, and thickened.

ED *abbr* effective dose.

ED$_{50}$ Symbol for median effective dose.

edaphon The organisms living in the soil.

EDC *abbr* expected date of confinement.

edema Accumulation of abnormally large amounts of fluid in the intercellular tissues, pericardial sac, pleural cavity, peritoneal cavity, or joint capsules. Causes of edema include increased capillary fluid pressure, venous obstruction (as in varicosities, thrombophlebitis, or pressure from casts or tight bandages), heart failure, renal disease, hepatic cirrhosis, hyperaldosteronism (as in Cushing's syndrome), excessive administration of parenteral fluids, corticosteroid therapy, and inflammatory reactions. Edema may also result from loss of serum protein in burns, draining wounds, fistulas, hemorrhage, nephrotic syndrome, or chronic diarrhea; allergic reactions; malnutrition; and lymphatic obstruction (as from cancer, filariasis, or other disorders).

TIME LINE Elderly patients are more likely to develop edema due to decreased cardiac and renal functioning or poor nutritional status. Use caution when giving I.V. fluids or medications that can raise sodium levels and possibly increase fluid retention.

Edsall's disease Cramps resulting from excessive exposure to heat. Also called *heat cramp.*

EDTA *abbr* edetate calcium disodium.

Edward's syndrome A congenital autosomal disorder marked by severe mental retardation, deafness, low-set ears, corneal opacities, skull abnormalities, jaw underdevelopment, small size and weight for gestational age, flexion deformities of fingers, and cardiovascular abnormalities. Affected infants seldom live longer than a few months. Also called *trisomy 18 s.*

EEE *abbr* eastern equine encephalitis.

EEG *abbr* **1.** electroencephalogram. **2.** electroencephalography.

effacement Shortening of the vaginal portion of the cervix and thinning of its walls during labor due to stretching and dilation caused by the fetus. Full effacement obliterates the constrictive neck of the uterus. The extent of effacement is expressed as a percentage of full effacement.

effect **1.** To cause. **2.** Result.

effective dose (ED) The dosage of a drug that may be expected to cause a specific degree of effect in the patient who receives it.

effective half-life In radiotherapy: the time required for a radioactive nuclide to diminish by 50% through the combined action of radioactive decay and biological elimination. The effective half-life equals the product of the biological half-life and the radioactive half-life divided by the product of the biological half-life and the radioactive half-life.

efferent Moving away from the center toward the periphery, as certain arteries, veins, nerves, and lymphatics.

efferent duct A passage through which a gland releases its secretions.

efferent neuron Any neuron conducting a nerve impulse that originated at the center and is heading toward the periphery.

efficacy **1.** The ability of a drug or treatment to produce the desired therapeutic effect regardless of dosage or potency. **2.** The ability of an intervention to produce the desired beneficial effect under ideal circumstances.

effleurage A massage technique using long strokes. In fingertip effleurage, the fingertips are used to stroke lightly in a pattern over one part of the body or to make long strokes over the back or an extremity.

effort syndrome An abnormal condition in which exercise or even slight effort produces palpitations, dyspnea, chest pain, dizziness, and fatigue. Diagnosis may require exercise electrocardiography. Also called *neurocirculatory asthenia.*

 CLINICAL TIP Signs and symptoms of effort syndrome — cold, moist hands; sighing respirations; and chest pain after exercise — commonly mimic angina pectoris but are more closely connected to anxiety states.

effraction A weakening or a breaking open.

effusion **1.** The escape of fluid from blood vessels (usually into a body cavity) caused by rupture or seepage. The condition is a common early sign of heart disease. **2.** An effused material, such as an exudate or transudate.

EFM *abbr* electronic fetal monitor.

egest To discharge undigested matter or waste material from a cell or organism, especially the evacuation of unabsorbed food residue from the intestines in defecation.

EHD *abbr* electrohemodynamics.

Ehlers-Danlos syndrome A hereditary disorder of the connective tissue marked by skin and joint hyperextensibility, easy bruising, friable tissues with bleeding and poor wound healing, pseudotumors, and tissue fragility. The syndrome occurs in at least 10 types.

eidetic Pertaining to or characterized by accurate recall, especially of visual images.

eidetic image An exceptionally vivid, elaborate, and apparently exact mental image resulting from a visual experience and arising as a memory, dream, or fantasy.

ejaculate **1.** To expel suddenly, especially semen. **2.** The semen discharged in a single emission.

ejaculation The sudden act of expulsion, as emission of semen from the male urethra during copulation, masturbation, or nocturnal emission. Usually, the fluid volume of the ejaculate ranges from 2 to 5 ml, with each milliliter containing 50 million to 150 million spermatozoa.

ejaculatory duct The passage formed by the union of the ductus deferens with the excretory duct of the seminal vesicle through which semen enters the urethra.

ejection click A high-pitched, clicking sound that follows the first heart sound in patients with high pulmonary resistance and hypertension, abnormalities of the semilunar heart valves, or dilatation of the aortic or pulmonary arteries. The sound may be described as aortic or pulmonic and as vascular or valvular.

 CLINICAL TIP In pregnant women, and many other healthy people, ejection clicks are common and without clinical significance.

ejection fraction Measure of ventricular contractility.

EKG *abbr* electrocardiogram.

elastance **1.** The quality of recoiling or returning to original form after removal of pressure. **2.** The degree to which an air-filled or fluid-filled organ, such as a lung or bladder, returns to its original dimensions after removal of a distending or compressing force. **3.** The measurement of the unit volume of change in such an organ per unit of decreased pressure change.

elastic band fixation Use of intermaxillary rubber bands attached to splints or appliances to stabilize fractured segments of the jaw. The rubber bands produce traction, bring the teeth into occlusion, and allow proper alignment while the fracture heals.

elasticity The condition or quality of regaining the original shape and size after being stretched, compressed, or otherwise distorted.

elbow The joint that connects the arm and forearm; it is covered by a protective capsule associated with three ligaments and an extensive synovial membrane. The elbow joint accommodates the radioulnar articulation and permits flexion and extension of the forearm.

electrically stimulated osteogenesis A process of bone regeneration induced electrically by surgically implanted electrodes, made possible by the different electric potentials within bone tissue. Nonstressed bone is electronegative over a fracture callus and in the metaphyseal regions, and electropositive in less active regions such as the diaphyses.

electroanalytical chemistry The branch of chemistry that deals with analysis of compounds using electric current to produce characteristic, observable changes in substances.

electrocardiogram (ECG, EKG) A graphic record produced by an electrocardiograph, showing variations in electrical potential, as detected at the body surface, resulting from excitation of the heart muscle. The P waveform of the ECG is produced by atrial excitation; the Q, R, S waveforms, by ventricular excitation. The T waveform indicates ventricular repolarization; it is sometimes followed by a U waveform.

electrocardiograph (EKG) A device used to record the electrical activity of the heart muscle to detect abnormal transmission of impulses through conductive tissues and thus diagnose specific cardiac abnormalities. Leads are affixed to certain points on the chest, arms, and legs, usually with an adhesive jelly that aids transmission of electrical impulses to the recording device.

electrocautery Application of a needle or snare heated by an electric current to destroy tissue, as for the removal of warts.

electrocoagulation A therapeutic form of electrosurgery that hardens tissue by the passage of high-frequency electric current.

electroconvulsive therapy (ECT) The induction of a brief seizure and loss of consciousness by application of a low-voltage alternating current to the brain via scalp electrodes. ECT is used in the treatment of affective disorders (primarily acute depression),

Normal ECG complex

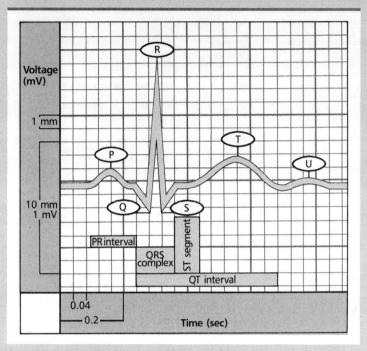

Voltage (mV)

1 mm

10 mm
1 mV

R

P

T

U

Q

S

PR interval

QRS complex

ST segment

QT interval

0.04
0.2

Time (sec)

---

especially in patients resistant to psychoactive drugs. On awakening, the patient has no memory of the shock.

electrodermal audiometry   A technique used to test hearing in which the subject is conditioned by harmless electric shock to pure tones; thereafter, he anticipates a shock when hearing a pure tone and reacts with a brief electrodermal response. The response is recorded, and the lowest intensity at which the response is elicited is considered the subject's hearing threshold.

electrodesiccation   A form of electrosurgery in which a high-frequency electric current destroys living tissue by burning. It is used primarily to remove small superficial growths but may be used along with curettage to eradicate abnormal tissue deeper in the skin.

electroencephalogram (EEG)   A graphic recording of the electrical potentials generated by currents emanating from the brain, as detected by electrodes placed on the scalp. The frequencies that are produced range from 2 to 12 cycles per second with an amplitude of up to 100 microvolts. Fluctuations in potentials result in different waveforms (called alpha, beta, delta, and theta waves). Variations in electroencephalographic brain-wave activity correlate with different neurologic conditions, psychological states, and levels of consciousness.

electroencephalograph   An instrument that performs electroencephalography.

electroencephalography (EEG)   The process of recording brain-wave activity, usually by means of electrodes applied to the scalp, to help diagnose seizure disorders, brain stem disorders, focal lesions, and impaired consciousness.

electrolyte   A substance that dissociates into ions when melted or dissolved in water or another solvent, thus becoming capable of conducting an electric current. Electrolytes differ in their concentrations in the blood plasma, interstitial fluid, and intracellular fluid, and affect the movement of substances between those compartments.

114 electrolyte balance

 CLINICAL TIP Adequate amounts of, and balance among, the principal electrolytes are essential for normal metabolism and function.

electrolyte balance A state of equilibrium among the electrolytes in the body.

electrolyte solution A solution containing electrolytes that is prepared for oral, parenteral, or rectal administration and used to restore or supplement specific ions necessary for homeostasis.

electromagnetic radiation Energy produced by the acceleration of electric charge and the associated electric and magnetic fields. The energy can be regarded as a continuous spectrum that includes energy with the shortest wavelength (gamma rays, which have a wavelength of 0.0011 angstrom) to that with the longest wavelength (long radio waves, which have a wavelength of more than 1 million km).

electromagnetic therapy A type of energy-based therapy that attempts to diagnose and treat illnesses believed to be the result of disturbances in the body's electromagnetic fields. Many different electric and magnetic devices are used to treat electromagnetic imbalances.

electromyogram (EMG) A record of the electrical activity of skeletal muscles, obtained by surface electrodes or needle electrodes and devices that amplify, transmit, and record the signals. The technique is helpful in diagnosing neuromuscular disorders, pinpointing motor nerve lesions, and measuring electrical potentials induced by voluntary muscle contraction.

electron A negatively charged elementary particle with a specific charge, mass, and spin. Electrons are present in all atoms in groupings called shells around the nucleus. The number of electrons circling the nucleus is equal to the atomic number of the substance.

electroneuromyography An electromyographic technique in which the nerve of a skeletal muscle being studied is stimulated by application of an electric current through needle electrodes. The procedure is used to study neuromuscular conduction, the extent of nerve lesions, and reflex responses.

electronic fetal monitor (EFM) A device that permits observation of the fetal heart rate and maternal uterine contractions. Applied externally, it detects the fetal heart rate through an ultrasound transducer on the abdomen and detects uterine contractions through a pressure sensor on the abdomen. Internal application is accomplished by an electrode clipped to the fetal scalp and an intrauterine catheter that detects the amplitude, frequency, and duration of uterine contractions.

electron microscope A microscope that uses a beam of electrons instead of a beam of light (as in an optical microscope) to form large images of very small objects; the images can then be photographed or viewed on a fluorescent screen. An electron microscope is used to study very thin sections of tissue.

electron microscopy Examination by means of an electron microscope to view and study an extremely thin tissue specimen.

electronystagmography The recording of the electrical activity of the extraocular muscles, as to obtain objective documentation of induced and spontaneous nystagmus.

electrophoresis A technique for analyzing and separating ionic solutes in response to changes in an applied electrical field, used widely to separate and identify serum proteins and other biological substances. Charged particles of a given substance migrate in a predictable direction and at a characteristic speed; the migration pattern can be recorded in bands on an electrophoretogram.

element In chemistry: one of more than 100 primary, simple substances that cannot be decomposed by chemical means into any other substance. Each atom of any element contains a specific number of electrons orbiting the nucleus.

elicit To draw forth or bring out.

Elliot's position A supine posture of a patient on the operating table that elevates the chest by placing a support under the lower costal margin. It is used in gallbladder surgery.

elliptocytosis A mild abnormal hematologic condition marked by increased numbers of elliptical or oval red blood cells (RBCs) with pale centers. Modest increases in the percentage of elliptical RBCs occur in a variety of anemias, including hereditary elliptocytosis, a rare congenital disorder.

emaciation A wasted condition or excessive leanness brought about by disease or lack of nutrition.

Embden-Meyerhof pathway A series of enzymatic reactions in the anaerobic conversion of glucose to lactic acid that yields energy in the form of adenosine triphosphate.

embolectomy Surgical removal of an embolus or a clot from a blood vessel.

embolism Obstruction of a blood vessel by an embolus. Types of embolisms include air embolism, fat embolism, blood clot, bone marrow embolism, and tumor cell embolism.

 CLINICAL TIP Signs and symptoms of embolism depend on the degree of occlusion, the nature of the embolus, and the size, nature, and location of the occluded vessel.

embolus, *pl.* **emboli**   A clot, foreign object, or mass of air or gas that migrates to another smaller vessel and, lodged there, causes an obstruction. Kinds of emboli include blood clots, bone marrow emboli, and tumor cell emboli.

embryo   1. An organism in the earliest stages of development. 2. In humans, the stage of prenatal development that extends from about 2 weeks after conception until the end of the 7th or 8th week. It is marked by rapid growth, differentiation of major organ systems, and development of primary external features.

embryology   The study of the origin, growth, development, and function of an organism from fertilized egg to birth.

embryomorph   A structure that suggests or resembles an embryo, particularly a mass of tissue that may represent an aborted conceptus.

embryonate   1. Of, pertaining to, or resembling an embryo. 2. Impregnated. 3. Containing an embryo.

embryonic disk   The thickened plate from which the embryo develops during the 2nd week of pregnancy. Scattered cells from the border of the disk migrate to the space between the trophoblast and yolk sac to become the embryonic mesoderm. The disk develops from the ectoderm and endoderm.

embryonic layer   One of the three layers of cells in the embryo from which all structures, organs, and parts of the body arise. In human zygotes, it is visible early in the second week.

emergence   A stage in the process of coming out of general anesthesia; includes spontaneous respiration, voluntary swallowing, and consciousness.

Emergency Medical Service (EMS)
A network of coordinated services that offers aid and medical assistance in an emergency. It is linked by a communications system that operates on both a local and regional level and involves personnel trained in the rescue, stabilization, transportation, and advanced treatment of trauma or medical emergency patients.

Emergency Medical Technician (EMT)
A person who is trained in and responsible for administering specialized emergency care and transporting victims of acute illness or injury to a medical facility. The EMT is trained in basic life support skills, extrication and disentanglement, emergency vehicle operation, basic anatomy, basic assessment of injury or illness, triage, care for specific injuries and illnesses, environmental emergen-

cies, childbirth, and transport of the patient. EMTs must qualify for recertification every 2 years.

Emergency Medical Technician-Advanced Life Support (EMT-ALS)   A third-level emergency medical technician who is certified in all skills of the basic-level EMT and EMT-I.V. An EMT-ALS is also trained in advanced life support systems, including electrical defibrillation equipment and may administer certain medications on the orders of a hospital physician, with whom radio contact is maintained.

Emergency Medical Technician-Intravenous (EMT-I.V.)   A second-level emergency medical technician who is certified in intravenous therapy, endotracheal intubation, and the use of medical antishock trousers, in addition to all skills of the basic-level EMT.

Emergency Medical Technician-Paramedic (EMT-P)   An advanced-level emergency medical technician who is certified in all skills of EMTs of all other levels and has additional training in pharmacology and administration of emergency drugs.

emergency medicine   A specialty of medicine that deals with the diagnosis and treatment of conditions resulting from trauma or sudden illness. After the patient's condition is stabilized, care of the patient is transferred to the primary physician or a specialist.

emergency nursing   Nursing care that is performed to prevent imminent severe damage or death or to prevent serious injury. Activities typically include basic life support, cardiopulmonary resuscitation, burn care, and control of hemorrhage.

emergency room (ER)   An area of a hospital specially designed to receive and initially treat patients suffering from sudden trauma or illness, such as hemorrhage, poisoning, fracture, myocardial infarction, and respiratory failure. Also called *emergency department.*

emergent evolution   The assumption that evolution takes place in a series of major changes at certain crucial stages and results from the total rearrangement of existing elements to produce something new that could not have been predicted.

emetic   1. Describing a substance that induces vomiting. 2. An agent that causes vomiting, such as syrup of ipecac, which is used in the emergency treatment of drug overdose and in certain cases of poisoning.

emetogenic potential   Likelihood that a drug or combination of drugs may cause nausea or vomiting. For example, cisplatin has a high emetogenic potential; more than 90% of patients on it will experience nausea

Effect of emphysema

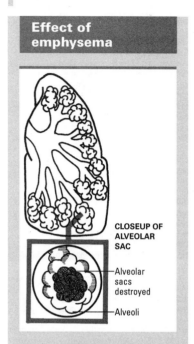

CLOSEUP OF
ALVEOLAR
SAC

Alveolar sacs destroyed

Alveoli

and vomiting. Bleomycin has a low potential; only 10% to 30% of patients are affected. Other factors contributing to emetogenic potential include the combination of drugs, doses and routes of administration, rates of administration, treatment schedules, and patient characteristics.

EMG *abbr* electromyogram.

emmetropia A state of normal vision characterized by the proper correlation between the refractive system of the eyeball and the eyeball's axial length. This correlation ensures that light rays entering the eye parallel to the optic axis are brought to a focus exactly on the retina.

empathy The capacity to be aware of and understand the emotions and mental state of another person.

emphysema A chronic, irreversible lung disorder marked by enlargement of air spaces distal to terminal bronchioles due to destruction of the alveolar walls; it results in decreased elastic recoil of the lungs. Types of emphysema are centriacinar, panacinar, and paraseptal. Emphysema of early onset is usually related to a rare genetic deficiency of serum alpha$_1$-antitrypsin. Acute emphysema may result from rupture of alveoli by severe

respiratory efforts, as in acute bronchopneumonia, suffocation, and occasionally during labor. Chronic emphysema usually accompanies chronic bronchitis, a major cause of which is cigarette smoking. In old age, the alveolar membranes atrophy and may collapse, producing large air-filled spaces with decreased total surface area of the pulmonary membranes.

CLINICAL TIP Signs and symptoms of emphysema include dyspnea, cough, cyanosis, orthopnea, unequal chest expansion, tachypnea, tachycardia, and an elevated temperature. Advanced emphysema may be accompanied by carbon dioxide narcosis with a decreased pH, increased partial pressure of carbon dioxide, restlessness, confusion, weakness, anorexia, heart failure, pulmonary edema, and respiratory failure.

empiric Describing a method of treating disease based on observations and experience. Empiric treatment of a new disease may be based on observations and experience gained in management of similar analogous disorders.

empiricism A form of treating disease that emphasizes observation, personal experience, and the experience of other practitioners.

emprosthotonos A body position characterized by forward, rigid flexure at the waist resulting from a prolonged, involuntary muscle spasm. It is most commonly associated with tetanus infection or strychnine poisoning. Also called *episthotonos.*

empyema Accumulation of pus in a body cavity.

EMS *abbr* Emergency Medical Service.

EMT *abbr* Emergency Medical Technician.

EMT-ALS *abbr* Emergency Medical Technician-Advanced Life Support.

EMT-I.V. *abbr* Emergency Medical Technician-Intravenous.

EMT-P *abbr* Emergency Medical Technician-Paramedic.

emulsify To disperse a liquid into another liquid, resulting in a colloidal suspension.

emulsion A preparation in which small particles of one liquid are dispersed throughout a second liquid.

enamel 1. A hard, smooth glossy coating. 2. The material that covers the dentin of the crown of a tooth.

enamel hypocalcification A hereditary defect in which the tooth enamel is soft and undercalcified but of normal quantity, resulting from defective ameloblastic maturation. The teeth have a chalky consistency, with surfaces that wear down rapidly; a yellow-to-brown stain appears where the underlying dentin of the teeth is exposed.

enamel hypoplasia A developmental defect in which the tooth enamel is incompletely formed, causing lack of contact between the teeth, rapid breakdown of occlusive surfaces, and a yellow-to-brown stain that appears where the dentin is exposed. The condition may be genetically transmitted or may result from environmental factors, vitamin deficiency, fluorosis, exanthematous diseases, congenital syphilis, or trauma to the mouth. Another cause of enamel hypoplasia is tetracycline use in the second half of pregnancy or during tooth development in the child.

enanthema An eruptive lesion on the surface of a mucous membrane.

encapsulated Of body parts: enclosed within a fibrous or membranous sheath.

encephalitis, *pl.* encephalitides An inflammatory condition of the brain, usually caused by an arbovirus infection transmitted by the bite of an infected mosquito. Other causes include hemorrhage and lead or other poisoning.

encephalocele Protrusion of part of the brain and meninges through a congenital or traumatic defect in the skull.

encephalogram A radiograph of the brain produced during encephalography.

encephalography Radiography showing the intracranial fluid-containing spaces of the brain after cerebrospinal fluid (CSF) is withdrawn and air or another gas is introduced. The technique is used mainly to locate the site of a CSF obstruction in hydrocephalus or to detect structural abnormalities of the posterior fossa. Types of encephalography are pneumoencephalography and ventriculography.

encephalomyelitis An inflammatory condition of the brain and spinal cord characterized by fever, headache, stiff neck, back pain, and vomiting; it sometimes leads to coma or even death. Severe inflammation that causes extensive damage to the nervous system may lead to such sequelae as seizure disorders or decreased mental ability.

encephalopathy An abnormal condition of the brain, especially one that is degenerative, chronic, or destructive.

enchondroma, *pl.* enchondromas, enchondromata A benign tumor of cartilage cells arising in the metaphysis of a bone, usually in the hands or feet.

encyst **1.** To enclose in a cyst or capsule. **2.** To form or become enclosed in a cyst or capsule.

endarterectomy Surgical excision of the tunica intima of an artery that has become thickened by atherosclerosis.

endarteritis An inflammatory disorder of the tunica intima of one or more arteries, possibly bringing about partial or complete arterial occlusion.

endemic Native or belonging to a particular population or geographic area.

endemic goiter Enlargement of the thyroid gland due to inadequate dietary intake of iodine, occurring occasionally in adolescents at puberty and widely in population groups in geographic areas with limited amounts of iodine in the soil, water, and food. Iodine deficiency results in diminished production and secretion of thyroid hormone; in response, the pituitary gland secretes increased amounts of thyroid-stimulating hormone, causing hyperplasia and hypertrophy of the thyroid. Initially, the goiter is diffuse but later becomes multinodular.

endemic typhus An acute, flea-borne infectious disease caused by *Rickettsia typhi* and transmitted by the bite of a rat flea. The disease is similar to but less severe than epidemic typhus. Permanent immunity follows infection.

endocarditis An abnormal condition of the endocardium and heart valves marked by vegetations on the valves and endocardium. It may occur as a primary disorder or arise in association with another disease.

endocardium, *pl.* endocardia The endothelial lining membrane of the cavities of the heart, consisting of small blood vessels and bundles of smooth muscle.

endocervicitis An inflammatory condition of the epithelium and glands of the canal of the uterine cervix.

endocervix **1.** The mucous membrane that lines the canal of the uterine cervix. **2.** The opening of the cervix into the uterine cavity.

endocrine **1.** Internal hormone secretion by glands. **2.** Describing an organ or structure that secretes products into the blood or lymph to catalyze specific effects at another location in the body.

endocrine system The system of ductless glands and other structures that elaborate and secrete hormones directly into the circulatory system to influence the function of specific target organs. Endocrine secretions affect various bodily processes, including metabolism and growth. Organs of the endocrine system include the hypothalamus; the pituitary, thyroid, parathyroid, adrenal, and pineal glands; the gonads; and the pancreas. Various other organs also have some endocrine function.

endocrinology The study of the endocrine system and the treatment of endocrine diseases and disorders.

endoderm In embryology: the innermost of the three primary germ layers of the embryo, comprising the lining of the cavities and passages of the body and the covering for many internal organs.

endogenous obesity Obesity caused by dysfunction of the metabolic or endocrine system.

endometrial Of or pertaining to the endometrium or uterine cavity.

endometrial hyperplasia An abnormal overgrowth of the endometrium resulting from sustained stimulation by estrogen without progesterone opposition.

endometrial polyp A projecting mass on the endometrium, usually benign, which may occur singly or in clusters and which commonly causes vaginal bleeding in perimenopausal women. Typically 1 cm ($^1/_2$″) or less in diameter, a polyp may grow and prolapse through the cervix and may be associated with endometrial hyperplasia, fibroids, or other uterine abnormalities.

endometriosis An abnormal condition in which endometrial tissue occurs in abnormal locations. It is more likely to affect women of higher socioeconomic status and women who defer pregnancy. Pregnancy seems to help prevent or ameliorate the disease.

endometrium The inner mucous membrane lining of the uterus, which has three layers — stratum compactum, stratum spongiosum, and stratum basale. Endometrial structure and thickness vary throughout the menstrual cycle.

endomorph A person whose body build is marked by a predominance of structures derived from the endoderm. Typically, an endomorph has a soft, round physique, a large trunk and thighs, fat accumulation throughout the body, and tapering extremities.

endoparasite A parasite that lives within the body of the host, such as a tapeworm.

endophyte A parasitic plant organism that lives within the body of its host.

endophytic 1. Pertaining to an endophyte. 2. Describing the tendency to grow inward or to proliferate on the inside of a structure, as a tumor that grows on the inside of an organ.

endoplasmic reticulum A network of membrane-enclosed cavities found throughout the cytoplasm of cells.

endorphins Endogenous opiates, produced in the brain, that act on the nervous system to reduce pain; include alpha endorphin, beta endorphin, and gamma endorphin.

endoscope An illuminated optical instrument, available in varying lengths, that is used to examine the interior of a body cavity or organ. It may be introduced through a natural opening in the body or inserted through an incision.

endoscopic retrograde cholangiography A radiographic technique used to examine the pancreatic ducts and hepatobiliary tree after injection of a contrast medium into the duodenal papilla.

endoscopy Visual inspection of a body cavity using an endoscope.

endothelium The layer of epithelial cells that is derived from the mesoderm and lines the cavities of the heart, blood and lymph vessels, and serous cavities.

endotoxin A heat-stable toxin, found in the outer membranes of some gram-negative bacteria, that is released only when the cells are disrupted. In large amounts, endotoxins can cause hemorrhagic shock and severe diarrhea; in smaller amounts, they can lead to fever, leukopenia, and other signs and symptoms.

endotracheal Within or through the trachea.

endotracheal anesthesia Anesthesia produced by passing a gas or a mixture of gases through an endotracheal tube; commonly used to induce general anesthesia.

endotracheal intubation Passage of a wide-bore tube through the mouth or nose into the trachea. It may be used to maintain a patent airway, to administer anesthesia, to aspirate secretions, to prevent aspiration of foreign material into the tracheobronchial tree of an unconscious or paralyzed person, or to administer positive pressure ventilation that cannot be given effectively by a mask.

endotracheal tube A flexible, large-bore catheter that is inserted through the mouth or nose into the trachea to a point above the bifurcation of the trachea proximal to the bronchi. It is used to control the airway and mechanically ventilate a patient.

endoxin A hormone that is an endogenous analogue of digoxin. It occurs naturally in humans and may regulate sodium excretion.

enema 1. A procedure in which a solution is introduced into the rectum for therapeutic or cleaning purposes. 2. The material used for introduction of an enema, available as a commercially packaged disposable unit or as reusable equipment assembled and prepared just before use.

 CLINICAL TIP Before an enema, the patient should be warned that some discomfort may occur because the colon tends to contract when distended by the fluid. Giving the enema slowly helps to prevent increased discomfort resulting from sudden distention.

energy The capacity to do work or to perform vigorous activity; the capacity to produce motion, overcome resistance, and induce physical changes.

enteric infection A disease of the small intestine resulting from infection.

enteritis Inflammation of the small intestine resulting from such causes as bacteria, viruses, or functional disorders. *Enterocolitis* refers to involvement of both the small and large intestines.

enteroanastomosis Surgical creation of an anastomosis between two sections of the intestine.

enterobiasis Infestation with nematodes (pinworms) of the *Enterobius* genus, especially *E. vermicularis*. The female worms deposit eggs in the perianal area, resulting in pruritus and insomnia.

enterocolitis Inflammation of the colon and small intestine.

enterocolostomy Surgical creation of an anastomosis between the small intestine and the colon.

enterogastritis Inflammation of the intestines and stomach.

enterohepatitis Inflammation of the intestines and liver.

enteropeptidase An enzyme secreted by the small intestine that activates the proteolytic enzyme in pancreatic fluid by converting trypsinogen to trypsin. Formerly called *enterokinase.*

enterostomal therapist A registered nurse who has at least 2 years of full-time clinical experience and has completed a continuing education course in caring for and teaching patients with stomas and draining wounds.

enterostomy 1. Creation of a permanent opening, as an artificial anus or fistula, into the intestine through the abdominal wall. 2. The permanent opening created by an incision made into the intestine through the abdominal wall.

enterovirus A virus of the genus *Enterovirus* that mainly inhabits the intestinal tract. Usually, infection is asymptomatic but sometimes results in one of several disease syndromes.

entrainment 1. A phenomenon in which a listener's body movements are coordinated with the rhythm of the sounds made by a speaker as the speaker moves several parts of the body. 2. A method used to identify the slowest pacing needed to terminate an arrhythmia. 3. Synchronization and control of the heart rhythm by an external stimulus.

entropion Turning inward of an edge or a margin, such as inward turning of the margin of the eyelid toward the eyeball. In *cicatricial entropion,* inversion of the eyelid margin results from scar tissue formation. *Spastic entropion* refers to eyelid inversion resulting from tonic spasm of the orbicularis oculi muscle.

enucleation Removal of an organ, a tumor, or another part so that it comes out in one piece.

eosin A group of rose-colored, acidic xanthine dyes that are bromine derivatives of fluorescein. They are commonly used in combination with a blue-purple basic dye such as hematoxylin to stain laboratory tissue slides.

eosinophil A granulocytic white blood cell (WBC) that stains readily with the acid dye eosin, characterized by a bilobed nucleus and cytoplasm containing a large number of coarse, refractile granules. Eosinophils constitute 1% to 3% of total WBCs. Allergy and certain infections increase the total eosinophil count; use of steroids, such as cortisone and prednisone, decrease it.

eosinophilia An abnormally large amount of eosinophils in the blood, as seen in many inflammatory conditions.

eosinophilic 1. Readily stainable by the dye eosin. 2. Describing an eosinophil.

eosinophilic leukemia A form of leukemia in which eosinophils are the predominant cells. It resembles chronic myelocytic leukemia but may take an acute course.

eosinophilic pneumonia An inflammation of the lungs in which eosinophils and large mononuclear cells infiltrate the alveoli, causing such signs and symptoms as pulmonary edema, cough, dyspnea, fever, night sweats, and weight loss.

ephemeral fever A febrile condition of unknown cause that lasts just 24 to 48 hours and is uncomplicated.

epicanthus A vertical fold of skin on either side of the nose that covers the canthus and the caruncle; it may be slight or pronounced. It is normal in people of certain races and may occur as a congenital anomaly in others.

epicardium The visceral portion of the pericardium that envelops the heart and folds back upon itself to form the parietal portion of the serous pericardium. It is composed of a single sheet of squamous epithelial cells overlying delicate connective tissue.

epicondyle A projection or eminence on the surface of a bone above its condyle.

epicranium The entire scalp, including the integument, aponeuroses, and muscular sheets.

epidemic   **1.** Affecting a disproportionately large number of people within a discrete population, region, or community at the same time. **2.** A disease that spreads rapidly through a demographic segment of the human population.

epidemiology   The branch of science that studies factors determining the incidence, distribution, and control of disease, injury, and other health-related events and their causes in a defined human population.

epidermis   The surface, or outermost, layer of the skin, composed of five layers — stratum basale, stratum spinosum, stratum granulosum, stratum lucidum, and stratum corneum.

epididymis   One of a pair of elongated, cordlike structures whose tightly coiled duct stores and conveys sperm from the seminiferous tubules of the testes to the vas deferens.

epididymitis   An inflammation of the epididymis. It may be acute or chronic and can result from urinary tract infection, sexually transmitted disease, prostatitis, trauma, or prostatectomy. Signs and symptoms include fever, chills, a tender, swollen epididymis, and pain in the groin.

epidural   On or outside the dura mater.

epidural anesthesia   Regional anesthesia of the pelvic, abdominal, genital, or other area by means of a local anesthetic that is injected into the epidural space of the spinal column.

epidural hematoma   A collection of blood in the epidural space.

epidural space   The space between the dura mater of the brain or spinal cord and the walls of the vertebral canal.

epigastric   Of or pertaining to the upper middle region of the abdomen within the infrasternal angle.

epigastric artery   One of three arteries that serve, respectively, the abdominal muscles and peritoneum; the abdominal muscles, skin, and diaphragm; and the skin of the abdomen, inguinal nodes, and superficial fascia.

epigastrium   The upper middle region of the abdomen within the infrasternal angle.

epiglottis   The lidlike, cartilaginous structure that overhangs the larynx and prevents food from entering the larynx and trachea during swallowing.

epiglottitis   An inflammation of the epiglottis. Acute epiglottitis, a severe form of the condition that primarily affects children, causes stridor, fever, sore throat, croupy cough, and a reddened, swollen epiglottis.

TIME LINE   A child with acute epiglottitis may require an emergency tracheostomy to maintain respiration.

epilating forceps   Small spring forceps used to remove unwanted hair.

epilepsy   A group of neurologic disorders marked by uncontrolled electrical discharge from the cerebral cortex and typically manifested by seizures with clouding of consciousness. Epilepsy is most commonly of unknown cause (idiopathic) but is sometimes associated with head trauma, intracranial infection, brain tumor, vascular disturbances, intoxication, or chemical imbalance.

epiphyseal fracture   A fracture at the juncture of the epiphysis and the shaft of the bone that leads to a separation in or fragmentation of the epiphyseal plate.

epiphysis, *pl.* epiphyses   The articular end of a bone, which is separated from the shaft by the epiphyseal plate until the bone stops growing, the plate is obliterated, and the shaft and head unite.

epiphysitis   Inflammation of the epiphysis of a bone or of the cartilage separating the epiphysis from the main bone.

episiotomy   Surgical incision into the perineum to enlarge the vaginal opening for delivery. It is performed to prevent traumatic tearing of the perineum, to hasten or promote delivery, or to prevent stretching of perineal muscles and connective tissue.

epispadias   The urethral opening on the dorsum of the penis.

epistaxis   Nosebleed; typically caused by local irritation of the nasal mucous membranes, nosepicking, chronic infection, trauma, hypertension, leukemia, or vitamin K deficiency.

   ALERT   If the patient has severe epistaxis he may be hypovolemic. Have him lie down and turn his head to the side to prevent blood from draining down the back of his throat, which could cause aspiration or vomiting. If he is not hypovolemic, have him sit upright and tilt his head forward. Constantly assess airway patency.

epithelioma   A neoplasm of epithelial origin; may be benign, as in adenoma or papilloma, or malignant, as in carcinoma.

epithelium   The covering of the internal and external body organs (including the lining of vessels), consisting of cells joined by connective material. Epithelium varies in the numbers of layers and the shapes of cells. Types of epithelium include simple squamous, simple cuboidal, and stratified columnar.

epitope   The simplest antigenic determinant of a complex antigenic molecule, consisting of a group of amino acids on the surface of the antigen.

epoöphoron A vestigial structure associated with the ovary; a persistent portion of the embryonic mesonephric duct. Located in the mesosalpinx between the ovary and the uterine tube, it is composed of a group of short tubules and a corresponding portion of the rudimentary each other.

EPSDT *abbr* Early and Periodic Screening, Diagnosis, and Treatment.

Epstein-Barr virus (EBV) A herpes-like virus that causes infectious mononucleosis; also associated with Burkitt's lymphoma and nasopharyngeal carcinoma.

Epstein's pearls Small, white cysts normally found on each side of the midline of the hard palate in the neonate. They usually disappear within a few weeks.

equilibrium A state of balance or repose between two or more opposing forces that exactly counteract each other.

Erb's palsy Paralysis of the upper brachial plexus, most commonly resulting from birth trauma. Signs and symptoms include loss of sensation in the affected arm and paralysis and atrophy of the deltoid, biceps, and brachialis muscles.

Erb's point Auscultation point on the precordium at the third intercostal space to the left of the sternum.

erectile Capable of erection; usually refers to the spongy tissue of the penis or clitoris when engorged with blood or, less commonly, to the epidermal tissue involved in the appearance of goose bumps (horripilation) in response to such stimuli as cold or fear.

erection The condition of being made hard, swollen, and elevated; observed in the penis and to a lesser extent in the clitoris when filled with blood. Erection usually results from sexual arousal but also may occur during sleep or certain types of physical stimulation.

ergonomics The study and analysis of human work, especially as it is affected by individual anatomy, physiology, psychology, and mechanics.

ergot The food storage body of a fungus, *Claviceps purpurea*, which commonly infects rye and other cereal grasses.

 CLINICAL TIP Some ergot alkaloids are used to treat migraines and as oxytoxic agents.

erosive gastritis Inflammation of the stomach characterized by multiple erosions of the mucous membrane lining the stomach. Signs and symptoms include pain, nausea, anorexia, and gastric hemorrhage.

ERT *abbr* external radiation therapy *or* estrogen replacement therapy.

eructation The act of bringing up air from the stomach through the mouth. Also called *belching.*

eruption 1. The act of breaking out, or becoming visible, as eruption of the teeth. 2. The rapid development of a skin lesion, especially one caused by a virus or drug reaction, and marked by redness and prominence.

ERV *abbr* expiratory reserve volume.

erysipelas An acute superficial cellulitis, usually caused by group A beta-hemolytic streptococci, characterized by redness, swelling, fever, pain, vesicles, bullae, and lymphadenopathy.

erysipeloid An infection acquired by handling meat or fish infected with *Erysipelothrix rhusiopathiae.* The disorder most commonly results in a self-limiting, localized cellulitis of the hands characterized by blue-red nodules or patches and, occasionally, by erythema.

erythema Redness or inflammation of the skin resulting from congestion of superficial capillaries, as in nervous blushes and mild sunburn.

 ALERT If your patient has sudden progressive erythema with rapid pulse, dyspnea, hoarseness, and agitation, quickly take vital signs as these may be signs of anaphylactic shock. Provide emergency respiratory support, and give epinephrine.

erythema marginatum Nonpruritic, macular, transient rash on the trunk or inner aspects of the upper arms or thighs that gives rise to red lesions with blanched centers.

erythema nodosum A hypersensitivity vasculitis characterized by bilateral, reddened, tender, subcutaneous nodules usually located on the shins. The condition is commonly associated with mild fever, malaise, and pains in muscles and joints.

erythrasma A chronic bacterial skin infection of the axillary or inguinal regions or toe webs characterized by sharply demarcated, red-brown, raised patches. Caused by *Corynebacterium minutissimum.*

erythroblastosis fetalis Hemolytic anemia of the newborn caused by placental transmission of maternally formed antibodies against the incompatible antigens of the fetal blood. It results from maternal-fetal blood group incompatibility, specifically involving the rhesus (Rh) factor and the ABO blood groups and is characterized by accelerated destruction of red blood cells and resulting jaundice. In Rh factor incompatibility, the hemolytic reaction appears only when the mother is Rh negative and the infant is Rh positive. Isoimmunization rarely occurs with the first pregnancy, but the risk increases with each succeeding pregnancy.

erythrocyte Red blood cell; the major cellular element of the circulating blood. Normally, an erythrocyte is a nonnucleated, yellowish, biconcave disk, adapted to transport oxygen. The count is usually maintained between 4.5 and 5 million cells per microliter in men and between 4 and 4.5 million cells per microliter in women. New erythrocytes are produced at a rate of slightly more than 1% a day; thus, a constant level is usually maintained.

erythrocyte sedimentation rate (ESR) The rate at which red blood cells settle in a tube of unclotted blood, expressed as the distance that the top of the column of red blood cells falls during a specified interval (as millimeters per hour).

 CLINICAL TIP An elevated ESR indicates inflammation but is not specific for any disorder.

erythropenia A deficiency of erythrocytes (red blood cells).

erythropoiesis The production of erythrocytes, involving maturation of a nucleated precursor into an erythrocyte that lacks a nucleus and is filled with hemoglobin. Erythropoiesis is regulated by the hormone erythropoietin.

erythropoietin A hormone secreted by the kidney in the adult and by the liver in the fetus. By acting on stem cells in the bone marrow to stimulate and regulate erythrocyte production, erythropoietin can increase the oxygen-carrying capacity of the blood.

eschar A thick scab or dry crust that appears after a thermal or chemical burn.

Escherichia A genus of gram-negative, motile or nonmotile, rod-shaped bacteria that occurs widely in nature and is occasionally pathogenic in humans.

Escherichia coli A species of coliform bacteria of the family Enterobacteriaceae, normally existing in the intestines. *E. coli* is the most common cause of urinary tract infection and of diarrhea in infants; it may also cause wound infection.

esophageal artery The branch of the thoracic aorta that supplies the esophagus.

esophageal lead A conductor connected to an electrocardiograph in which the electrode is placed within the esophagus. Such a lead is used to help detect large atrial deflections by identifying cardiac arrhythmias.

esophageal varices Enlarged, tortuous veins in the lower esophagus, resulting from portal hypertension.

 ALERT Esophageal varices are particularly vulnerable to ulceration and hemorrhage.

esophagectomy Surgical excision of all or part of the esophagus, such as to treat severe, bleeding esophageal varices or esophageal cancer.

esophagitis Inflammation of the mucous membrane that lines the esophagus, caused by such conditions as gastric reflux, infection, or irritation from a nasogastric tube or caustic chemical ingestion.

esophagus The muscular passage that extends from the pharynx to the stomach, measuring about 24 cm (9″) long. Beginning at the cricoid cartilage, opposite the sixth cervical vertebra, the esophagus descends to the cardiac sphincter of the stomach.

esophoria A form of strabismus in which the visual axis of one eye deviates toward that of the other eye in the absence of visual stimuli for fusion.

esotropia Cross-eye; a form of strabismus characterized by inward deviation of the visual axis of one eye relative to the other eye.

ESR *abbr* erythrocyte sedimentation rate.

essential amino acid Any of the nine amino acids needed for protein synthesis that is not synthesized by the human body, including histidine, isoleucine, leucine, lysine, methionine, phenylalanine, threonine, tryptophan, and valine. Essential amino acids are required for nitrogen equilibrium in adults and for optimal growth in children.

essential fatty acid A polyunsaturated fatty acid that cannot be synthesized by the body and must be obtained from the diet. Examples include linoleic, linolenic, and arachidonic acids. Precursors of prostaglandins, essential fatty acids play an important role in fat transport and metabolism, maintenance of cell membranes, and normal functioning of the reproductive and endocrine systems.

essential fever Any fever of unknown cause.

essential hypertension An elevated arterial blood pressure for which no organic cause can be found.

essential nutrient A substance that is necessary for growth, normal function, and body maintenance, such as carbohydrates, proteins, fats, minerals, and vitamins. Most of these substances cannot be synthesized by the body and therefore must be obtained from the diet.

ester An organic compound formed by reaction between alcohols and acids. Examples of esters include fats, which are formed by the bonding of the alcohol glycerol with fatty acids.

estrogen Any of a group of hormonal steroid compounds that promote the development of female secondary sex characteristics and, during the menstrual cycle, render the female genital tract suitable for fertilization, implantation, and nutrition of the early embryo. Estrogen is formed in the ovaries, adrenal cortices, testes, and fetoplacental unit.

estrogen receptor test   A test that predicts the usefulness of hormonal therapy in the treatment of cancer by measuring the response of the patient's cancer cells to estrogen.

estrus   The cyclical period of sexual receptivity in female mammals (except humans), characterized by an intense sexual urge.

ethmoid bone   The light, spongy bone located at the base of the cranium that forms most of the walls of the superior part of the nasal cavity.

ethnic   Pertaining to a group of people sharing social customs, language, religion, or physical traits.

ethnocentrism   A tendency to consider other ethnic groups in terms of the standards of one's own ethnic group, especially when done with a belief in the superiority of one's own group.

etiology   1. The study of the factors that may cause or contribute to the development of a disease, including the patient's susceptibility, the disease agent, and the way in which the agent is introduced into the patient's body. 2. The cause or origin of a disease.

eukaryocyte, eucaryocyte   An organism whose cells have a true nucleus; includes the cells of higher plants and animals, fungi, protozoa, and most algae.

euploid   1. Of or pertaining to an individual or a strain with a balanced set of chromosomes that is an exact multiple of the haploid number characteristic of the species, as diploid, triploid, tetraploid, or polyploid. 2. Such an individual or strain.

eustachian tube   The channel, measuring about 36 mm (1¼″) long, that connects the tympanic cavity with the nasopharynx and adjusts air pressure in the middle ear to the external pressure. Also called *auditory tube.*

eustachitis   Inflammation of the eustachian tube.

euthanasia   The act of actively bringing about or passively allowing the death of a hopelessly ill or injured person for reasons of mercy.

euthyroid   Having normal thyroid gland function.

evacuate   1. To remove or discharge a substance from the body as waste. 2. A substance removed or discharged from the body.

evaporation   The change of a liquid to a vapor at a temperature below the boiling point of the liquid. Evaporation occurs at the surface of the liquid, hastened by an increase in temperature and a decrease in atmospheric pressure.

eversion   Turning outward.

evisceration   1. Pushing out or removal of the viscera, especially through a surgical incision. 2. In ophthalmology: excision of the contents of the eyeball (except the sclera).

evoked potential   The brain waveforms recorded during stimulation of a nerve, muscle, sensory receptor, or area of the central nervous system. Types of evoked potentials include auditory, somatosensory, and visual.

CLINICAL TIP Evoked potential testing is used to detect neurologic lesions and to evaluate multiple sclerosis and various vision and hearing disorders.

Ewing's sarcoma   A malignant, metastatic tumor of the bone, usually occurring in long bones, characterized by pain, swelling, fever, and leukocytosis. Histologically, this tumor is difficult to distinguish from a neuroblastoma or a reticulum cell sarcoma. Also called *Ewing's tumor.*

exacerbation   An increase in the seriousness of a disease or disorder, or in its signs and symptoms.

exanthem, *pl.* exanthemata   1. A skin eruption or rash. 2. Any of the common infectious diseases of childhood in which rash is present, including scarlet fever, measles, roseola infantum, and rubella.

excise   To remove completely by cutting.

excision   1. Operative removal of an organ. 2. In molecular biology: removal of a genetic element from a strand of deoxyribonucleic acid.

excitability   Ability of a cardiac cell to respond to electrical stimuli.

exciting eye   The eye having the primary injury and whose influence involves the other eye in sympathetic ophthalmia (inflammation of the uveal tract after a wound involving the uveal tract of the other eye). Also called *primary eye.*

excoriation   An injury to the skin resulting from abrasion or scratching.

excrete   To eliminate a waste substance, commonly by means of a normal secretion.

excretion   1. The act or process of eliminating substances by body organs or tissues through natural metabolic activity. 2. A substance that is excreted.

excretory   Relating to the process of excretion.

excretory duct   A conductive, nonsecretory duct.

excretory urography   A diagnostic test in which a radiopaque dye is injected intravenously and a series of X-rays are taken over a period of time, as the dye clears from the kidneys and ureters, to identify abnormalities in urinary system structure or function.

exercise electrocardiogram (exercise ECG) A stress test in which an electrocardiogram is recorded as the patient walks on a treadmill or pedals a stationary bicycle for a given length of time at a specific rate of speed. The test helps to diagnose cardiac abnormalities that were absent during rest.

exfoliation Peeling and sloughing off in layers, as of dead skin; exaggerated in certain skin diseases.

exfoliative cytology Microscopic examination of desquamated cells to determine the presence of malignancy or microbiologic changes or to measure levels of one or more substances. The cells are obtained from lesions, secretions, and other material by aspiration, scraping, smear, or washings.

exfoliative dermatitis An inflammatory skin disorder characterized by widespread excessive peeling or shedding of skin. The condition may occur secondary to an underlying skin disorder or may be idiopathic.

exhale To eliminate from the lungs by breathing.

exit dose In radiotherapy: the intensity of the radiation emerging at the surface of the body opposite that where radiotherapy is directed.

exocrine Of or relating to outward secretion through a duct to the surface of an organ or tissue or into a vessel.

exocrine gland Any gland that opens onto the surface of the skin through a duct or ducts in the epithelium, as the sweat glands and sebaceous glands. Simple exocrine glands have one duct; compound glands have more than one duct.

exophoria Deviation of the visual axis of one eye away from that of the other eye, in the absence of visual fusional stimuli.

exophthalmia Abnormal protrusion of the eyeballs, usually caused by orbital inflammation, edema, tumor, trauma to the extraocular muscles, or cavernous sinus thrombosis. Less commonly, it results from hyperthyroidism and Graves' disease.

exophytic Growing outward, as a tumor that grows on the surface or exterior epithelium of an organ or other structure.

exophytic carcinoma A malignant, epithelial neoplasm with marked outward growth, resembling a papilloma or wart.

exostosis An abnormal, benign, bony growth projecting from the surface of a bone.

exotoxin A toxic, heat-labile substance secreted or excreted by species of certain bacteria. Exotoxins are the most poisonous substances known.

exotropia Walleye; strabismus characterized by outward deviation of one eye relative to the other, resulting in diplopia.

expectation of life Life expectancy; the number of years that a person of a given age will live, as determined by statistical averages of mortality in a specific geographic area and, possibly qualified by certain demographic factors specific to the individual.

expected date of delivery (EDD) The predicted date of delivery of a fetus, considered to occur 280 days, or 40 weeks, after conception. To calculate EDD, 3 months are counted back from the first day of the woman's last menstrual period and then 7 days are added.

 CLINICAL TIP The EDD is only an estimate. Typically, the expectant woman is advised that she is likely to give birth within 2 weeks before or after the calculated date.

expectorant 1. Of or relating to a substance that aids the elimination of mucus or other exudates from the lungs and trachea. 2. An agent that promotes expectoration by reducing the viscosity of pulmonary secretions or by stimulating secretion of mucus.

expectoration The ejection of mucus or other exudates from the trachea and lungs by coughing and spitting.

experimental design A study design used in research to test cause-and-effect relationships between variables. An independent variable is given to an experimental group but not to the control group; then both groups are measured on the same dependent variable.

experimental embryology The analysis through experimental techniques of the factors and relationships that influence prenatal development.

experimental psychology The study of mental processes and behaviors in a controlled clinical environment using various experiments, manipulations, and tests.

expert witness A person who has special knowledge of a subject about which a court requests testimony. Special knowledge may be acquired by experience, education, observation, or study and isn't possessed by the average person. An expert witness gives expert testimony or expert evidence. This evidence usually serves to educate the court and the jury about the subject under consideration.

expiration The act of breathing out.

expiratory reserve volume (ERV) The maximum volume of gas that can be expired from the lungs. ERV is equal to functional residual capacity minus residual volume.

expired gas (E)   Any gas expired from the lungs.

expressivity   In genetics: the extent to which a genetic trait is expressed in an individual. Expression of a trait may vary in degree but is never completely unexpressed in persons of the same genotype; for example, polydactyly may be expressed as extra fingers in one generation and extra toes in the next.

expulsive stage of labor   The second stage of labor, which begins after full dilation of the cervix and ends in delivery of the neonate. During this stage, a bearing-down reflex accompanies the uterine contraction.

extended-care facility   An institution whose staff provides medical and nursing care for an individual over a prolonged period, as during the course of a chronic illness or during rehabilitation. Types of extended-care facilities include skilled nursing facility and intermediate-care facility.

extension   Movement permitted by a joint that increases the angle between two adjoining bones.

extension tubing   Small-bore tubing that attaches to any I.V. tubing and joins it with the venipuncture device; allows I.V. tubing to be changed away from the insertion site, thereby reducing risk of contamination.

extensor carpi radialis brevis   A short radial extensor muscle of the wrist that serves to extend and abduct the hand. It arises from the lateral epicondyle of the humerus, inserts into the dorsal surface of the third metacarpal bone, and is innervated by a branch of the radial nerve.

extensor muscles   Muscles that extend a body part.

extern, externe   A student or recent graduate in medicine, osteopathy, podiatry, or dentistry who assists in the care of patients in a health care facility while not residing there.

external   **1.** Situated on, occurring on, or acting from the outside or exterior of the body or an organ. **2.** Relating to outward appearances.

external absorption   The taking up of drugs, poisons, nutrients, or other substances through the skin or mucous membranes.

external acoustic meatus   The S-shaped passage of the external ear that extends from the auricle to the tympanic membrane. Also called *external auditory canal.*

external carotid artery   Either of a pair of arteries that arise from the common carotid artery and channel blood to the neck, face, and skull.

external ear   The outer structure of the ear. Made up of the pinna and the external

acoustic meatus, it funnels sound waves to the middle ear.

external fistula   An abnormal passage between an organ and the body surface.

external jugular vein   One of a pair of large vessels in the neck that arise in the parotid gland at the level of the angle of the jaw and are formed by the junction of the retromandibular vein and the posterior auricular vein. It receives most of the blood from the exterior skull and the deep tissues of the face, passes down the neck, and opens into the subclavian vein, the internal jugular vein, or the brachiocephalic vein.

external pin fixation   A method for stabilizing fractures by means of metal pins transfixed through the fragments of the fractured bone, with an external compression device attached to the pins. The pins are removed after the fracture has healed.

 CLINICAL TIP Pin care includes regular cleaning of the skin around the pins and, commonly, applying antibiotic solutions or ointments.

external radiation therapy (ERT)   Therapeutic application of ionizing radiation from an external beam; used in the treatment of cancer, keloids, and certain other dermatologic conditions as well as to combat rejection of transplanted organs.

external rotation   The movement of a body part away from the midline, as when the hip turns a leg outward.

extracapsular fracture   Any fracture of the humerus or femur occurring near the joint but outside the joint capsule. Such a fracture typically occurs in the hip.

extracellular   Outside a cell or cell tissue or in spaces between groups or layers of cells. In the human body, extracellular fluids account for about 40% of the total water content.

extracellular fluid (ECF)   Body fluids located outside the cells, including the interstitial fluid and blood plasma. The adult body contains about 11.2 liters of interstitial fluid (about 16% of body weight) and about 2.8 liters of plasma (about 4% of body weight). ECF helps to control the movement of water and electrolytes through the body and provides a constant external environment for the cells. Important ionized components of ECF include protein, magnesium, potassium, chlorine, and calcium.

extrapyramidal   **1.** Describing the tissues and structures of the brain located outside the pyramidal tract, not running through the medullary pyramid — excluding the motor neurons, motor cortex, and corticospinal and corticobulbar tracts. **2.** Of or relating to the function of these tissues and structures.

extrapyramidal disease   Any of a group of conditions involving lesions of the extrapyramidal tracts and characterized by involuntary movement, changes in muscle tone, and abnormal posture, as in chorea, tardive dyskinesia, and Parkinson's disease.

extrapyramidal system   A complex of upper motor neurons that connects the basal ganglia, substantia nigra, and thalamic and subthalamic nuclei to each other and to parts of the cerebellum, cerebrum, and reticular formation. Working with the pyramidal system, it controls and coordinates movement and posture and integrates motor impulses originating in the cortex.

extrapyramidal tracts   The tracts of those motor nerves outside the pyramidal tracts that run from the brain to the anterior horns of the spinal cord. In the brain, the extrapyramidal tracts comprise relays of motor neurons between motor areas of the cerebral cortex, basal ganglia, thalamus, cerebellum, and brain stem.

extrasystole   A premature contraction of the heart that does not change the fundamental heart rhythm.

 CLINICAL TIP Extrasystole arises from a site other than the sinoatrial node.

extravasation   Escape, usually of blood, lymph, or intravenous solution, from a vessel into surrounding tissues.

extrinsic   Not inherently part of the cardiac electrical system.

extrinsic asthma   A type of asthma in which attacks are triggered by environmental stimuli, usually allergens. Initial onset usually occurs before age 30.

exudate   Fluid, cells, or other substances that have escaped from cells or blood vessels through small breaks or pores in cell membranes and have been deposited in tissues or on tissue surfaces.

exudative   Pertaining to the escape of fluid, cells, and cellular debris from cells and tissues, usually as a result of inflammation.

eye   The organ of vision, located within the bony orbit at the front of the skull and innervated by the optic nerve. Within the eye, the cornea refracts light through the pupil in the iris and onto the lens, which focuses images onto the retina. Light-sensitive cells in the retina — called cones and rods — receive the images and transmit impulses to the brain via the optic nerve.

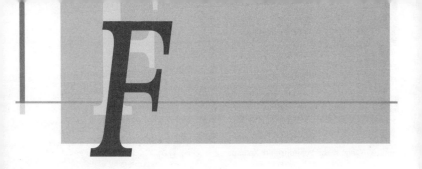

F₁ In genetics: the first filial generation; the heterozygous offspring produced by the mating of two unrelated individuals.

F₂ In genetics: the second filial generation; the offspring produced by mating two members of the first filial generation.

FAAN *abbr* Fellow of the American Academy of Nursing.

FACCP *abbr* Fellow of the American College of Chest Physicians.

facial Pertaining to the face.

facial diplegia A rare neuromuscular condition characterized by paralysis of both sides of the face.

FACOG *abbr* Fellow of the American College of Obstetricians and Gynecologists.

FACS *abbr* Fellow of the American College of Surgeons.

FACSM *abbr* Fellow of the American College of Sports Medicine.

factor IV Calcium as an element in the process of blood coagulation.

factor V Proaccelerin; an unstable procoagulant needed to rapidly convert prothrombin to thrombin. Functions in both intrinsic and extrinsic pathways of blood coagulation.

factor VII Proconvertin; acts in the extrinsic pathway of coagulation; synthesized in the liver by the action of vitamin K.

factor VIII Antihemophilic factor; a coagulation factor that functions in the intrinsic pathway of coagulation. Deficiency of this factor causes hemophilia A.

factor IX Plasma thromboplastin component; a coagulation factor that functions in the intrinsic pathway of coagulation. Deficiency of this factor causes hemophilia B, or Christmas disease.

factor IX complex A systemic hemostatic containing partially purified factor IX fraction and concentrated factors II, VII, and X fractions; used to treat factor IX deficiency.

factor X Stuart factor; a coagulation factor synthesized in the liver by vitamin K. Active in both the intrinsic and extrinsic pathways of coagulation.

factor XI Plasma thromboplastin antecedent; a stable coagulation factor active in the intrinsic pathway of coagulation.

factor XII Hageman factor; initiates the intrinsic pathway of coagulation. Triggers the formation of bradykinin and associated enzymatic reactions.

factor XIII Fibrin stabilizing factor; acts with calcium to enable fibrin strands to form a firm blood clot.

facultative aerobe Microorganism able to grow under both anaerobic and aerobic conditions but develops most rapidly in an aerobic environment.

Faget's sign A slow pulse associated with a high fever; an unusual sign that suggests yellow fever.

Fahrenheit A temperature scale in which the boiling point of water is 212° and the freezing point of water is 32° at average atmospheric pressure.

fallopian tube Uterine tube; one of a pair of tubes extending from the uterus and opening at the other end into the peritoneal cavity near the ovary.

false negative A test result that incorrectly excludes the presence of a finding, condition, or disease.

false positive A test result that incorrectly indicates the presence of a disease or other condition.

falx, *pl.* **falces** A sickle-shaped structure.

falx cerebelli A small sickle-shaped fold of dura mater attached to the occipital bone and projecting into the posterior cerebellar notch between the two cerebellar hemispheres.

falx cerebri A sickle-shaped fold of dura mater that extends into and follows along the longitudinal fissure separating the two hemispheres of the cerebrum.

family nurse practitioner (FNP) A registered nurse possessing specialty skills necessary for the detection and management of acute self-limiting conditions and management of chronic stable conditions; provides primary, ambulatory care in collaboration with primary care physicians.

family practice physician A medical specialist who offers comprehensive primary health care to all members of a family.

Fanconi's syndrome 1. Fanconi's anemia; a rare, usually congenital disorder, characterized by aplastic anemia, bone marrow abnormalities, and patchy brown skin discoloration; associated with abnormalities of the musculoskeletal and genitourinary systems. 2. A group of diseases marked by cystinosis and abnormalities of renal tubular function.

 TIME LINE Children who undergo kidney transplantation and do not develop immunologic problems will have return of kidney function. The transplanted kidney does not develop the functional abnormalities of Fanconi's syndrome, but the patient may continue to accumulate cystine in the cornea.

Farber test Microscopic examination of newborn meconium for presence of vernix cells; absence of these cells suggests intestinal obstruction or atresia.

farmer's lung A respiratory disorder caused by inhalation of actinomycetes or other spores from moldy hay.

fascia, *pl.* fasciae Sheets or bands of fibrous tissue that envelop the body under the skin and enclose muscles and muscle groups.

fascial Pertaining to the fascia — a sheet or band of fibrous tissue.

fasciculation A localized, uncontrollable contraction of a single muscle group innervated by a single motor nerve filament; may be seen under the skin.

 CLINICAL TIP A fasciculation may result from an adverse drug reaction or from such disorders as dietary deficiency, cerebral palsy, fever, or uremia.

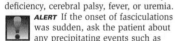 *ALERT* If the onset of fasciculations was sudden, ask the patient about any precipitating events such as exposure to pesticides. Pesticide poison, although uncommon, is a medical emergency requiring prompt and vigorous intervention.

fasciculus, *pl.* fasciculi A small bundle of fibers, usually of muscle or nerve.

fascioliasis Infection with the liver fluke *Fasciola hepatica;* may result in obstruction of the biliary passages and invasion of the liver.

fastigium 1. The highest point in the course of an illness, as of fever. 2. The highest point of the roof of the fourth ventricle of the brain.

fat 1. A substance composed of lipids or fatty acids. 2. Adipose tissue; rounds out body contours and serves as a reserve source of energy.

fatigue fever A benign episode of fever caused by accumulation of metabolic waste products after overexercise.

fatigue fracture Any fracture that results from prolonged walking or exercise rather than from trauma, as commonly occurs in the metatarsal bones of runners.

fat metabolism The biochemical process by which fats are broken down to simpler compounds by digestion; catabolism of 1 g of fat provides 9 kilocalories of energy.

fatty acid Any of several organic acids derived from fats by hydrolysis.

fatty liver A liver affected by infiltration of fats.

fauces The throat; passage from the mouth into the pharynx.

favism An acute condition caused by ingestion of the beans or inhalation of pollen from the *Vicia faba* plant; occurs in people with glucose-6-phosphate dehydrogenase deficiency.

 CLINICAL TIP Favism is marked by severe hemolytic anemia, fever, headache, abdominal pain, and coma.

favus A ringworm infection of the scalp, usually caused by *Trichophyton schoenleinii.*

FCAP *abbr* Fellow of the College of American Pathologists.

FDA *abbr* Food and Drug Administration.

Fe Symbol for iron.

febrile Feverish; pertaining to or characterized by an elevated body temperature.

fecal fistula An abnormal passage from the colon that opens on the body surface or into another hollow organ and discharges feces.

fecal impaction An accumulation of hardened feces in the rectum or sigmoid colon that the person cannot evacuate.

fecalith A hard, impacted mass of feces.

feces Waste or excrement formed in the intestine and expelled through the rectum.

fecundity Pronounced fertility; the ability to produce offspring, especially in large numbers and rapidly.

Federation Licensing Examination (FLEX) The standardized examination for state licensure of physicians.

Fehling's solution A solution containing cupric sulfate, sodium hydroxide, and potassium sodium tartrate; used to test for the presence of glucose and other reducing substances in the urine.

Fellow of the American Academy of Nursing (FAAN) A member of the American Academy of Nursing.

Fellow of the American College of Chest Physicians (FACCP) A board-certified member of the American College of Chest Physicians.

Fellow of the American College of Surgeons (FACS)   A member of the American College of Surgeons, recognized by that professional organization as qualified to practice surgery.

Fellow of the College of American Pathologists (FCAP)   A member of the College of American Pathologists.

Felty's syndrome   A syndrome characterized by hypersplenism, chronic rheumatoid arthritis, splenomegaly, leukopenia, and pigmented spots on the lower extremities.

feminizing adrenal tumor   A rare, usually malignant neoplasm of the adrenal cortex, characterized in males by gynecomastia, a high level of estrogen in urine, and loss of potency.

femur   The thigh bone; the largest bone in the body, extending from the pelvis to the knee.

fenestra, *pl.* **fenestrae**   Any windowlike opening, including an opening in a bandage or cast, to relieve pressure or to administer skin care.

fenestration   1. The act of opening by perforation. 2. A surgical procedure in which a new opening is created in the labryinth of the ear to restore hearing in otosclerosis.

fermentation   The anaerobic conversion of organic compounds, especially carbohydrates, to simpler compounds by the action of an enzyme; results in energy in the form of adenosine triphosphate. Used in production of alcohol, bread, vinegar, and other products.

fermium (Fm)   An artificial radioactive element. Its atomic number is 100; its atomic weight is 253.

ferritin   An iron compound essential for hematopoiesis; found in the intestinal mucosa, spleen, liver, bone marrow, and reticuloendothelial cells, it is one of the chief forms of iron stored in the body.

fertile   Fruitful; able to produce offspring.

fertilization membrane   A strong membrane that forms around the fertilized ovum, preventing penetration of additional spermatozoa.

fertilizin   A glycoprotein found on the ovum plasma membrane in various species; believed to bind the spermatozoon to the ovum.

fetal age   The age of the conceptus from the time elapsed since fertilization.

fetal attitude   The relationship of the parts of the fetal body to each other; in normal attitude, joints are moderately flexed, back curved forward, head bent with the chin on chest.

fetal circulation   The pathway of blood flow in the fetus. Oxygenated blood from the placenta travels through the umbilical vein and ductus venosus to the inferior vena cava and right atrium; then it bypasses the lungs by following one of two paths: through the foramen ovale to the left atrium and then to the aorta or through the right ventricle, pulmonary artery, and ductus arteriosus to the aorta and the rest of the body. Shortly after birth, the ductus arteriosus and foramen ovale close, allowing normal circulation. See the illustration on page 130.

fetal distress   Compromised condition of the fetus, usually signaled by changes in fetal heart rate or rhythm during labor or by biochemical changes in amniotic fluid.

fetal heart rate (FHR)   The number of fetal heartbeats occurring in a given timeframe, usually 120 to 160 beats/minute. Varies in cycles of fetal rest and activity and is affected by many factors, including maternal fever and uterine contractions.

fetal heart tones (FHT)   Vibrations of the fetal heart heard by Doppler stethoscope through the maternal abdomen in pregnancy, as early as the 12th week.

fetal hydantoin syndrome (FHS)   Birth defect linked with prenatal maternal ingestion of hydantoin analogues such as phenytoin; characterized by craniofacial and skeletal abnormalities, mental and physical retardation, and cardiac defects.

   TIME LINE About 10% of infants whose mothers take hydantoin during pregnancy develop FHS in some form.

fetal hydrops   Massive edema of the fetus or newborn, occurring in severe hemolytic disease of the newborn.

fetal position   A description of the relationship of the presenting part of the fetus to the quadrants of the maternal pelvis, identified with the initials L (left), R (right), A (anterior), and P (posterior); the presenting part is identified by the initials O (occiput), M (mentum), and S (sacrum).

fetal presentation   The presenting part of the fetus; the part that enters the inlet of the maternal pelvis first; includes cephalic, which may be vertex, brow, or chin; breech, which may be frank, complete, or footling; and shoulder.

fetal stage   In human embryology: interval in the development of the fetus in utero lasting from the end of the embryonic stage (end of the 7th week of gestation) to birth (38 to 42 weeks' gestation).

fetology   The branch of medicine associated with the fetus in utero.

Fetal circulation

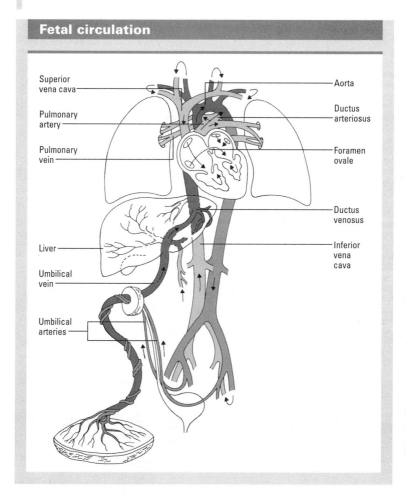

Superior vena cava

Pulmonary artery

Pulmonary vein

Liver

Umbilical vein

Umbilical arteries

Aorta

Ductus arteriosus

Foramen ovale

Ductus venosus

Inferior vena cava

fetometry   Estimation of the size of the fetus, especially the diameter of the head and circumference of the trunk, before delivery.

fetoprotein   A fetal protein antigen found in adults. Alpha-fetoprotein, when found in maternal blood during pregnancy, is an indicator of neural tube defects in the fetus; other forms, when found in adults, are associated with liver disease and neoplasms.

fetor hepaticus   Musty, sweet-smelling breath characteristic of hepatic disease.

fetoscope   **1.** A stethoscope designed for auscultating fetal heartbeat through the mother's abdomen. **2.** An endoscope that permits visualization of the fetus in utero.

fetoscopy   Direct observation of the fetus in utero, using a fetoscope introduced through a small abdominal incision.

FEV   *abbr* forced expiratory volume.

F factor   In bacterial genetics: a conjugating plasmid found in male bacterial cells but not in female cells.

FHR   *abbr* fetal heart rate.

FHS   *abbr* fetal hydantoin syndrome.

FHT   *abbr* fetal heart tones.

fiberoptics   A process that uses coated glass or plastic fibers to transmit light by internal reflections, thereby allowing visualization of an internal organ.

fiberscope   A flexible endoscope with an inner lumen coated with light-conveying glass or plastic fibers that have special optic properties.

fibrillation   A small, involuntary muscle contraction that is not visible externally and that results from activation of a single muscle cell or muscle fiber.

fibrin   The insoluble protein that makes up a blood clot; formed by thrombin from fibrinogen during normal clotting.

fibrinogen   Coagulation factor I; a plasma protein that is converted into fibrin by thrombin in the presence of calcium; essential to the process of coagulation.

fibrinokinase   An enzyme derived from animal tissue that activates plasminogen.

fibrinolysin   Plasmin; a proteolytic enzyme that occurs as plasminogen in plasma; converts fibrin to soluble products.

fibrinolysis   The enzymatic dissolution of fibrin by fibrinolysin.

fibrinopeptide   One of two peptides released by the action of thrombin on fibrinogen.

fibroadenoma, *pl.* fibroadenomas, fibroadenomata   A benign tumor composed of glandular epithelial and fibrous tissue; especially seen in the breast.

fibroangioma, *pl.* fibroangiomas, fibroangiomata   A tumor composed of a mass of blood vessels and fibrous tissue.

fibroblast   A long, flat connective tissue cell; gives rise to various precursor cells, such as chondroblasts, collagenoblasts, and osteoblasts, that form the fibrous tissue of the body.

fibrocartilage   The type of cartilage seen in the intervertebral disks, consisting of a dense matrix of collagenous fibers.

fibrocystic disease of the breast
Mammary dysplasia marked by formation of single or multiple fluid-filled cysts in the breasts; caused by exaggerated tissue response to normal cyclic changes.

CLINICAL TIP   Although the cysts are benign, they must be observed for growth or change.

fibromyositis   Inflammation of muscle and fibrous connective tissues; any of a group of disorders marked by such inflammation and by stiffness and pain in muscles and joints.

fibrosarcoma, *pl.* fibrosarcomas, fibrosarcomata   A malignant neoplasm that contains connective tissue; arises from fibroblasts that produce collagen.

fibrosis   Formation of fibrous connective tissue; occurs normally in the formation of scar tissue.

fibrositis   Inflammation of fibrous connective tissue, especially of the muscle

sheaths and fascia; usually characterized by pain and stiffness.

fibrous capsule   An anatomic structure made of fibrous elements that encloses an organ or body part.

fibrous joint   Any immovable joint in which the bones are connected by a continuous fibrous tissue, as in the sutures of the skull.

fibrous tissue   The connective tissue of the body, consisting of closely woven elastic fibers.

fibula   The outer bone of the lower leg, lateral to and smaller than the tibia.

Fick principle   Based on the law of conservation of mass and used for making indirect measurements of cardiac output; holds that the difference between the oxygen concentrations of arterial and mixed venous blood is equal to the amount of oxygen taken up by each unit of blood as it passes through the lungs. So cardiac output can be calculated if the oxygen uptake for a given period — as well as the oxygen saturation of arterial and mixed venous blood — is known.

Fick's law   In physics: an observed law stating that the rate at which a substance diffuses through an area depends on the difference in its concentration at two given points, called the concentration gradient.

field   In data processing: a particular area in which the same type of data is entered; one unit of data, such as the patient's name.

field fever   A disorder caused by strains of *Leptospira interrogans,* affecting primarily agricultural workers, characterized by fever, abdominal pain, diarrhea, vomiting, stupor, and conjunctivitis; forms include cane-field fever and harvest fever.

FIGLU   *abbr* formiminoglutamic acid.

figure-eight bandage   A bandage that crosses over and around itself like the figure eight.

filiform bougie   An extremely thin cylindrical instrument used for exploration of or passage through a narrow stricture or a sinus tract.

filiform catheter   A tubular flexible instrument with a slender, threadlike tip that is used to dilate urethral strictures and can bypass obstructions caused by calculation or angulations.

film badge   A small packet of photographic film, sensitive to ionizing radiation, used to indicate exposure to radiation of personnel working with X-rays and other radioactive sources.

fish tapeworm infection   A disorder that produces mild gastrointestinal symptoms and pernicious anemia and that is caused by the tapeworm *Diphyllobothrium latum;* transmitted to humans by consumption of contaminated freshwater fish. Common in temperate zones, including the Great Lakes region of the United States.

fission 1. The act or process of splitting. 2. A type of asexual reproduction common in single-celled organisms, such as bacteria, in which the cell divides into two or more equal parts, each of which eventually develops into a complete organism. 3. The splitting of an atomic nucleus and subsequent release of energy.

fissural angioma A hemangioma, composed of a cluster of dilated blood vessels, found in an embryonal fissure of the lip, face, or neck.

fissure 1. A cleft or groove on the surface of an organ, especially that in the cerebral cortex. 2. A cracklike skin lesion. 3. A deep cleft on a tooth surface, occurring during the development of tooth enamel.

fissure fracture Any fracture in which a crack extends from the surface into the cortex of the bone but not through the bone.

fistula, *pl.* **fistulas, fistulae** An abnormal communication between an internal organ and the body surface or between two hollow internal organs.

fixating eye In strabismus, the eye that can be focused on the object of vision.

fixative Fluid used to preserve cytologic or histologic specimens for later examination.

fixed bridgework A partial denture incorporating artificial teeth permanently attached to the natural teeth.

fixed coupling An abnormal pulse in which premature heartbeats follow normal ones at identical intervals.

fixed dressing A dressing impregnated with a hardening agent, such as plaster of Paris, sodium silicate, or starch, applied to immobilize the body part being treated.

fixed drug eruption A circumscribed inflammatory skin lesion recurring in the same location, caused by exposure to a sensitizing drug.

fixed idea A persistent, obsessional thought or notion, especially a delusional idea that dominates mental activity and persists despite contrary evidence or rational refutation. Also called *idée fixe.*

flaccid Relaxed, soft, and flabby; lacking muscle tone.

flaccid paralysis Type of paralysis characterized by loss of muscle tone in the affected part and lack of tendon reflexes.

flagellate Any microorganism that possesses a whiplike organelle by which it propels itself; examples include *Trypanosoma, Leishmania, Trichomonas,* and *Giardia* species.

flail chest A condition in which the chest wall moves paradoxically with breathing, contracting on inspiration and bulging on expiration; caused by multiple rib fractures.

 ALERT Flail chest can also cause tension pneumothorax, a life-threatening condition in which air enters the chest but cannot be ejected during exhalation. Thoracic pressure buildup causes lung collapse and subsequent mediastinal shift.

flame photometry Measurement of the wavelength of light emitted by a substance exposed to a flame, used to identify clinical specimens of body fluids; in the clinical laboratory, used to measure sodium, potassium, calcium, and lithium levels.

flare reaction A local, venous inflammatory response to infusion of an irritant, with or without accompanying skin reaction. Redness may be observed surrounding the venipuncture site or along the vein path. Patient complaints may include burning, pain, aching along the vein, or itching.

flask closure In dentistry: the bringing together of the two halves of a flask that encloses and forms a denture base.

flat electroencephalogram A chart on which no tracings of brain waves are recorded during electroencephalography, indicating absence of brain activity.

flatus Air or gas in the gastrointestinal tract that may be passed through the anus.

flexion 1. Bending of a joint between two bones of the skeleton that decreases the angle between the bones. 2. Raising an arm or leg forward by movement at the shoulder or hip joint.

floaters Spots that appear to drift in front of the eye, caused by vitreous debris; usually benign.

flow regulator A supplemental I.V. device that ensures accurate delivery of I.V. fluids by regulating the number of milliliters delivered per hour.

fluid balance Constant and approximately equal distribution of fluids between intracellular and extracellular compartments.

fluke A flatworm of the class *Trematoda,* including the genus *Schistosoma,* which in the adult stage are internal parasites.

fluorescence The property of emitting light of one wavelength (usually ultraviolet) when exposed to light of a slightly shorter wavelength.

fluorescence microscopy Examination of naturally fluorescent materials or of specimens that have been stained with fluorescent dye using a microscope equipped to emit ultraviolet light.

fluorescent antibody test (FA test) A test in which a fluorescent dye is used to stain an antibody, to identify clinical specimens, for example, under the fluorescent microscope; used in diagnosis of hepatitis, mononucleosis, and biliary cirrhosis.

Fluorescent Treponemal Antibody Absorption Test (FTA-ABS test) The standard serologic test for syphilis.

fluoridation The process of adding fluoride to a public water supply to reduce the incidence of dental caries.

fluoride A compound of fluorine; introduced into drinking water and applied directly to the teeth to prevent dental caries.

fluorine (F) An element of the halogen family. Its atomic number is 9; its atomic weight is 19. It is part of the structure of bones and teeth in the form of fluoride.

fluoroacetic acid A colorless, water-soluble, highly toxic compound that blocks the Krebs citric acid cycle, causing convulsions and ventricular fibrillation.

fluorometry Identification of small amounts of a substance by measuring the characteristic wavelength of light it emits under fluorescence.

fluoroscope A device used for examining deep structures by X-ray; the images are projected on a fluorescent screen for visual examination.

fluoroscopy A radiologic technique for visually examining a deep structure of the body using a fluoroscope.

FMET *abbr* formylmethionine.

FMG *abbr* foreign medical graduate.

FNP *abbr* family nurse practitioner.

focal seizure A convulsive episode that begins with transient motor, sensory, or psychic abnormality; the type of activity reflects the affected part of the cerebral hemisphere. The seizures commonly begin as localized spasmodic movements or visual or olfactory hallucinations. Focal seizures may spread progressively to end in a generalized convulsion; focal manifestations immediately preceding a generalized seizure constitute an aura.

 TIME LINE More likely in children than adults, focal seizures can spread and become generalized. Typically, they cause the child's eyes, or his head and eyes, to turn to the side; in neonates, they cause mouth twitching, staring, or both.

folinic acid A derivative of folic acid used to treat megaloblastic anemias caused by folic acid deficiency and to reverse the toxic effects of folic acid antagonists such as methotrexate.

follicle **1.** A spherical mass of cells that usually contains a cavity, as an ovarian follicle. **2.** A pouchlike depression, as the hair follicle.

follicle-stimulating hormone (FSH) A gonadotropic hormone of the anterior pituitary; stimulates growth and maturation of graafian follicles in the ovary, induces the endometrial changes of the proliferative phase of the menstrual cycle, and promotes spermatogenesis in the male.

fomentation Treatment with a warm, moist application; the substance or poultice applied.

fontanel, fontanelle A soft spot, such as the spaces covered by tough membranes remaining between the bones of an infant's skull.

Food and Drug Administration (FDA) The federal agency responsible for the enforcement of federal regulations regarding food, drugs, and cosmetics.

food exchange list A grouping of foods that enables calculation of proper diet and selection of foods by patients with various diseases and deficiency states such as diabetes. Common foods are divided into six lists in which the carbohydrate, fat, and protein values are equal for the items listed; these lists include milk, vegetables, fruits, bread, meat, and fats.

food poisoning A group of illnesses resulting from the ingestion of a food contaminated by bacteria and their toxins or of a food that is in itself chemically toxic. Varies in severity from mild to life-threatening.

 CLINICAL TIP The bacterial form of food poisoning usually is manifested as acute gastroenteritis, whereas toxic ingestion can cause neurologic signs.

foot The distal extremity of the leg, consisting of the tarsus, metatarsus, phalanges, and related structures and tissue that envelops them.

foot-and-mouth disease A common viral disease of farm animals, which occasionally affects humans exposed to infected products; marked by eruption of vesicles on the tongue, oral mucous membranes, hands, and feet.

footling breech An intrauterine presentation of the fetus during labor in which one or both feet precede the body into the inlet of the maternal pelvis.

foot-pound A unit of measurement for work or energy; the amount of work required to raise one pound a distance of one foot against gravity.

foramen, *pl.* foramina An opening or passage in a membranous structure or bone.

foramen magnum Great foramen; a passage in the occipital bone that connects the spinal column and the cranial cavity; the spinal cord passes through it.

foramen of Monro   The interventricular foramen; a passage between the lateral and third ventricles of the brain.

foramen ovale   The opening in the septum secundum of the fetal heart between the right and left atria.

Forbes-Albright syndrome   An endocrine disease characterized by amenorrhea, prolactinemia, and galactorrhea, caused by an adenoma of the anterior pituitary.

force   Energy that initiates or arrests motion, changes an object's speed or direction, or alters an object's size or shape.

forced expiratory volume (FEV)   Volume of air that can be forcibly expelled in a unit of time after full inspiration; usually measured as forced expiratory volume in 1 second.

forceps   A surgical instrument with two handles or sides, each attached to a blade, used to grasp tissues or to handle sterile surgical supplies.

forceps delivery   Extraction of the infant from its mother using instruments applied to the infant's head; usually performed to quickly deliver a fetus experiencing distress or to shorten normal labor.

foreign body obstruction   A disturbance in normal function caused by an object lodged in a body orifice or passage that interferes with the patency of the passage.

forensic medicine   A branch of medicine dealing with the application of medical knowledge to the purposes of law.

forensic psychiatry   The branch of psychiatry that deals with the legal aspects of mental disorders, especially the determination of insanity for the purposes of law.

foreskin   The prepuce; a loose fold of skin that covers the glans penis.

formalin   A 37% solution of formaldehyde in water; used to preserve specimens for pathologic and histologic examination.

formiminoglutamic acid (FIGLU)   An intermediate compound formed in the metabolism of histidine to glutamic acid; occurs in urine in elevated levels in folic acid deficiency.

formulary   A listing of pharmaceuticals and a collection of formulas for medicinal preparations; health care facilities maintain formularies that list all drugs commonly stocked in their pharmacies.

fornix, *pl.* fornices   An archlike structure or the space created by the arch, as the fornix cerebri or the vaginal fornices.

fossa, *pl.* fossae   A usually longitudinal depression on the surface of a body part, especially on the end of a bone, as the olecranon fossa.

Foster bed   A special bed used in the care and treatment of severely injured patients, especially those with spinal injuries.

four-point gait   A crutch gait in which the patient moves forward by advancing one crutch, then the opposite leg, followed by the other crutch, then the other leg, and so on.

Fowler's position   A posture assumed when the head of the bed is raised 18" to 20" (46 to 51 cm) and the individual's knees are elevated.

fractionation   1. In chemistry: the separation of a substance into its basic constituents using such procedures as distillation. 2. In bacteriology: isolation of a pure culture by successive culturing of a small portion of a colony of bacteria. 3. In histology: isolation of the different components of living cells by centrifugation. 4. In radiology: administration of smaller units of radiation over an extended period rather than in a single large dose to minimize tissue damage. Also called *dose fractionation* or *fractionation radiation*.

fracture   A traumatic injury leading to a break or rupture in a bone; classified according to the bone involved, the part of that bone, and the nature of the break. Kinds include avulsion, comminuted, compound, dislocation, extracapsular, greenstick, impacted, intracapsular, longitudinal, oblique, simple, and transverse fractures.

fracture-dislocation   A fracture of a bone near a joint, with associated dislocation of the joint.

fractured rib   A break in one of the bones of the thoracic skeleton; caused by a blow or injury or by violent coughing or sneezing. Most commonly broken are the fourth to eighth ribs. Complications occur when sharp bone fragments pierce the lung, causing hemothorax or pneumothorax.

Franceschetti's syndrome   A hereditary disorder characterized by facial anomalies, including slanting palpebral fissures, absence of the lower eyelid and pinna, micrognathia, and hypoplasia of the zygomatic arch.

francium (Fr)   An element (atomic number 87; atomic weight 223) formed from the decay of actinium; all isotopes are radioactive and short-lived.

frank   Unmistakable; clinically evident, as the obvious presence of a condition or a disease.

frank breech   Presentation of the fetus in labor in which the buttocks precede the body into the maternal pelvic inlet, with the legs straight in front of the body, and the feet against the face.

Frank-Starling relationship The ventricular function curve; a mechanism for determining cardiac output, based on the relationship between the length of myocardial fibers at the onset of contraction and the ability of the ventricles to pump. The force exerted per heartbeat is directly proportional to the degree of stretch of the myocardial fiber; improved performance results from a longer initial fiber length or a larger diastolic ventricular volume. End-diastolic pressure is used as an index of volume or myocardial stretch and is plotted against measures of ventricular strength, such as systolic pressure, stroke volume, and cardiac work. A normal curve can be described; in heart failure, the curve shifts to the right and down.

fraud Intentional deception resulting in damage to another, whether to his person, rights, property, or reputation. Fraud usually consists of a misrepresentation, concealment, or nondisclosure of a material fact or at least misleading conduct, devices, or contrivance.

FRC *abbr* functional residual capacity.

FRCS *abbr* Fellow of the Royal College of Surgeons.

freckle A benign, small brown or tan macule on the skin, usually resulting from exposure to sunlight, especially in children. Tendency to freckling is inherited.

free association Encouragement of spontaneous verbalization of thoughts and emotions entering the consciousness during psychoanalysis.

free clinic A community-run health program that provides ambulatory health care for patients at nominal or no cost.

free-floating anxiety Severe, generalized, persistent fear that is not attributable to any specific object, situation, or idea.

free radicals Molecules containing an odd number of electrons. These substances may play a role in cancer formation by interacting with deoxyribonucleic acid and impairing normal cell function.

free thyroxine The amount of the active thyroid hormone, thyroxine (T_4), circulating in the blood that is not bound to tissue proteins.

Freiberg's infarction An abnormal condition of the second metatarsal, characterized by thickening of the shaft and aseptic necrosis of bone tissue at its head; it causes pain in the joint when standing.

Frei test A skin test to confirm diagnosis of lymphogranuloma venereum in which reaction to an injection of killed antigen is compared to a control.

Frejka pillow splint A corrective device that is used to maintain abduction and artic-

ulation of the head of the femur with the acetabulum in congenital dislocation of the hip.

fremitus A vibration that can be perceived through palpation during physical examination, especially a palpable vibration of the chest wall, as in bronchial fremitus, tactile fremitus, or vocal fremitus.

frenum, *pl.* frenums, frena A small fold of skin or mucous membrane that limits or restrains movement of a structure. Also called *frenulum.*

frequency 1. The number of occurrences of any recurrent phenomenon within a fixed period, as the number of heartbeats per minute. 2. The number of occurrences of a particular event or the number of persons in a statistical sample having a particular characteristic.

Freudian 1. Of or pertaining to Sigmund Freud; his psychological theories, which stress the unconscious repression of instinctual drives and sexual desires during the formative years as the basis for later psychoneurotic disorders; and his method of psychotherapy, which uses psychoanalysis to treat such disturbances. 2. Anything interpreted according to Freud's theories or in psychoanalytic terms. 3. Of or pertaining to the school of psychiatry based on Freud's theories. 4. An adherent to Freud's school of psychiatry.

Freudian fixation Arrested psychosexual development characterized by a suffocating attachment to another person or object, especially one's mother or father; hence, father fixation and mother fixation are forms of this disorder.

Freudianism, Freudism The school of psychiatry based on the psychoanalytic theories and methods of Sigmund Freud and his followers.

friction The act of one surface rubbing against another.

friction burn A wound caused by abrasion of the skin from violent rubbing, as, for example, from a rope slipping through the hands.

friction rub A dry, grating sound heard during auscultation that is caused by the rubbing of two serous surfaces.

 CLINICAL TIP When auscultated over the pericardial area, friction rub suggests pericarditis; when over the lungs, it may be produced by pleurae and suggests heart or lung disease.

Friedländer's bacillus A bacterium of the species *Klebsiella pneumoniae* that is the cause of acute bacterial pneumonia.

Friedreich's ataxia A hereditary condition, usually manifesting in childhood or youth, characterized by pronounced sclerosis of the posterior columns of the spinal cord, ataxia, speech impairment, muscular weakness or paralysis of the lower extremities, and an abnormal gait. There is no curative treatment for Friedreich's ataxia, although spinal fusion may correct the associated scoliosis.

frolement 1. The sound often heard when auscultating the chest in diseases of the pericardium. 2. Massage that uses a light brushing stroke with the palm of the hand.

frontal lobe The anterior portion of the cerebral hemisphere, lying beneath the frontal bone and extending posteriorly to the central sulcus and inferiorly to the lateral fissure. It influences personality and is associated with the higher mental activities, such as planning, judgment, and conceptualizing.

frontal lobe syndrome Behavioral and personality changes observed after destruction or interference with the function of the gray matter in the frontal lobes, such as occurs with tumors or trauma. Emotion is blunted, inhibitions weakened, and judgment impaired; also marked by inability to concentrate and by inappropriate euphoria (although some patients instead demonstrate apathy).

frontal plane Any plane passing through the body from the head to the feet, perpendicular to the sagittal planes, dividing the body into front and back parts. Also called *coronal plane.*

frontal sinus One of a pair of small paranasal cavities in the frontal bone of the skull that communicates with the nasal cavity; measures approximately 3 cm (1¼″) in height, 2.5 cm (1″) in width, and 2.5 cm in depth and is lined with a mucous membrane continuous with that of the nasal cavity.

frontal vein One of a pair of superficial veins of the face, arising in the plexus of the forehead. Each frontal vein communicates with the frontal tributaries of the superficial temporal vein and lies near the vein of the opposite side as it courses toward the root of the nose. The two frontal veins communicate by a transverse vessel before joining the supraorbital veins.

frostbite Damage to tissues as a result of exposure to extreme cold, characterized by distinct pallor of exposed skin surfaces, particularly the nose, ears, fingers, and toes; results from vasoconstriction and damage to blood vessels, which impair local circulation, resulting in anoxia, edema, and necrosis.

frottage Sexual gratification obtained by rubbing up against another person who is unaware of the activity, as can occur in a crowd.

frozen-section method A method used to prepare a portion of tissue for pathologic examination, in which the tissue is moistened, rapidly frozen, and cut by a microtome.

fructokinase An enzyme that catalyzes the reaction of adenosine triphosphate and D-fructose that forms fructose 6-phosphate.

fructose A sugar present in honey and many fruits; a preparation of the sugar in crystalline form, administered in an intravenous solution as a source of carbohydrate calories and fluid.

fructosuria Presence of the sugar fructose in the urine; sometimes caused by absence of the enzyme fructokinase, which occurs as a hereditary disorder. Also called *levulosuria.*

FSH *abbr* follicle-stimulating hormone.

FTC *abbr* Federal Trade Commission.

fubernaculum Fibromuscular band that connects the testes to the scrotal floor.

fugue A state of dissociative reaction during which the person appears normal and acts and wanders as though conscious but has no recollection afterward of the actions or behavior. The syndrome appears to be caused by inability to cope with severe conflict or with a chronically stressful life situation.

fulcrum The stable point or position on which a lever turns in moving an object.

fulguration Destruction of tissue by high-frequency electricity.

full bath One in which the patient's body is immersed in water up to the neck.

full liquid diet A diet given to patients immediately following surgery or to those with acute or chronic conditions that leave them unable to chew or consume even soft foods; consists of liquids and any food that can be served in strained or liquid forms, including custards, ice cream, and soft-cooked eggs.

fulminating Sudden, severe; said of a disease or condition that occurs suddenly and with great intensity.

function 1. The normal physiologic activity of an organ or body part. 2. To perform an activity or to work normally.

functional differentiation In embryology: specialization or diversification that results from the particular function of a cell or tissue.

functional disease 1. A disease that affects function but produces no tissue damage. 2. A disorder with no known organic basis; some symptoms, such as headache, impotence, certain heart murmurs, and constipation, may be symptoms of either organic or functional disease.

functional dyspepsia   Impaired digestion due to atony or to a neurologic problem.

functional imaging   In nuclear medicine: a diagnostic procedure in which a radioactive tracer administered to the patient delineates a physiologic process in a sequence of radiographic or scintillation camera images.

functional residual capacity (FRC)
The volume of air in the lungs at the end of a normal expiration.

fundal height   The height of the uterine fundus, measured in centimeters, from the top of the symphysis pubis to the highest point in the midline at the top of the uterus; measured at each prenatal visit to determine size and age of the fetus; can also reveal a multiple pregnancy. From the 20th to the 32nd week of pregnancy, the height in centimeters is normally equal to the gestation in weeks.

fundus, *pl.* **fundi**   The base of an organ; the portion of a hollow organ farthest from its mouth, as the fundus of the uterus.

funduscopy   Ophthalmoscopy; the examination of the fundus of the eye using an ophthalmoscope.

fungal infection   An inflammatory condition caused by a fungus, including aspergillosis, blastomycosis, candidiasis, coccidioidomycosis, and histoplasmosis. Most are superficial and mild inflammations of the skin or nails, but systemic disease is possible, especially as opportunistic infections in immunocompromised patients.

fungate   Funguslike growth or growing rapidly, like a fungus.

fungemia   Fungal infection disseminated through the blood.

fungicide   A drug that destroys fungi.

fungus, *pl.* **fungi**   A simple parasitic plant, including mushrooms, yeasts, rusts, and molds, that lacks chlorophyll and has rigid cell walls; unable to make its own food, it is dependent on other life forms. May reproduce by budding or by spore formation.

funiculitis   **1.** An abnormal inflammatory condition of the spermatic cord. **2.** Inflammation of a spinal nerve root within the spinal cord.

FUO   *abbr* fever of undetermined origin.

furosemide   A loop diuretic used to treat hypertension and edema.

furuncle   A boil; a painful nodule in the skin caused by localized staphylococcal infection that originates in a gland or hair follicle. Necrosis in the center of the inflamed area forms a core of dead tissue. Treatment may include antibiotics, local moist heat, or incision and drainage.

furunculosis   Persistent occurrence of successive crops of boils that are caused by staphylococci or streptococci.

fusimotor   Pertaining to the motor nerve fibers that innervate the intrafusal fibers of the muscle spindle.

fusion   **1.** Coordination of the separate images of the object of vision into a single entity. **2.** The operative consolidation of a joint. **3.** The operative joining together of spinal vertebrae to stabilize a segment of the spinal column injured by severe trauma, a herniated disk, or degenerative disease.

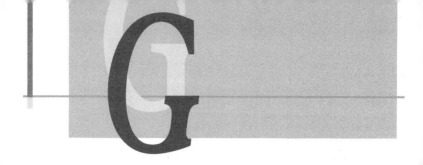

g *abbr* gram.

G *abbr* gauge.

GABA *abbr* gamma-aminobutyric acid.

gadolinium (Gd) A rare element (atomic number, 64; atomic weight, 157.25).

gag reflex A normal reflex elicited by touching the soft palate or the back of the pharynx; response is elevation of the palate, retraction of the tongue, and contraction of the constrictor muscle of the pharynx. Also called *pharyngeal reflex.*

 ALERT If you detect an abnormal gag reflex, immediately stop the patient's oral intake to prevent aspiration. Quickly evaluate his LOC, and if it is decreased, place him in a side-lying position to prevent aspiration.

gait ataxia Unsteady, uncoordinated walk, with a wide base and turned out feet; coming down first on the heel and then on the toes with a double tap.

galactokinase An enzyme that catalyzes the initial step of galactose use; deficiency can result in accumulation of galactitol in the lens and the development of cataracts in infants.

galactokinase deficiency An inborn error of metabolism in which galactokinase is deficient or absent; results in galactosemia, cataracts, hepatomegaly, and mental deficiency.

galactophorous duct Lactiferous duct; a passage that carries milk secreted by the lobes of the breast to and through the nipples.

galactorrhea Excessive flow of milk; lactation not associated with childbirth or nursing.

galactose A simple sugar obtained from lactose by enzymatic action; dextrorotatory form found in lactose, nerve cell membranes, and sugar beets; levorotatory form found in flaxseed mucilage.

galactosemia Any of three inherited disorders of galactose metabolism. Classic galactosemia, the most common of the three, is caused by deficiency of the enzyme galactosy-1-phosphate uridyl transferase and is characterized by cirrhosis of the liver, hepatomegaly, retardation, and cataracts.

Galant reflex A deep abdominal reflex in which the abdominal muscles contract when the top front of the iliac crest is tapped.

gallbladder A pear-shaped excretory sac lodged in a hollow on the surface of the liver; serves as a reservoir for bile; contracts during digestion of fats, ejecting bile through the common bile duct into the duodenum.

gallium A metallic element that is liquid at room temperature; its atomic number is 31; its atomic weight is 69.72.

gallop A cardiac arrhythmia in which one or two extra sounds are heard in diastole on auscultation of the heart; these are related to atrial contraction, early rapid filling of a ventricle, or to a concurrence of these two events.

TIME LINE An atrial gallop may occur normally in children, especially after exercise. However, it may also result from congenital heart disease, such atrial septal defect, ventricular septal defect, patent ductus arteriosis, and severe pulmonary valvular stenosis.

gamete **1.** A mature male or female germ cell. **2.** The ovum or spermatozoon; haploid reproductive cells that unite to initiate the development of a new individual.

gametogenesis Development of the male and female reproductive cells, occurring through meiosis.

gamma-aminobutyric acid (GABA) An amino acid that is the principal inhibitory neurotransmitter in the brain.

gamma efferent fiber A thin axon of a gamma motor nerve fiber that innervates the intrafusal fibers of a muscle spindle.

gamma radiation Electromagnetic emission of high-energy photons from the nucleus of an atom during nuclear reactions.

gamogenesis Sexual reproduction occurring through the fusion of gametes.

ganglion, *pl.* **ganglia** **1.** A knot or knotlike mass. **2.** A group of nerve cells, chiefly those collected in groups outside the central nervous system. **3.** A benign cystic tumor, usually developing on a tendon; consists of a fluid-filled capsule.

gangrene   Death of tissue, usually resulting from ischemia followed by bacterial invasion and putrefaction.

gap junctions   Channels through which ions and other small molecules pass.

Gardner-Diamond syndrome   A condition, usually appearing in women, believed to result from sensitization to one's own erythrocytes, marked by painful, transient bruises that enlarge and involve adjacent tissues.

 CLINICAL TIP The bruises appear without apparent cause but may accompany emotional stress, various collagen disorders, and abnormalities of protein metabolism.

Gardner's syndrome   An inherited disorder marked by development of multiple tumors, including polyposis of the large bowel, fibrous dysplasia of the skull, extra teeth, osteomas, fibromas, and epidermal cysts. Bowel polyps predispose to carcinoma of the colon.

Gardner-Wells tongs   An instrument used to exert traction on the skull and immobilize the cervical vertebrae after injury to the cervical spine.

gas chromatography   A technique used to separate and analyze mixtures of different substances according to differences in their affinities for standard absorbents. The mixture being tested is dissolved, vaporized, and carried by an inert gas through a column containing the sorbent, which may be either an inert porous solid or a nonvolatile liquid coated on a solid support. The speed at which each substance moves depends on its vapor pressure and on its affinity for the sorbent; these differences are graphed by a chart recorder.

gas embolism   Occlusion of a blood vessel by expanding bubbles of gas; may occur after trauma or surgery. Also called *air embolism.*

gastrectomy   Excision of all or part of the stomach.

gastric analysis   Examination of the stomach contents; measures pH and acid output and can also detect presence of blood, bile, bacteria, and abnormal cells.

 ALERT Antacids, anticholinergics, and cimetidine may interfere with test results due to a decrease in gastric secretions or acidity that lowers intraesophageal pH. Likewise, alcohol, cholinergics, reserpine, adrenergic blockers, and corticosteroids may elevate intraesophageal pH as a result of reflux from a relaxed lower esophageal sphincter or increased gastric secretions.

gastric juice   The digestive fluid secreted by the gastric glands in the stomach, consisting chiefly of pepsin, hydrochloric acid, mucin, and intrinsic factor; strongly acid (pH 0.9 to 1.5).

gastric lavage   The irrigation or washing out of the stomach with sterile water or a saline solution.

gastric motility   The spontaneous movements of the stomach, which aid in digestion by moving food through the stomach itself and out through the pyloric sphincter into the duodenum.

gastric node   One of the nodes from two groups along the left and right gastric arteries that receive lymph from the stomach, spleen, pancreas, liver, and duodenum.

gastritis   Inflammation of the stomach and stomach lining.

gastrocnemius   A large superficial muscle in the posterior of the leg; arises from two points of origin on the back and side of the knee and unites with the soleus tendon to form the Achilles tendon; acts to produce plantar flexion of the ankle and to flex the knee.

gastroenteritis   Inflammation of the lining of the stomach and intestines that accompanies numerous gastrointestinal disorders; characterized by anorexia, weakness, abdominal pain, nausea, and diarrhea.

gastroenterologist   A physician who specializes in diseases of the digestive tract.

gastroenterology   The study of the stomach, intestines, gallbladder, and bile duct and of diseases affecting them.

gastroenterostomy   Surgical formation of an anastomosis between the stomach and the intestines, usually at the jejunum.

gastroesophageal reflux   A backflow of the contents of the stomach and duodenum into the esophagus; may occur normally, as after a heavy meal, or may result from incompetence of the lower esophageal sphincter.

gastroschisis   A congenital defect characterized by incomplete abdominal wall closure and usually accompanied by protrusion of parts of the small and large intestines outside the body.

gastroscope   A fiberoptic endoscope used to examine the stomach's interior.

gastrostomy   Creation of an opening into the stomach for the purpose of administering food or fluids.

Gatch bed   A bed that has divided sections, allowing the knees to be flexed with the legs supported or allowing the head to be raised.

Gaucher's disease   A group of rare, familial disorders of fat metabolism that result from deficiency of the enzyme glucocerebrosidase, leading to widespread accumulation of glucocerebroside in the storage cells of the liver, spleen, lymph nodes, alveolaer capillaries, and bone marrow; in its most severe form, presents in infancy and is associated with hepatosplenomegaly, central nervous system impairment, and death.

gauge   Diameter of a needle.

gauntlet bandage   A figure-eight bandage that covers the hand and fingers like a glove.

gavage   Feeding a patient through a stomach tube, either for the purpose of force-feeding or to deliver a high-potency diet.

Gay-Lussac's law   A law that states that under constant pressure, the volume of a specific mass of a gas will increase at a constant rate as the temperature is increased.

Geiger-Müller counter   An electronic device that uses a gas-filled tube to indicate the level of radioactivity of any substance by measuring the emission of ionizing particles.

gel   A colloid with a firm consistency even though it contains a large amount of liquid, used in many medicines as, for example, a vehicle for other drugs, an antacid, or an astringent.

gender   Sex; the classification of a person as male, female, or intersexual.

gene   The biological unit of heredity; a segment of deoxyribonucleic acid containing information required for synthesis of a product.

gene library   In molecular genetics: a random collection of the genetic information from a specific species, obtained from cloned fragments.

general anesthesia   A state marked by absence of pain sensation and unconsciousness, induced by various anesthetic agents given primarily by inhalation or intravenous injection.

generalized anaphylaxis   Anaphylactic shock; a severe manifestation of hypersensitivity in which exposure to an antigen results in life-threatening respiratory distress that may be followed by vascular collapse and shock; accompanied by itching, edema, and urticaria.

generalized tonic-clonic seizure   Grand mal seizure; an epileptic seizure, frequently preceded by an aura, that is characterized by loss of consciousness and muscle spasm (tonic phase), followed by convulsive movement of the limbs (clonic phase).

generation   **1.** Procreation; the process of reproduction. **2.** A group of individuals that are the same number of life cycles from a common ancestor. **3.** The period between the birth of one individual and the birth of its offspring.

generic   **1.** Of or pertaining to a genus. **2.** Of or pertaining to a nonproprietary product or drug, one not protected by trademark. **3.** Of or pertaining to a drug name that is descriptive of the drug's chemical structure.

genesis   **1.** The origin, generation, or development of something; coming into being. **2.** The act of procreating or originating.

gene splicing   Attaching a segment of deoxyribonucleic acid (DNA) from one organism to a strand of DNA from another organism.

genetic   **1.** Pertaining to reproduction, origin, or heredity. **2.** Produced by a gene; inherited.

genetic code   The way in which information is carried by the deoxyribonucleic acid (DNA) molecules to determine the specific amino acids and their arrangement in the polypeptide chain of each protein; represents the sequence of nucleotides along the DNA molecule of each chromosome in the cell. During transcription, this arrangement is carried by messenger ribonucleic acid from the nucleus to the cytoplasm of the cell, where it is translated into protein at the ribosomes.

genetic colonization   The propagation of genetic information by a host into which a gene has been introduced; may be done artificially or by a parasite.

genetic counseling   The process by which an expert in hereditary diseases provides appropriate information to parents or relatives in families with genetic disorders and advice about available courses of action.

genetic homeostasis   The mechanisms that maintain genetic variability within a population through adaptation to changing environments and conditions of life; corrects disturbances in the genetic makeup of the population.

geneticist   One who specializes in the study of genetics.

genetic load   The aggregate of accumulated detrimental genes in the genome of an individual; may be hidden but can be transmitted to descendants and cause disorders. These genes may appear in the genome by mutation and selection within a recent generation or by inheritance.

genetic map   A graphic representation showing the position of genes on a chromosome and the relative distances between them.

genetic marker   A gene with a simple mode of inheritance that produces a readily recognizable genetic trait; can be used in family and population studies or in linkage analysis.

genetics The science of heredity, specifically the means by which traits are passed from parents to offspring.

genome The complete gene complement in the chromosomes of an organism.

genotype 1. The complete genetic constitution of an organism, as determined by the combination and location of the genes on the chromosomes. 2. The alleles situated at one or more sites; each pair of alleles determines a specific characteristic or trait, usually designated by a letter or symbol, such as AA when the alleles are identical and Aa when they differ. 3. A group or class of organisms having the same genetic makeup.

genupectoral position The knee-chest position, in which the patient is prone, kneeling so that the weight of the body is supported by the knees and chest, with the abdomen raised. The arms are flexed and the upper part of the body is supported in part by the elbows.

genu valgum Knock-knee; a deformity in which the knees are close together, knocking as the person walks, and the ankles are widely separated.

genu varum Bowleg; a deformity in which the knees are bent outward and the lower extremities bow inward.

geriatrician A medical specialist in geriatrics.

geriatrics The branch of medicine dealing with aging and the diagnosis and treatment of problems affecting the aged, including senility.

germ 1. A microorganism, especially a pathogenic one. 2. Living matter able to develop into a self-sufficient organism, such as a seed, spore, or egg.

germanium (Ge) A rare metallic element (atomic number, 32; atomic weight, 72.59).

germ cell The cell of an organism whose function is reproductive; any stage of development of such a cell, such as an ovum or spermatozoon or any of their preceding forms.

germination Sprouting of a seed; the initial growth of an organism from the time of fertilization to the formation of the embryo.

germ layer One of the three primordial cell layers — the ectoderm, endoderm, and mesoderm — formed in the early stages of embryonic development from which all body tissues are derived.

gerontology The study of the aging process and of all aspects of the problems of aging

gestate 1. To carry a developing fetus in the womb. 2. To grow and develop slowly toward maturity.

gestation The length of pregnancy in animals that give birth to live young, from fertilization of the ovum until birth. Varies with the species; in humans the average duration is 266 days or approximately 280 days from the onset of the last menstrual period.

gestational age The duration of a pregnancy, usually expressed in completed weeks from the first day of the mother's last menstrual period.

GFR *abbr* glomerular filtration rate.

GH *abbr* growth hormone.

GHRF *abbr* growth hormone releasing factor.

GI *abbr* gastrointestinal.

giant cell myeloma A bone tumor that contains multinucleated giant cells that resemble osteoclasts scattered in a matrix of spindle cells; may cause local pain and tenderness, functional disability, and pathologic fractures.

giant chromosome 1. A large chromosome found in the oocytes of certain lower animals. Also called *lampbrush chromosome*. 2. A stage in the division of chromosomes, in which large bundles of unseparated chromonemata occur; seen in the salivary glands of some insects. Also called *polytene chromosome*.

giant follicular lymphoma A nodular, malignant lymphoma characterized by clusters of lymphomatous cells in multiple nodules within the lymph nodes.

giardiasis A common inflammation of the intestine caused by the protozoan *Giardia lamblia*, spread by person-to-person contact or via contaminated water.

Gibson murmur Continuous murmur heard throughout systole and diastole in older children and adults due to shunting of blood from the aorta into the pulmonary artery.

Giemsa's stain An azure dye used in the microscopic examination of the blood to detect protozoan parasites, such as *Plasmodium* and *Trypanosoma*, viral inclusion bodies, and *Chlamydia*; also used routinely in the preparation of a smear for a differential white cell count.

gigantism A condition characterized by abnormal stature or overgrowth of the body or any of its parts; caused most frequently by oversecretion of pituitary growth hormone.

Gilbert syndrome An inborn error of metabolism that results in benign hyperbilirubinemia and jaundice.

Gilles de la Tourette's syndrome An abnormal condition with onset in childhood characterized by facial and verbal tics and involuntary arm and shoulder movements that can progress to generalized jerking movements.

gingiva, *pl.* gingivae The gums; portion of the oral mucosa that acts as supportive tissue for the teeth; covers the crowns of unerupted teeth and encircles the necks of erupted teeth.

gingivitis Inflammation of the gums characterized by swollen appearance and bleeding.

gland A group of specialized cells that secrete or excrete materials not related to their ordinary metabolic needs.

glans, *pl.* glandes A small, rounded mass, or glandlike body.

glans of clitoris A small mass of erectile tissue at the end of the clitoris, continuous with the intermediate part of the vaginal vestibular bulbs.

glans penis The conical tip of the penis; an expansion of the corpus spongiosum that covers the head of the penis.

Glasgow coma scale A scale used to determine a patient's level of consciousness; It is used primarily on head trauma or stroke patients.

glaucoma A group of eye diseases characterized by abnormally elevated pressure within the eye due to obstruction of the outflow of aqueous humor.

gliding joint A plane joint; a type of synovial joint that allows only gliding movements of the opposing bones, as in the intermetacarpal joints.

glioma, *pl.* gliomas, gliomata 1. A tumor made of neuroglial tissue. 2. Any of the primary tumors of the brain, including astrocytoma, ependymoma, glioblastoma multiforme, medulloblastoma, and oligodendroglioma.

gliosarcoma, *pl.* gliosarcomas, gliosarcomata A tumor composed of immature spindle-shaped cells with large nuclei in the supporting connective tissue of nerve cells.

Glisson's sling An apparatus used to apply traction to the cervical spine; made up of a leather collar for the neck and chin, which is attached to weights and a pulley.

globulin One of a class of proteins that precipitate from plasma on saturation with ammonium sulfate; may be fractionated by solubility, electrophoretic mobility, and size into many subgroups.

glomerulonephritis A bilateral inflammation of the glomeruli, often following a streptococcal infection.

glossitis Inflammation of the tongue; results in pain or a burning sensation and sensitivity to hot foods.

glossopharyngeal Of or pertaining to the tongue and pharynx.

glossoplasty A surgical procedure on the tongue performed to correct a congenital anomaly, repair an injury, or restore function after excision of a malignant lesion.

glossopyrosis A burning sensation in the tongue with no lesions apparent in the painful area.

glossorrhaphy The suturing of a tongue wound.

glossotrichia Hairy tongue; a condition of the tongue in which the filiform papillae elongate, resulting in a furry appearance.

glottis, *pl.* glottises, glottides The vocal apparatus, made up of the true vocal cords and the slitlike opening between them.

glucagon A hormone secreted by the alpha cells of the islets of Langerhans in the pancreas that stimulates the conversion of glycogen to glucose in the liver.

glucagonoma syndrome A disorder resulting from a glucagon-secreting tumor of the pancreatic islet cells, characterized by hyperglycemia, stomatitis, anemia, weight loss, and a characteristic migratory rash.

glucocorticoid A corticosteroid that primarily affects carbohydrate metabolism by promoting gluconeogenesis, liver glycogen deposition, and increased blood glucose; also affects muscle tone, helps maintain arterial pressure, exerts anti-inflammatory effects, and influences many other body functions.

gluconeogenesis The formation of glucose from noncarbohydrate molecules, such as amino acids or lactate.

glucose A simple sugar found in certain foods, especially fruits; the end product of carbohydrate metabolism and the chief energy source in living organisms.

glucose-6-phosphate dehydrogenase (G6PD) deficiency The most common of the inborn errors of metabolism; an inherited disorder in which red blood cells are partially or completely deficient in glucose-6-phosphate dehydrogenase, a critical enzyme in the metabolism of glucose; causes a hemolytic anemia.

glucosuria Abnormal presence of glucose in the urine; may result from ingestion of large amounts of carbohydrate or from a kidney or metabolic disease.

glutamic acid A nonessential amino acid found in proteins; acts as an excitatory neurotransmitter.

glutamic-oxaloacetic transaminase (GOT) Aspartate aminotransferase; an enzyme that catalyzes a reaction in the liver that transfers excess nitrogen into aspartate for disposal; it is also normally present in most body cells and is released into the blood when tissue damage occurs.

glutamic-pyruvic transaminase (GPT) Alanine aminotranferase; an enzyme that acts to catalyze a reaction that results in nitrogen transfer; normally found in the serum and body tissues, especially the liver; activity is increased in presence of liver disease.

gluteal tuberosity A ridge on the lateral posterior surface of the femur; the point of insertion of the gluteus maximus.

gluten The protein constituent of wheat and other grains that makes dough elastic.

glycerol The alcohol component of fats, soluble in ethyl alcohol and water; formed in the metabolism of fatty acids.

glycine Aminoacetic acid; a nonessential amino acid that occurs as a component of many proteins; believed to be a neurotransmitter.

glycogen A polysaccharide found in the liver that is the chief form of carbohydrate stored in animal cells.

glycogenesis The formation or synthesis of glycogen from glucose.

glycogenolysis In metabolism, the body's mobilization and conversion of glycogen to glucose.

glycolic acid Hydroxyacetic acid; an intermediate active in the conversion of serine to glycine; aids digestion and fat absorption.

glycolysis The anaerobic enzymatically catalyzed reactions by which glucose and other sugars are converted to lactic acid or pyruvic acid, releasing energy in the form of adenosine triphosphate.

glycoside Any compound containing a sugar, especially those that yield a sugar and a nonsugar component on hydrolysis.

glycosuria Abnormal presence of glucose in the urine; can result from ingesting large amounts of carbohydrate or from endocrine or renal disorders.

 ALERT High dietary vitamin C intake may give a false negative for the presence of glucose in the urine.

glycosuric acid Homogentisic acid; an intermediate product of phenylalanine and tyrosine metabolism present as a melanin-like material in the urine of people who have alkaptonuria.

goblet cell A specialized mucus gland of the epithelium of the respiratory passages, stomach, and intestine; shaped like a goblet because droplets of mucigen collect in one end of the cell and distend it.

goiter Enlarged thyroid gland, usually evident as a pronounced swelling in the front of the neck.

gold (Au) A yellow, soft metallic element that occurs naturally as a free metal. Its

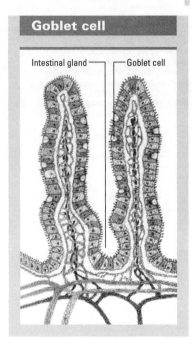

Goblet cell

Intestinal gland ——— Goblet cell

atomic number is 79; its atomic weight is 197. Compounds of the element are used to treat arthritis.

Golgi apparatus A complex membranous system within cells, composed of several flattened sacs, vacuoles, and vesicles; the sites of formation of the carbohydrate side chains of glycoproteins, mucopolysaccharides, and other substances. Also called *Golgi complex.*

Golgi-Mazzoni corpuscles Thin capsules found in the subcutaneous tissue of the fingers; they envelop the terminal nerve fibrils.

gonad An organ that produces gametes, such as an ovary or a testis.

gonadotropin, gonadotrophin Any hormone that stimulates gonadal function, such as follicle-stimulating hormone and luteinizing hormone.

gonorrhea A common sexually transmitted disease most often affecting the genitourinary tract and, occasionally, the pharynx, conjunctiva, or rectum; caused by *Neisseria gonorrhoeae.*

gonorrheal conjunctivitis A destructive form of purulent conjunctivitis caused by infection by *Neisseria gonorrhoeae;* can be seen bilaterally in newborns of infected mothers. May result in corneal scarring and blindness if untreated.

Goodell's sign   Softening of the cervix, a probable sign of pregnancy.

Goodpasture's syndrome   Glomeru-lonephritis associated with hemoptysis; produces pulmonary hemosiderosis, progressive renal failure, and death.

Gordon reflex   **1.** An abnormal variation of the Babinski reflex, elicited by compressing the calf muscles, characterized by extension of the great toe and fanning of the other toes. It is evidence of disease of the pyramidal tract. **2.** An abnormal reflex, elicited by compressing the forearm muscles, characterized by flexion of the fingers or of the thumb and index finger. It is seen in diseases of the pyramidal tract.

Gordon's elementary body   A particle found in all tissues that contain eosinophils; once thought to be the viral cause of Hodgkin's disease.

GOT   *abbr* glutamine-oxaloacetic transaminase.

gout   A group of disorders associated with inborn errors of metabolism that affect purine and pyrimidine use; results in increased production of uric acid or interferes with its excretion. Manifested by hyperuricemia, recurrent acute inflammatory arthritis, deposition of urate crystals in the joints of the extremities, and uric acid urolithiasis.

GP   *abbr* general practitioner.

GPT   *abbr* glutamic-pyruvic transaminase.

gr   *abbr* grain.

graafian follicle   A mature ovarian vesicle containing an ovum; ruptures during ovulation to release the ovum.

grace period   In general, any period specified in a contract during which payment is permitted, without penalty, beyond the due date of the debt.

gracile   Slender and graceful.

graft   **1.** Any tissue or organ taken from one site or person and implanted into another to repair a defect. **2.** To implant or transplant tissue.

graft-versus-host (GVH) reaction   An immune response of donor cells against the host tissue; occurs commonly in bone marrow transplant and maternal-fetal blood transfusion. Also called *graft-versus-host disease*.

grain (gr)   The smallest unit of mass in avoirdupois, troy, and apothecaries' weights, equal to 0.06479891 gram. The troy and apothecaries' ounces contain 480 grains; the avoirdupois ounce contains 437.5 grains.

gram (g)   The basic unit of mass in the metric system; equal to 1/1000 of a kilogram, 15.432 grains, and 0.03 ounce avoirdupois.

gram-negative   Being decolorized or losing the stain in Gram's method of staining microorganisms; characteristic of bacterial cell wall composed of a thin peptidoglycan layer covered by a lipoprotein and lipopolysaccharide layer.

gram-positive   Resisting decoloration or retaining the violet color of the stain used in Gram's method of staining microorganisms.

Gram stain   The method of differential staining of microorganisms using a violet stain followed by an iodine solution, decolorizing with an alcohol or acetone solution, and counterstaining with safranin.

grandfather clause   A provision permitting persons engaged in an activity before passage of a law affecting that activity to receive a license without having to meet the new requirements.

granulocyte   A cell containing granules, especially a leukocyte that contains basophil, eosinophil, or neutrophil granules in its cytoplasm.

granulocytopenia   A severely low granulocyte level.

granuloma, *pl.* **granulomas, granulomata**   A mass of nodular granulation tissue that represents a chronic inflammatory response to injury or infection.

grasp reflex   A reflex induced by stroking the palm or sole; the fingers or toes flex in a grasping motion.

Graves' disease   A disorder of the thyroid characterized by pronounced thyrotoxicosis usually associated with an enlarged thyroid gland, exophthalmos, or pretibial myxedema.

> **ALERT** Carefully monitor cardiac function if the patient is elderly or has coronary artery disease. If heart rate is more than 100 beats/minute, check blood pressure and pulse often.

gravid   Pregnant; carrying developing young.

gravity   The force of attraction at the surface of the earth or other object.

grievance   A complaint about working conditions or contract violations brought by an employee or union against an employer.

Groshong catheter   A common tunneled catheter, which has a pressure-sensitive valve in the tip that keeps the lumen closed when not in use; also opening inward during blood aspiration and outward during blood or fluid administration, eliminating the need for heparin flushes.

gross   Large; visible to the naked eye, as gross anatomy (the study of organs or parts of the body) or gross pathology (the study of tissue changes without the use of magnification).

gross negligence   The flagrant and inexcusable failure to perform a legal duty in reckless disregard of the consequences.

growth hormone (GH)   Somatotropin; a protein hormone secreted by the anterior pituitary in response to growth hormone releasing factor from the hypothalamus; promotes body growth and fat mobilization and inhibits glucose utilization.

Grünfelder's reflex   Dorsal flexion of the great toe with a fanlike spreading of the other toes, caused by continued pressure on the posterior lateral fontanel; seen in young children with middle-ear disease.

grunting   Short, audible breaks in exhalation that are sometimes associated with severe chest pain. The grunt occurs when the glottis briefly stops airflow, halting movement of lungs and surrounding structures.

ALERT Grunting respirations indicate intrathoracic disease with lower respiratory involvement. Though most common in children, they sometimes occur in adults during severe respiratory distress. They demand immediate medical attention, especially when combined with wheezing, tachycardia, accessory muscle use, hypotension, cyanosis, and decreased LOC.

gtt   *abbr* drops.

GTT   *abbr* glucose tolerance test.

GU   *abbr* genitourinary.

guide wire   A device that stiffens a catheter to ease its advancement through a vein. This device can damage the vein if used incorrectly.

Guillain-Barré syndrome   An acute febrile polyneuritis that occurs after a viral infection; marked by rapidly ascending paralysis that begins as paresthesia of the feet.

gynecology   The branch of medicine concerned with the health care of women, including sexual and reproductive function and diseases of the reproductive organs.

gynecomastia, gynecomasty   Enlargement and development of the mammary glands in men, usually temporary and benign.

TIME LINE In newborns, gynecomastia may be associated with galactorrhea ("witch's milk"). This sign usually disappears within a few weeks but may persist until age 2. Most males have physiologic gynecomastia at some time during adolescence, usually around age 14. It is typically asymmetrical and tender, resolving within 2 years and rarely persisting beyond age 20.

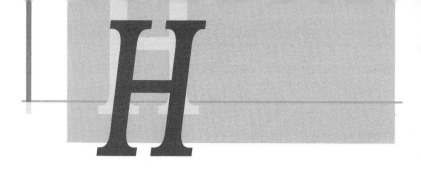

habituation 1. A decrease in responsiveness resulting from repeated exposure to a stimulus. 2. Tolerance to the effects of a drug from repeated or continuous use. 3. Psychological dependence on a substance or other stimulus.

Haemophilus A genus of nonmotile, gram-negative bacteria that are aerobic or facultatively aerobic. *Haemophilus* bacteria grow best or can only thrive in media containing blood. These organisms may cause disease but are also found as part of the normal flora in the respiratory tracts of vertebrates.

Haemophilus influenzae A species of *Haemophilus* bacteria found in the respiratory tract. In humans, the bacillus causes respiratory tract infections, conjunctivitis, and purulent meningitis.

hafnium (Hf) A metallic element with an atomic weight of 178.49 (atomic number 72) that readily absorbs neutrons.

Hagedorn needle A curved surgical needle with flat sides and an exceptionally large eye.

hairy-cell leukemia A rare form of lymphocytic leukemia characterized by the appearance of malignant cells with numerous hairlike projections in the blood, bone marrow, and spleen.

halitosis Foul-smelling breath that may be caused by inadequate cleaning of the mouth and teeth, infections in the mouth, the ingestion of pungent foods (such as garlic), the use of alcohol or tobacco, or certain gastrointestinal problems.

TIME LINE In children, halitosis commonly results from thumb or blanket sucking or mouth breathing. However, phenylketonuria (PKU), a metabolic disorder that affects infants, may produce a musty or mousy breath odor.

Halsted's forceps A small, straight or curved hemostat used for clamping small blood vessels to halt bleeding or to hold delicate tissue.

hamartoma Benign, tumorlike nodule composed of an overgrowth of mature cells

and tissues normally present in the affected part.

hanging drop preparation A laboratory technique in which a drop of culture medium is placed on a coverslip and is suspended over the depression in a specially designed glass slide.

haploid Having half the number of chromosomes that are normally found in somatic cells (in humans, the diploid number is 46 and the haploid number is 23). Germ cells, eggs, and sperm are haploid cells.

haptoglobin A group of proteins found in human blood that combine with free hemoglobin.

hard palate The bony, front portion of the roof of the mouth.

harelip A congenital malformation in which the maxillary and median nasal processes fail to close normally at one or more sites on the lip (usually the upper lip). Also called *cleft lip.*

Hashimoto's disease An inflammation of the thyroid gland, caused by an autoimmune disorder, in which lymphocytes infiltrate the thyroid and cause destruction of thyroid tissue and hypothyroidism.

haversian canal Any one of the small canals or channels in the haversian system of compact bone.

Hawthorne effect An observed improvement in the quantity or quality of output of an individual or group of people that is stimulated by the mere fact that they are being observed.

Hb A *abbr* hemoglobin A.
Hb C *abbr* hemoglobin C.
Hb F *abbr* hemoglobin F.
HBIG *abbr* hepatitis B immune globulin.
Hb S *abbr* hemoglobin S.
HBsAG *abbr* hepatitis B surface antigen.
Hb S-C *abbr* hemoglobin S-C.
HCG *abbr* human chorionic gonadotropin.
HCl *abbr* hydrochloric acid.
HCT *abbr* hematocrit.
HDL *abbr* high-density lipoprotein.
He Symbol for helium.

Heaf test A tuberculin skin test using a multiple-puncture technique.

Healing Touch A form of energetic healing, developed by nurses in the 1980s, based on the concept of a human energy field. By moving her hands over the patient's body, the nurse theoretically realigns the patient's energy flow and reactivates the mind-body-spirit connection that ultimately allows self-healing.

health maintenance organization (HMO) An organization that provides basic and supplemental health maintenance and treatment services to voluntary enrollees who prepay fixed, periodic fees set without regard to the amount or kind of services received. HMO enrollees are cared for by member primary physicians with limited referral to outside specialists.

heart murmur An abnormal heart sound, detectable on auscultation with a stethoscope, that results from the flow of blood through one of the openings between the heart's chambers.

CLINICAL TIP A murmur may (but does not always) indicate a health problem, such as a narrowing of the openings or failure of the valves to close completely.

heart rate The number of times the heart beats in one minute.

heart sound A sound that can be detected on auscultation with a stethoscope that results from the closure of the heart valves. The first and second heart sounds (heard as "lub" and "dub" sounds) are normal; additional sounds may indicate the presence of a cardiac disorder.

heart valve One of the four structures located at the openings between the chambers of the heart that control the flow of blood from one chamber to the next and prevent the backflow of blood into the previous chamber. The four valves are the atrial, pulmonic, tricuspid, and mitral.

heat cramp A painful spasm of a muscle (usually in the arms, legs, or abdomen) caused by overexertion in hot weather; in some cases, cramping is related to dehydration and salt deficiency caused by excessive sweating.

heat exhaustion Extreme weakness, dizziness, heat cramps, and sometimes loss of consciousness caused by severe dehydration during exposure to intense heat (as during spells of extremely hot, dry weather).

heat hyperpyrexia A severe and, in many cases, fatal condition caused by prolonged exposure to excessively high atmospheric temperatures, particularly when overexertion is a factor. The signs and symptoms include headache, dizziness, confusion, and hot, dry skin; in severe cases, collapse, coma, and tachycardia may develop. Also called *heat apoplexy, heatstroke, malignant hyperpyrexia.*

Heberden node A hard, pea-sized growth that occurs at the tip of a finger, usually seen in patients with osteoarthritis.

HEENT *abbr* head, eyes, ears, nose, and throat.

Hegar's sign A softening of the lower portion of the uterus that occurs at about the seventh week of pregnancy and is considered an early sign of possible pregnancy.

height The distance between the bottom and top of an object, structure, or organ measured in an upright position.

helium (He) An extremely light (atomic weight 4, atomic number 2), colorless, nonflammable, odorless gas that is mixed with air and oxygen in the treatment of various respiratory disorders.

helix 1. A line in the shape of a spring, the form in which many organic molecules are organized (such as the double-helix formation of deoxyribonucleic acid). 2. The rim of cartilage that forms the margin of the external portion of the ear.

HELLP *abbr* hemolysis, elevated liver enzymes, low platelets.

helminth An intestinal parasitic worm, primarily a roundworm, tapeworm, or fluke.

hemadsorption The adherence of a substance or agent to the surface of a red blood cell.

hemangioma, *pl.* hemangiomas, hemangiomata A congenital malformation in which a mass of small blood vessels proliferate and form a tumorlike mass, usually in the skin or subcutaneous tissue.

hemapheresis Collection and removal of specific blood components from the blood, then return of the remaining constituents to the patient.

hematemesis The vomiting of blood.

hematinic 1. Of or relating to an improvement in the condition of the blood. 2. An agent that increases the number of red blood cells, increases the hemoglobin concentration, or both.

hematochezia The passage of bloody stools.

hematocrit 1. The solid contents of the blood. 2. The volume of packed blood cells in a given amount of blood, measured after centrifugation; the hematocrit value is expressed as a percentage of total blood volume. The normal range for men is 40% to 54%; for women, 37% to 47%.

hematologist A person who specializes in the study of blood and blood-forming tissues.

hematology The study of blood and blood-forming tissues.

hematoma, *pl.* **hematomas, hematomata** A mass of blood that has accumulated in an organ, tissue, or space after a break in a blood vessel, resulting from an injury or bleeding following surgery.

hematopoiesis The process in which blood cells and other blood elements form and develop. Also called *hemopoiesis, sanguification.*

hematuria The presence of blood in the urine.

heme The oxygen- and pigment-carrying portion of hemoglobin.

hemicrania **1.** A migraine headache. **2.** Any headache that is felt in only one side of the head.

hemisphere **1.** One-half of any sphere or globular object or structure. **2.** In the brain: one side of the cerebrum or cerebellum.

hemochromatosis A rare disorder in which iron accumulates in the tissues and organs, especially the liver, pancreas, and skin. This may result in cirrhosis of the liver, diabetes, and heart failure.

 CLINICAL TIP Hemochromatosis also may be acquired by excessive ingestion or injection of iron.

hemodialysis A procedure, most commonly used in treating patients with defective or absent kidney function, in which chemical substances or wastes are removed from the blood. Hemodialysis is also used to clear toxic chemicals or drugs from the blood.

hemolysis The destruction of red blood cells and the release of hemoglobin into the fluid medium surrounding them, which may occur after exposure to bacterial toxins, the venom of certain snakes, or certain immune bodies, or following injection of hypotonic saline solutions.

hemolytic anemia Anemia resulting from the breakdown of red blood cells.

hemolytic reaction A life-threatening reaction to a blood transfusion that occurs as a result of incompatible ABO or Rh factors or improper blood storage.

hemolytic uremic syndrome A rare disease characterized by hemolytic anemia, thrombocytopenia, and acute renal failure.

hemophilia A bleeding disorder characterized by a failure of the blood clotting mechanism. It is an inherited condition occurring almost exclusively in males.

hemoptysis The coughing or spitting up of blood caused by hemorrhage in the lungs

or bronchi. Minor amounts of blood may appear in the sputum of individuals with bronchitis or upper respiratory tract infections.

 ALERT Massive hemoptysis can cause airway obstruction and asphyxiation. If the patient coughs up copious amounts of blood, endotracheal intubation may be required. Monitor blood pressure and pulse to detect hypotension.

hemorrhage The loss of blood from internal or surface blood vessels. The term is usually used to denote significant, rapid bleeding.

hemorrhagic fever A disease caused by infection with an arbovirus, characterized by a variety of flulike symptoms that may be followed by scattered bleeding from the capillaries and other internal bleeding, kidney damage, and neurologic complications; the disease is sometimes fatal.

hemorrhagic shock Shock resulting from the acute, severe loss of blood, characterized by physical collapse, tachycardia, hypotension, and skin that is pale, cold, and clammy.

hemorrhoid Bulging of the external vein of the rectum or anus, which results in swelling and pain.

hemosiderosis An accumulation of the blood protein hemosiderin in the tissues.

hemostasis The cessation of bleeding, either through the natural process of coagulation or by mechanical or chemical intervention.

hemostat **1.** A device used to clamp blood vessels to halt bleeding, usually during surgery. **2.** Any mechanical or chemical agent that stops the flow of blood from a vessel.

hemostatic Of or relating to natural hemostasis or to any mechanical or chemical agent that stops the flow of blood from a vessel.

hemothorax The accumulation of blood in the pleural cavity, resulting from a traumatic injury or from the rupture of small blood vessels in individuals with inflammatory or malignant diseases of the lungs.

Henry's law In physics: a law stating that the solubility of a gas in a liquid is proportional to the pressure of the gas if the temperature is constant and if the gas does not chemically react with the liquid.

hepatic coma A coma occurring in individuals with severe liver disease or damage, including cirrhosis, hepatitis, and poisoning.

hepatitis Inflammation of the liver, usually due to a viral infection but may also result from exposure to toxic agents.

hepatitis A Inflammation of the liver from infection with the hepatitis A virus, typically involving the gradual onset of signs and symptoms.

hepatitis B Inflammation of the liver from infection with the hepatitis B virus, typically involving the rapid onset of signs and symptoms.

hepatitis B immune globulin (HBIG) An agent that provides passive immunity after an individual has been exposed to the hepatitis B virus.

hepatitis B surface antigen (HBsAG) An antigen that develops in individuals who become infected with the hepatitis B virus or who are carriers of the virus. Also called *Australia antigen*.

hepatization A process by which loose tissue is converted into a solid mass of the consistency of the liver. The term is usually used in reference to lung tissue that undergoes such a transformation due to pneumonia.

hepatojugular reflux Distention of the jugular vein induced by manual pressure over the liver.

hepatoma Any tumor of the liver.

hepatomegaly Enlargement of the liver.

hepatotoxicity The ability of any substance, including ethyl alcohol and certain drugs, to damage the liver.

herbal medicine The use of plants for healing purposes, dating back to the ancient cultures of Egypt, China, and India, and possibly prehistoric time. Currently, more than 25% of conventional drugs are derived from herbs; about 80% of the world's population uses herbal remedies.

heredity The transmission from ancestors to descendants, through the genes, of realized or potential traits or characteristics.

herniated disk The abnormal protrusion of a portion of a degenerated or fragmented intervertebral disk into the spinal canal or the intervertebral foramen.

herniation The rupture of a structure or part of a structure through the tissue in which it is normally enclosed.

herpes An infection caused by a virus; usually used as a shorthand term referring to herpes simplex infections.

herpes genitalis Herpes simplex occurring on the skin and mucous membranes of the genitals, considered to be a sexually transmitted disease. Most commonly, infection is with herpesvirus type 2 (also called type 2 herpes simplex virus, or HSV-2), but infection with herpesvirus type 1 is not unusual.

herpes simplex An infection caused by herpesvirus type 1 or type 2, characterized by painful, itching lesions consisting of tiny blisters. The most common sites are the areas on and around the mouth and on the skin and mucous membranes of the genitals. Recurrences of lesions are common and have been associated with physiologic events, such as sunburn and fever, and emotional stress. Also called *fever blisters, fever sores*.

herpes zoster An acute infection characterized by pain resulting from the inflammation of ganglia and dorsal nerve roots as well as the eruption of painful blistering lesions that occur on one side of the body, following the course of a nerve. The infectious agent is a herpesvirus, the varicella-zoster virus (V-ZV). Commonly called *shingles*.

herpetiform 1. Resembling herpes. 2. A lesion characterized by clusters of blisters, similar to the lesions that occur in individuals with herpes simplex.

hertz (Hz) A unit frequency that equals 1 cycle per second.

hesperidin A crystalline glycoside found in unripe citrus fruits, particularly in the peel of an orange.

heteroallele One of a pair of genes at a specific locus on homologous chromosomes that differs from the other of the pair, resulting in a mutation.

heterochromatin That portion of chromosome material that is inactive in gene expression but may function in controlling metabolic activities, transcription, and cell division.

heterogeneous Characterized by variety and dissimilarity in characteristics or properties.

heterozygosis Development of a zygote by the joining of two gametes with dissimilar pairs of genes.

heterozygous Genes with different alleles at the same site (locus).

Hf Symbol for hafnium.

HF *abbr* Hageman factor.

HFPPV *abbr* high-frequency positive-pressure ventilation.

Hg Symbol for mercury.

HHNS *abbr* hyperosmolar hyperglycemic nonketotic syndrome.

hiatal hernia Rupture of part of the stomach through the esophageal opening in the diaphragm.

hidrosis The production and excretion of sweat.

high-density lipoprotein (HDL) A fraction of the lipid and protein complexes found in the blood that is cholesterol-poor and protein rich, compared with lower-density fractions. A high level of high-density lipoprotein is associated with a reduced risk for atherosclerosis.

high-energy phosphate compound A chemical compound containing a high-energy bond between phosphoric acid residues and certain organic substances.

high forceps delivery   A procedure in which obstetric forceps are applied to a baby's head before it is engaged in the birth canal; not an accepted procedure.

high Fowler's position   Placement of the patient in a semisitting position by raising the head of the bed more than 20" (51 cm).

hilum, *pl.* hila   The area in an organ at which nerves and vessels enter and leave.

hinge joint   A joint in which the convex end of one bone corresponds to the concave end of another bone, allowing motion in only one plane. The elbow is an example of a hinge joint. Also called *ginglymus.*

hirsutism   The presence, especially in women, of excess hair on the face and body, usually in a male pattern; may be a normal, inherited trait, or may occur from a metabolic or hormonal disorder or from exposure to certain drugs.

 TIME LINE Hirsutism can occur after menopause if peripheral conversion of estrogen is poor.

histamine   A chemical compound found in all tissues that causes capillary dilation, smooth-muscle contraction, reduction in blood pressure, and secretion of gastric acid. Histamine is formed and released during allergic reactions.

histocompatibility   A state in which tissues are sufficiently similar to allow a successful transplant of an organ or tissue.

histogram   A column or bar graph that compares variables by frequency of occurrence.

histography   The process of describing tissues and cells.

histologist   A specialist in histology.

histology   The microscopic study of the structure of cells, tissues, and organs in relation to their function.

HIV   *abbr* human immunodeficiency virus.

HLA-A   *abbr* human leukocyte antigen A.

HLA-B   *abbr* human leukocyte antigen B.

HLA-D   *abbr* human leukocyte antigen D.

HLA-L   *abbr* human leukocyte antigen L.

HMO   *abbr* health maintenance organization.

Ho   Symbol for holmium.

H$_0$ Symbol for null hypothesis.

Hodgkin's disease   Cancer of the lymphoid cells, characterized by the progressive enlargement of the lymph nodes, spleen, and sometimes the liver and by gradually worsening anemia.

Hoffmann's reflex   The flexion of the tip of the thumb and of the second and third phalanges of one or more of the fingers when the nail on the first, second, or third fingers is flicked.

holism   The belief that an integrated whole has a reality independent of and greater than the sum of the parts; the basis for holistic nursing.

Homan's sign   The occurrence of pain in the calf or back of the knee when the ankle is slowly dorsiflexed, which may indicate the presence of a thrombosis in a leg vein or inflammation of a calf muscle.

homeopathy   Based on the theory that "like cures like," a method of healing in which minute quantities of a substance that produces certain symptoms in a healthy person are given to a sick person to cure those same symptoms. Homeopathic remedies are thought to stimulate the body's ability to heal itself.

homeostasis   A state of equilibrium in bodily functions and in the chemical composition of the fluids and tissues.

homeotypic, homeotypical   Of or relating to the usual type.

homogenesis   The production of offspring that resemble the parents; the opposite of heterogenesis.

homogeny   Homogenesis.

homolog, homologue   A body structure, chemical compound, tissue, or serum that has the quality of being homologous.

homologous   1. Relating to biological structures that are similar in form and origin, although not necessarily in function. 2. Pertaining to chemical compounds in a series that differ from each other in specific increments. 3. Denoting tissue or serum obtained from members of the same species.

homologous chromosomes   Members of any pair of chromosomes.

homoplasy   A corresponding likeness in parts or organs that results from parallel evolution or exposure to similar environments rather than from a common ancestry.

homozygosis   1. The formation of a zygote by the joining of two gametes that have one or more pairs of identical genes. 2. The production of purebred organisms or strains through inbreeding.

hordeolum   The inflammation of the sebaceous gland of the eyelid that results in a pus-filled lesion. Also called *sty.*

hormone   A chemical substance produced in the body that has a specific regulatory effect on activities of target cells or organs.

hospice   A system of family-centered care designed to assist the chronically ill person to be comfortable and to maintain a satisfactory lifestyle through the terminal phases of dying. Hospice care is multidisciplinary and includes home visits, professional medical help on call, teaching and emotional support of the family, and physical care of the client. Some hospice programs provide care in a nursing center, as well as at home.

host An organism on which a parasite lives and from which the parasite obtains its nourishment.

Howell-Jolly bodies Spherical or ovoid granules that may occasionally be seen on microscopic examination of red blood cells that have been stained with dyes.

 CLINICAL TIP Howell-Jolly bodies are observed most commonly in individuals who have undergone splenectomy.

HPL *abbr* human placental lactogen.

HSV *abbr* herpes simplex virus.

Hubbard tank A large tank used for underwater exercise and burn debridement.

human leukocyte antigen (HLA) The gene products of any of four loci on the sixth chromosome (designated HLA-A, HLA-B, HLA-C, and HLA-D) that are linked to certain diseases as well as histocompatibility.

 ALERT Recent blood transfusions may interfere with tests results.

human placental lactogen (HPL) An agent found in human placentas that is structurally similar to the growth hormone, somatotropin, and resembles somatotropin and prolactin in biological activity.

humoral immunity Immunity that develops in response to exposure to antigens and that is associated with antibodies that circulate in serum.

humoral response One of a broad category of hypersensitivity reactions. Humoral responses are mediated by B-cell lymphocytes and occur in type I, type II, and type III hypersensitivity reactions.

Hutchinson's triad The three signs that indicate the presence of congenital syphilis: inflammation of the middle and posterior layers of the corneas (parenchymatous keratitis); disease of the inner ear that results in hearing loss; and malformed, characteristically notched teeth.

hyaline cartilage The smooth, translucent cartilage that covers the ends of bones at the joints. Also called *true cartilage.*

hybrid **1.** The offspring of two plants or animals of different races, breeds, genera, or species. **2.** Of or relating to such offspring.

hydatid mole, hydatidiform mole A usually benign neoplasm that occurs at the end of a degenerating pregnancy and arises from enlarged chorionic villi and the proliferation of trophoblastic tissue.

hydramnios Presence of an excess volume of amniotic fluid during pregnancy.

hydrocarbon One of a group of hydrogen-carbon compounds; usually associated with environmental pollution because many hydrocarbons are released into the atmosphere as a result of combustion of petroleum-derived automotive and other fuels.

hydrocephalus, hydrocephaly A condition in which fluid accumulates within the skull, causing dilation of the ventricles of the cerebrum and separation of the cranial bones; also associated with thinning brain tissue.

hydrogen (H) A colorless, odorless, highly inflammable gas; the simplest and lightest element, with an atomic number of 1 and an atomic weight of 1.008.

hydrometer An instrument that measures the specific gravity (and, therefore, the strength) of a liquid by comparing its weight with that of the same amount of water.

hydronephrosis The dilation of the renal pelvis and calyx as a result of obstructed urinary flow in a ureter.

hydrops An accumulation of excess clear, watery fluid in any body cavity or tissue.

hydrops fetalis An abnormal accumulation of serous fluid in the tissues of a fetus, such as in erythroblastosis fetalis.

hymen A thin fold of membranous tissue that partly covers the vaginal opening.

hyoid bone A U-shaped bone that is suspended from the styloid processes of the temporal bones and lies between the mandible and the larynx. See illustration on page 152.

hyperbilirubinemia An abnormally increased amount of bilirubin in the blood, resulting in jaundice when the concentration is high enough.

hypercalcemia An abnormally increased amount of calcium compounds or an elevated level of calcium ions in the blood.

hypercapnia An abnormally increased amount of carbon dioxide in the blood.

hypercholesterolemia A disorder characterized by an abnormally increased amount of cholesterol in the blood.

hyperchromic **1.** Having increased chromatin. **2.** Having an abnormally high color or being overpigmented. **3.** Showing increased staining capacity.

hypercoagulability A tendency of the blood to coagulate more readily than is normal.

hyperemesis gravidarum Severe and prolonged vomiting during pregnancy to such a degree that weight loss and an imbalance of fluids and electrolytes occur.

hypergenesis Excessive development or the development of redundant (supernumerary) organs or body parts.

Hyoid bone

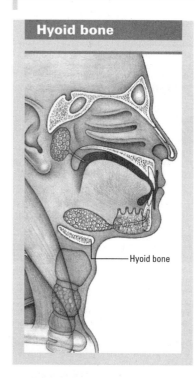

Hyoid bone

hyperglycemia   An abnormally increased amount of glucose in the blood. The term is usually associated with diabetes mellitus.

hyperhidrosis   Excessive secretion of sweat.

hyperkalemia   Excessive serum potassium level.

hyperlipoproteinemia   One of a number of disorders characterized by an abnormally increased concentration of lipoproteins in the blood.

hypermagnesemia   An abnormally increased concentration of magnesium in the blood.

hypernatremia   An abnormally increased concentration of sodium in the blood, resulting from excess loss or inadequate intake of fluid and an imbalance of serum electrolytes.

hyperopia   A problem with visual refraction that results in clearer vision for distant rather than near objects.

hyperosmolar hyperglycemic nonketotic syndrome (HHNS)   A complication of diabetes mellitus in which the level of blood glucose is increased but ketosis does not occur; coma results when the high con-

centration of blood glucose causes dehydration of brain tissues.

hyperphosphatemia   Excess phosphorus in the extracellular fluid; occurs when the serum phosphorus level is above 2.6 mEq/L.

hyperpigmentation   Excess pigmentation or coloration of a tissue or part; usually used to denote an abnormal darkening of the skin.

 TIME LINE Bizarre arrangements of linear or streaky hyperpigmented lesions on a child's sun-exposed lower legs suggest phytophotodermatitis. Advise parents to protect the child's legs with long pants and socks.

hyperplasia   An abnormal increase in the number of cells in a tissue or organ, resulting in an increase in the organ or tissue's bulk but not in the formation of a tumor.

hyperpnea, hyperpnoea   An increase in the depth and frequency of respiration when an individual is at rest.

ALERT Carefully examine the patient with hyperpnea for related signs of life-threatening conditions, such as increased intracranial pressure (ICP), metabolic acidosis, diabetic ketoacidosis, and uremia. Be prepared for rapid intervention.

hyperpyrexia   A severe increase in body temperature; an extremely high fever.

hypersensitivity   An exaggerated response to a stimulus; commonly refers to allergic hypersensitivity or a hypersensitivity reaction.

hypersensitivity reaction   An exaggerated immune system response upon exposure to an antigen.

hypersomnia   Excessively long periods of sleep, with normal functioning during waking periods.

hypertension   A persistent, abnormal elevation in blood pressure, usually defined as systolic pressure exceeding 140 mm Hg or diastolic pressure exceeding 90 mm Hg.

hyperthermia   A severe elevation in body temperature induced for therapeutic purposes.

hypertonic   1. A solution that has greater osmotic pressure compared to another solution; a fluid in which cells shrink. 2. In reference to muscles or arteries, having a greater than normal degree of tension.

hypertrichosis   Excessive hair growth.

hypertrophy   Increase in the volume of a tissue or organ due to enlargement of existing cells.

hyperventilation   Respiration that is deeper and more frequent than normal, resulting in the loss of excessive carbon dioxide from the blood.

hypervolemia Abnormal increase in the volume of circulating fluid in the body

hypesthesia An abnormally diminished sensitivity to sensory nerve stimulation.

hypocalcemia An abnormally low concentration of calcium in the blood; serum calcium deficiency.

hypochromic A deficiency of pigmentation, generally used with reference to hypopigmented erythrocytes.

hypochromic anemia Anemia characterized by an abnormal decrease in the mean corpuscular volume, mean corpuscular hemoglobin content, and mean corpuscular hemoglobin concentration.

hypodermoclysis, hypodermatoclysis The subcutaneous injection of a saline or other solution; commonly used to describe the injection of large amounts of fluid, electrolytes, and nutrients.

hypokalemia A condition characterized by an abnormally low concentration of potassium ions in the blood.

hypokalemic alkalosis A pathologic condition resulting from the accumulation of base or the loss of acid from the body associated with a low level of serum potassium.

hypolipoproteinemia A group of rare, hereditary defects of lipid metabolism that result in varying complexes of signs.

hypomagnesemia An abnormally low concentration of magnesium in the blood plasma, resulting in nausea, vomiting, muscle weakness, tremors, tetany, and lethargy.

hyponatremia A less than normal concentration of sodium in the blood, caused by inadequate excretion of water or by excessive water in the circulating bloodstream.

hypophosphatemia Deficit of phosphorus in extracellular fluid; occurs when the serum phosphorus level falls below 1.8 mEq/L.

hypoplasia Incomplete development or underdevelopment of an organ or tissue.

hypopnea Abnormally slow or shallow breathing.

hypoproteinemia Abnormally decreased level of total protein in the blood.

hypoprothrombinemia Abnormally decreased level of clotting factor (factor II, or prothrombin) in the circulating blood.

hypospadias A congenital abnormality in males in which the urethral opening is on the underside, rather than at the tip, of the penis; in females, the defect is manifested by a urethral opening into the vagina.

hypotension An abnormal decrease in blood pressure, which results in inadequate blood perfusion, and therefore in a decreased oxygen and nutrient supply, to the tissues throughout the body.

ALERT If a patient's systolic blood pressure is less than 80 mm Hg, or 30 mm Hg below his baseline pressure, suspect shock immediately. Quickly assess the patient's LOC, apical pulse (for tachycardia), and the presence of cool, clammy skin.

hypothermia A body temperature that is significantly below normal. Accidental hypothermia may occur upon prolonged exposure to cold weather.

hypothermia therapy The deliberate reduction of body temperature to significantly below normal; used chiefly in individuals with extremely high fevers, and sometimes during surgical procedures involving the brain or heart.

hypotonic 1. A solution that has a decreased osmotic pressure compared to another solution; a fluid in which cells swell. 2. In reference to muscles or arteries, having a less than normal degree of tension.

hypoventilation Respiration that is more shallow and less frequent than normal, resulting in an abnormal increase of carbon dioxide in the blood.

hypovolemic shock A significantly diminished volume of blood in the circulation, usually resulting from hemorrhage or dehydration, characterized by physical collapse, tachycardia, diminished urinary excretion, and pale, cold, clammy skin.

hyypoxemia A decreased level of oxygen in the arterial blood, although not as severe as anoxia.

hypoxia A decreased level of oxygen in inspired air, the arterial blood, or the tissues, although not as severe as anoxia.

hysterectomy A surgical procedure in which the corpus of the uterus and cervix are removed.

hysterosalpingography A diagnostic procedure in which X-ray films of the uterus and fallopian tubes are obtained after injection, through the cervix, of a radiopaque substance.

hysteroscopy Direct endoscopic visual examination of the uterine cavity.

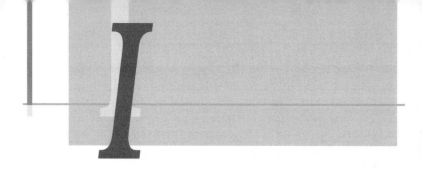

IADH *abbr* inappropriate secretion of antidiuretic hormone.

IADR *abbr* International Association for Dental Research.

IAET *abbr* International Association for Enterostomal Therapy.

iatrogenic Introduced inadvertently by a medical practitioner or resulting from a diagnostic procedure or treatment.

iatrogenic protein-energy malnutrition A form of malnutrition, common during hospitalization, in which a patient's nutritional status deteriorates; most common in patients hospitalized longer than 2 weeks.

IC *abbr* inspiratory capacity.

ICCU *abbr* intensive coronary-care unit.

ICD *abbr* 1. International Classification of Diseases. 2. Intrauterine contraceptive device. 3. Implantable cardioverted defibrillator.

ICDA *abbr* International Classification of Disease, adapted for use in the United States.

ICF *abbr* intracellular fluid.

ichthyosis A congenital skin disorder characterized by dryness and keratinization resulting in an appearance resembling fish scales; the disorder appears at birth or in early infancy.

ichthyosis vulgaris A form of ichthyosis characterized by the appearance of fine scales on the trunk, arms, and legs but sparing the flexural areas; onset is usually in childhood.

ICN *abbr* International Council of Nurses.

ICP *abbr* intracranial pressure.

ICS *abbr* International Congress of Surgeons.

ICSH *abbr* interstitial cell-stimulating hormone.

ICU *abbr* intensive care unit.

ID *abbr* identification, immunodiffusion, infective dose, initial dose, intradermal, infectious disease.

IDDM *abbr* insulin-dependent diabetes mellitus.

ideational apraxia The misuse of objects due to a loss of ability to identify them, in the absence of sensory or motor impairment.

ideomotor apraxia The inability to translate an idea into motion, resulting from some interference with the transmission of the appropriate impulses from the brain to the motor centers.

idiopathic Having no known cause.

idiopathic disease A disease that has no identifiable cause.

idiopathy A primary disease that has no identifiable cause.

idiosyncrasy, idiocrasy A behavioral, mental, physical, or physiologic characteristic or mannerism that is unique or peculiar to an individual or group.

idiosyncratic reaction A hypersensitivity reaction to a drug, food, or other agent that is unique to a particular individual.

Ig *abbr* immunoglobulin.

IgA *abbr* immunoglobulin A.

ileal conduit Use of a segment of the ileum for diversion of urinary flow from the ureters.

ileocecal valve A cone-shaped structure with a star-shaped opening that lies between the ileum of the small intestine and the cecum of the large intestine whose function is to allow the intestinal contents to continue through the intestinal tract in a forward direction.

ileocolic lymph node One of the nodes that lie along the ileocolic artery that drain lymphatic fluid from the ascending colon to the superior mesenteric nodes.

ileostomy A surgical procedure in which a channel is formed that allows passage of intestinal contents from the ileum of the small intestine directly to the outside of the body.

ileum Distal portion of the small intestine, extending from the jejunum to the cecum.

ileus Failure of appropriate forward movement of bowel contents.

iliac muscle A muscle located in the iliac fossa, innervated by the lumbar plexus; its function is to allow flexion and internal rotation of the thigh.

ilium, *pl.* ilia The broad, flaring section of the hip bone that fuses with the ischium and pubis during early childhood.

I.M. *abbr* intramuscular.

IMA *abbr* Industrial Medical Association.

imagery The process of imagining or visualizing an image using any of the five senses; used to change attitudes and behaviors, as well as physiologic reactions.

imbricate To create a surface from overlapping layers, in the manner of laying shingles; imbrication is a surgical technique in which overlapping layers of tissue are used to close wounds or to repair defects.

iminoglycinuria An inherited defect in the transport of amino acids characterized by the excretion of glycine, proline, and hydroxyproline in the urine; considered to be a benign condition.

immersion 1. The submerging of a body under water or another liquid. 2. In microscopy: a technique in which the space between the microscope lens and the cover glass is filled with a liquid, primarily water or oil, to improve resolution under certain circumstances.

immobilize To cause to be fixed in one position or to render incapable of motion. Casts, splints, or surgical fixation may be used to immobilize body parts.

immune complex hypersensitivity An immunoglobulin G (IgG) or IgM complement-dependent, immediate-acting humoral hypersensitivity to certain soluble antigens.

immune cytolysis The destruction of a cell associated with an immune response.

immune gamma globulin Passive immunizing agents obtained from pooled human plasma. It is prescribed for immunization against measles, poliomyelitis, chickenpox, serum hepatitis following transfusion, hepatitis A, agammaglobulinemia, and hypogammaglobulinemia.

immune human globulin A sterile solution of globulins, used as a passive immunizing agent, derived from adult human blood.

immune response The defensive reaction of the body to substances or agents that the immune system perceives as foreign or to aberrant cells that form in the body. The immune response involves the production and release of antibodies. See illustration on page 156.

immune system A complex consisting of cellular, molecular, and genetic components that, working in interrelationship, allow the body to mount a defensive immune response.

immunity A state of protection against a disease, especially one of infectious origin.

immunization 1. The process of acquiring or enhancing immunity. 2. The administration of agents that induce immunity.

immunodeficient A state characterized by a defect in the functioning of the immune system and immune response, reducing an individual's resistance to infection.

immunodiagnosis A process by which certain immunologic characteristics of cells, serum, or other specimens are determined.

immunodiffusion A method of studying antigen-antibody reactions to identify and quantify any immunoglobulins that may be present.

immunoelectrophoresis A test that uses both electrophoresis and immunodiffusion to separate and, therefore, identify antigens and antibodies.

immunofluorescence A technique in which antibodies are labeled with fluorescein or rhodamine stains and are used to locate specific antigens in tissues.

immunoglobulin One of the five classes of structurally related glycoproteins that function as antibodies.

immunology Study of all aspects of immunity, induced sensitivity, and allergy.

immunomodulation Alteration of the immune response to a desired level.

immunosuppression The inhibition of the body's immune response, which may occur naturally or may be induced by disease or by the administration of a chemical, biological, or physical agent.

immunotherapy Any of several methods used to produce or enhance immunity to specific antigens or allergens.

impedance plethysmography A type of plethysmography in which changes are recorded in electrical impedance between two electrodes that are placed on opposite sides of an organ or other body structure, as a means of determining changes in volume of that organ or structure.

imperforate Of an organ or body passage: without the normal opening.

imperforate anus The congenital absence of a normal orifice at the distal portion of the intestines.

impetigo A contagious, inflammatory skin infection, which usually occurs on the face, characterized by the appearance of small, itchy blisters that rupture and form a crusty scab; usually caused by streptococcal or staphylococcal bacteria or a combination of both types of organisms.

implant 1. To graft or transplant material into tissues. 2. In dentistry: a prosthesis inserted into the jawbone to which artificial crowns or bridges are attached, as a means of replacing one or more teeth. 3. In orthopedics: a metal or plastic device used in joint reconstruction. 4. In radiotherapy: a radioactive material inserted into tissue as a treat-

Immune response

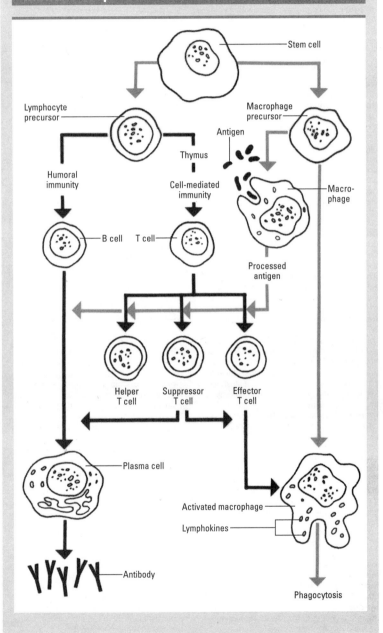

Incisors

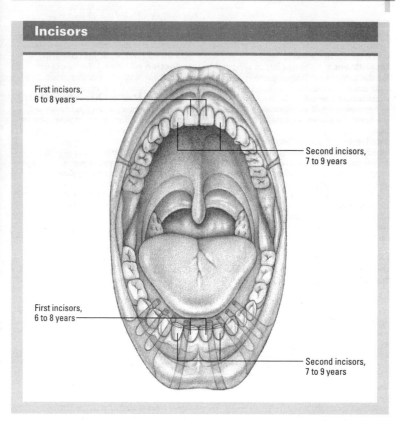

First incisors,
6 to 8 years

Second incisors,
7 to 9 years

First incisors,
6 to 8 years

Second incisors,
7 to 9 years

ment for certain types of cancer, including prostate and cervical cancer.

implantation dermoid cyst A cystic mass formed from epidermal cells that have been forced beneath the surface of the skin as a result of traumatic injury.

impotence 1. Lacking strength or power. 2. Inability of an adult male to achieve or maintain penile erection and, therefore, to engage in sexual intercourse.

IMV *abbr* intermittent mandatory ventilation.

INA *abbr* International Neurological Association.

inanition fever An abnormal elevation in temperature that is seen in infants who are dehydrated because of reduced fluid intake or prolonged diarrhea or vomiting. Also called *thirst fever.*

inborn error of metabolism Any of a number of conditions that result from an inherited malfunction of a protein essential to a metabolic process.

inbreeding The mating of humans or animals (or fertilization of plants) that are more closely genetically related than would be expected through random selection.

incident An event that is inconsistent with ordinary routine, regardless of whether injury occurs.

incident report A formal, written report that informs hospital administration (and the hospital's insurance company) about an incident; serves as a contemporary, factual statement in the event of a lawsuit.

incision 1. The division of soft parts with a sharp instrument such as a knife or scalpel. 2. A surgical wound.

incisor One of the four teeth at the front of each jaw; the cutting teeth at the front of the mouth.

incompetent cervix In obstetrics: a condition characterized by dilation of the cervical os of the uterus before term without labor or contractions of the uterus.

incomplete abortion   The loss or deliberate termination of a pregnancy in which some products of conception, usually the placenta, remain in the uterus.

incontinence   The inability to prevent the discharge of any body excretions, specifically urine or feces.

incubation period   The time that elapses between entry of an infectious agent and the onset of signs and symptoms of an infection.

incubator   1. An enclosed container in which temperature, humidity, and the oxygen concentration in the air can be controlled, used to maintain a newborn. 2. An apparatus in which microorganisms are cultured under controlled conditions, especially temperature.

incudectomy   A surgical procedure in which the incus is removed.

incus   One of the three small bones in the middle ear whose function is to conduct sound vibrations; the common name for this bone, because of its shape, is the anvil.

independent practitioner organization (IPO)   A hybrid form with characteristics of both IPAs and medical associations; they're often organized by community physicians as a mechanism to evaluate and negotiate participation in HMOs.

indeterminate cleavage   Cell division in a fertilized ovum that results in the development of blastomeres, each of which has the same potential (if separated from the rest) to produce a complete embryo.

Index Medicus   A listing, by subject and author, of articles published in medical journals throughout the world.

index myopia   A type of nearsightedness that results from increased refractivity of the lens in the eye.

Indian Health Service   A division of the U.S. Department of Health and Human Services that is dedicated to providing public health services and medical care to Native Americans.

indicator   A substance that changes color or in any other way visibly demonstrates that a chemical reaction has been completed.

indirect calorimetry   The determination of the amount of heat produced by an oxidation reaction through calculations derived from measurements of oxygen uptake or the liberation of carbon dioxide and the excretion of nitrogen.

indoleacetic acid   One of several indolic acids, which are metabolites of tryptophan, an amino acid. Small amounts of indoleacetic acid are normally present in the urine.

induced fever   An elevation of body temperature that is deliberately produced through physical means (the application of

heat) or injection with an infectious organism for the purpose of destroying pathogenic organisms that are highly sensitive to heat. Also called *therapeutic hyperthermia*.

induction of labor   The use of oxytocics or other methods to artificially produce uterine contractions in a pregnant woman.

Industrial Medical Association (IMA)   An organization of medical scientists and clinicians whose work concerns health care issues specifically related to technology and industry.

indwelling catheter   A catheter, usually one with a balloon end, designed to remain in the urinary bladder for a prolonged time.

inert gas   The group of highly stable gases that demonstrate extremely low chemical reactivity. They are, in order of atomic weight, helium, neon, argon, krypton, xenon, and radon.

inertia   A physical law which states that matter at rest tends to remain at rest unless acted upon by an outside force, and matter in motion remains in motion, moving in the same direction, unless acted upon by an outside force.

infant mortality   An accounting of deaths during the first year of life, expressed as the number of deaths per live births.

infarct   An area of tissue necrosis that results from a sudden interruption of the flow of arterial or venous blood in that area.

infection   The invasion and multiplication of pathogenic organisms within the body.

inferior   Anatomically, lying beneath or lower than a specific reference point.

inferior mesenteric node   One of a number of lymph nodes situated along the inferior mesenteric artery and branches whose function is to provide lymph drainage from the descending colon, sigmoid colon, and upper portion of the rectum.

inferior orbital fissure   A cleft at the apex of the orbit that provides space for the passage of the trigeminal nerve's maxillary division and orbital branch, the infraorbital and zygomatic nerves, and the infraorbital arteries and veins.

inferior phrenic artery   One of a pair of vessels that branch from the abdominal aorta below the diaphragm.

inferior sagittal sinus   One of the six venous channels of the posterior dura mater that drains blood from the brain into the internal jugular vein.

inferior vena cava   A central vein; venous return from the legs enters the inferior vena cava, returning blood to the right atrium; blood enters the inferior vena cava from the legs through the femoral venous system and abdominal accessory veins.

infertile   Having a diminished capacity to produce offspring; not necessarily sterile.

infertility   Of or relating to the condition of being infertile.

infiltration   Infusion of I.V. solution into surrounding tissues instead of the blood vessel. Symptoms include discomfort, decreased skin temperature around the site, blanching, absent backflow of blood, and slower flow rate.

inflammation   The cytologic and histologic reactions that occur in the blood vessels and tissues near the site of an injury or irritation caused by physical, chemical, or biological agents.

 CLINICAL TIP Signs of inflammation include redness (rubor), heat (calor), swelling (tumor), pain (dolor), and loss of function (functio laesa).

influenza   An acute, highly contagious, viral infection of the upper respiratory tract, acquired by inhalation of airborne droplets containing the virus. The characteristic signs and symptoms include the sudden onset of fever, chills, headache, muscle aches, severe prostration, and a dry cough; secondary bacterial infection is a risk, particularly among elderly or debilitated individuals. Also called *flu, grippe.*

informed consent   Permission obtained from a patient to perform a specific test or procedure after the patient has been fully informed about the methods and risks involved.

infrared radiation   The emission of invisible, extremely short waves of heat, ranging in length from 700 to 1,000 nanometers.

infrared therapy   The application of infrared radiant heat for the relief of pain and the stimulation of blood circulation, transmitted through incandescent lights or other specialized equipment.

infusion   In medication administration: the introduction of any substance other than blood into a vein, usually in relatively large quantities (e.g., 250 ml), in contrast to injection, which is the administration of small quantities of a substance. Infusion requires the use of a needle that is connected to rubber or plastic tubing, which, in turn, is connected to a container filled with the substance to be infused.

infusion pump   A device that automatically provides the delivery of medication into the venous circulation according to a preset dosage schedule. Surgical implantation of some infusion pumps is possible.

inguinal   Of or relating to the groin.

inguinal falx   The conjoined or conjoint tendon that forms the beginning of the transverse and internal oblique abdominal muscles.

inguinal node   One of the deep (lymphonodi inguinales profundi) or superficial (lymphonodi inguinales superficiales) nodes in the groin area that drain lymph from the tissue and vessels in the upper thigh.

inhalation analgesia   The blunting of pain perception, without the induction of loss of consciousness, produced by the administration of a gas or vapor, such as nitrous oxide, that depresses the central nervous system; used especially during labor and in dental procedures.

inhalation anesthesia   General anesthesia produced by the administration of an anesthetic gas or airborne liquid anesthetic agent.

inhalation therapy   The administration of nebulized or aerosolized drugs, water vapor, or oxygen or other gases, which reach the respiratory tract along with inspired air.

inhale   **1.** To draw air into the body. **2.** To draw in an airborne substance along with inspired air.

inherent   A part, condition, or consequence that occurs naturally; inborn.

inheritance   The complete array of what was acquired by the transmission of genetic material from both parents.

inherited disorder   A condition or disease that is transmitted to offspring by genetic transmission from either or both parents. Also called *genetic disorder.*

inhibiting hormone   A hypothalamus-produced chemical substance that inhibits the secretion of some anterior pituitary hormones.

inion   The protruding portion of the occipital bone; the area at the back of the head that is most prominent.

injection   The introduction into the body of a small amount of a drug or nutritional substance with a syringe and, commonly, a needle. Injection may be into dermal or subcutaneous tissue, muscle, veins, or arteries or into any of the canals or cavities of the body.

in-line filter   A filter in the fluid pathway between the I.V. tubing and the venipuncture device that removes pathogens and particles and helps prevent air from entering the vein.

in loco parentis   Latin phrase meaning "in the place of the parent"; assumption of the parental obligations of caring for a child by a person or institution without adoption.

innate   Inborn; belonging to an individual at birth.

innervation   Distribution and action of the nervous system.

innocent   In clinical medicine: not dangerous; not malignant.

inoculate   **1.** To confer or stimulate an increase in immunity to a certain disease by introducing the infectious agent or other antigenic substance into the body. **2.** In laboratory medicine: to introduce a microorganism, usually a pathogen, into or onto a culture medium.

inorganic   Not pertaining to living matter or organisms; not formed by living organisms.

inorganic acid   An acid composed of molecules that contain no organic radicals.

inorganic chemistry   The study of chemical compounds that do not involve covalent bonds, or of chemical elements other than hydrocarbons.

inorganic dust   Fine particles composed of inorganic elements or compounds.

insemination   The introduction of seminal fluid into the vagina, either naturally (during sexual intercourse) or artificially (to achieve conception by any means other than sexual intercourse).

insensible perspiration   **1.** Perspiration that evaporates from the skin before it is felt as moisture. **2.** The evaporation of moisture from the lungs.

in situ   **1.** Located in the expected position. **2.** Not extending beyond the area of origin; commonly used to describe a malignant tumor that has not begun to spread to tissue beyond the original site of development.

insoluble   Incapable of being dissolved in a liquid.

insomnia   The inability to fall asleep, premature wakening, or the occurrence of periods of wakefulness during sleep time; a term usually reserved for chronic, rather than occasional, sleep disturbance.

ALERT Be alert for the use of herbal medicines, such as ginseng and green tea, which can cause adverse reactions, including insomnia.

inspection   The close visual examination and observation of the body surface, posture, and movements.

inspiration   The act of inhaling air into the lungs.

inspiratory capacity   The sum of the tidal volume and inspiratory reserve volume; the amount of air that can be drawn into the lungs after normal expiration.

inspiratory reserve volume (IRV)
The inspiratory capacity minus the tidal volume; the greatest amount of air that can be drawn into the lungs after normal inspiration.

inspissate   To make thicker or to condense by the evaporation or absorption of fluid.

instillation   The dropping of a fluid onto or into a part, such as the instillation of liquid medication into the eyes with an eyedropper.

insufflate   **1.** To blow a gas or a medicated powder, aerosol, or vapor into a cavity. **2.** To blow air into the airway, especially of a newborn.

insulin   A hormone that is used by the body in the regulation of glucose, the synthesis of protein, and the production and storage of certain lipids. Endogenous (natural) insulin is produced in the pancreas by beta cells in the islets of Langerhans; insulin that is prepared from the pancreatic tissue of animals is used in the treatment of individuals with diabetes mellitus, in whom insulin production and secretion is insufficient.

insulin kinase   An enzyme that activates the hormone insulin.

insulinogenic   That which enhances or promotes the synthesis and secretion of insulin from the pancreatic beta cells.

insulinoma, *pl.* **insulinomas, insulinomata**   An adenoma originating in the cells of the islets of Langerhans in the pancreas. Also called *insuloma.*

insulin shock   Shock caused by severe hypoglycemia (low blood glucose), resulting from an excess level of insulin in the circulation.

integral dose   In radiotherapy: energy that a patient or object absorbs during radiation exposure. Also called *volume dose.*

integrating dose meter   In radiotherapy: an ionization chamber, commonly placed on the patient's skin, that measures the amount of radiation administered during exposure.

integumentary system   The skin (dermis and epidermis) and all structures derived from it, including hair, nails, sweat glands, and sebaceous glands.

intellectualization   In psychiatry: the unconscious focusing of the intellect, through the use of tools such as reasoning and logic, to avoid confronting an impulse, emotion, or circumstance that an individual perceives as stressful.

intention tremor   Tremor occurring on attempts at voluntary movement.

intensive care unit (ICU)   A specially staffed hospital unit that treats patients who require close monitoring and intensive care with highly technical, sophisticated equipment.

intercalary   Pertaining to that which occurs between two others, such as two abnormal pulse strokes separated by two normal beats.

intercostal   Between the ribs.

intercostal bulging The visible protrusion of soft tissue between the ribs; most commonly seen in individuals with chronic asthma or other respiratory disorders, resulting from increased effort on expiration.

interferon (IFN) A class of glycoproteins that are produced after cells are exposed to a virus; the fact that interferon prevents viral replication in noninfected cells makes interferon therapy a potentially valuable treatment for a variety of viral infections.

intermediate care A level of medical care for certain chronically ill or disabled individuals in which room and board are provided without skilled nursing care.

intermittent fever A cyclically recurrent fever, with intervening periods of normal body temperature.

intermittent infusion device A device that maintains venous access in patients who must receive regular or intermittent I.V. medications but don't require continuous infusion. Commonly called a saline or heparin lock because it's kept patent with periodic saline or heparin solution flushes.

intermittent mandatory ventilation (IMV) The use of a mechanical respirator to provide positive pressure at specified intervals in a patient who is otherwise breathing independently for the purpose of increasing tidal volume.

intermittent positive pressure breathing (IPPB) The use of a mechanical respirator to assist in respiration, in which positive air pressure is used to periodically inflate the lungs; exhalation occurs passively, through a valve.

internal carotid artery Either of two arteries that arise from either of the common carotid arteries at the upper border of the thyroid cartilage and end in the interior cranial fossa, where they divide into the anterior and middle cerebral arteries.

internal ear The area of the ear that comprises the canals, the vestibule, and the cochlea. Also called *inner ear, labyrinth.*

internal fertilization The joining of gametes within the female's body following insemination.

internal fixation The stabilization of fragments of fractured bones by the use of such methods as wires, plates, screws, or surgical cement and without external devices.

internal iliac artery An artery that arises at the common iliac artery and brances into arterial vessels that supply walls and organs of the pelvis, the genital organs, and a section of the thigh. Also called *hypogastric artery.*

internal iliac node One of a number of lymph nodes that lie along the iliac artery and branches, which drain lymph from the organs in the pelvis and the tissue in the perineum and gluteal region.

internal iliac vein A vein that runs from the upper portion of the greater sciatic notch to the top of the pelvis and joins the external iliac vein to form the common iliac vein. Also called *hypogastric vein.*

internal rotation Movement of part of the body toward the midline.

internal thoracic artery One of two arteries that originate at the subclavian arteries and supply the pericardium and the muscles of the chest, breasts, and abdomen.

International Association for Dental Research (IADR) A worldwide organization dedicated to dental research and the dissemination of information from that research.

International Classification of Disease, Adapted (ICDA) A system for classifying diseases derived by the Health Resource Services Administration, from classifications developed by the World Health Organization, that is currently in use in the United States.

International Congress of Surgeons (ICS) A worldwide professional organization of medical doctors who specialize in surgery.

International Council of Nurses (ICN) A worldwide organization of nursing professionals.

International System of Units A system developed to standardize measurements of some substances, such as vitamins, enzymes, hormones, and some antibiotics. Measurements of such substances are expressed in International Units (IU).

International Unit (IU, I.U.) In the International System of Units, the amount of a substance that has been shown to yield a particular biological result.

interoceptive Of or relating to the interoceptors or to the information they transmit to the spinal cord and the brain.

interoceptor One of a number of forms of receptors, or sensory end organs, which lie within the cells lining the respiratory and gastrointestinal tracts and in other visceral structures and which convey information regarding the functioning of these systems and structures to the spinal cord and the brain.

interphase The period of time in the life cycle of a cell during which it is not dividing, chromatin is replicating, and the normal biochemical and physiologic functions of the cell are taking place.

interstitial cystitis A chronic condition of the bladder characterized by inflammation of the mucosa and muscular tissue, pain when the bladder is not empty, a reduction in the capacity of the bladder, and irritative symptoms.

interstitial emphysema   A type of emphysema characterized by the presence of air or gas in the pulmonary interstitial or connective tissue, resulting from a traumatic injury in which the lung is penetrated or from the rupture of alveolar cells.

interstitial fluid   Lymphlike fluid in the spaces between the cells of the body tissues, accounting for approximately 16% of an individual's body weight.

interstitial growth   Growth from numerous centers within an area, as in hyperplasia or hypertrophy.

interstitial nephritis   A type of acute or chronic nephritis in which the interstitial connective tissue of the kidney and tubules is affected.

interstitial pneumonia   Chronic, diffuse lung inflammation beyond the terminal bronchioles, associated with fibrosis and collagen formation in the alveolar walls and with large mononuclear cells in the alveolar spaces.

intertrigo   Dermatitis that occurs at moist, warm sites where skin surfaces rub together, such as the armpits, the inner surfaces of the thighs, and between the buttocks; caused by an overgrowth of normal flora.

intertrochanteric line   A line that separates the neck and the shaft of the femur, passing down and across from the greater trochanter and terminating at the linea aspera.

intervillous space   A space between any two or more villi.

intestinal absorption   The process by which the body takes in nutrients and other essential products from ingested foods or other substances as this material passes through the gastrointestinal system.

intestinal angina   Abdominal pain that is intermittent and usually occurs a certain amount of time after eating, caused by arterial disease in the mesenteric circulation. Also called *abdominal angina.*

intestinal apoplexy   The sudden occurrence of hemorrhage, thrombosis, or embolus involving the mesenteric or abdominal circulation. Also called *abdominal apoplexy.*

intestinal dyspepsia   Impaired digestion associated with a problem that arises in the intestines.

intestinal fistula   An abnormal passage leading from the lumen of the bowel to the surface of the body; sometimes surgically created for feces to exit after a malignant or severely ulcerated bowel segment has been removed.

intestinal obstruction   A blockage, clogging, or stricture of the lumen in any area of the bowel that prevents the normal passage of intestinal contents.

intra-aortic balloon pump   A device consisting of a balloon attached to a catheter that is introduced into the descending thoracic aorta via the femoral artery. Alternating inflation (during diastole) and deflation (during systole) of the balloon alters resistance to aortic blood flow and both decreases the heart's workload and increases the supply of blood to the coronary arteries.

ALERT   When a patient is on IAPB, don't flex the patient's "ballooned" leg at the hip, as this may displace or fracture the catheter. Assess pedal pulses and skin temperature to make sure circulation to the leg is adequate.

intra-articular injection   The injection of a drug into a joint; commonly the injection of an anti-inflammatory medication such as a corticosteroid preparation.

intracatheter   A thin, plastic tube, usually attached to a puncturing needle, that is introduced into a blood vessel to permit infusion, injection, or the monitoring of pressure.

intracavitary therapy   The placement of radioactive pellets or other sources within a body cavity to provide radiation therapy to specifically targeted tissues within the body.

intracellular fluid (ICF)   The fluid contained inside body tissue cells; accounts for 30% to 40% of body weight.

intradermal injection   Injection of any substance into the skin between the dermis and epidermis. The technique is typically used to produce a local drug effect (as in local anesthesia for procedures such as suturing wounds) or during allergy testing. Also called *intracutaneous injection.*

intradermal test   A type of allergy test in which minute amounts of suspected allergens or their products are injected into the skin to confirm the presence of allergic sensitivity.

intradural lipoma   A benign tumor composed of mature fat cells that develops in or beneath the dura mater, usually in the spine.

CLINICAL TIP   Although benign, an intradural lipoma may interfere with the normal function of the patient's spinal nerves, thereby causing pain and motor dysfunction.

intramuscular injection   The injection of medication into muscle tissue.

intraocular pressure   The pressure of the fluid within the eye, which is measured in millimeters of mercury (mm Hg) by a device called a manometer; normal intraocular pressure ranges from 12 to 20 mm Hg, and above-normal measurements are caused by increased resistance to the flow of aqueous humor within the trabecular network.

intraosseous infusion   An emergency procedure for fluid resuscitation or infusion of medication or blood in children under age 6; an intraosseous needle is placed in the bone's medullary cavity, allowing direct access.

intraparietal sulcus   The groove that separates the parietal lobe of the cerebrum into the superior and inferior parietal lobules.

intrathecal   Within the spinal canal.

intrauterine device (IUD)   A device made of plastic or metal (usually copper) that is inserted into the uterus for the purpose of altering the uterine environment and making it unfavorable for implantation of a fertilized egg. Some types of IUDs also contain contraceptive hormones, which are released over time.

intrauterine growth curve   A graphic representation of the weight of a fetus throughout its gestational age, from conception to birth.

intrauterine growth retardation   An abnormal condition characterized by an infant's weight measuring below the 10th percentile for gestational age, resulting from insufficient growth within the uterus because of genetic disorders, maternal disease, or fetal malnutrition. A newborn so affected is often referred to as a small-for-gestational-age infant.

intravenous bolus   A relatively large dose of a drug or a volume of fluid given intravenously and over a short period of time.

intravenous catheter   A thin, plastic tube, attached to a puncturing needle that is inserted into a vein and through which medications and therapeutic fluids are administered.

intravenous infusion   The introduction of a solution into a vein.

intravenous injection   The introduction of a hypodermic needle into a vein to administer a dose of a drug.

intravenous pyelography (IVP)   A diagnostic test in which a radiopaque dye is injected intravenously and a series of X-rays are taken over a period of time, as the dye clears from the kidneys and ureters, to identify abnormalities in urinary system structure or function. Also called *excretory urography.*

intraventricular   Of or relating to the area within either the right or left ventricle of the heart.

intraventricular (I-V) block   A conduction delay within the ventricles or myocardium; types of I-V blocks include hemiblocks,

bundle-branch blocks, and peri-infarction blocks.

intrinsic asthma   A form of asthma that is not associated with any identifiable causes but is presumably due to some inherent process, possibly allergic in origin.

introitus   Entrance to a canal or cavity, such as the vagina.

intubation   1. The insertion of a tube into a body passage, hollow organ, or cavity. 2. The passage of a tube through the nose or mouth and through the larynx for ventilation or to administer anesthetic gas.

inulin clearance   A test to measure the rate of filtration through the renal glomeruli, in which inulin is infused intravenously; the clearance rate is calculated based on the time it takes for inulin to appear in the urine after infusion.

invagination   The insertion of one part of a structure into another part of the same structure; ensheathing or infolding.

invasion   1. The beginning of a disease process. 2. The spread of a cancerous tumor into adjacent tissue.

invasive   1. Pertaining to invasion. 2. Pertaining to a diagnostic or therapeutic procedure that requires insertion of an instrument or device into the body through the skin or an orifice.

invasive carcinoma   A malignant neoplasm in which epithelial cells infiltrate or destroy tissue in the area adjacent to the malignancy.

inverse square law   A law which states that the intensity of radiation that reaches a surface is inversely proportional to the square of the distance from the radiation source.

inversion   In physiology: the turning of a structure inward.

involuntary   Independent of or contrary to one's will.

involution   1. The folding inward of the edges of a structure. 2. The return of an enlarged organ to its normal size.

iodine (I)   A nonmetallic element with the atomic number 53 and an atomic weight of 128.9. Compounds containing iodine are used in the manufacture of a variety of diagnostic and therapeutic agents, including topical anesthetics, reagents, stains, and drugs for treating thyroid disease.

iodize   To administer or impregnate with iodine.

ion   A single atom or group of atoms that carries an electrical charge because of the loss or gain of one or more valence electrons.

ionization   1. The process of dissociation of compounds into ions. 2. The production of ions resulting from exposure of matter to radiation.

ionize To dissociate atoms or molecules into ions; to separate into ions.

IPPB *abbr* intermittent positive pressure breathing.

iralgia, iridalgia Pain in the iris of the eye.

iridectomy Surgical removal of a portion of the iris.

iridocyclitis Inflammation of both the iris and ciliary body.

iridotomy A surgical procedure in which some of the fibers of the iris are divided, forming an artificial pupil.

iris A circular diaphragm in the eye composed of contractile tissue, perforated by the pupil, and located between the cornea and the lens; regulates the entrance of light into the eye by contracting and dilating.

iritis Inflammation of the iris of the eye.

iron (Fe) A metallic element, with the atomic number 26 and an atomic weight of 55.847, found widely in nature. It occurs in the human body as part of the hemoglobin molecule and is administered as a treatment for certain types of anemia.

iron-deficiency anemia Anemia characterized by an insufficient amount of iron in the serum, decreased stores of iron in the bone marrow, and elevated serum iron-binding.

iron-rich food Food containing a large amount of iron, such as certain shellfish, animal organs (liver, heart, kidneys), and lean meats.

iron transport The physiologic process in which iron is carried from the point at which it is absorbed by the intestines to the many sites in the body where it is used or stored.

irradiation The therapeutic application of electromagnetic radiation, such as heat, light, or radium, to a body part.

irrigation 1. The use of a fluid to wash out a body cavity or wound. 2. The cleaning, using a stream of fluid, of a tube or drain inserted into the body.

irrigator An instrument with a flexible tube used for irrigation.

irritable bowel syndrome A condition characterized by diarrhea resulting from increased bowel motility; although the cause is unknown, many clinicians believe this condition is associated with emotional stress.

irritant An agent that produces a local inflammatory reaction.

IRV *abbr* inspiratory reserve volume.

ischemia The temporary loss of adequate blood supply in a localized area resulting from obstruction of the blood supply from any cause, including constriction of the blood vessels, atherosclerosis, embolism, and thrombosis.

ischemic pain Pain or other discomfort, including angina pectoris, that results from ischemia.

isoagglutinogen An isoantigen that induces agglutination of the cells to which it is attached when its specific isoantibody is present.

isoantibody An antibody, which occurs in only some individuals, that reacts only with a corresponding isoantigen.

isoantigen An antigen, such as a blood group antigen, that interacts with isoantibodies in other members of the same species.

isobar One of two or more nuclides that have different atomic numbers but the same atomic weight.

isodose In radiotherapy: a radiation dose of the same strength to more than one area of the body.

isoenzyme One of a group of enzymes that share catalytic properties but differ in other physical properties.

isogamete A somatic cell that is identical in size and structure to another to which it unites for reproduction.

isometric exercise Exercise characterized by the contraction of muscles without movement of the body part that would normally be affected by the contraction of those muscles; the contraction produces tension over the entire length of the muscle and the energy is liberated as heat.

isometric growth An increase in size of different organs or parts of an organism at the same rate.

isotonic Of or relating to a solution that has the same osmotic pressure as another solution; a solution in which cells neither swell nor shrink.

isotonic exercise Exercise characterized by the shortening of a muscle against a constant weight load, as in weight lifting.

isotope A chemical element that shares with at least one other element an atomic number, virtually identical chemical properties, and the same number of nuclear protons but which differs from the other element in both atomic weight and in the number of neutrons contained in the nucleus.

ITP *abbr* idiopathic thrombocytopenic purpura.

IU, I.U. *abbr* International Unit.

IUCD *abbr* intrauterine contraceptive device.

IUD *abbr* intrauterine device.

I.V. 1. *abbr* intravenous. 2. *Informal.* The equipment required to administer fluids intravenously. **3.** The intravenous administration of fluids.

IVAC pump   The brand name of a portable, electronic, intravenous pump used for automatically regulating and monitoring the administration of intravenous fluids.

IVP   *abbr* intravenous pyelogram; intravenous pyelography.

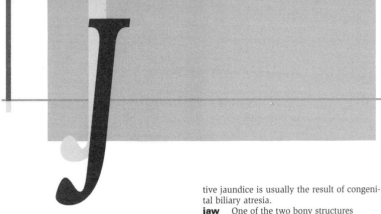

jackknife position A position used for rectal surgery or rectal examination in which the patient is placed face down with the buttocks raised. Also called *Kraske position.*

jacksonian epilepsy A form of epilepsy characterized by focal motor seizures with unilateral clonic movements that begin in one group of muscles and then spread to adjacent groups, reflecting the progression of seizure activity through the motor cortex.

Jacob's membrane A layer of the retina, composed of rods and cones.

JAMA *abbr Journal of the American Medical Association.*

Janeway lesion A small, erythematous or hemorrhagic macule, usually on the palms or soles, sometimes seen in patients with subacute bacterial endocarditis. Also called *Janeway spots.*

 TIME LINE In children, Janeway lesions or spots commonly stem from endocarditis related to congenital heart defects or rheumatic fever.

Japanese encephalitis An epidemic form of encephalitis caused by a flavovirus, transmitted by infected mosquitos, that is seen in eastern and southern Asia. It may occur as an asymptomatic subclinical infection or as an acute encephalitis with cortical damage and spinal cord lesions.

JAPHA *abbr Journal of the American Public Health Association.*

Jarisch-Herxheimer reaction A transient immunologic reaction that sometimes follows antibiotic treatment of syphilis, leptospirosis, or relapsing fever, characterized by fever, chills, headache, myalgia, and exacerbation of skin lesions.

jaundice A yellow appearance of the skin, mucous membranes, and sclerae of the eyes, resulting from elevated serum bilirubin levels.

 TIME LINE Physiologic jaundice is common in neonates, developing 3 to 5 days after birth. In infants, obstruc-

tive jaundice is usually the result of congenital biliary atresia.

jaw One of the two bony structures (mandible and maxilla) that hold the teeth and form the framework of the mouth.

jaw reflex Closure of the mouth elicited by a downward blow on the lower jaw while it hangs passively open; usually indicates a corticospinal tract lesion. Also called *jaw jerk reflex, chin reflex.*

jejunum, *pl.* **jejuna** One of the three portions of the small intestine, extending from the duodenum to the ileum.

Jendrassik's maneuver A diagnostic procedure in which the patient hooks the fingers of both hands together and tries to pull them apart.

Job-Basedow phenomenon Thyrotoxicosis occurring after dietary iodine administration to a patient with endemic goiter who lives in an area of environmental iodine deficiency.

joint An articulation, or place of union, between two or more bones.

 CLINICAL TIP Joints are classified according to structure and movability as fibrous, cartilaginous, or synovial.

Joint Commission on Accreditation of Healthcare Organizations (JCAHO) A private, nongovernmental agency that establishes guidelines for the operation of hospitals and other health care facilities, conducts accreditation programs and surveys, and encourages the attainment of high standards of institutional medical care. Members include representatives from the American Medical Association, American College of Physicians, and American College of Surgeons.

jugular foramen One of a pair of openings formed on the jugular notches between the temporal and occipital bones of the skull, which channel various blood vessels and nerves.

jumping gene In genetics: a unit of genetic information associated with a deoxyribonucleic acid segment capable of moving from one position in the genome to another.

junction nevus A small, discrete, flat or slightly raised macule arising from pigment cells at the epidermal-dermal junction.

just cause A lawful, rightful, proper reason to act; a defendant establishes a cause for action in his favor.

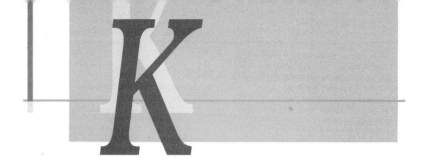

Kaposi's sarcoma   A malignant tumor that begins as soft, brownish or purple nodules, usually on the feet. It spreads slowly in the skin, metastasizing to the lymph nodes and internal organs. A particularly severe form of the disease occurs in patients with compromised immune systems, specifically transplant recipients and individuals with acquired immunodeficiency syndrome.

karyokinesis   The process in early cell division during which the nucleus divides and nuclear material is equally distributed. This four-stage process, known as mitosis, includes the prophase, metaphase, anaphase, and telophase, and occurs before the division of the cytoplasm.

karyolymph   The clear, usually nonstaining, liquid part of the cell nucleus.

karyolysis   The swelling and breakdown of the cell nucleus.

karyomere   1. A saclike structure containing only a small portion of the typical nucleus, usually following atypical mitosis. 2. A chromomere, or segment, of the chromosome.

Katz index   Assessment tool that evaluates a patient's ability to perform basic activities of daily living, such as bathing, dressing, toileting, transfer, continence, and feeding.

Kayser-Fleischer ring   A gray-green to red-gold discolored ring at the outer margin of the cornea. It is a characteristic symptom of Wilson's disease, a rare, progressive, degenerative liver disorder caused by a defect in copper metabolism and transmitted as an autosomal recessive trait.

kcal   *abbr* kilocalorie.

Kellgren's syndrome   A form of osteoarthritis affecting the joints of the fingers and toes, the arch of the foot, the hand and wrist, the knees, and the spine.

keloid, cheloid   A scar resulting from the overgrowth of collagen in the tissue at the site of a wound of the skin. The progressively enlarging scar is elevated, rounded, and firm, with irregular, clawlike margins.

keratectomy   Surgical removal of a small, superficial lesion of the cornea. The surgery,

usually performed for anterior staphyloma, does not warrant a corneal graft.

keratoconjunctivitis   An inflammation of the cornea and the conjunctiva.

keratoconus   A noninflammatory, usually bilateral, protrusion of the central part of the cornea. Also called conical cornea.

keratolytic   An agent that promotes the softening and dissolution, or peeling, of the horny layer of the epidermis.

keratomalacia   A condition, associated with vitamin A deficiency, characterized by the abnormal dryness of the conjunctiva and ulceration of the cornea.

keratopathy   A noninflammatory disease of the cornea.

keratosis   Any skin condition in which there is a thickening or horny growth, such as a callus or wart.

kerion   An inflamed, spongy, exuding nodule that occurs as an immune reaction to a superficial fungus infection such as tinea capitis of the scalp.

Kernig's sign   Sign of meningitis in which a patient in the supine position can easily and completely extend the leg; but in a sitting position (or lying with the thigh flexed upon the abdomen) the patient can't completely extend the leg.

ketoacidosis   Acidosis accompanied by ketosis, resulting from faulty carbohydrate metabolism. May result from diabetes or starvation.

ketone bodies   The normal intermediate products of the metabolism of fatty acids and carbohydrates in the liver; include beta-hydroxylbutyric acid, acetoacetic acid, and acetone.

ketonuria   Excess ketones in the urine.

ketosis   The abnormal accumulation of ketone bodies in the body fluids and tissues resulting from the incomplete metabolism of fatty acids; a condition associated with uncontrolled diabetes mellitus, starvation, and alcoholism.

kg   *abbr* kilogram.

kidney   One of a pair of bean-shaped urinary organs located on either side of the vertebral column in the lumbar region of the abdomen.

kilogram (kg)   A unit for the measurement of mass in the metric system. One kilogram is equal to 1,000 grams or 2.2046 pounds avoirdupois.

kinase   An enzyme that catalyzes the transfer of a high-energy phosphate group from a donor molecule, such as adenosine triphosphate, to an acceptor molecule.

kinematics   In physiology: the geometry of the motion of the body without regard to the forces acting to produce the motion.

kinetics   In physiology: the study of the forces that produce, arrest, or modify the motions of the body.

kinetotherapeutic bath   A bath in which underwater exercises are performed to strengthen weak or partially paralyzed muscles.

knee   A complex joint formed by the femur, tibia, and patella where the thigh connects with the lower leg.

koilonychia   Abnormally thin nails that are concave from side to side, with turned up edges.

Korotkoff sounds   Sounds heard while measuring blood pressure using a sphygmomanometer and stethoscope.

Kraske position   An anatomic position in which the patient is prone, with buttocks raised and head and feet down.

kraurosis vulvae   A disease found most often in older women and characterized by the atrophy, dryness, and severe itching of the external genitalia.

Krause's corpuscles   A type of small, encapsulated nerve ending found in the skin, conjunctiva of the eye, mucous membranes of the lips and tongue, the penis and clitoris, and the synovial membranes of certain joints.

Krebs citric acid cycle   A complicated series of enzymatic reactions involving the oxidative metabolism of carbon chains of sugars, fatty acids, and amino acids to yield high-energy phosphate bonds, carbon dioxide, and water.

Krukenberg's tumor   A cancer of the ovary usually resulting from a metastasis of stomach cancer or other gastrointestinal malignancy.

Kupffer's cells   Large, phagocytic cells lining the walls of the hepatic sinusoids.

Kussmaul respirations   Abnormally deep, gasping type of respirations, resulting from air hunger, associated with severe diabetic acidosis and coma.

Kussmaul's sign   Increased jugular venous distention on inspiration due to restricted right-sided filling.

kwashiorkor   A malnutrition disease resulting from severe protein deficiency and characterized by retarded growth, changes in hair and skin pigment, edema, and pathological changes in the liver. It primarily affects children in undeveloped countries, mainly in the tropics and subtropics.

kyphoscoliosis   Forward and lateral curvature of the spine.

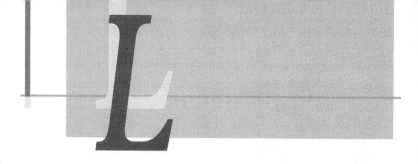

label In radiology: a substance, such as a radioactive tracer, that tends to become deposited and fixed in a certain type of organ, tissue, cell, or microorganism.

labeled compound A compound containing a radioactive or stable isotope; through radioactive tracing, the compound or its fragments can be followed through various physical, chemical, or biological processes.

labia, *sing.* labium 1. A fleshy edge or border. 2. The liplike folds of skin at the vaginal opening.

labia majora, *sing.* labium majus Two raised folds of adipose and connective tissue covered by skin, one on either side of the vaginal orifice outside the labia minora, that taper down and back from the mons pubis to the perineum.

labia minora, *sing.* labium minus Two moist folds of skin between the labia majora that taper down and back from the clitoris along both sides of the vaginal orifice.

labor The time and processes occurring from the onset of cervical effacement and dilation to delivery of the placenta.

laboratory medicine The branch of medicine that studies specimens of body substances, such as fluid and tissue, outside of the patient, usually in the laboratory.

laboratory test A procedure performed in a laboratory that detects, identifies, or measures a significant substance, analyzes organ functions, or evaluates the nature of a condition or disease.

labored breathing Abnormal respiration with evidence of increased work of breathing, such as use of accessory chest wall muscles, grunting, stridor, or nasal flaring.

labyrinthectomy Excision of the labyrinth of the ear.

labyrinthine deafness Deafness caused by a disease or defect of the labyrinth.

lacrimal apparatus A network of eye structures (the lacrimal glands, upper and lower canaliculi, lacrimal sac, and nasolacrimal duct) that secretes and circulates tears from the surface of the eyeball.

lacrimal bone A small, thin, fragile bone of the face, located at the anterior part of the medial wall of the orbit and joining the frontal and ethmoidal bones and the maxilla and inferior nasal concha.

lacrimal caruncle The small, fleshy, red protuberance at the medial angle of the eye, which houses sebaceous and sudoriferous glands and secretes a white substance.

lacrimal duct One of two short passages in the eyelid, extending from the lacrimal lake to the lacrimal sac, through which tears pass.

lacrimal fistula An abnormal passage connecting a lacrimal duct or sac to the surface of the eye or eyelid.

lacrimal gland One of a pair of glands situated at the upper outer angle of each orbit that secretes tears.

lacrimal nerve The sensory branch of the maxillary division of the trigeminal nerve that supplies the lacrimal gland, conjunctiva, and upper eye.

lacrimal papilla A small, nipple-shaped projection in the conjunctiva near the medial angle of each eye through which tears emerge.

lacrimal sac The dilated upper end of the nasolacrimal duct of the eye.

lactalbumin A protein, similar to albumin, that occurs in milk.

lactase An enzyme, found in the intestinal mucosa, kidney, and liver, that catalyzes the hydrolysis of alpha-D-galactoside to D-galactose.

lactase deficiency A congenital or acquired deficiency in or absence of lactase activity in the intestinal mucosa, leading to inability to digest lactose.

lactate dehydrogenase (LD) An enzyme, found in almost all body tissues, that catalyzes the reversible conversion of muscle lactic acid into pyruvic acid as the final step in glycolysis.

 ALERT Recent surgery, pregnancy, prosthetic heart valve, or use of anabolic steroids, anesthetics, alcohol, narcotics, or procainamide may increase LD levels.

lactation   The secretion of milk from the mammary glands. It is controlled by hormones, notably prolactin and oxytocin.

lacteal gland   A blind-ended lymphatic capillary in each villus of the small intestine that opens into the lymphatic vessels in the submucosa. During absorption, the gland turns white from the influence of digested fat. Also called *lacteal.*

lactic acid   A clear, odorless, three-carbon organic acid, produced from pyruvic acid in active muscle tissue when the oxygen supply is limited and then removed for conversion to glucose by the liver. During strenuous exercise, lactic acid may build up in the muscles, causing cramps.

lactiferous duct   One of the many ducts that drain milk from the lobes of the breast onto the nipple surface.

lactose   A disaccharide found in milk that consists of one glucose molecule linked to a galactose molecule.

lactose intolerance   An intolerance for lactose that interferes with the ability to digest lactose. It usually results from an inherited deficiency of lactase activity in the intestinal mucosa.

 CLINICAL TIP Many adults suffer from lactose intolerance, the more common hereditary form of lactase deficiency. The rare hereditary form, called congenital lactose intolerance, is marked by vomiting, diarrhea, and failure to thrive.

lacuna, *pl.* **lacunae**   1. A gap or cavity within the tissues, especially bony tissue. 2. A defect or gap, as in the field of vision (scotoma).

lacus lacrimalis   The triangular space at the medial angle of the eye where tears collect and where the lacrimal caruncle is found.

Laënnec's catarrh   Bronchial asthma with expectoration of small, viscous beads of sputum.

lagophthalmos   Inability to close the eye completely, resulting from a muscular or neurologic disorder.

lambdoid suture   The line of juncture between the parietal and occipital bones of the skull (named for its resemblance to the Greek letter lambda.)

lamina, *pl.* **laminae**   1. A thin, flat plate or layer. 2. The lamina of the vertebral arch.

laminated thrombus   A thrombus made up of layers, which apparently formed at different times.

laminectomy   Surgical removal of the bony arches of one or more vertebrae, performed to relieve spinal cord compression or to remove a displaced intervertebral disk.

laminotomy   Division of lamina of a vertebra.

Lancefield's classification   A serologic classification of hemolytic streptococci based on antigenic characteristics; groups A through O have been identified.

lancet   1. A small, pointed, two-edged surgical knife. 2. A short, pointed blade used to puncture the skin and collect a drop of blood for a capillary sample.

lancinating   Darting, tearing, sharply cutting, as lancinating pain.

Landau reflex   Formation of a convex upward arc by the entire body, with the head raised and legs slightly flexed. It is a normal response seen in infants held in a prone position.

Landsteiner's classification   Classification of human blood into groups A, B, AB, or O based on the presence or absence of the agglutinogens A and B on red blood cells.

lanthanum (La)   A rare metallic element. Its atomic number is 57; atomic weight, 138.91.

lanugo   The soft, fine hair covering the face, shoulders, and back of the fetus or neonate before 28 weeks' gestation.

laparoscope   An instrument with an illuminated tube, inserted through an incision in the abdominal wall, to visually examine the interior of the peritoneal cavity.

laparoscopy   1. Examination of the interior of the peritoneal cavity by means of a laparoscope. 2. A surgical procedure involving laparoscopy, especially one done under laparoscopic guidance to remove the ova or to sterilize a female.

laparotomy   Surgical incision through the flank to gain access to the peritoneal cavity, commonly performed on an exploratory basis.

large-for-gestational-age newborn   A newborn whose birth weight exceeds the 90th percentile for gestational age on the Colorado intrauterine growth chart (whether delivered prematurely, at term, or later than term).

large intestine   The portion of the gastrointestinal tract that extends from the pyloric opening of the stomach to the anus, consisting of the cecum, colon, rectum, and anal canal. Its primary functions are to absorb water and form feces.

laryngeal nerve   Nerve with sensory and motor branches that supplies the laryngeal, pharyngeal, and tracheal structures.

laryngeal veins   Inferior and superior veins of the larynx.

laryngectomy   Partial or total removal of the larynx, commonly performed to treat cancer of the larynx.

CLINICAL TIP A partial laryngectomy removes only the vocal cords, not the entire larynx.

laryngitis Inflammation of the larynx, typically accompanied by sore throat, hoarseness, cough, and difficulty swallowing. The condition may be acute, as from a respiratory infection, or chronic, as from heavy smoking or excessive use of the voice.

larynx A structure located between the root of the tongue and the upper end of the trachea, just below and in front of the lowest part of the pharynx. Composed of numerous cartilages and muscles, the larynx serves as the organ of voice and protects the airway from the entrance of liquids or solids during swallowing.

Lasègue's sign In sciatica, pain in the back and leg elicited by passively raising the heel from the bed with the knee straight.

Lassa fever An acute, highly contagious disease caused by a virulent arenavirus. Endemic throughout West Africa, it is spread by interpersonal contact with the multimammate rat (*Mastomys natalensis*) or by contact with its urine. Signs and symptoms include fever, headache, dry cough, vomiting, diarrhea, sore throat, and facial edema. With severe disease, blood pressure drops suddenly on the seventh day; shock, peripheral vasoconstriction, hypovolemia, and anuria may lead to death.

latent period A seemingly inactive interval between the time of exposure to an infection or injurious agent (such as a high dose of radiation) and the development of an obvious response.

latent phase The first part of the first stage of labor, preceding active labor. It is characterized by short, irregular, mild contractions and cervical dilation to 3 or 4 cm.

lateral Pertaining to the side.

lateral aortic node Any of the lymph nodes in the two chains of the left lumbar group, located on the left side of the aorta, that drain the pelvis and abdomen.

lateral aperture of the fourth ventricle An opening between the end of each lateral recess of the fourth ventricle and the subarachnoid space, through which the ventricular cavity communicates with the subarachnoid space. Also called *foramen of Magendie*.

lateral recumbent position Position in which the patient lies on the left side with the right thigh and knee drawn up.

lateral umbilical fold A fold in the peritoneum on either side of the inferior part of the anterior abdominal wall, overlying the inferior epigastric vessels. Also called *epigastric fold*.

latex agglutination test An antibody test used to aid diagnosis of rheumatoid arthritis in which antigen to a given antibody is adsorbed to latex particles and mixed with a solution to observe for latex agglutination. Also called *latex fixation test*.

latissimus dorsi One of a pair of large, triangular muscles in the thoracic and lumbar region of the back. It extends the upper arm and adducts the upper arm posteriorly.

lavage The therapeutic washing out or irrigation of an organ, such as the bowel or bladder.

law of definite proportions In chemistry: a law stating that any compound always contains the same kinds of elements in the same proportion.

law of universal gravitation In physics: a law stating that bodies attract other bodies with a force directly proportional to the masses of the objects and inversely proportional to the square of the distance separating them.

Lawton scale Assessment tool used to evaluate a patient's ability to perform relatively complex tasks, such as using a telephone, cooking, managing finances, and taking medications.

laxative 1. Cathartic or purgative. 2. A substance that promotes evacuation of the bowel by a mild action.

LBW *abbr* low birth weight.

LD *abbr* 1. lethal dose. 2. lactate dehydrogenase.

LD50 Lethal dose 50, or the median lethal dose; the amount of a toxic or pharmacologic substance that kills 50% of test subjects.

LDL *abbr* low-density lipoproteins.

LE *abbr* lupus erythematosus.

lead (Pb) A heavy, dull gray, soft, ductile, metallic element with many uses. Its atomic number is 82; atomic weight, 207.2.

lead equivalent In radiology: the thickness of pure lead that would provide the same shielding effect against radiation, under specified conditions, as would a material under consideration.

lead pipe fracture A fracture in which the cortex of the bone is slightly compressed at the point of impact, resulting in a linear fracture on the opposite side of the bone.

lead poisoning Poisoning caused by the ingestion or absorption of lead or one of its salts. Signs and symptoms include loss of appetite and weight, anemia, constipation, insomnia, headache, dizziness, irritability, a blue line at the margin of the gums, and peripheral neuropathy.

Leber's congenital amaurosis A rare type of blindness or severe vision impairment that is transmitted as an autosomal recessive trait and manifests at birth or shortly thereafter. Also called *congenital amaurosis.*

lecithin Any of a group of waxy phospholipids commonly found in animals and plants, possessing wetting, emulsifying, and antioxidant properties.

Lee-White test A technique used to determine the length of time needed for a clot to form in a test tube of venous blood.

left common carotid artery The longer of the two common carotid arteries. It arises from the aortic arch and has cervical and thoracic portions.

left coronary artery Either of a pair of branches from the ascending aorta, originating in the left posterior aortic sinus and branching into the left interventricular artery and the circumflex branch. It provides blood to both of the ventricles and to the left atrium.

left hepatic duct A duct that emerges from the undersurface of the liver and drains bile from the left lobe. It immediately joins the right hepatic duct to form one hepatic duct, which then merges with the cystic duct from the gallbladder to form the common bile duct.

left pulmonary artery The shorter and smaller of the two arteries that carry deoxygenated blood from the right side of heart to the lungs. Rising from the pulmonary trunk, it typically has more separate branches than does the right pulmonary artery.

left-sided heart failure Impairment of the left ventricle of the heart, marked by inability to contract forcefully enough to maintain normal cardiac output and peripheral perfusion. Typically, the condition causes pulmonary congestion and edema, leading to dyspnea and orthopnea.

left ventricle The thick-walled, lower chamber of the heart that pumps blood through all the vessels of the body except those to and from the lungs.

leg cylinder cast An orthopedic device made of fiberglass, plaster, or synthetic material, used to immobilize and support the leg in treating fractures extending from the ankle to the upper thigh.

legal guardian An officer or agent of the court who's appointed to protect the interests of minors or incompetent persons and provide for their welfare, education, and support.

Legionella pneumophila A gram-negative, rod-shaped bacterium that causes legionnaire's disease. It is found in numerous environmental sites as well as in blood and certain body tissues.

legionnaire's disease An acute, flulike disease caused by *Legionella pneumophila.*

Signs and symptoms include high fever, GI distress, headache, pneumonia and, occasionally, involvement of the liver, kidneys, and nervous system.

leiomyoma, *pl.* **leiomyomas, leiomyomata** A benign tumor derived from smooth muscle — usually of the uterus or, less commonly, the stomach, esophagus, or small intestine.

leiomyoma uteri A benign tumor of the smooth muscle of the uterus that usually occurs in multiples and is firm, well-circumscribed, round, and gray-white. Also called *fibroid* (colloquially), *uterine myoma.*

lens 1. A transparent piece of glass or plastic that is shaped to converge or scatter light rays in a specific way, as in eyeglasses. 2. The transparent, biconvex, crystalline lens of the eye, located between the posterior chamber and the vitreous body.

lens capsule The clear, elastic envelope surrounding the lens of the eye. Also called *crystalline capsule, capsule of the lens.*

lens implant An artificial lens made of clear polymethylmethacrylate, typically implanted at the time of cataract extraction to correct vision.

CLINICAL TIP A lens implant can correct vision to 20/20 in some people. It also provides normal depth perception and peripheral vision without distortion.

LE prep *abbr* lupus erythematosus preparation.

lepromin test A skin sensitivity test in which a suspension of heat-killed *Mycobacterium leprae* is injected intradermally to help distinguish between the lepromatous and tuberculoid forms of leprosy.

leprosy A chronic and slowly progressive communicable disease caused by *Mycobacterium leprae*, characterized by the development of granulomatous or neurotrophic lesions of the skin, mucous membranes, nerves, bones, and viscera. It occurs in two major clinical forms — lepromatous and tuberculoid. Also called *Hansen's disease, lepra.*

leptonema The threadlike chromosome formation in the first stage of meiosis before synapsis begins.

Leriche syndrome A vascular disorder caused by obstruction of the terminal aorta, characterized by intermittent claudication in the hips, thighs, or calves; absent pulses in the femoral arteries; pallor and coolness of the legs; fatigue; and, in men, impotence.

Lesch-Nyhan syndrome A hereditary disorder of purine metabolism that is transmitted as a recessive, sex-linked trait, characterized by physical and mental retardation, compulsive biting of the fingers and lips, impaired renal function, and spastic cerebral palsy.

lesion Any abnormal change in the structure of an organ or a part as a result of trauma or disease, especially one that is circumscribed and well defined. Types of lesions include wounds, sores, tumors, and rashes.

lesser omentum A membranous fold of peritoneum that joins the lesser curvature of the stomach and the first part of the duodenum with the hepatic portal.

lesser trochanter A short, conical projection, located at the base of the neck of the femur, that provides insertion of the tendon of the psoas major muscle.

lethal equivalent Any recessive gene carried in the heterozygous state that, if homozygous, would result in the death of the individual or organism.

lethal gene Any gene carried in the heterozygous state that, if homozygous, would cause death of the organism.

lethargy Slowed responses, sluggish speech, and slowed mental and motor processes in a patient oriented to time, place, and person.

Letterer-Siwe disease Hyperplasia of the reticuloendothelial tissue, characterized by hemorrhaging, eczema, progressive anemia, hepatosplenomegaly, and lymph node enlargement.

leucine An essential amino acid, obtained through the digestion or hydrolytic cleavage of protein, that is needed by infants for optimal growth and by adults for nitrogen equilibrium.

leukapheresis Electrophoretic separation and removal of selected leukocytes from a blood sample, followed by transfusion of the remainder of the blood into the donor.

leukemia A progressive malignant disease of the blood-forming organs characterized by abnormal numbers and forms of immature circulating white blood cells, with infiltration of the lymph nodes, liver, spleen, and other sites.

 CLINICAL TIP Leukemia may be classified as acute or chronic based on the degree of cell differentiation or as myelogenous or lymphocytic based on the predominant cell type involved.

leukemia cutis A cutaneous manifestation of leukemia in which malignant white blood cells infiltrate the skin.

leukemoid reaction A clinical syndrome that resembles leukemia based solely on the morphologic appearance of blood cells.

leukocyte A white blood cell; one of the formed elements of the circulating blood. Originating in the lymph nodes and red bone marrow, leukocytes can produce antibodies and migrate to an injury site, where they surround and isolate foreign matter, dead tissue, and bacteria. The two major types of leukocytes are granulocytes (those with granules in the cytoplasm) and agranulocytes (those lacking granules in the cytoplasm). Also called *white blood cell.*

leukocytosis An abnormal increase in the number of circulating white blood cells, commonly resulting from such conditions as fever, hemorrhage, infection, or inflammation. It commonly accompanies bacterial infections.

leukopenia An abnormal reduction in the number of circulating white blood cells to fewer than 5,000 cells/μl.

leukoplakia A precancerous, white, thickened, firmly attached, and sharply circumscribed patch on a mucous membrane.

leukopoiesis The production of white blood cells.

leukorrhea A whitish discharge from the vagina.

leukotrienes Group of compounds derived from unsaturated fatty acids; extremely potent mediators of immediate hypersensitivity reactions and inflammation.

levator, *pl.* levators 1. A muscle that elevates the structure into which it is inserted. 2. A surgical instrument used to raise depressed osseous fragments in fractures of the skull and other bones.

levator ani One of a pair of muscles of the pelvic diaphragm that form the floor of the pelvic cavity and support the pelvic organs.

LeVeen shunt A surgically implanted plastic tube used to shunt ascites fluid or other fluid from the peritoneal cavity to the jugular vein.

level of consciousness (LOC) The degree of wakefulness and orientation.

 TIME LINE The primary cause of decreased LOC in children is head trauma, which often results from a motor vehicle accident or physical abuse. Others include accidental poisoning, hydrocephalus, and meningitis or brain abscess following an ear or respiratory infection.

lever In physiology: any of the bones and associated joints that act together as a lever, or rigid bar, free to turn about a fixed point (its fulcrum). As a muscle contracts, it applies a pulling force on a bone lever at the point where the muscle attaches to the bone, causing the bone to move about its joint fulcrum.

Leydig cell tumor A tumor, usually benign, that derives from the Leydig cells of the testis. In adults, it may cause gynecomastia;

if it develops before puberty, it may cause precocious sexual development. Also called *interstitial cell tumor.*

Leydig's cells Epithelioid cells of the interstitial tissue of the testis. These testosterone-secreting cells constitute the endocrine tissue of the testes. Also called *interstitial cells, interstitial cells of Leydig.*

LFT *abbr* liver function test.

LGA *abbr* large for gestational age.

LGV *abbr* lymphogranuloma venereum.

LH *abbr* luteinizing hormone.

Lhermitte's sign Sudden, brief, electric-like shocks that pass down the body when the head is flexed forward. This sign appears in multiple sclerosis and in compression disorders of the cervical spinal cord.

LH-FSH *abbr* luteinizing hormone–follicle-stimulating hormone.

LH-RF *abbr* luteinizing hormone–releasing factor.

LH-RH *abbr* luteinizing hormone–releasing hormone.

Li Symbol for lithium.

licensed practical nurse (LPN) A person trained in basic nursing techniques and direct patient care who practices under supervision of a registered nurse or other health care provider. LPNs typically complete 1 or 2 years of training, must pass the NCLEX-PN examination, and meet requirements set forth by the state board of nursing. In Canada, LPNs are called nursing assistants. Also called *licensed vocational nurse* (U.S.).

licensure The granting of permission by a competent authority (usually a governmental agency) to an organization or person to engage in a practice or activity that would otherwise be illegal. Issued licenses include those for operation of general hospitals or nursing homes; for health care professionals, such as doctors; and for the production or distribution of biologic products. Licensure is usually granted on the basis of education and examination rather than performance. It's usually permanent, but a periodic fee, demonstration of competence, or continuing education may be required. Licensure may be revoked by the granting agency for incompetence, criminal acts, or other reasons stipulated in the rules governing the specific area of licensure.

lichenification Thickening and hardening of the skin.

lichen nitidus A chronic inflammatory skin disorder characterized by numerous pale, flat-topped, glistening, discrete, smooth papules, which typically appear on the lower abdomen, inner thighs, penis, wrists, forearms, breasts, and buttocks.

lichen planus A chronic, pruritic, inflammatory skin disease of unknown cause, marked by flat-topped, angular papules with a shiny, fine scale and whitish lines. The lesions, which dissolve on their own, may be discrete or may coalesce to form plaques or other configurations.

life science Science that deals with living organisms and life processes. Types of life sciences include anatomy and biology.

ligament A shiny, flexible band of fibrous tissue, predominantly white, that supports and strengthens joints and connects bones or cartilages.

ligation Application of a ligature, such as wire or thread, to tie off a blood vessel or duct in an effort to prevent or halt bleeding or to prevent material from passing through a duct (as in tubal ligation).

ligature A substance, such as silk, cotton, wire, or catgut, used to tie off a vessel or other part.

ligature needle A long, thin, steel needle with an eye in its curved end, used for passing a ligature underneath an artery.

light bath Exposure of the body to the sun or to artificial light rays for therapeutic purposes.

light diet A diet of moderate quantities of soft-cooked and easily digested foods, appropriate for convalescent patients who take little or no exercise.

lightening A subjective sensation reported by some women as the fetus descends into the pelvic inlet and changes the shape and position of the uterus near term.

light reflex Contraction of the pupil of the eye in response to direct or consensual pupillary stimulation.

limb 1. An arm or a leg. 2. A branch of an internal organ that resembles an arm or a leg.

limbic system A group of brain structures situated below the cerebral cortex that are involved in feelings, motivation, and sexual arousal.

linea alba The whitish median line in the anterior abdominal wall formed by the union of the aponeuroses of the three flat abdominal muscles. It extends from the symphysis pubis to the xiphoid process.

linea arcuata The tendinous band in the sheath of the rectus abdominis muscle below the umbilicus.

linea aspera The broad, posterior crest of the thigh bone, which extends into three ridges to which the gluteus maximus, pectineus, iliacus, and several other muscles are attached.

linear accelerator A type of particle accelerator in which charged particles are accelerated in a straight line, either by a steady electrical field or by means of radiofrequency electrical fields. The particles are used in radiotherapy and radionuclide production as well as in physics research.

linear fracture   A fracture that runs along the length of a bone without displacing the bone tissue.

linea semilunaris   A curved line on the ventral abdominal wall, roughly parallel to the median line and situated about halfway between the median line and the side of the body.

lingual artery   One of a pair of arteries originating from the external carotid arteries and branching into the suprahyoid, sublingual, dorsal lingual, and deep lingual arteries. It supplies the tongue, epiglottis, tonsil, and sublingual gland.

linitis   Inflammation of cellular gastric tissue, as in adenocarcinoma of the stomach.

linkage group   In genetics: a group of genes located on the same chromosome and inherited as a unit.

linked genes   Genes that are located on the same chromosome and transmitted together as a unit.

linoleic acid   A polyunsaturated fatty acid found in certain plant oils, such as soybean and linseed oils, that is one of the essential fatty acids.

lipase   An enzyme secreted by the pancreas and the small intestine that catalyzes the breakdown of fats into fatty acids and glycerol.

lipemia   A condition marked by an abnormal elevation in the plasma concentration of any or all of the lipids. Also called *hyperlipidemia.*

lipid   Any of a diverse group of organic compounds found in living organisms that are insoluble in water but soluble in such organic solvents as benzene, alcohol, and chloroform. Major lipids include fats, phospholipids, and steroids.

lipidosis   A general term for several lysosomal storage diseases characterized by abnormal buildup of lipids in the reticuloendothelial cells. Also called *lipid storage disease.*

lipochrome   Any of the naturally occurring fat-soluble pigments, such as carotene, which, when ingested, impart a yellowish or orange-red tinge to lipid-containing tissues.

lipodystrophia progressiva   A disturbance in fat metabolism characterized by loss of subcutaneous fat on the face and upper body, with the lower part of the body appearing enlarged. The condition may be associated with renal disease, insulin-resistant diabetes, or hypertriglyceridemia. Also called

partial lipodystrophy, progressive lipodystrophy.

lipodystrophy   Any disturbance in fat metabolism.

lipoid   Resembling a lipid.

lipoma, *pl.* lipomas, lipomata   A benign, soft, encapsulated tumor usually consisting of mature fat cells.

lipoma arborescens   A fatty tumor of a joint, usually the knee, characterized by treelike projections of fatty tissue.

lipoma capsulare   A benign tumor caused by an increase in fat within the capsule of an organ.

lipomatosis   Abnormal localized or tumorlike accumulations of fat in body tissues.

lipomatosis dolorosa   Lipomatosis in which the fatty accumulations are painful or tender. Also called *lipoma dolorosa.*

lipoprotein   One of a group of compounds consisting of a lipid combined with a protein. Lipoproteins transport lipids in the blood and lymph and are the main structural components of cell membranes. Synthesized primarily in the liver, they contain varying amounts of triglycerides, cholesterol, phospholipids, and protein.

liposome   A chemical vehicle for transmitting chemotherapeutic drugs directly to a cancerous tumor; consists of ring-shaped layers, usually phospholipids, with aqueous fluid in between. Drugs bind with the lipid layers (or aqueous solution, if water soluable) and are then carried as part of the liposome to specific tumor cells.

liquefaction   The conversion of a material, such as a solid or a gas, into a liquid.

liquid diet   A diet consisting of foods served in liquid form.

> **CLINICAL TIP** A liquid diet is commonly prescribed for preoperative and postoperative patients and for those who have acute GI inflammatory conditions or oral or esophageal lesions.

Lisfranc's dislocation   A dislocation of the foot involving all of the proximal metatarsals.

Listeria   A genus of bacteria of small, coccoid, gram-positive rods found in human and animal feces and on vegetation.

Listeria monocytogenes   A common species of *Listeria* that causes listeriosis and sometimes results in meningitis, perinatal septicemia, and other diseases.

listeriosis   An infectious disease caused by *Listeria monocytogenes.* In utero infection may result in spontaneous abortion, stillbirth, or preterm birth. In adults, infection can cause meningitis and endocarditis.

lithopedion, lithopedium   A dead fetus that has become calcified or petrified.

Lipoprotein synthesis and metabolism

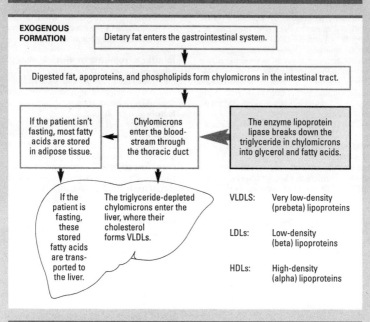

EXOGENOUS FORMATION

Dietary fat enters the gastrointestinal system.

Digested fat, apoproteins, and phospholipids form chylomicrons in the intestinal tract.

If the patient isn't fasting, most fatty acids are stored in adipose tissue.

Chylomicrons enter the blood-stream through the thoracic duct

The enzyme lipoprotein lipase breaks down the triglyceride in chylomicrons into glycerol and fatty acids.

If the patient is fasting, these stored fatty acids are transported to the liver.

The triglyceride-depleted chylomicrons enter the liver, where their cholesterol forms VLDLs.

VLDLS: Very low-density (prebeta) lipoproteins

LDLs: Low-density (beta) lipoproteins

HDLs: High-density (alpha) lipoproteins

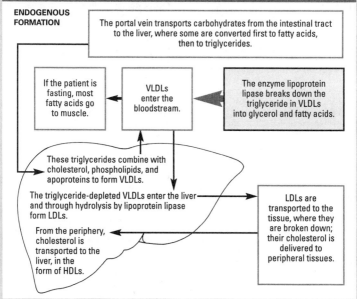

ENDOGENOUS FORMATION

The portal vein transports carbohydrates from the intestinal tract to the liver, where some are converted first to fatty acids, then to triglycerides.

If the patient is fasting, most fatty acids go to muscle.

VLDLs enter the bloodstream.

The enzyme lipoprotein lipase breaks down the triglyceride in VLDLs into glycerol and fatty acids.

These triglycerides combine with cholesterol, phospholipids, and apoproteins to form VLDLs.

The triglyceride-depleted VLDLs enter the liver and through hydrolysis by lipoprotein lipase form LDLs.

From the periphery, cholesterol is transported to the liver, in the form of HDLs.

LDLs are transported to the tissue, where they are broken down; their cholesterol is delivered to peripheral tissues.

lithotomy forceps   A forceps used to extract calculi, usually from the urinary bladder.

lithotomy position   A position in which a patient lies on the back with the hips and knees flexed and the thighs abducted and externally rotated.

lithotrite   An instrument used to crush a stone in the urinary bladder.

litmus paper   Absorbent paper soaked in litmus solution that is used to determine pH. It turns red under acid conditions and blue under alkaline conditions.

live birth   The birth of a newborn showing any sign of life, such as respiration, pulse, umbilical pulsation, or voluntary muscle movement.

livedo reticularis   A vascular reaction to various disorders marked by blue or red skin mottling. The condition worsens in cold weather.

liver   A large, dark red gland located in the right side of the abdomen, immediately below the diaphragm and partially anterior to the stomach. Consisting of a right lobe, left lobe, caudate lobe, and quadrate lobe, the liver has many digestive, metabolic, and regulatory functions.

liver biopsy   Introduction of a Menghini needle into the liver under local anesthesia to obtain a tissue specimen for histologic analysis.

liver cancer   A malignant neoplasm of the liver, most commonly occurring as a metastasis from a cancerous tumor elsewhere in the body.

liver disease   Any disease of the liver, such as cirrhosis, cholestasis, and hepatitis.

liver function test   Any of a group of tests used to evaluate the function of the liver. Includes Kinberg's test, the lipase test, Macdonald's test, and Quick's test.

liver scan   A noninvasive diagnostic technique used to examine the liver after intravenous administration of a radioactive colloid that is taken up by Kupffer's cells in the liver.

LMP   *abbr* last menstrual period.

lobar bronchus   An air passage that arises from the primary bronchus and passes into one of the lobes of the right or left lung.

lobar pneumonia   An acute disease characterized by inflammation of one or more lobes of the lung and consolidation of lung tissue. Signs and symptoms include chills, sudden high fever, coughing, dyspnea, tachypnea, and blood-stained expectoration.

lobe   1. A curved or rounded projection. 2. A relatively well-defined portion of an organ, such as the brain, liver, or lungs, that is bounded by sulci, fissures, or connective tissue.

lobectomy   Surgical excision of a lobe, usually of a lung.

lobotomy   1. Incision into a lobe. 2. In neurosurgery: severing of the white matter of the frontal lobe of the brain, usually performed to alter the patient's affective responses.

lobular carcinoma in situ   A slowly progressive, precancerous neoplasm of the breast, usually too small and widely dispersed to be palpated. It accounts for a small percentage of breast tumors.

lobule   A small lobe.

LOC   *abbr* level of consciousness.

local anesthesia   Administration of an anesthetic to a confined part of the body to cause loss of sensation in that part.

local anesthetic   A substance whose pain-reducing action is confined to a limited part of the body. Typically, such an anesthetic produces its effect by blocking nerve conduction.

localization film   In radiotherapy: a diagnostic film obtained to verify a treatment portal or to visualize the position of an interstitial or intracavitary implant. It is most commonly taken to compute the dose delivered.

lochia   The vaginal discharge present during the first several weeks after delivery.

CLINICAL TIP Lochia occurs in three distinct stages. Lochia rubra, present during the first 3 to 4 postpartal days, is bloody and may contain mucus, tissue, debris, and small clots. Lochia serosa, persisting for 5 to 7 days postpartum, is a pink or brownish discharge. Lochia alba is a creamy white, brown, or colorless discharge consisting mainly of serum and white blood cells. Lochia typically stops flowing at about 6 weeks postpartum.

lock-out interval   A time set on a patient controlled analgesia device during which the device can't be activated.

loculate   Divided into cavities or small spaces.

loculus   A small chamber, pocket, or cavity.

locus of infection   The site of origin of an infection.

Löffler's syndrome   A condition characterized by episodes of pulmonary eosinophilia and transient lung opacities, with dyspnea, fever, anorexia, and weight loss.

long arm cast   An orthopedic cast made of plaster, fiberglass, or synthetic material that is used to immobilize the upper extremity from the hand to the upper arm.

long leg cast   An orthopedic cast made of plaster, fiberglass, or synthetic material that is used to immobilize the leg from the toes to the upper thigh.

loop of Henle   The long, U-shaped portion of a renal tubule, consisting of a descending limb and an ascending limb.

loose fibrous tissue   A type of connective tissue consisting of elastic fibers, collagen fibers, and fluid-filled areolae.

lordosis   An increased anterior concavity in the curvature of the lumbar and cervical spine when the person is viewed from the side.

LOS   *abbr* length of stay.

low-birth-weight (LBW) newborn   A newborn who weighs 2,500 g (5.5 lb) or less at birth.

low-calcium diet   A diet that restricts calcium intake and prohibits most dairy foods, all deep green leafy vegetables, and breads made with milk or dry skim milk.

low-calorie diet   A diet that restricts the intake of calories to a level below that needed to maintain the patient's current weight.

low cervical cesarean section   Surgical delivery of a newborn through a transperitoneal or extraperitoneal transverse incision made in the lower uterine segment.

low-cholesterol diet   A diet that limits the intake of foods containing saturated fatty acids and animal fats.

low-density lipoprotein (LDL)   A class of lipid-protein complexes that transports cholesterol to extrahepatic tissues. High blood levels of LDLs are thought to increase the risk of coronary artery disease.

lower extremity suspension   An orthopedic technique for treating fractures and correcting certain musculoskeletal abnormalities of the lower limbs.

lower motor neuron paralysis   Paralysis resulting from a spinal cord lesion that damages the peripheral neurons whose cell bodies lie in the ventral gray columns of the cord and that terminate in the skeletal muscles.

CLINICAL TIP A patient with a partially transected spinal cord loses some degree of voluntary muscle function, depending on the areas innervated by the nerves involved. A patient with complete transection loses all voluntary muscle control.

low-fat diet   A diet that restricts fat intake and consists primarily of easily digestible, high-carbohydrate foods.

low-fat milk   Milk containing 1% to 2% fat, giving it a higher fat content than skim milk but a lower fat content than whole milk.

low forceps   Delivery in which forceps are used when the leading point of the fetal

skull has reached the perineum (+ 2 station) and rotation is necessary.

Lown-Ganong-Levine syndrome   A cardiac conduction syndrome in which the accessory pathway bypasses the atrioventricular node and links the atrium with the His bundle, causing atrial tachycardia. On electrocardiography, the PR interval is short and the QRS complex is normal.

low-residue diet   A diet that leaves the least possible residue in the lower GI tract. It consists primarily of such foods as sucrose, dextrose, gelatin, broth, meat, liver, cottage cheese, and rice.

low-sodium diet   A diet that restricts the intake of sodium chloride, used primarily to treat hypertension and some forms of edema.

LP   *abbr* lumbar puncture.

LPN   *abbr* licensed practical nurse.

LTB   *abbr* laryngotracheobronchitis.

Lu   Symbol for lutetium.

lucid lethargy   A mental state in which a person exhibits loss of will despite normal intellectual and conscious function.

Ludwig's angina   Severe streptococcal cellulitis of the floor of the mouth, typically caused by infection in the mandibular molar area or a penetrating injury. Signs and symptoms include fever, tachypnea, tongue elevation, dysphagia, and a swollen glottis.

luer-lock injection cap   An I.V. device, possibly attached to the end of an extension set, with a clamping mechanism that provides ready access for intermittent infusions. This reduces the discomfort of reaccessing the port and prolongs the port septum's life by decreasing needle punctures.

Lugol's solution   An aqueous solution of iodine (4.5% to 5.5%) and potassium iodide (9.5% to 10.5%) in purified water, used as a thyroid hormone antagonist. Also called *iodine strong solution*.

lukewarm bath   A bath in water that is between 92° and 97° F (33.3° and 36.1° C).

lumbago   Pain in the lower back (lumbar) region, commonly resulting from muscle strain, rheumatoid arthritis, osteoarthritis, or a herniated intravertebral disk. Ischemic lumbago, marked by pain in the lower back and buttocks, stems from vascular insufficiency (as from terminal aortic obstruction).

lumbar   Of or relating to the loins, or the part of the body between the thorax and the pelvis.

lumbar nerves   The five pairs of spinal nerves that originate in the lumbar region.

lumbar node   A node in one of the seven groups of parietal lymph nodes that drain the abdomen and pelvis.

lumbar plexus   A network of spinal nerves formed by the ventral branches of the

Needle position for lumbar puncture

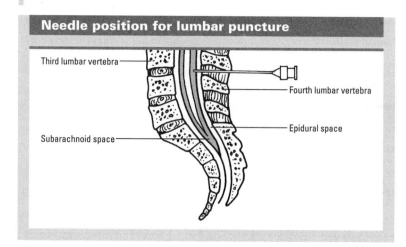

Third lumbar vertebra

Fourth lumbar vertebra

Epidural space

Subarachnoid space

second to fifth lumbar nerves in the lumbar region of the back in the psoas major muscle. (Some authorities include the first lumbar nerve.)

lumbar puncture Fluid withdrawal from the subarachnoid space of the lumbar region of the spinal canal, usually between the third and fourth lumbar vertebrae, for diagnostic or therapeutic purposes. Also called *spinal tap.*

lumbar subarachnoid peritoneostomy Surgical incision into the peritoneal cavity for the purpose of draining cerebrospinal fluid, most commonly performed in newborns to treat hydrocephalus.

lumbar subarachnoid ureterostomy Surgical creation of a fistula to drain excess cerebrospinal fluid though the ureter to the bladder, most commonly performed in newborns to treat hydrocephalus.

lumbar vertebra One of the five bones of the spinal column located in the lumbar (lower back) region, which support the small of the back. Lumbar vertebrae have a body without facets and lack a foramen in the transverse process.

lumbosacral plexus A collective term for the lumbar and sacral nerve plexuses together.

lumen, pl. lumina, lumens. **1.** The space enclosed by a vessel, duct, or other tubular or saclike organ. **2.** The unit of luminous flux equal to the flux emitted in a unit solid angle by a uniform point source of one candle intensity.

lunate bone The crescent-shaped carpal bone located in the proximal row of carpal bones between the scaphoid and triangular bones.

lung One of a pair of spongy, highly elastic respiratory organs situated in the lateral cavities of the chest, separated from each other by the heart and mediastinal structures. The thin, moist membrane in the lung is the site of gas exchange. The lungs lack muscle and are ventilated by respiratory movements.

lung compliance A measure of the ease with which the lungs and thorax expand during respiratory movements, expressed as unit of volume change per unit of pressure change.

lupus erythematosus cell preparation A laboratory test used to help diagnose systemic lupus erythematosus (SLE) or to monitor SLE treatment. In a positive result for SLE, large, spherical, phagocytized inclusions appear within neutrophils that have been incubated with a specimen of the patient's serum.

luteal phase The second half of the menstrual cycle from ovulation to menstruation, marked by stimulation of the corpus luteum by luteinizing hormone to produce progesterone.

lutein A yellow-red, crystalline pigment, or lipochrome, found in the corpus luteum, in plants with carotenes and chlorophylls, and in animal fats and egg yolk.

luteinizing hormone (LH) A hormone produced by the anterior pituitary that stimulates ovulation, progesterone synthesis, and development of the corpus luteum in females and androgen production in males.

lycopene The red, unsaturated hydrocarbon that is the carotenoid pigment of tomatoes and various fruits and berries.

Lyme disease An acute, recurrent multisystemic disorder transmitted by the spiro-

The lungs

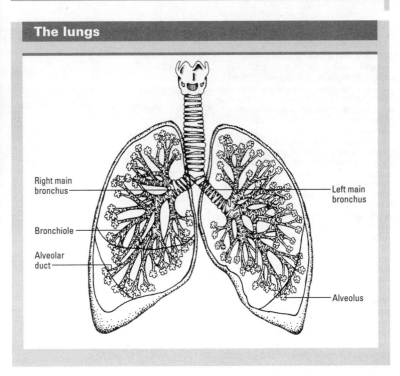

Right main bronchus

Left main bronchus

Bronchiole

Alveolar duct

Alveolus

chete *Borrelia burgdorferi,* which is carried by ticks in the Ixodidae family.

 CLINICAL TIP Typically, Lyme disease begins in the summer with the classic skin lesion, erythema chronicum migrans. Weeks or months later, cardiac or neurologic abnormalities may develop, possibly followed by arthritis.

lymph A colorless liquid found in the lymphatic system, into which it drains from the spaces between cells. Lymph resembles blood plasma, and consists mainly of water with dissolved salts and protein. It circulates through the lymphatic vessels and is filtered by the lymph nodes.

lymphadenitis Inflammation of one or more lymph nodes, usually caused by a primary infection elsewhere in the body or by a systemic neoplastic disease.

lymphangiectasia Dilatation of the intestinal lymphatic vessels, arising either as a congenital condition or secondary to inflammation, cancer involving the major intestinal lymphatic ducts, or increased lymphatic pressure. Signs and symptoms include diarrhea, steatorrhea, and protein malabsorption.

lymphangioma, *pl.* lymphangiomas, lymphangiomata A benign lymphatic tumor caused by congenital malformation of the lymphatic system. In simple lymphangioma, skin lesions may be slightly raised or nodular, or they may be deeper and sharply circumscribed.

lymphangitis Inflammation of one or more lymphatic vessels, usually resulting from beta-hemolytic streptococcal infection of an arm or a leg.

lymphatic capillary plexus One of a network of lymphatic capillaries that drain lymph from intercellular fluid.

lymphatic system A specialized component of the circulatory system that produces, filters, and conveys lymph and produces various blood cells. Besides lymph, the lymphatic system includes a group of vessels called lymphatics that return the lymph to the blood; lymph nodes, located along the paths of the collecting vessels; isolated nodules of lymphatic tissue, such as Peyer's patches in the intestinal wall; specialized lymphatic organs, such as the thymus, spleen, and tonsils; valves; and ducts.

lymphedema   Edema of an arm or a leg caused by the buildup of interstitial fluid as a result of lymphatic inflammation or obstruction or a lymph node disorder.

lymph node   One of many small masses of lymphoid tissue that filter out bacteria and other foreign particles to prevent them from entering the bloodstream and causing infection. Lymph nodes also produce lymphocytes, monocytes, and plasma cells.

lymphocyte   A type of white blood cell with a large nucleus and scant cytoplasm, which serves as an immunologically competent cell. The two general categories are B lymphocytes and T lymphocytes.

lymphocytopenia   A reduction in the normal number of lymphocytes in the peripheral circulation. The condition may occur as a primary hematologic disorder or may arise secondary to cancer, a nutritional deficiency, or infectious mononucleosis.

lymphokine   A soluble chemical factor secreted by T lymphocytes that mediates the activities of lymphoid cells. Examples include interleukin-2 and macrophage migration inhibition factor.

lymphoma, *pl.* **lymphomas, lymphomata**   A neoplastic disorder of lymphoid tissue, usually malignant.

lysine   A hydrolytic product of protein that is an essential amino acid required by infants for optimal growth and by adults for maintenance of nitrogen balance.

lysosome   A membrane-bound sac within the cytoplasm that contains various hydrolytic enzymes responsible for the digestion of material in food vacuoles, dissolution of bacteria and other foreign particles entering the cell, and, on cell death, the breakdown of all cell structures.

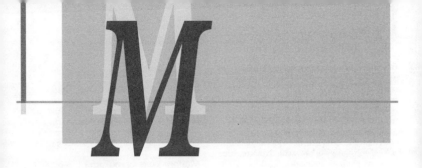

M 1. Symbol for molar solution. 2. *abbr* metastasis in the TNM system for staging malignant neoplastic disease.

Ma *abbr* milliampere.

MA *abbr* 1. mental age. 2. Master of Arts.

MAC *abbr* minimum alveolar concentration

macerate To make a solid soft by wetting or soaking.

macrobiotic diet The most widely followed alternative nutritional program in the United States, macrobiotics emphasize consumption of specific whole grain cereals, organic vegetables, beans, and sea vegetables to balance the body's *yin* and *yang* energies. After classification of their cancer as *yin* or *yang* (according to location and characteristics), many cancer patients use the diet therapeutically, eating *yang* foods for *yin* cancers, and vice versa.

macroblepharia A condition in which the eyelids are abnormally large.

macrobrachia A condition characterized by abnormally large arms.

macrocephaly, macrocephalia A congenital deformity in which the head and brain are disproportionately large; this anomaly results in some mental and growth retardation.

macrocheilia A condition characterized by excessively large lips.

macrocyte A mature erythrocyte with a diameter of 10 to 12 microns. This unusually large erythrocyte is common in megaloblastic anemia.

macrocytic anemia A blood disorder in which erythropoiesis is impaired. Patients suffering from this condition have large, fragile red blood cells that aren't normally present in the circulation.

macrogamete The larger, less active female gamete of certain thallophytes and sporozoa (especially the malarial parasite).

macroglobulinemia A condition in which clones of a plasma B cell react to an antigenic signal, thereby overproducing a large immunoglobulin M.

ALERT This increase of macroglobulins in the blood can impair the patient's circulatory system and cause weakness, fatigue, and neurologic disorders.

macroglossia A congenital defect in which the tongue is unusually large, as in Down syndrome.

macronutrient An element that is essential for the normal physiological processes. These nutrients, which are required in relatively large amounts, include calcium, chloride, magnesium, phosphorus, potassium, carbon, hydrogen, oxygen, sulfur, sodium, and nitrogen.

macrophage Any of the many forms of mononuclear phagocytes found in tissues. They arise from hematopoietic stem cells in the bone marrow. Among the cells now recognized as macrophages are Kupffer cells in the liver and histiocytes in the loose connective tissue.

macropodia A condition characterized by abnormally large feet.

macrostomia A condition characterized by an abnormally large mouth.

macula, *pl.* maculae A general term for an area in which color distinguishes it from its surrounding tissue.

maculopapular A skin eruption consisting of macules and papules, characterized by discolored areas of the skin that are elevated less than 1 cm.

maculopathy Degeneration of the retinal macula.

Maffucci's syndrome Enchondromatosis associated with cutaneous or visceral hemangiomas. Also called *Kast's syndrome.*

magnesium (Mg) A light silvery metallic element; atomic number, 12; atomic weight, 24.312. Its salts are essential in nutrition and are required for the activity of many enzymes.

magnetic resonance imaging (MRI) Noninvasive method of scanning the body by using an electromagnetic field and radio waves to provide visual images on a computer screen and magnetic tape recordings.

magnetoencephalography (MEG) A measure of the magnetic field produced by the brain's electrical activity.

malabsorption Insufficient intestinal absorption of nutrients.

malabsorption syndrome Disorders resulting from insufficient absorption of dietary nutrients and excessive loss of nonabsorbed substances in the stool. Symptoms include weight loss, abdominal bloating, anorexia, bone pain, muscle cramps, and steatorrhea.

malacia A softening or softness in a part or tissue of the body as a result of disease.

malaise A feeling of discomfort and fatigue, often occurring at the beginning of an illness.

malaria An infectious disease that results from being bitten by an infected *Anopheles* mosquito. Endemic in parts of Africa, Asia, Turkey, the West Indies, and Central and South America, malaria is caused by four species of the protozoan genus *Plasmodium.* Symptoms include chills, fever, anemia, and an enlarged spleen; this disease has a tendency to recur.

malathion poisoning A condition that results from eating or absorbing malathion, an organophosphorus compound used as an insecticide. Such poisoning is characterized by vomiting, nausea, abdominal cramps, headache, dizziness, weakness, confusion, convulsions, and respiratory difficulties.

male 1. a. An organism of the sex that fertilizes the female to beget young, or that produces spermatozoa. b. Masculine. 2. A male person.

malformation A defect of an organ or larger part of the body, resulting from abnormal development.

malignant hyperthermia A condition in which general anesthesia (particularly halothane, succinylcholine chloride, and methoxyflurane) causes a sudden rapid rise in temperature, associated with sweating, cyanosis, increased carbon dioxide production and, usually, muscle rigidity. Affected people carry an autosomal dominant trait.

malignant neoplasm Any new and abnormal growth, especially where growth is uncontrolled and progressive. The tumor is often irregular and tends to invade and metastasize.

malignant tumor A growth that invades, metastasizes, and shows a greater degree of anaplasia than benign cells.

malleotomy Surgical procedure used in ankylosis of the ossicles of the middle ear that divides the malleus.

mallet fracture A break or rupture in the dorsal base of a distal phalanx of the hand or foot, involving the associated extensor apparatus, and caused by tearing or pulling a ligament. This causes dropped flexion of the distal segment.

malleus The outermost of the three auditory ossicles in the middle ear. Attached to the tympanic membrane, its club-shaped head articulates with the incus. Also called *hammer.*

Mallory-Weiss syndrome A condition in which one or more lacerations in the mucous membrane at the esophagogastric junction result in prolonged severe vomiting and massive bleeding.

malnutrition Any nutritional disorder resulting from an unbalanced or insufficient diet or from defective absorption or utilization of foods.

malocclusion Abnormal position of the teeth of the upper jaw in relation to the teeth of the lower jaw, resulting in less efficient mastication and jaw movement.

malpighian corpuscle One of many renal corpuscles; small, deep-red bodies in the kidney, each communicating with a renal tubule.

malpractice A professional's wrongful conduct, improper discharge of professional duties, or failure to meet standards of care that results in harm to another person.

malt worker's lung An occupational hazard in which exposure to fungi-laden particles of moldy barley grain or malt causes respiratory disorders.

mamillary body A part of the hypothalmus containing two small round masses of gray matter. The two masses are near each other in the interpeduncular space.

mamilliplasty Surgical repair of the nipple.

mamillitis Inflammation of the nipple.

mammaplasty Plastic reconstruction of the breast, which may be performed to increase or reduce its size, or which may be necessary after removal of a tumor.

mammary gland An accessory gland of the skin of female mammals that secretes milk in mature females. These glands are also present, although not functional, in children and in males.

mammectomy Excision of the breast.

mammogram A radiograph of the breast, used for diagnostic purposes.

mammography Radiography of the mammary gland to identify benign and malignant neoplastic processes.

mammothermography A technique that uses an infrared camera to portray surface temperature of the body to diagnose breast tumors.

managed-care organizations   Systems that integrate the financing and delivery of appropriate health care services to covered individuals by means of contracts with selected providers.

mandible   The bone of the lower jaw.

manganese (Mn)   A metallic element; atomic number, 25; atomic weight, 54.938. Manganese occurs throughout the body and is necessary to synthesize mucopolysaccharides and to activate a number of enzymes.

manometer   An instrument that measures the pressure or tension of liquids or gases (e.g., blood). It uses a tube marked with a scale, containing a relatively incompressible fluid.

Mantoux test   A test for tuberculosis whereby tuberculin is administered intradermally using a needle and syringe. Raised skin (an area of 10 mm or more) at the injection site 24 to 72 hours later indicates a reaction.

manual rotation   A procedure in which the fetus's head is turned by hand within the birth canal from a transverse to an anteroposterior position; this is done to facilitate delivery.

manubriosternal articulation   The connection between the manubrium and the sternum; this often closes by age 25.

manubrium   A general term for a handle-like structure or part; the cranial portion of the sternum, which articulates with the clavicles and first two pairs of ribs.

MAO   *abbr* monoamine oxidase.

MAP   *abbr* mean arterial pressure.

maple bark disease   An inflammation of the lungs caused by the mold *Cryptostroma corticale*, found in maple tree bark.

maple syrup urine disease   A condition characterized by a missing enzyme that results in an inability to break down the amino acids lysine, leucine, and isoleucine. This inherited disorder has symptoms that include a maple-syrup odor of the urine and hyperreflexia; it's usually diagnosed in infancy.

mapping   In genetics: identifying the relative position of genes on chromosomes by analyzing new combinations of genes.

marasmus   A form of malnutrition that chiefly occurs in the first year of life. Although symptoms include growth retardation and progressive wasting of subcutaneous tissue and muscle, the child usually has an appetite and is mentally alert.

Marburg disease, virus   A disorder marked by acute fever, rash, prostration, hemorrhages, pancreatis, and hepatitis.

march hemoglobinuria   The presence of hemoglobin in the urine; a rare, abnormal condition that occurs after strenuous or prolonged physical exercise.

Marcus Gunn pupil sign   During ophthalmologic examination, the paradoxical dilation of the pupils in response to afferent visual stimuli.

Marfan's syndrome   A congenital disorder in which the extremities (especially the fingers and toes) are elongated and other deformities of the eyes and the cardiovascular system exist.

 TIME LINE To avoid sudden death due to dissecting aortic aneurysm or other cardiac complications, high school and college athletes (particularly basketball players) who fit the criteria for Marfan's syndrome should undergo a careful clinical and cardiovascular examination before being allowed to play.

marginal placenta previa   A condition in which the placenta develops in the lower uterine segment so that it covers or adjoins the internal os.

Marie Strümpell disease   A form of arthritis of the spinal column. Also called *spondylitis.*

Marseilles fever   A disease caused by *Rickettsia conorii* transmitted by the brown dog tick *(Rhipicephalus sanguineus)*. It occurs around the Mediterranean and in Africa, the Crimea, and India.

marsupialize   A way to treat a cyst when it cannot be removed. A pouch is created surgically by resection of the anterior wall and suture of the cut edges to establish a pouch from what was initially an enclosed cyst. After several months, granulation tissue will close the wound.

masculine   Pertaining to the male sex; possessing qualities or characteristics of a male.

mass   1. The characteristic property of matter that gives it weight and inertia. 2. In pharmacy: a cohesive mixture from which pills are made. 3. An aggregate of cells clustered together.

masseter   The thick, rectangular cheek muscle that acts to raise the mandible and close the jaw.

mass reflex   Occurring in patients with spinal cord injury, this condition is characterized by widespread nerve discharge, resulting in flexor muscle spasms, urinary and fecal incontinence, priapism, hypertension, and diaphoresis.

mass spectrometer   An analytic instrument that identifies a substance by sorting a stream of charged particles (ions) depending on their mass.

MAST   *abbr* medical anti-shock trousers.

mastalgia Pain in the mammary gland caused by infection, fibrocystic disease, advanced cancer, congestion during lactation, and before or during menstruation.

mast cell A connective tissue cell consisting of large basophilic granules that contain heparin, serotonin, bradykinin, and histamine.

mast cell leukemia A type of leukemia characterized by large numbers of connective tissue mast cells in circulating blood.

mastectomy The surgical resection of a breast, usually performed to remove a malignant tumor.

Master "two-step" exercise A standardized, electrocardiographic test for detecting coronary artery disease in which the patient repeatedly steps on and off two 9″ steps.

mastication The process of chewing, tearing, or grinding food and mixing with saliva in preparation for swallowing and digestion.

mastitis Inflammation of the mammary gland, usually caused by streptococcal or staphylococcal infection and infrequent breast-feeding.

mastocytosis A rare disease caused by local or systemic overproduction of mast cells that infiltrate the tissues and other organs.

mastodynia Pain in the breast.

mastoidectomy Surgical removal of part of the mastoid process of the temporal bone, usually to treat chronic suppurative otitis media or mastoiditis when antibiotics are ineffective.

mastoid process A conical projection of the caudal, posterior portion of the temporal bone from which several muscles are attached, including the sternocleidomastoideus and splenius capitis. A hollow section contains air cells that are characterized by a large, irregular tympanic antrum in the superior anterior portion of the process.

mastopexy, mastoplasty Surgical reconstruction of a pendulous breast.

mastoptosis Condition characterized by pendulous breasts.

mastotomy Incision of the breast.

materia medica 1. The study of drugs and other substances used in medicine, their sources, preparation, uses, and effects (pharmacology). 2. A drug or substance used in medical treatment.

maternal deprivation syndrome A condition caused by physical or emotional deprivation, resulting in developmental retardation.

matrix 1. An intracellular substance. 2. A basic substance from which a specific structure or tissue develops. Also called *ground substance*. 3. A mold used for shaping a tooth surface in dental procedures.

matter 1. Anything that has mass and occupies space. 2. Substance whose constituents aren't otherwise identified, such as gray matter or pus.

maturation The stage or process of becoming completely developed.

maturity 1. A state of completed growth or development, usually designated as the period of life between adolescence and old age. 2. The time when an organism is capable of reproduction.

maxilla, *pl.* **maxillae** One of a pair of large bones that form the upper jaw. It consists of a pyramidal body and four processes: the zygomatic, frontal, alveolar, and palatine.

maxillary sinus One of a pair of large cells that form an air cavity in the maxillary body.

maxillary vein One of a pair of deep facial veins, accompanying the maxillary artery and passing between the condyle of the mandible and the sphenomandibular ligament.

maxillomandibular fixation The temporary stabilization of maxillary or mandibular fractures with wires, elastic bands, or metal splints.

maximal breathing capacity Quantity of exchanged gas per minute with maximal rate and depth of respiration.

maximal expiratory flow rate (MEFR) Rate of the most rapid flow of gas from the lungs during expiration.

maximum inspiratory pressure (MIP) Maximum pressure within the lung alveoli that occurs during inspiration.

maximum permissible dose equivalent In radiotherapy: maximum radiation that a person or specific body part should receive in a defined time period.

Mayer's reflex Reflex elicited by taking the ring finger and flexing it at the metacarpophalangeal joint of a person whose hand is relaxed with thumb abducted. The normal response is adduction and apposition of the thumb.

May-Hegglin anomaly A rare inherited hematologic disorder that is characterized by leukopenia, giant platelets, and Döhle's bodies inclusion.

MBC *abbr* maximal breathing capacity.

MBD *abbr* minimal brain dysfunction.

mC *abbr* millicoulomb.

McArdle's disease An inherited metabolic condition in which excessive amounts of glycogen occur in skeletal muscle.

MCAT *abbr* Medical College Aptitude Test.

McBurney's point An extremely sensitive site in acute appendicitis; it occurs in the

Maxillary sinus

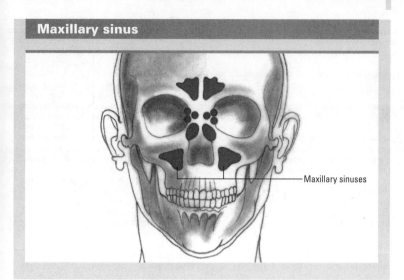

Maxillary sinuses

appendix area about 2″ (5 cm) below the right anterior superior spine of the ilium, on a line between the spine and the umbilicus.

McBurney's sign Signifies appendicitis; a patient's reaction suggesting severe pain and extreme tenderness when McBurney's point is palpated.

 TIME LINE In elderly patients, McBurney's sign (as well as other peritoneal signs) may be decreased or absent.

mcg *abbr* microgram.

MCH *abbr* **1.** mean corpuscular hemoglobin. **2.** maternal and child health.

MCHC *abbr* mean corpuscular hemoglobin concentration.

MCi *abbr* megacurie, a unit of one million curies, which is a measure of radioactivity.

mCi *abbr* millicurie.

MCL *abbr* midclavicular line.

McMurray sign An audible click that occurs when rotating the tibia on the femur, suggesting meniscal structure injury.

 TIME LINE McMurray sign in children is usually elicited by meniscal tear due to sports injury. It may also be elicited in children with congenital discoid meniscus.

MCTD *abbr* mixed connective tissue disease.

MCV *abbr* mean corpuscular volume.

MD *abbr* Doctor of Medicine.

mean **1.** A position occurring midway between two extremes of a set of values or data. **2.** Arithmetic mean: a number that is derived by dividing the total of a set of values by the number of items in that set. **3.** Geometric mean: a number that lies between the first and last of a set of values arranged in a geometric progression.

mean arterial pressure (MAP) An arithmetic mean of blood pressure in arterial portion of circulation.

mean corpuscular hemoglobin (MCH) The average hemoglobin content of a red blood cell, obtained from the ratio between the hemoglobin amount and number of red blood cells in a specimen. Normal value is 28 to 32 picograms of hemoglobin per red blood cell.

mean corpuscular hemoglobin concentration (MCHC) An average hemoglobin concentration in grams per 100 ml of packed red blood cells, obtained from the ratio of hemoglobin to hematocrit. Normal value is 32% to 36%.

mean corpuscular volume (MCV) An average volume of each red blood cell, obtained from the ratio of hematocrit to the number of red blood cells. Normal value is 82 to 92 cubic microns.

measles An acute, highly infectious, viral disease that involves the respiratory tract and is characterized by a spreading maculopapular cutaneous rash.

measles and rubella virus vaccine, live An active immunizing agent that is administered to induce resistance measles and rubella.

measles, mumps, and rubella virus vaccine, live   An active immunizing agent that is administered for the simultaneous protection against measles, mumps, and rubella.

 ALERT Conditions prohibiting the use of live measles, mumps, and rubella virus vaccine include immunosuppression, concomitant administration of corticosteroids, tuberculosis, hypersensitivity to neomycin, neoplasms of the lymphatic system or of the bone marrow, known or suspected pregnancy, or acute infection.

measurement   The numerical value of the extent or quantity of a substance, energy, or time.

meatorrhaphy   Suture of the cut end of the urethra to the glans penis after incision to enlarge the urethral meatus.

meatoscopy   Visual inspection of any meatus, especially the urethra, usually with the help of a speculum.

meatus, *pl.* meatus   An opening or passage in the body, such as the external acoustic meatus that leads from the external ear to the tympanic membrane.

mechanical advantage   In physiology: the ratio of the output force developed by muscles to the input force applied to the structures moved by the muscles, especially the ratio of these forces associated with structures that act as levers.

mechanoreceptor   A sensory nerve ending that is excited by mechanical stimuli, such as touch, pressure, and muscular contractions.

Meckel's diverticulum   An anomalous sac extending from the ileum wall between $11^{3}/_{4}''$ and $35^{1}/_{2}''$ (30 to 90 cm) from the ileocecal sphincter.

meconium   A dark, greenish black material that occurs in the intestines of a fetus that forms the first stools of a newborn. The fluid is thick and sticky and is composed of intestinal gland secretions, some amniotic fluid, and intrauterine debris.

meconium ileus   Obstruction of the small intestine in a newborn caused by firmly packed thick, dry, tenacious meconium at or near the ileocecal valve.

meconium plug syndrome   Obstruction of the large intestine in a newborn caused by thick, rubbery meconium filling the colon and part of the terminal ileum.

MED   *abbr* **1.** minimal effective dose. **2.** minimal erythema dose.

Medex   An American Medical Association–accredited educational program for military personnel with medical experience to qualify as physician's assistants.

medial   Pertaining to the middle.

medial cuneiform bone   The largest of three cuneiform bones of the foot, situated on the medial side of the tarsus, between the scaphoid bone and the first metatarsal.

medial malleolus   Bony prominence on the inside of the ankle.

medial pectoral nerve   A branch of the brachial plexus that, together with the lateral pectoral nerve, supplies the pectoral muscles.

median   In statistics: the middle number of the scores in a sample. In an odd number of scores arrayed in ascending order, it's the middle score; in an even number of scores so arrayed, the median is the average between the two middle scores.

median aperture of fourth ventricle   An opening that exists between the lower part of the roof of the fourth ventricle and the subarachnoid space.

median cubital veins   Veins of the elbow and forearm that are most commonly used for venipuncture.

median effective dose   The drug dosage that may cause a specific intensity of effect in 50% of subjects to whom it's given.

median lethal dose (MLD)   In radiotherapy: quantity of radiation that kills 50% of individuals in a large group of animals or organisms within a specified time period.

median plane   A vertical plane that separates the body into right and left halves and passes through the sagittal suture of the skull.

median toxic dose (TD$_{50}$)   The drug dosage that may cause a toxic effect in 50% of subjects to whom it's given.

mediastinum, *pl.* mediastina   Part of the thoracic cavity in the middle of the thorax, between the pleural sacs that contain the two lungs.

Medicaid   A program that subsidizes medical care for low-income women and children, some men, and people with certain disabilities. Although passed by Congress in 1965, Medicaid is a state-level program; each state defines income levels and other standards of eligibility, and the federal government subsidizes a portion of expenses.

Medical College Aptitude Test (MCAT)   Taken by applicants to medical school, the score on this examination is an important criterion for acceptance.

medical model   Traditionally, the diagnosis and treatment of disease as practiced by physicians in the western world since the time of Koch and Pasteur. The physician focuses on the dysfunction within the person, using a problem-solving approach. Based on the medical history, physical examination, and diagnostic tests, a specific disease may be identified and treated. The medical model focuses on the physical and biological aspects of specific disorders. Nursing is different from the medical model because the patient is perceived primarily as a social person relating to the environment; nursing care is based on a nursing assessment that assumes multiple causes for the person's problems.

medical record A written, legal record of every aspect of a patient's care; includes illnesses and treatment.

medical release form The form an institution asks a patient to sign on refusal of medical treatment; protects both the institution and health care professionals from liability if the patient's condition worsens because of his refusal.

Medical Women's International Association (MWIA) An international organization of women doctors.

Medicare Federally funded national health insurance authorized by the Social Security Act for persons age 65 and older.

medicine 1. A drug or remedy for illness. 2. The art and science of the diagnosis, treatment, and prevention of disease and the maintenance of good health. 3. The nonsurgical treatment of disease.

MEDLARS A computerized literature retrieval service of the National Library of Medicine.

MEDLINE A National Library of Medicine computer database covering about 1 million biomedical journal articles published in the current and preceding 3 years.

medulla, *pl.* **medullae** The innermost part of a structure or organ.

medulla oblongata The most important part of the brain, continuing as the bulbous portion of the spinal cord just above the foramen magnum and separated from the pons by a horizontal groove.

medullary artery An artery that supplies nutrients (blood) to the bone marrow.

medullary cavity The innermost part of the bone shaft that contains yellow marrow.

medullary cystic disease A chronic familial disease of the kidney that is characterized by the slow onset of uremia.

medullary pyramids Small, cone-shaped structures on the walls of the renal sinuses that make up the medulla of the kidney.

medullary sponge kidney An inborn kidney defect that leads to cystic dilatation of the collecting tubules.

medullated nerves Nerves that are covered with a white, fatty sheath of material known as myelin.

medulloblastoma A poorly differentiated, malignant neoplasm composed of tightly packed cells of spongioblastic and neuroblastic lineage.

MEFR *abbr* maximal expiratory flow rate.

magacephaly Excessively large head size.

megacolon An abnormally large or dilated colon that may be congenital, toxic, or acquired.

megakaryoblasts Cells in the red bone marrow where platelets originate.

megakaryocyte An oversized bone marrow cell that has a diameter of 35 to 160 cubic microns and a nucleus with several lobes.

megakaryocytic leukemia A rare malignancy of blood-forming tissue in which megakaryocytes multiply excessively in the bone marrow and circulate in the blood.

megalencephaly Overgrowth of the head and brain.

megaloblast A large, nucleated, immature red blood cell that develops in excessive numbers in the bone marrow and occurs in the circulation in many anemias caused by deficiency of vitamin B_{12}, folic acid, or intrinsic factor.

megaloblastic anemia A hematologic disorder that is characterized by the production and peripheral proliferation of megaloblasts.

megalocornea Developmental anomaly characterized by a large cornea.

megalocystis Abnormally enlarged and thin-walled bladder that mainly occurs in female children.

megalogastria Abnormally large stomach.

megaloglossia Excessively large lips. Also called *macrochalia.*

megalopthalmos Abnormally large eyes.

megaloureter Congenital ureteral dilation without demonstrable cause.

meibomian gland One of many sebaceous glands located in the tarsal plate of each eyelid that secrete sebum from their ducts on the posterior margin of each eyelid.

meiosis A method of cell division that occurs in germ cells (sperm or ova) and results in four daughter cells containing half the number of chromosomes characteristic of the species.

melanin A dark pigment that occurs in the hair, skin, and in the iris and choroid of the eye.

melanocyte A melanin-producing cell.

melanocyte nevus Pigmented overgrowth of skin.

melanocyte-stimulating hormone (MSH) Hormone secreted by the pituitary gland.

melanoderma   Abnormal darkening of the skin caused by excessive deposits of melanin and iron or silver salts.

melanoma   Malignant neoplasms, mainly of the skin, that are composed of melanocytes.

melatonin   Secreted by the pineal gland, melatonin has marked diurnal rhythm; blood levels are up to 10 times greater at night than during the day.

melena   Black, tarry stool containing digested blood. It usually results from bleeding in the upper gastrointestinal tract and often signifies peptic ulcer or small bowel disease.

TIME LINE   Newborns may experience melena neonatorum due to extravasation of blood into the alimentary canal. In older children, melena usually results from peptic ulcer, gastritis, and Meckel's diverticulum.

membrana tectoria   The broad, strong ligament that helps connect the axis to the occipital bone of the skull.

membrane   A thin layer of tissue that covers a surface, lines a cavity, or divides a space.

menarche   The first menstruation and the beginning of cyclic menstrual function, occurring usually between ages 9 and 17.

Mendel's laws, mendelian laws   The principles of inheritance, based on the breeding experiments of garden peas by Gregor Mendel, usually expressed as two laws: the law of segregation and the law of independent assortment.

Mendelson's syndrome   A respiratory disorder caused by the chemical pneumonia that results from the pulmonary aspiration of acidic gastric contents.

Mèniére's disease   A chronic inner ear disease that is characterized by recurrent episodes of vertigo, progressive unilateral nerve deafness, and tinnitus.

meninges, *sing.* **meninx**   The three membranes (dura mater, pia mater, and arachnoid) that enclose the brain and spinal cord.

meningocele   A saclike protrusion of the meninges through a congenital defect in the skull or vertebral column that forms a hernial cyst and is filled with cerebrospinal fluid but not neural tissue.

meniscectomy   Surgical removal of a crescent-shaped cartilage of the knee joint, usually done when a torn cartilage results in chronic pain and instability or locking of the joint.

meniscus   **1.** The crescent shape of fluid occurring at the interface between liquid and air. Liquid measurements should be read from the meniscus base. **2.** A lens with both convex and concave aspects. **3.** A curved, fibrous cartilage in the knees and other joints.

Menkes' syndrome   A familial disorder caused by defective copper absorption and is characterized by the growth of sparse, kinky hair. Infants suffer cerebral degeneration, retarded growth, and early death.

menometrorrhagia   Excessive menstrual and uterine bleeding other than that caused by menstruation. The disorder is a combination of metrorrhagia and menorrhagia and may signify urogenital malignancy.

menopause   The cessation of menses, but may also be used to refer to the female climacteric. Menses stop naturally with the decline of cyclic hormonal production and function between ages 45 and 60 but may stop earlier because of illness or the surgical removal of the uterus or both ovaries.

menorrhagia   Abnormally heavy or long menstruation.

menses   The monthly flow of blood and decidua that occurs during menstruation. The first day of menstrual flow is also the first day of the menstrual cycle.

menstrual cycle   The recurring cycle in the endometrium during which the decidual layer of the endometrium is shed, then regrows, proliferates, is maintained for several days, and sheds again at menstruation. Menstruation normally lasts 5 days; the average length of the cycle, from the first day of bleeding of one cycle to that of another, is 28 days. The length, duration, and character of cycles vary among women. Menstrual cycles begin at menarche and end with menopause.

menstrual phase   The final of the four phases of the menstrual cycle, the one in which menstruation occurs. The necrotic mucosa of the endometrium is shed, leaving the stratum basale; bleeding, primarily from spiral arteries, occurs. The average blood loss is 30 ml (1 oz).

mental age   Age level at which a person functions intellectually, as determined by standardized psychological and intelligence tests; expressed as the age at which that level is average.

mental competence   The ability to understand information and act reasonably; a mentally competent person comprehends explanations and the results of his decisions.

mental health   A state of mind in which a healthy person copes with and adjusts to the stresses of daily living in an acceptable manner.

Mental Health Association (MHA)   A voluntary, nonprofessional agency focused on improving mental health facilities and services in community clinics and hospitals, recruiting and training volunteers, and promoting mental health legislation.

mental incompetence   The inability to understand the nature and effect of one's actions; a mentally incompetent person is incapable of understanding explanations or the results of his decisions. Compare *adjudicated incompetent* and *incompetence.*

mental status   The degree of competence exhibited by a person in intellectual, emotional, psychological, and personality functioning as measured by psychological testing with reference to a statistical normal value.

mental status examination   A diagnostic procedure to determine the mental status of a person; a trained interviewer poses certain questions in a carefully standardized manner, then evaluates verbal responses and behavioral reactions.

mEq   *abbr* milliequivalent.

mercurial   1. Of or referring to mercury, particularly a medicine containing the element mercury. 2. An adverse effect associated with mercurial medication, such as a mercurial tremor due to mercury poisoning.

mercury (Hg)   A metallic element (atomic number, 80; atomic weight, 200.59) that is liquid at room temperature and occurs naturally almost entirely as its sulfide, cinnabar.

merozoite   Stage in the life cycle of the malaria parasite.

mesencephalon   A part of the brain stem, located between the cerebrum and the pons, that consists primarily of white substance with some gray substance around the cerebral aqueduct.

mesenteric node   A node in one of three groups of superior mesenteric lymph glands that serve part of the intestine.

mesentery   A peritoneal fold attaching the stomach, small intestine, pancreas, and other abdominal organs to the dorsal body wall.

mesoderm   In embryology: the middle cell layer of the developing embryo; it lies between the ectoderm and the entoderm.

mesorchium   Fold in the tissue between the testes and epididymis.

MET   *abbr* metabolic equivalent.

metabolic acidosis   Acidosis resulting from accumulation of keto acids in the blood at the expense of bicarbonate.

metabolic alkalosis   Shift in acid-base status towards the alkaline due to uncompensated loss of acids, ingestion or retention of excess bases, or potassium depletion.

metabolic respiratory quotient (R)   The ratio of carbon dioxide production to oxygen consumption. The values of R change depending on the fuel being burned; because fat contains less oxygen compared with glucose, the R of fat is lower than that of glucose, whereas the R of protein lies between that of glucose and fat.

metabolism   The sum of all chemical processes that occur in living organisms, resulting in growth, release of energy, waste removal, and other body functions related to the distribution of nutrients in the blood after digestion.

metacarpus   The middle portion of the hand that consists of five slender bones numbered from the thumb side, metacarpals I through V.

metal   An element that conducts heat and electricity, is malleable and ductile, and forms positive ions (cations) in solution.

metal fume fever   An occupational disorder, occurring in welders or other metallic workers, caused by inhaling metallic oxide fumes and characterized by influenza-type symptoms.

metamorphosis   A change in shape or structure, especially that from one stage of development to another, such as the transition from larva to adult form.

metaphase   The second stage of cell division in mitosis and meiosis during which the chromosomes become arranged in the equatorial plane of the spindle to form the equatorial plate, with the centromeres attached to the spindle fibers in preparation for separation.

metaplasia   Change in adult cells to an abnormal form for that tissue.

metastasis, *pl.* metastases   The transfer of tumor cells to distant parts of the body. Because malignant tumors aren't enclosed, cells may escape, embolize, and be transported to sites distant from the primary tumor via the lymphatic circulation or blood.

metatarsal   1. Of or relating to the metatarsus of the foot. 2. One of five bones comprising the metatarsus.

metatarsal stress fracture   A break of a metatarsal bone caused by prolonged running or walking that is commonly difficult to diagnose radiographically.

metatarsus   Part of the foot, consisting of five bones numbered I to V from the medial side.

methemoglobin   A form of hemoglobin in which the iron component has been oxidized to the ferric state. It cannot carry oxygen and thus does not contribute to the oxygen-transporting capacity of blood.

metralgia   Pain in the uterus.

metric system   A decimal system of measurement based on the meter (39.37 inches) as the unit of length, on the gram (15.432 grains) as the unit of weight or mass, and on the liter (0.908 U.S. dry quart or 1.0567 U.S. liquid quarts) as the unit of volume.

metrorrhagia   Uterine bleeding other than menstruation.

 ALERT Herbal medicines, such as ginseng, can cause postmenopausal bleeding.

Meynet's node   One of several nodules that may develop within the capsules surrounding joints and in tendons affected by rheumatic diseases, especially in children.

Mfd   *abbr* microfarad.

MFD   *abbr* minimal fatal dose.

mg   *abbr* milligram.

Mg   Symbol for magnesium.

MHA   *abbr* Mental Health Association.

MI   *abbr* myocardial infarction.

microaggregates   Small particles formed after a few days of blood storage from degenerating platelets, leukocytes, and fibrin strands; may contribute to formation of microemboli (small clots that obstruct circulation) in the lungs. Microaggregates can pass through a 170-micron filter; microaggregate filters remove these smaller particles, but cost more and may slow the infusion rate.

microcurie (μc)   A unit of radiation that equals one millionth (10^{-6}) of a curie.

microcyte   A small erythrocyte with a mean corpuscular volume of below 80 microns, often occurring in iron deficiency and other anemias.

microencapsulation   A procedure used in the bioassay of hormones in which some antibodies are encapsulated with a perforated membrane, resembling a whiffle ball.

microgram (mcg, μg)   A measurement of mass that equals one millionth (10^{-6}) of a gram.

microliter (μl)   A unit of liquid volume that equals one millionth (10^{-6}) of a liter.

microlith   A small, round mass of mineral matter or calcified stone.

micrometer   An instrument used for the measurement of small angles or distances on objects observed through a microscope or telescope.

micron (μ)   **1.** A metric unit of length equal to one millionth (10^{-6}) of a meter. **2.** In physical chemistry: a colloidal particle with a diameter of 0.2 to 10 microns.

micronucleus   **1.** A small or minute nucleus. **2.** In protozoa: the smaller of two nuclei in each cell; it functions in sexual reproduction.

micronutrient   An essential dietary element or compound required only in minute amounts for normal physiological processes of the body. Also called *microelement, minor element, trace element.*

microorganism   A microscopic organism that may be pathogenic, such as bacteria, fungi, protozoa, and viruses.

micropodia   A developmental anomaly characterized by abnormally small feet, usually associated with other congenital malformations or bone disorders.

microscopic anatomy   The study of the microscopic structure of tissues and cells.

microscopy   A technique for examining minute objects using a microscope.

micturition reflex   Response to increased pressure in the bladder, resulting in contraction of the bladder wall and relaxation of the urethral sphincter.

midclavicular line   In anatomy: an imaginary vertical line on the front surface of the chest passing through the midpoint of the clavicle and the center of the nipple that divides each side of the anterior chest into two parts.

middle ear   An irregular-shaped opening in the temporal bone containing the tympanic cavity with its auditory ossicles and the auditory tube which carries air from the posterior pharynx into the middle ear.

middle lobe syndrome   Incomplete expansion of the middle lobe of the right lung, characterized by chronic infection, cough, dyspnea, wheezing, and obstructive pneumonitis.

middle mediastinum   The widest part of the mediastinum containing the heart enclosed in the pericardium, ascending aorta, lower half of the superior vena cava, pulmonary arteries and veins, and phrenic nerves.

migraine   Recurring vascular headache characterized by unilateral onset, severe pain, sensitivity to light, and autonomic disturbances during the acute phase.

 CLINICAL TIP Migraine attacks, which may last for hours or even days, are often preceded by an aura.

migratory thrombophlebitis   An abnormal condition in which thromboses occur at multiple sites in the superficial peripheral veins and sometimes in the deep veins.

Mikulicz's syndrome   A chronic bilateral enlargement of the salivary, parotid, and lacrimal glands, found in a variety of diseases, including leukemia, lupus erythematosus, sarcoidosis, and tuberculosis.

milia   Tiny, firm white to yellow cysts of the epidermis caused by obstruction of hair follicles and eccrine sweat glands. One type is seen on each side of the hard palate seam in newborn infants, usually disappearing within a few weeks.

miliaria   An eruption of tiny vesicles caused by obstruction of the ducts of the sweat glands, usually accompanied by inflammation.

milk-ejection reflex The release of milk from the milk glands into the ducts, a normal reflex in lactating women that is controlled by a combination of hormones and tactile stimulation of the nipple.

milker's nodule Purple nodules on the fingers or palm, transmitted by the paravaccinia virus, acquired from lesions on the udder of an infected cow. The lesions usually break down and heal without scarring.

milliampere (mA) A unit of electrical current equal to one thousandth (10^{-3}) of an ampere.

millicoulomb (mC) A unit of electrical charge equal to one thousandth (10^{-3}) of a coulomb.

millicurie (mCi) A unit of radioactivity equal to one thousandth (10^{-3}) of a curie, or 3.7×10^7 disintegrations/second.

milliequivalent (mEq) The number of grams of solute dissolved in one milliliter of a normal solution.

milligram (mg) A unit of weight equal to one thousandth (10^{-3}) of a gram.

milliliter (ml) A unit of volume equal to one thousandth (10^{-3}) of a liter.

millimeter (mm) A unit of length equal to one thousandth (10^{-3}) of a meter.

millimicrogram (mμg) A unit of weight equal to one thousandth (10^{-3}) of a microgram, or one billionth (10^{-9}) of a gram. More commonly referred to as a nanogram.

millimole (mmol) A unit of mass equal to one thousandth (10^{-3}) of a mole. Also called *gram molecule.*

milliosmol (mOsm) The concentration of an ion in a solution, expressed in milligrams per liter divided by atomic weight.

millipede A many-legged, wormlike arthropod characterized by having two pairs of short legs on most of its body segments. Certain species squirt irritating fluids that may cause dermatitis.

millirad (mrad) A unit of measurement of the absorbed dose of ionizing radiation equal to one thousandth (10^{-3}) of a rad.

milliroentgen (mr) A unit of radiation equal to one thousandth (10^{-3}) of a roentgen.

millivolt (mV) A unit of electromotive force equal to one one-thousandth (10^{-3}) of a volt.

mineral 1. An inorganic substance occurring naturally in the earth's crust, having a characteristic chemical composition and usually of definite crystalline structure. 2. In nutrition: any of the inorganic elements, such as sodium, potassium, calcium, and iron, generally obtained from foods and necessary for the proper functioning of the human body.

mineral deficiency The inability to use one or more of the mineral elements essential to human body function due to a genetic defect, poor absorption, or the lack of that mineral in the diet.

mineralization The addition of any mineral to the body.

mineralocorticoid Any of a group of hormones, secreted by the adrenal cortex, that regulate electrolyte and water balance by effecting ion transport in epithelial cells. They maintain normal blood volume, promote sodium and water retention, and increase urinary excretion of potassium and hydrogen ions.

miner's elbow An enlargement of the olecranon bursa, caused by inflammation resulting from resting the weight of the body on the elbow, as is done in mining.

Minerva jacket A cast covering both the trunk and the head, leaving the face and ears exposed, applied for support and immobilization of the cervical and thoracic spine, especially in cases of fracture.

minim (m) A measurement of volume equal to $1/60$ of a fluid dram (about 0.06 ml). In the apothecaries' system, originally one drop (of water).

minimum alveolar concentration The smallest amount of an anesthetic gas at a pressure of one atmosphere that produces immobility in 50% of subjects exposed to a noxious stimulus.

miosis Contraction of the iris, causing the pupil to become smaller.

TIME LINE Miosis occurs frequently in the neonate simply because he's asleep or drowsy most of the time. Bilateral miosis occurs in congenital microcoria.

miotic 1. Of or pertaining to miosis. 2. Causing constriction of the pupil of the eye. 3. Any agent that causes constriction of the pupil of the eye; for example, an increase in light, or instillation of the drug pilocarpine.

MIP *abbr* maximum inspiratory pressure.

miracidium, *pl.* **miracidia** The ciliated, first-stage larva of a parasitic trematode, which further develops within the body of a host snail.

misdemeanor An offense considered less serious than a felony, with a lesser penalty (usually a fine or imprisonment for less than 1 year).

misfeasance An improper performance of a normally lawful act, especially in a way that might cause injury or damage.

mitochondrion, *pl.* **mitochondria** A small, round to rod-shaped organelle within the cytoplasm of cells. Its principal function is in cellular metabolism and respiration.

mitogenetic radiation, mitogenic radiation The specific energy that is supposedly given off by cells undergoing mitosis, which may, in turn, stimulate the process of mitosis in other cells.

mitogenic factor A kind of lymphokine that is released from activated T lymphocytes and stimulates the production of normal unsensitized lymphocytes.

mitolactol An orally administered antineoplastic agent used in the treatment of invasive ovarian cancer.

mitome The thready, reticular network of protoplasm found within the cell.

mitosis The division of the cell nucleus during which the daughter nuclei receive identical complements of the diploid number of chromosomes characteristic of the species.

mitotane An orally administered antineoplastic agent used in inoperable cancer of the adrenal cortex.

mitotic index The ratio of the number of cells in a population undergoing mitosis to the number of cells not undergoing mitosis, used to estimate the tissue growth rate.

mitral 1. Of or referring to the mitral, or bicuspid, valve of the heart. 2. Shaped like a miter.

mitral gradient The difference in pressure between the left atrium and left ventricle of the heart during diastole.

mitral valve The valve connecting the left atrium and the left ventricle of the heart. Of the four heart valves, it's the only one with two cusps (or flaps) rather than three. Also called *bicuspid valve.*

mitral valve stenosis A narrowing of the mitral valve of the heart caused by adhesions, usually resulting from rheumatic endocarditis.

mittelschmerz Abdominal pain usually occurring in the middle of the menstrual cycle and associated with ovulation.

mixed-cell malignant lymphoma A cancer of the lymphatic system containing both lymphocytes and histiocytes (macrophages).

mixed-cell sarcoma A tumor composed of two or more cellular elements, excluding fibrous tissue as one of the elements. Also called *malignant mesenchymoma.*

mixed connective tissue disease A systemic disease characterized by the combined symptoms of various collagen diseases, such as scleroderma, myositis, systemic lupus erythematosus, and rheumatoid arthritis.

mixed dentition A phase of dentition during which some of the permanent teeth have emerged before all of the deciduous teeth have been shed.

mixed glioma A tumor of the brain or spinal cord composed of more than one glial cell type; the most common form includes oligodendroglioma cells in an otherwise typical astrocytoma.

mixed-lymphocyte culture (MLC) reaction An assay in which lymphocytes from two individuals are cultured together to determine compatible donors for bone marrow transplant or grafting; also used in the diagnosis of immunodeficiency diseases.

mixed tumor A tumor composed of more than one kind of neoplastic tissue, particularly a tumor (either benign or malignant) of the salivary gland.

mixture 1. In chemistry: an aggregate composed of two or more substances that aren't chemically combined and do not exist in fixed proportions. 2. In pharmacology: a combination of different drugs either as a liquid or suspension.

ml *abbr* milliliter.

MLC *abbr* mixed lymphocyte culture.

MLD *abbr* 1. median lethal dose. 2. minimum lethal dose.

mm *abbr* millimeter.

MMEF *abbr* maximal midexpiratory flow.

mm Hg *abbr* millimeters of mercury.

mmol *abbr* millimole.

Mn Symbol for manganese.

mode The most frequently occurring value in a statistical sampling or population.

moderator band A bundle of muscle at the apex of the right ventricle of the heart. It's believed to prevent overdistention of the ventricle.

Moeller's glossitis A chronic inflammation characterized by superficial, red lesions on the tip and edges of the tongue.

moiety 1. A half or equal part. 2. Any portion.

molar 1. Any one of the 12 posterior teeth, 6 in each dental arch, used for grinding food and also to support the dental arch. 2. Of or referring to the gram molecular weight of a substance.

molar pregnancy An abnormal pregnancy in which a fertilized ovum develops into a hydatid mole in the early embryonic stage of development.

molar solution (M) A solution containing one mole of solute per liter of solution.

mold 1. A fungus or a growth of fungi. 2. A cast or form which gives shape to an object.

molding The shaping of a baby's head during labor as it adjusts to the shape and size of the birth canal.

mole (mol) The amount of a substance containing the same number of elementary particles as there are atoms in 12 grams of carbon 12 (6.023 × 10²³, Avogadro's number).

molecule   The smallest amount of a substance that can exist alone and still exhibit the characteristic chemical properties of the element or compound; a combination of two or more atoms held together by chemical forces and forming a specific chemical substance.

molluscum contagiosum   A common, benign disease of the skin and occasionally the mucous membranes caused by a poxvirus.

molybdenum (Mo)   A silvery-white metallic element with an atomic number of 42 and an atomic weight of 95.94. It's an essential trace element.

mongolian spot   A benign, blue-gray to gray-brown patch occurring most often over the sacrum and on the buttocks of some newborns.

 CLINICAL TIP Mongolian spots occur primarily in dark-skinned patients, including those of East Asian descent, and usually disappear during early childhood.

monoamine   An amine molecule containing only one amine group. Serotonin, dopamine, epinephrine, and norepinephrine are examples of monoamines.

monoamine oxidase (MAO)   An enzyme that catalyzes the oxidation of amines. Also called *amine oxidase.*

monobasic acid   An acid with only one replaceable atom of hydrogen; for example, hydrochloric acid.

monobenzone   A depigmenting agent applied topically to the skin.

monoblast   A large, immature monocyte not normally seen in peripheral blood or bone marrow, but may be present in monocytic anemia.

monoclonal   Of or referring to a group of identical cells or clones derived from a single cell.

monoclonal antibodies   Antibodies cloned in quantity from a single cell to make a vaccine.

monocyte   A leukocyte with a single kidney-shaped or ovoid nucleus. Monocytes are formed in the bone marrow from promonocytes and then transported to tissues, such as the lung and the liver, where they develop into macrophages.

 ALERT Monocytes are increased by infection, collagen vascular disease, carcinomas, lymphomas, and monocytic leukemia; but decreased by hairy cell leukemia, human immunodeficiency virus infection, rheumatoid arthritis, and prednisone therapy.

monocytic leukemia   A cancer of the blood-forming tissues in which the predominant cells are identified as monocytes.

monocytopenia   A decrease in the proportion of monocytes in the blood.

monocytosis   An increase in the proportion of monocytes in the blood.

monohybrid cross   The mating of two parent organisms or strains each having a different homozygous gene pair for only one specific trait. The offspring of the monohybrid cross will be heterozygous for the specific trait.

monohydric alcohol   An alcohol containing only one hydroxyl group.

monomorphic   Form of ventricular tachycardia in which the QRS complexes have a uniform appearance from beat to beat.

mononeuropathy   A disease affecting a single nerve.

mononucleosis   An abnormally high level of monocytes in the blood.

monorchism   A condition in which only one testicle is present in the scrotum.

monosomy   The absence of one chromosome from the normal diploid complement.

monozygotic twins   Two offspring that develop from a single fertilized ovum that splits into equal halves during an early phase in embryonic development, resulting in two separate and identical fetuses. Such twins, also referred to as identical, are always of the same sex, have the same genetic makeup, possess identical blood groups, and closely resemble each other physically, psychologically, and mentally.

Monteggia's fracture   Fracture in the proximal half of the shaft of the ulna, coupled with a dislocation of the radius; often results from attempts to use the forearm to defend oneself from blows.

Montgomery's tubercles   The enlargement during pregnancy of Morgagni's tubercles on the areola of the breast.

moon face   A condition characterized by a rounded, puffy face, occurring in people treated with large doses of corticosteroids, such as those with rheumatoid arthritis or acute childhood leukemia.

Moore's fracture   A fracture of the lower part of the radius with dislocation of the head of the ulna.

morbidity   A diseased or abnormal condition.

morbidity rate   In statistics: the rate at which a disease or abnormality occurs in an area or population, calculated by dividing the number of affected people by the total area or population.

Morgagni's globule   Small, round cell fragments that may form between the eye lens and its capsule; a sign of a mature cataract.

Morgagni's tubercles Small nodules on the surface of the areola of the mammary gland. The tubercles are produced by the large sebaceous glands just beneath the skin of the areolae.

Moro's reflex A defensive reflex in infants elicited by a sudden loud noise or by striking the table on which the infant lies, resulting in flexion of the thighs and knees, clenching of the fingers, an embracing posture of the arms and, usually, a brief cry. It's a normal reflex exhibited by infants up to age 4 months.

morphea Condition in which connective tissue replaces skin and sometimes subcutaneous tissues.

morphogenetic In embryology: of or referring to a substance or hormone that stimulates growth and differentiation.

morphology The study of the form and structure of an organism, organ, or part.

Morquio's disease A familial form of mucopolysaccharidosis in childhood resulting primarily in abnormal musculoskeletal development with secondary nervous system involvement.

mortality 1. The condition of being subject to death. 2. The death rate, the ratio of deaths per unit of population in a specific region, age-group, disease, or other classification.

mortar A cup-shaped vessel made of glass, iron, porcelain, or other material, in which drugs are ground or crushed with a pestle.

Morton's neuralgia A severe, throbbing foot pain resulting from the compression of a branch of the plantar nerve by the metatarsal heads.

morula, *pl.* morulas, morulae The solid mass of cells formed by the cleavage of the fertilized ovum during an early embryonic development stage.

mosaicism In genetics: the presence of two or more cell populations that differ in genetic constitution in an individual, organism, or cell culture derived from a single zygote.

Mossbauer spectrometer An instrument used in chemical-physical research that can detect small changes in the interaction between an atomic nucleus and its environment caused by changes in chemical state, pressure, or temperature.

motor 1. Of or referring to motion, the body apparatus that produces movement, or the brain functions that control purposeful action. 2. Of or referring to a muscle, nerve, or brain center that produces or promotes motion.

motor aphasia The inability to speak or write remembered words due to a lesion in the area of the brain that controls motor speech.

motor apraxia The inability to perform skilled movements or to handle small objects, although the proper use of the object is understood. The patient appears clumsy rather than weak.

motor area Any area of the cerebral cortex primarily involved in controlling or stimulating the contraction of voluntary muscles.

motor end plate A broad band of terminal fibers of the motor nerves of the voluntary muscles. Motor nerves derived from the cranial and spinal nerves enter the sheaths of striated muscle fibers, lose their myelin sheaths, and ramify like the roots of a tree.

motor fiber A spinal nerve fiber that conducts impulses to muscle fibers.

motor image The visual concept of the possible movements of the body.

motor nerve A peripheral efferent nerve that conducts impulses away from the brain or the spinal cord to motor end plates, resulting in the stimulation of muscle contractions.

motor neuron paralysis An injury to the spinal cord that causes damage to the motor neurons and results in various degrees of functional impairment depending on the site of the lesion.

motor point The point at which a motor nerve enters the muscle.

motor seizure A transitory disturbance in brain function caused by abnormal neuronal discharges that arise initially in a localized motor area of the cerebral cortex.

motor unit A functional structure formed by a motor nerve cell and the muscle fibers it innervates.

mouse-tooth forceps Dressing forceps with one or more fine teeth on the tip of each blade. The tips turn in, and the delicate teeth interlock.

mouth The opening at the anterior end of the digestive tube, containing the tongue and the teeth and bounded anteriorly by the lips.

mouth-to-nose resuscitation An artificial resuscitation technique in which the patient's mouth is held closed and the air is breathed through the patient's nose into the lungs.

MPD *abbr* maximum permissible dose.

MPH *abbr* Master of Public Health.

MPS *abbr* 1. mononuclear phagocyte system. 2. mucopolysaccharidosis.

MPS I *abbr* mucopolysaccharidosis I.

MPS II *abbr* mucopolysaccharidosis II.

mR *abbr* milliroentgen.

MRI *abbr* magnetic resonance imaging.

mRNA *abbr* messenger ribonucleic acid.

Motor end plate

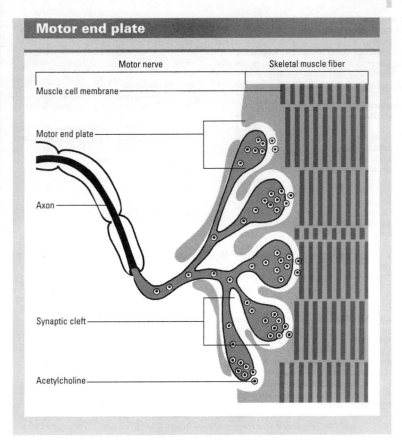

Motor nerve   Skeletal muscle fiber

Muscle cell membrane

Motor end plate

Axon

Synaptic cleft

Acetylcholine

MS *abbr* **1.** multiple sclerosis. **2.** Master of Science. **3.** Master of Surgery.

MSH *abbr* melanocyte-stimulating hormone.

MSN *abbr* Master of Science in Nursing.

MT *abbr* Medical Technologist.

mu *abbr* micron.

Much's granules Gram-positive, nonacid-fast rods and granules found in tuberculosis sputum.

mucin A mucopolysaccharide that is the main ingredient in mucus. It's the lubricant that protects body surfaces from friction and erosion and is present in most glands that secrete mucus.

mucocele Cyst or polyp that contains mucus.

mucocutaneous Of or referring to the mucous membrane and skin.

mucoid Of, referring to, or resembling mucus.

mucolytic Agent that destroys mucus.

mucopolysaccharidosis (MPS), *pl.* **mucopolysaccharidoses** Any of a group of genetic lysosomal storage diseases characterized by greater than normal accumulations of mucopolysaccharides in the tissues.

mucoprotein A compound present in connective and supporting tissue that contains mucopolysaccharides as prosthetic groups and is resistant to denaturation.

mucopurulent Containing a combination of mucus and pus.

mucositis Inflammation of mucous membranes.

mucous membrane Any one of four major kinds of thin sheets of tissue that line bodily passages and cavities that communicate with the air.

mucus The viscous, slimy secretions of mucous membranes and glands, composed of mucin, white blood cells, water, inorganic salts, and exfoliated cells.

mucus plug In obstetrics: a plug formed by mucus secretions in the cervix that closes the cervical canal during pregnancy; usually expelled at the onset of dilation of the cervix, just before labor begins.

MUGA scan *abbr* multiple gated acquisition scan.

müllerian duct One of a pair of embryonic ducts that develop into the fallopian tubes and uterus in females and that either atrophy or develop into a vestigial structure in males.

multifactorial inheritance The development of a characteristic, disease, or condition that is determined by multiple factors, including both genetic and nongenetic (environmental) factors.

multiform Type of premature ventricular contractions with differing QRS configurations due to originations from different irritable sites in the ventricle. Also called *multifocal*.

multiphasic screening Examination of a group of individuals using various diagnostic procedures in the same screening program.

multiple fission A form of asexual reproduction in certain unicellular organisms such as bacteria in which the cell divides into a number of daughter cells.

multiple lipomatosis A rare, genetic disorder characterized by abnormal localized accumulations of subcutaneous fat in the tissues of the body.

multiple myeloma A widely distributed cancer of the bone marrow which results in bone pain and pathological fractures.

multiple peripheral neuritis Widely distributed inflammation of the peripheral nerves, characterized initially by numbness and tingling in the extremities, progressing to pain, weakness, diminished reflexes, and possible paralysis.

multipolar mitosis A type of cell division in which the spindle has more than two poles, resulting in the formation of as many daughter cells.

mummified fetus A dead fetus that has shriveled and dried up in the uterus.

mumps An acute infectious disease caused by a paramyxovirus and characterized by swelling of one or both of the parotid glands.

mumps virus vaccine, live A live, attenuated virus vaccine prescribed for immunization of adolescents and adults who have either never had mumps or never been immunized with live mumps vaccine. Since the virus is incubated in chick embryos, the virus should not be given to anyone with a known hypersensitivity to chicken proteins. Immunosuppression, concomitant use of corticosteroids, acute infection, pregnancy, or a sensitivity to neomycin or this drug prohibits its use.

murine typhus An acute, endemic infectious disease caused by *Rickettsia typhi*, which is transmitted from rats to humans by the bite of an infected flea.

murmur A low-pitched blowing or fluttering sound of cardiac or vascular origin heard on auscultation.

TIME LINE Innocent murmurs, such as Still's murmur, are frequently heard in young children and often disappear in puberty. Pathognomonic heart murmurs in infants and young children usually result from congenital heart disease, such as atrial and ventricular septal defects.

Murray Valley encephalitis An acute inflammation of the brain caused by a mosquito-borne virus. The name is derived from an epidemic in the early 1950s in Australia's Murray Valley.

muscarine A chemical substance found in some poisonous mushrooms that produces a characteristic toxic syndrome when ingested.

muscarinic Of or referring to the effects of muscarine or acetylcholine on postganglionic parasympathetic receptor cells and in the central nervous system.

muscle A body tissue composed of fibers that are capable of contracting, thus causing movement of the parts and organs of the body.

muscular dystrophy A group of degenerative genetic diseases characterized by weakness and the progressive atrophy of skeletal muscles with no evidence of involvement of the nervous system.

muscular sarcoidosis A sarcoidosis of the skeletal muscles with sarcoid tubercles, interstitial inflammation with fibrosis, and atrophy damage of the muscle fibers.

musculocutaneous nerve A terminal branch of the brachial plexus forms this lateral cutaneous nerve of the forearm and muscular branches.

mushroom worker's lung A type of hypersensitivity lung inflammation found in workers in the mushroom-growing industry.

mutagen A chemical or physical agent that induces or increases the rate of genetic mutations.

mutant gene Any gene in which the loss, gain, or exchange of genetic material results in a change in function that is genetically transmittable.

mutation A permanent and transmissible change in genetic material that alters the original expression of the gene.

muton In molecular genetics: the smallest unit of deoxyribonucleic acid, possibly one nucleotide, whose alteration can produce a mutation.

mV *abbr* millivolt.

mVO$_2$ *abbr* myocardial oxygen consumption.

MVV *abbr* maximal voluntary ventilation.

MWIA *abbr* Medical Women's International Association.

myalgia *abbr* Diffuse muscle pain or tenderness associated with many infectious diseases.

myalgic asthenia A condition characterized by a feeling of general fatigue and muscular pains.

myasthenia Any abnormal weakness of a muscle or group of muscles resulting from any of several causes.

myasthenia gravis An abnormal muscle weakness and fatigability, especially in the muscles of the face and throat, resulting from a defect in the conduction of nerve impulses at the myoneural junction.

 ALERT Be alert for signs of impending crisis, such as increased muscle weakness, respiratory distress, and difficulty talking or chewing.

mycetoma A serious fungal infection involving skin, subcutaneous tissue, fascia, and bone, usually of the foot or leg.

mycobacteria Plural of mycobacterium.

mycobacteriosis A disease caused by a mycobacteria other than *Mycobacterium tuberculosis. Also called **atypical tuberculosis.***

Mycobacterium A genus of acid-fast, gram-positive, rod-shaped aerobic bacteria. The genus contains many different species, including the bacteria that cause tuberculosis (*M. tuberculosis*) and leprosy (*M. leprae*).

mycology The science and study of fungi and the diseases they cause.

mycoplasmal pneumonia A contagious respiratory disease caused by *Mycoplasma pneumoniae*, characterized by a sore throat, dry cough, fever, malaise, and myalgia.

mycosis Any disease resulting from a fungus infection.

mycotic aneurysm A stretching of the wall of a blood vessel caused by the growth of a bacterium or fungus in the vessel wall. The infection may arise in a preexisting arteriosclerotic aneurysm.

mydriasis Pronounced or abnormal dilation of the pupil, such as from a drug.

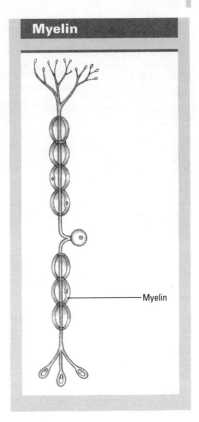

Myelin

Myelin

 TIME LINE Mydriasis occurs in children as a result of ocular trauma, drugs, Adie's syndrome and, most frequently, increased intracranial pressure.

myectomy Excision of a muscle.

myelin A white, creamy substance composed primarily of lipids with some protein that forms an insulating sheath around various nerve fibers throughout the body.

myelinic neuroma A tumor composed of myelinated nerve fibers.

myelinolysis A demyelination or pathological process that destroys myelin. For example, central pontine myelinolysis is a widespread demyelination of the pons occurring in alcoholics.

myelin sheath The cylindrical covering on the axons of some nerves that acts as an electrical insulator to speed the transmission of nerve impulses. It's composed of concentric layers of myelin formed in the peripheral nerves by Schwann cells.

myelitis   Any inflammation of the spinal cord that may involve motor or sensory dysfunction; usually a symptom of a more specific disease process.

myeloblast   An immature cell found primarily in the bone marrow; one of the most primitive precursors of granular leukocytes. The cytoplasm appears light blue, scanty, and nongranular when seen in a stained blood smear through a microscope.

myeloblastic leukemia   A cancer of the blood-forming tissues, characterized by the presence of many myeloblasts in the circulating blood and tissues.

myeloblastomatosis   The presence of multiple malignant tumors composed of myeloblasts.

myeloblastosis   The abnormal presence of an excess of myeloblasts in the circulation.

myelocele   A saclike protrusion of the spinal cord through a defect in the vertebral column.

myeloclast   A cell which breaks down the myelin sheath.

myelocyst   A benign cyst that develops from the rudimentary medullary canals that form the vertebral canal during embryonic development.

myelocystocele   A protrusion of a cystic tumor containing spinal cord substance through a defect in the vertebral column.

myelocyte   An immature cell found primarily in the bone marrow; one of the intermediate precursors of granular leukocytes. Differentiation into specific cytoplasmic granules can be noted.

myelocythemia   The presence of an excess of myelocytes in the circulating blood, as in myelocytic leukemia.

myelocytic leukemia   A cancer of the blood-forming tissues, characterized by the unregulated and excessive production of myelocytes of the granulocytic series.

myelogenesis   1. The prenatal development of the nervous system, in particular the brain and spinal cord. 2. The development of the myelin sheath around nerve fibers.

myelogenous   Referring to the cells produced in the bone marrow or to the tissue from which such cells are produced.

myelography   Radiography of the spinal cord and the spinal subarachnoid space following the injection of a contrast medium. It's used to identify and study spinal lesions caused by trauma or disease.

myeloid   1. Of, referring to, or derived from the bone marrow. 2. Of or referring to the spinal cord. 3. Having the appearance of myelocytes, but not originating in the bone marrow.

myeloma   Osteolytic neoplasm consisting of a protrusion of cells typical of the bone marrow.

myelomatous cells   Increased number of immature plasma cells.

myelomeningocele   The protrusion of a hernial sac containing a portion of the spinal cord, its meninges, and cerebrospinal fluid through a congenital defect in the vertebral column.

myelomere   Any of the segments of the developing brain or spinal cord during prenatal development.

myelophthisic anemia   A disorder in which lesions of the bone marrow displace the blood-forming tissues; characterized by the presence of a variable number of immature red blood cells and myeloid cells in the circulation.

myelopoiesis   The formation of the bone marrow or the cells that originate from it.

myelosuppression   Interference with, and suppression of the blood-forming stem cells in the bone marrow; a possible complication of chemotherapy.

myesthesia   Muscle sense or the consciousness of touch or muscle contraction.

myolysis   Degeneration of muscle tissue.

myocardial infarction (MI)   A gross necrosis of the myocardium resulting from an interruption of the blood supply to that area; usually caused by atherosclerosis or an embolism of the coronary artery.

myocarditis   An inflammation of the myocardium which may arise from a number of conditions, including viral, bacterial, or fungal infection; serum sickness; rheumatic fever; a chemical agent; or a complication of a collagen disease.

myocardium   A thick, contractile, middle layer of the heart wall composed of cardiac muscle cells.

myodynia   Pain in a muscle.

myogelosis   A condition in which there is an area of hardening or nodules within muscles, especially the gluteus muscle.

myoglobin   A respiratory pigment in muscle tissue responsible for its red color and its ability to store oxygen. It consists of one heme molecule containing one iron molecule attached to a single globin chain.

myolysis   Degeneration of muscle tissue.

myoma, *pl.* **myomas, myomata**   A common, benign tumor of the smooth muscle, most commonly of the uterus.

 CLINICAL TIP   Myoma develops most frequently after age 30 in women, especially black women, who have never been pregnant. Symptoms may include menorrhagia, backache, constipation, dysmenorrhea, and dyspareunia, among others.

myomalacia   Softening of a muscle.

myomectomy   Removal of tumors in the uterine muscle.

myomelanosis   Area of black pigment in a muscle.

myometritis   Inflammation or infection of the myometrium of the uterus.

myometrium, *pl.* **myometria**   The muscular layer of the uterine wall.

myonecrosis   The death, or necrosis, of individual muscle fibers.

myopathy   Any disease of the skeletal muscle. Generally characterized by muscle weakness, wasting, and histological changes within muscle tissue, such as is found in any of the muscular dystrophies.

myopia   A condition of nearsightedness in which parallel rays are focused in front of the retina. It's usually caused by the elongation of the eyeball or an error of refraction.

myosarcoma   A malignant tumor derived from muscle tissue.

myosclerosis   Hardening of muscle tissue.

myosin   The most abundant protein in muscle tissue. The interaction between myosin and actin is responsible for the contraction and relaxation of muscle.

myositis   Inflammation of voluntary muscle tissue.

myositis fibrosa   An inflammation of the muscles, characterized by the formation of connective tissue within the muscle.

myositis purulenta   Any bacterial infection of muscle tissue. This condition may result in the formation of pus and ultimately gangrene.

myotenotomy   The surgical division of a muscle tendon.

myotome   That part of an embryonic somite that develops into somatic, or voluntary, muscle.

myotomic muscle   Any of the muscles of the trunk of the body, derived from myotomes and divided into the deep muscles of the back, chest, and abdomen.

myotomy   Cutting or dissection of a muscle.

myotonia   A condition marked by increased muscle contractibility and irritability coupled with a decrease in the ability of the muscle or group to relax.

myotonic muscular dystrophy   A rare, degenerative, hereditary form of muscular dystrophy characterized by weakness of the muscles, primarily of the face and neck, followed by atrophy. A person with this condition may exhibit slurred speech, cataracts, frontal balding, and cardiac abnormalities.

myringectomy   Surgical removal of the eardrum.

myringitis   An inflammation or infection of the eardrum.

myringoplasty   Surgical restoration of a perforated eardrum with a tissue graft, performed to correct hearing loss.

myringotomy   Surgically puncturing the eardrum to drain fluid and relieve pressure from the middle ear.

myxedema   A condition associated with primary hypothyroidism and characterized by dry, waxy swelling of the skin with abnormal deposits of mucin in the skin (mucinosis) and other tissues, and a nonpitting type of edema.

myxoma   A benign tumor of the connective tissue, composed of star-shaped cells in a loose mucoid matrix crossed by delicate reticulum fibers.

myxosarcoma   A sarcoma containing some myxomatous tissue.

myxovirus   Family of medium-sized ribonucleic acid viruses, including those that cause influenza, that are further divided into orthomyxoviruses and paramyxoviruses.

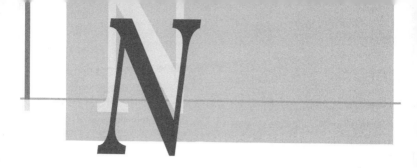

n, 2n, 3n, 4n   Symbols for the haploid, diploid, triploid, and tetraploid chromosome number of any cell, organism, strain, or individual.

N   1. Symbol for normal. 2. *abbr* node in the TNM (tumor, node, metastasis) system for staging malignant neoplastic disease.

N₂O   Symbol for nitrous oxide.

Na   Symbol for sodium.

NAACOG   *abbr* Nurses Association of the American College of Obstetrics and Gynecology.

nabothian cyst   Cyst formed in the nabothian gland.

nabothian gland   One of several small glands of the uterine cervix that secrete mucus.

nadir   Lowest point on a curve or scale, often related to blood counts.

Nägele's rule   A system used to estimate the date of delivery based on a mean length of gestation. Subtract 3 months from the 1st day of the last normal menstrual period, and add 7 days to that date.

Nahrungs Einheit Milch (nem)   A nutritional unit in Pirquet's feeding method that equals 1 g of breast milk.

nail   A flattened, horny, elastic structure at the end of a finger or toe.

NAMH   *abbr* National Association for Mental Health.

nandrolone decanoate, nandrolone phenpropionate   Anabolic steroids.

nanism   Dwarfism; a small-sized or underdeveloped body. Types of nanism are mulibrey nanism, Paltauf's nanism, pituitary nanism, renal nanism, senile nanism, symptomatic nanism. Also called *nanosomia.*

nanocephaly, nanocephalia, nanocephalism   A developmental anomaly characterized by a small-sized head.

nanocormia   A developmental anomaly characterized by an abnormal and disproportionately small trunk compared with the head and limbs.

nanocurie (nCi)   A unit of radiation that is equivalent to one billionth of a curie.

naphthalene poisoning   Toxicity caused by ingesting naphthalene or paradichlorobenzene.

 CLINICAL TIP   Symptoms of naphthalene poisoning include nausea, vomiting, headache, abdominal pain, spasm, and convulsions.

napkin-ring tumor   A tumor encircling a tubular structure, typically impairing its function and constricting its lumen.

NAPNES   *abbr* National Association for Practical Nurse Education and Services.

narcoleptic   Of or related to a condition or substance that causes an uncontrollable desire to sleep.

narcosis   A state of insensibility or stupor caused by narcotic drugs.

nasal   Of or pertaining to the nose and nasal cavity.

nasal cavity   A pair of cavities that open on the face through the pear-shaped anterior nasal aperture and communicate with the pharynx.

nasal glioma   A tumorlike mass in the nasal cavity that is composed of ectopic neural tissue.

nasalis   One of three muscles of the nose that is divided into a transverse and alar part.

nasal septum   The partition separating the nostrils that is composed of bone and cartilage covered by mucous membrane.

nasal sinus   One of many cavities in various skull bones that is lined with ciliated mucous membrane continuous with that of the nasal cavity.

nasal turbinates   The ledges that form the side and lower wall of each nasal cavity.

nascent   1. Just born; starting to exist; incipient. 2. In chemistry: related to a substance released during a chemical reaction which, because of its uncombined form, is more reactive.

nasion   1. The anthropometric point at the front of the skull where the midsagittal plane intersects a horizontal line tangential to the highest points in the superior palpebral sulci. 2. The depression at the root of the nose below the eyebrows that indicates the frontonasal suture.

nasogastric intubation The placement of a nasogastric tube through the nose into the stomach to relieve gastric distention by removing gas, gastric secretions, or food; to instill medication, food, or fluids; or to obtain a specimen for laboratory analysis.

nasogastric tube A tube inserted into the stomach through the nose.

nasolabial reflex A sudden backward head movement, arching of the back, and extension and stretching of the limbs when infants respond to a touch to the tip of the nose with an upward sweeping motion.

nasolacrimal duct A channel carrying tears from the lacrimal sac to the nasal cavity.

nasomandibular fixation Type of maxillomandibular fixation used to stabilize jaw fractures in which maxillomandibular splints are connected to a wire through a hole drilled in the anterior nasal spine of the maxillary bone.

nasopharyngeal angiofibroma A benign tumor of the nasopharynx composed of fibrous connective tissue with many vascular spaces.

nasopharyngitis Inflammation of the nose and pharynx.

nasopharynx One of three regions of the throat, located behind the nose and extending from the posterior nares to the level of the soft palate.

nasotracheal tube A tube inserted through the nasal cavity and pharynx into the trachea.

NATA *abbr* National Athletic Trainers Association.

National Association for Practical Nurse Education and Services (NAPNES) A national professional organization focused on educating practical nurses and the services provided by licensed practical nurses.

National Bureau of Standards (NBS) A federal agency in the United States Department of Commerce that determines measurement standards for commerce, industry, and science.

National Eye Institute (NEI) A division of the National Institutes of Health, the NEI supports research in the functioning of the human eye and visual system, pathology of visual disorders, and rehabilitation of the visually handicapped.

National Formulary (NF) A publication listing the official standards for the preparation of several pharmaceuticals not listed in the United States Pharmacopoeia.

National Institute of Child Health and Human Development (NICHHD) Institute within the National Institutes of Health that is focused on all aspects of the growth, development, and health of children in the United States.

National Institutes of Health (NIH) An agency within the Health Resource Services Administration composed of many institutions and constituent divisions, including the Bureau of Health Manpower Education, the National Library of Medicine, the National Cancer Institute, the National Institute on Aging, and several research institutes and divisions.

natriuresis The excessive excretion of sodium in urine, such as from the effects of natriuretic diuretics or metabolic or endocrine disorders.

natriuretic 1. Of or related to natriuresis. 2. A substance that inhibits sodium ion resorption from the glomerular filtrate in the kidneys, allowing more sodium to be excreted in the urine.

natural childbirth Labor and parturition achieved by a mother with minimal or no medical assistance. It's often considered the ideal method of giving birth — safest for the baby and most satisfying for the mother.

natural dentition The entire arrangement of teeth in the dental arch, consisting of deciduous or permanent teeth or a mixture of both.

natural immunity A usually inbuilt and permanent form of immunity to a specific disease.

natural selection The natural evolutionary processes by which organisms best adapted to the environment tend to survive and propagate the species whereas those unfit are eliminated.

naturopathy An alternative system of medical practice that combines mainstream understanding of human physiology and disease with alternative remedies such as herbal and nutritional therapies, acupuncture, hydrotherapy, and counseling. Naturopathic physicians eschew drugs and surgery in favor of natural treatments designed to stimulate the body's own healing ability.

nausea Unpleasant sensation with the tendency to vomit.

Nb Symbol for niobium.

NBS *abbr* National Bureau of Standards.

NBS standard In nuclear medicine: a radioactive source standardized or certified (or both) by the National Bureau of Standards.

nCi *abbr* nanocurie.

NCI *abbr* National Cancer Institute, an institute of the National Institutes of Health.

Nd *abbr* neodymium.

Jet nebulizer

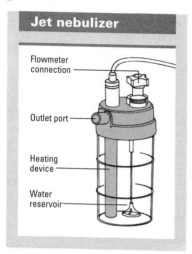

- Flowmeter connection
- Outlet port
- Heating device
- Water reservoir

NDA *abbr* National Dental Association.

Ne Symbol for neon.

nebula, *pl.* nebulae 1. A corneal opacity or scar that rarely obstructs vision and can be seen only by oblique illumination. 2. A murkiness in urine. 3. An oily concoction applied with an atomizer.

nebulize To vaporize or disperse a liquid into a fine spray.

nebulizer A device that employs a baffle to produce a fine aerosol spray consisting of particles less than 30 micrometers in diameter.

neck A constricted section, such as part of the body connecting the head and trunk.

neck-righting reflex An involuntary response in which turning the head to one side while a neonate is lying down causes rotation of the shoulders and trunk in the same direction.

necrobiosis lipoidica A skin disorder that is characterized by thin, shiny, yellowish red plaques on the shins or forearms.

necrolysis Disintegration or exfoliation of dead tissue.

necrosis Localized tissue death that occurs in groups of cells because of disease or injury.

necrotizing enteritis Acute inflammation of the small and large intestine by *Clostridium perfringens* characterized by severe abdominal pain, bloody diarrhea, and vomiting.

ALERT Be alert for signs or symptoms of gastric distention and perforation, including apnea, cardiovascular shock, sudden drop in temperature, brady-

cardia, sudden listlessness, rag doll limpness, increasing abdominal tenderness, edema, erythema, or involuntary abdomenal rigidity.

necrotizing vasculitis An inflammation of blood vessels, characterized by necrosis, fibrosis, and proliferation of the inner vascular wall, sometimes resulting in occlusion and infarction.

needle biopsy The removal of part of living tissue for microscopic study by inserting a hollow needle through the skin or the external surface of an organ or tumor and rotating it within the underlying cellular layers.

negative 1. Of a laboratory test: suggesting that a substance or reaction is absent. 2. Of a sign: indicating that a finding is not present, often meaning that there is no pathologic change. 3. Of a substance: tending to carry a negative chemical charge.

negative catalysis A decreased rate of a chemical reaction that is caused by a substance that is not part of the process or consumed or affected by the reaction.

negative pi meson (pion) A form of electromagnetic radiation released from a proton linear accelerator.

negative pi meson (pion) radiotherapy A type of radiotherapy that uses a negative pi meson beam emitted by a proton linear accelerator. Pion radiotherapy requires fewer rad and has a 60% greater biological effect than usual X-radiation methods.

negative pressure Less-than-ambient atmospheric pressure, such as in a vacuum, at an altitude above sea level, or in a hypobaric chamber.

negligence Failure to act as an ordinary prudent person would under similar circumstances. Conduct that falls below the standard established by law for the protection of others under the same circumstances.

NEHA *abbr* National Environmental Health Association.

NEI *abbr* National Eye Institute.

Neisseria gonorrhoeae Gram-negative, nonmotile, diplococcal bacteria, commonly observed microscopically as flattened pairs within the cytoplasm of neutrophils, that cause gonorrhea.

NEJM *abbr New England Journal of Medicine.*

Nelson's syndrome An endocrine disorder that may occur after adrenalectomy for Cushing's disease.

nematode A multicellular parasite belonging to the phylum Nematoda. All roundworms belong to the phylum, including Ancylostoma duodenale, Ascaris lumbricoides, Enterobius vermicularis, Necator americanus, and Strongyloides stercoralis.

neoantigen   A new specific antigen that develops in a cell infected by oncogenic virus.

neoblastic   Of or related to new tissue or development within a new tissue.

neodymium (Nd)   A rare earth element with atomic number 60 and atomic weight 144.24.

neon (Ne)   A colorless, odorless, gaseous element with atomic number 10 and atomic weight 20.183; it's one of the inert gases.

neonatal intensive care unit (NICU)   A hospital unit containing several sophisticated mechanical devices and special equipment for managing and caring for premature and seriously ill newborn infants.

neonatal mortality   The statistical rate of infant death during the first 28 days after birth, expressed as the number of such deaths per 1,000 live births in a specific geographic area or institution in a defined time period.

neonatal period   The interval between birth and age 28 days. It represents the time of the greatest risk to the infant; about 65% of all deaths that occur in the first year occur during this time period.

neonatal pustular melanosis   A temporary skin disorder affecting neonates that is characterized by vesicles that become pustular.

neonatal thermoregulation   The regulation of a neonate's body temperature, which may be affected by evaporation, conduction, radiation, and convection.

neonate   An infant from birth to age 4 weeks.

neonatology   The branch of medicine that specializes in the care of the neonate, especially the diagnosis and treatment of disorders.

neoplasm   An abnormal growth of new tissue, benign or malignant.

neoplastic fracture   A fracture occurring as a result of weakened bone tissue caused by neoplasm or a malignant growth.

nephrectomy   The surgical removal of a kidney, usually done to remove a tumor, drain an abcess, or treat hydronephrosis.

nephritis   Inflammation and abnormal function of the kidneys.

nephroangiosclerosis   Necrosis of the renal arterioles, usually occurring with hypertension.

nephrogenic diabetes insipidus   A disorder in which the kidneys do not concentrate the urine, resulting in polyuria, polydipsia, and very dilute urine.

nephrogenous   Of or related to the formation and development of the kidneys.

nephrolith   The presence of a calculus (stone) in a kidney.

nephrolithiasis   A disorder characterized by the presence of calculi in a kidney.

nephrology   The study of the structure and function of the kidney.

nephrolytic   Of or related to the destruction of the structure and function of a kidney.

nephromegaly   Enlargement of the kidney.

nephron   A structural and functional unit of the kidney, similar to a microscopic funnel with a long stem and two convoluted sections.

nephropathy   Any disorder of the kidney, including inflammatory, degenerative, and sclerotic conditions.

nephroptosis   A downward displacement of a kidney.

nephrorrhagia   Hemorrhage from or into the kidney.

nephrorrhaphy   A surgical procedure that sutures a floating kidney in place.

nephrostomy   Creation of a permanent passage leading directly into the kidney's pelvis.

nephrotic syndrome   A clinical classification including all kidney diseases characterized by marked proteinuria, hypoalbuminemia, and edema.

nephrotomy   A surgical procedure in which the kidney is incised.

nephrotoxic   Any substance that is toxic or destructive to a kidney.

nephrotoxin   A toxin with specific destructive properties against kidney cells.

neptunium (Np)   A metallic element with atomic number 93 and atomic weight 237 that is obtained by bombarding uranium with neutrons.

nerve   A bundle of fibers lying outside the central nervous system that connect the brain and spinal cord with various parts of the body.

nerve compression   A disorder that causes harmful pressure on nerve trunks, resulting in nerve damage and muscle weakness or atrophy.

nerve entrapment   A type of mononeuropathy that is characterized by nerve damage and muscle weakness or atrophy.

nerve fibers   Threadlike dendrites and axons.

nerve pathways   Tracts that conduct sensory and motor impulses throughout the nervous system.

nerve trunk   White, glistening, cordlike bundle of formed nerve fibers running together.

Neurohypophysis

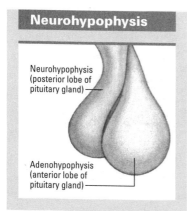

Neurohypophysis (posterior lobe of pituitary gland)

Adenohypophysis (anterior lobe of pituitary gland)

nervous breakdown   *Informal.* A mental condition that significantly disrupts normal functioning.

nervous system   A system of extensive and intricate structures that activates, coordinates, and controls all bodily functions. It's divided into the central nervous system (brain and spinal cord) and the peripheral nervous system (cranial and spinal nerves).

Neufeld nail   An orthopedic nail with a V-shaped tip and shank that is used to fix an intertrochanteric fracture. The nail is driven into the femur neck until it reaches a round metal plate screwed on the side of the femur; it's then secured to a receptacle on the plate.

neural crest   Band of ectodermally derived cells that lies along the outer surface of each side of the neural tube during the early development of an embryo.

neuralgia   Severe stabbing pain caused by several disorders affecting the nervous system.

neural groove   The longitudinal depression occurring between the neural folds when the neural plate invaginates to form the neural tube during early embryonic development.

neural plate   A thickened layer of ectodermal tissue that occurs along the central longitudinal axis of an early developing embryo and gives rise to the neural tube and subsequently the brain, spinal cord, and central nervous system tissue.

neural tube   The longitudinal tube, located along the central axis of an early developing embryo, from which the brain, spinal cord, and other central nervous system tissue are derived.

neural tube defect   A congenital malformation involving the skull and spinal column that is mainly caused by the failure of the neural tube to close during embryonic development.

neurenteric canal   A tubular canal between the posterior neural tube and archenteron in early embryonic development of lower animals.

neurilemma, neurolemma   A cell layer, composed of Schwann cells, that encloses the segmented myelin sheaths of peripheral nerve fibers.

neuritis, *pl.* **neuritides**   Inflammation of a nerve.

neuroblast   An embryonic cell that will develop into a neuron; an immature nerve cell.

neuroblastoma, *pl.* **neuroblastomas, neuroblastomata**   A malignant tumor composed of neuroblasts and affecting infants and children.

neurocoele, neurocele, neurocoel   A system of cavities in the central nervous system of humans and other vertebrates.

neurofibroma, *pl.* **neurofibromas, neurofibromata**   A fibrous tumor of peripheral nerves resulting from the abnormal proliferation of Schwann cells.

neurofibromatosis   An autosomally dominant trait that is characterized by several neurofibromas of the nerves and skin, café-au-lait spots on the skin and, sometimes, developmental anomalies of the muscles, bones, and visceral tissue.

neurogenesis   The development of nervous system tissue.

neurogenic arthropathy   Neural damage that is characterized by the gradual and usually painless degeneration of a joint.

neurogenic bladder   Urinary bladder dysfunction caused by a lesion of the nervous system.

neurogenic fracture   A fracture caused by the weakening of a bone as its nerve supply is destroyed.

neuroglia   A type of cell occurring in the nervous system.

neurohormonal regulation   The joint effect of nervous system and hormonal action to regulate the function of an organ or gland.

neurohypophysis   The posterior lobe of the pituitary gland that releases antidiuretic hormone (ADH) and oxytocin when stimulated by the hypothalamus. ADH acts on the cells of the distal and collecting tubules of the kidneys, enhancing water permeability and reducing the volume of urine. Oxytocin produces strong contractions of the pregnant uterus and causes milk to flow from lactating breasts. Stimulation of the nipples by a nursing infant also triggers the release of oxytocin.

neuroleptanesthesia Anesthesia achieved by the administration of a neuropharmacologic agent, a narcotic analgesic, and nitrous oxide in oxygen.

neurology The branch of medicine focused on the nervous system and its disorders.

neurolysis Surgical freeing of perineural adhesions.

neuroma, *pl.* **neuromas, neuromata** A benign neoplasm that is mainly made up of neurons and nerve fibers, usually arising from a nerve tissue.

neuroma cutis A skin neoplasm containing nervous tissue that may be extremely sensitive to painful stimuli.

neuromuscular junction The space between the end of a large myelinated nerve fiber and a skeletal muscle fiber.

neuromuscular spindle A small bundle of delicate muscular fibers, enclosed by a capsule, in which sensory nerve fibers terminate.

neuromyal transmission The transmission of impulses from a motor neuron to a muscle fiber at the myoneural junction.

neuromyelitis Inflammation of the spinal cord and peripheral nerves.

neuron, neurone A nerve cell of the nervous system, containing a nucleus within a cell body and extending one or more processes. Classification of neurons is based on the direction in which they conduct impulses and the number of processes they extend.

neuropathy Inflammation and degeneration of the peripheral nerves.

neuroplasty Plastic repair of a nerve.

neuroplegia Nerve paralysis caused by disease, injury, or effect of neuroleptic drugs.

neuropore The open ends of the neural tube of the early embryo.

neurorrhaphy Suturing of a nerve.

neurosarcoma A malignant neoplasm containing nervous, connective, and vascular tissues.

neurosurgery Surgery involving the brain, spinal cord, or peripheral nerves.

neurotendinous spindle A capsule containing enlarged tendon fibers, occurring mainly near the junctions of tendons and muscles.

neurotoxic Something that is poisonous or destructive to nerve cells.

neurotoxin A toxin that attacks and destroys nerve cells or tissues; examples include *Clostridium botulinum, Clostridium tetani,* and *Corynebacterium diphtheriae.*

neurotransmitter Any one of a group of substances that act on a target nerve cell to excite or inhibit transmission of nerve im-

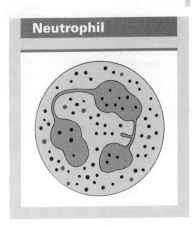

Neutrophil

pulses; substances include norepinephrine, acetylcholine, and dopamine.

neurotripsy Surgical crushing of a nerve.

neutral A state of being indifferent. In chemistry: a substance that is neither an alkali nor an acid. In electricity: a state in which something has neither a positive nor a negative charge.

neutralization The act of making something neutral; the process by which an antibody neutralizes the infectivity of a virus.

neutral thermal environment An environment created to maintain a normal body temperature in order to reduce caloric expenditure and oxygen consumption.

neutrocytopenia Decrease of neutrophils in the blood.

neutron In physics: an electrically neutral particle about the size of a proton, existing in all known atomic nuclei except the hydrogen isotope.

neutron activation analysis The review of elements in a sample after the sample has been exposed to neutron irradiation to convert its elements to a radioactive form in order to measure and identify the element's radiation emissions.

neutropenia An unusual decrease in the quantity of neutrophil cells in the blood.

neutrophil Any cell, especially blood cells, that stains easily with neutral dyes. Neutrophils are one of three types of leukocytes (white blood cells) and are essential for the ingestion and destruction of bacteria and small particles.

neutrophilia An increase in the quantity of neutrophil cells in the blood.

 CLINICAL TIP A common form of leukocytosis, neutrophilia has many causes, including acute infections, hemorrhage, and rapidly growing cancers.

nevus A benign birthmark or congenital skin blemish. Bleeding, itching, or changes in color, size, or texture of the blemish should be investigated for cancer.

nevus flammeus A common facial birthmark that is usually found on the face and neck. It varies in color from faint pink to dark red-purple; light varieties usually fade during childhood; dark ones, also known as *port-wine stains*, persist.

New England Journal of Medicine (NEJM) A professional journal devoted to publishing the findings of medical research; also publishes articles and editorials related to political and ethical issues in medicine.

next of kin One or more persons in the nearest degree of relationship to another person.

Nezelof's syndrome An immunodeficiency disorder in which patients are susceptible to life-threatening infections from everyday pathogens such as *Candida albicans*. The condition may be inherited. Also called *cellular immunodeficiency with immunoglobulins*.

NF *abbr National Formulary.*

ng *abbr nanogram.*

NGF *abbr nerve growth factor.*

NHSC *abbr National Health Service Corps.*

Ni Symbol for nickel.

niacin A B-complex vitamin. Niacin is used to prevent and to treat pellagra and it acts as a vasodilator and can reduce blood levels of cholesterol. Also called *vitamin B_3, nicotinic acid.*

NICHHD *abbr National Institute of Child Health and Human Development.*

nick In molecular genetics: a break in a single strand of double-stranded deoxyribonucleic acid caused by a missing bond.

nickel (Ni) A silver-white metallic element. Its atomic number is 28; its atomic weight, 58.71; specific gravity, 8.9.

nickel dermatitis An allergic contact dermatitis caused by exposure to nickel. Items containing nickel include jewelry (rings, earrings, necklaces), watches, metal clasps, and coins.

nicotine A poisonous, colorless, substance with a burning taste; found in tobacco and is a contributor to the health problems associated with smoking.

NICU *abbr neonatal intensive care unit.*

nidation The implantation of the fertilized ovum into the endometrium of the uterus.

Niemann-Pick disease An inherited disease characterized by an enlarged liver and spleen; bone marrow cells have foamy cytoplasm; onset of disease is in early infancy.

night vision The ability to see poorly lit objects. The retinal rods in the eye contain a light-sensitive chemical that is essential for conducting optic impulses in low-light conditions.

NIH *abbr National Institutes of Health.*

90-90 traction An orthopedic apparatus combining traction, suspension, and a short leg cast or splint to immobilize and position a leg. The device is used mostly in pediatrics to treat a displaced fractured femur.

niobium (Nb) A chemical element. Its atomic number is 41; its atomic weight is 92.906.

nipple A pigmented projection in the front of the mammary gland (breast); allows for the discharge of milk. Also called *papilla mammae, mamilla, thelium.*

nipple discharge Exudation of fluid from the nipple. The fluid may be normal, as colostrum in pregnancy, or it may be a sign of cancer or an endocrine or infectious disease.

TIME LINE Infants of both sexes may experience a milky breast discharge beginning 3 days after birth and lasting up to 2 weeks.

nipple inversion Inward turning or depression of the central portion of the nipple.

Nissl bodies Large granular bodies found in the cytoplasm of nerve cells. The bodies can be stained with basic dyes. Also called *chromatic granules, Nissl's granules, Nissl's substance.*

nitrite A salt or ester of nitrous acid. Amyl or organic nitrites are used as vasodilators and antispasmodics in the treatment of angina pectoris. Sodium nitrites are often used in the preservation of meats such as bacon.

nitrogen (N) A colorless, gaseous element. Its atomic number is 7; atomic weight, 14.007; specific gravity, 0.9713.

nitrogen balance The relationship between the intake and excretion of nitrogen. Nitrogen is usually taken into the body as food and excreted in urine and feces.

nitrous oxide (N_2O) A colorless, odorless, nonflammable gas. Nitrous oxide may be used as an anesthetic in childbirth, dentistry, and surgery, where it's administered with oxygen and provides light anesthesia.

NMR *abbr nuclear magnetic resonance.*

No Symbol for nobelium.

nobelium (No) A chemical element obtained by bombardment of curium. Its atomic number is 102; atomic weight, 253.

no-code order An order, written in the patient record and signed by a physician, instructing staff not to attempt to resuscitate a patient if he suffers cardiac or respiratory failure.

nocturia   Excessive urination during the night.

 TIME LINE Postmenopausal women have decreased bladder elasticity, but urine output remains constant, resulting in nocturia.

nocturnal   Occurring or happening at night; an animal that is active at night.

nocturnal paroxysmal dyspnea   An abnormal respiratory condition in which shortness of breath, profuse sweating, tachycardia, and wheezing awaken a person.

node   A small mass of tissue similar to a knot or swelling. Specific nodes include lymph nodes.

nodes of Ranvier   Interruptions in the myelin sheath of axons, separating the sheath into segments.

nodular   Like a node; small, rounded, firm.

nodular circumscribed lipomatosis
A condition in which encapsulated lipomas circle the neck like a collar. They may be distributed symmetrically or randomly.

nodular melanoma   A uniformly pigmented melanoma that is usually bluish-black and nodular; it may be surrounded by a halo of unpigmented skin.

noma   A severe process in which a small ulcer in the mouth or on the genitalia becomes necrotic.

nomenclature   A classified, systematic method for naming structures and organisms. In biology it's called binomial nomenclature; in chemistry, chemical nomenclature.

Nomina Anatomica   The International Congress of Anatomists' official book of international nomenclature for anatomy.

nomogram   A graphic representation of numerical relationships, with three or more straight or curved lines. Also called *alignment chart*.

non-A, non-B hepatitis   Viral hepatitis that is neither hepatitis A nor hepatitis B; caused by an antigenically different strain from those viruses.

nonbacterial thrombic endocarditis
A type of endocarditis that affects heart valves; can be identified by the kind of lesions.

noncoring needle   Vascular access port needle with an angled or deflected point that slices the septum on entry, rather than coring it like a conventional needle. When the noncoring needle is removed, the septum reseals itself.

nondisjunction   The failure of a pair of chromosomes to separate properly during

meiosis. The result is one daughter cell has too many chromosomes, and the other, too few.

nongonococcal urethritis   An infection of the urethra in males in which there is mild dysuria and minimal to moderate penile discharge.

noninvasive   In health care: a diagnostic or therapeutic technique that does not require entering the body or breaking the skin; for example, listening to breath sounds using a stethoscope.

nonosteogenic fibroma   A common, sometimes painful bone lesion similar to fibrous cortical defect; it usually appears in the long bones of the lower extremities in late childhood or adolescence. Also called *metaphyseal fibrous defect*.

nonparametric test of significance
In statistics: one of numerous mathematical tests that analyze rank order and incidence data.

nonproductive cough   A sudden, loud expulsion of air from the lungs that does not remove material from the respiratory tract; the cough may be caused by an irritation or inflammation.

nonulcerative blepharitis   A type of blepharitis in which greasy scales form along the margins of the eyelids around the lashes; there may also be swelling and thickening of the skin.

nonvesicant   An agent that doesn't cause blisters.

Noonan's syndrome   A male disorder characterized by webbed neck, ptosis, hypogonadism, congenital heart disease, and short stature.

norepinephrine   An adrenergic hormone that is a vasoconstrictor (and can therefore raise blood pressure) and has little effect on cardiac output.

norm   Normal; the ideal standard for a group.

norma basilaris   The outline of the base of the skull, as viewed from above.

normal   1. In chemistry: a solution in which 1 liter contains 1 gram equivalent of the solute. 2. A standard, average, or typical example of a set of objects. Something that performs properly.

normal human serum albumin   A preparation of human serum albumin for treating shock, hypoproteinemia, and hypovolemia.

normoblast   A nucleated red blood cell that is similar in size to the adult circulating erythrocyte.

nose   A specialized structure on the face that serves as a passageway for air to and from the lungs. It also serves as the organ of the sense of smell. The term includes the external nose and the nasal cavity. Also called *nasus.*

nosocomial   Originating in a hospital. The term usually refers to an infection not present before a patient entered a hospital.

nosocomial infection   An infection acquired during a hospital stay. Common nosocomial infections include those caused by *Candida albicans, Escherichia coli,* hepatitis viruses, herpes zoster virus, *Pseudomonas,* and *Staphylococcus.*

nosophilia   Abnormal desire to be ill.

notomelus   A malformation in which a fetus has accessory limbs on its back.

nourish   To provide the essential nutrients for maintaining life; to nurture.

Np   Symbol for neptunium.

NPO   *abbr nil per os,* a Latin phrase meaning "nothing by mouth."

N-propyl alcohol   A colorless liquid used as a solvent.

NREM   *abbr* nonrapid eye movement.

NSAIDs   *abbr* nonsteroidal anti-inflammatory drugs.

nucha, *pl.* nuchae   The back, or nape, of the neck.

nuchal cord   A condition in which the umbilical cord is wrapped around a fetus's neck in the uterus or during delivery.

nuchal rigidity   A characteristic sign of meningitis; the involuntary muscle stiffening at the nape of the neck that accompanies cervical spine injury, meningeal irritation, or bleeding after a head injury.

 ALERT   After eliciting nuchal rigidity, attempt to elicit Kernig's and Brudzinski's signs, quickly evaluate level of consciousness, and take vital signs. If you note signs of increased intracranial pressure — such as increased systolic pressure, bradycardia, and widened pulse pressure — start an I.V. line for drug administration and administer oxygen, as necessary.

nuclear isomer   One of two or more nuclides with the same number of neutrons and protons in the nucleus but existing in different energy states.

nuclear magnetic resonance   Phosphorus nuclear magnetic resonance instruments measure and image spectra emitted by phosphorus in body tissues.

nucleic acid   A high-molecular-weight nucleotide polymer found in the cells of all living things; the most important structures are deoxyribonucleic acid and ribonucleic acid.

nucleocapsid   In a virus: a protein coat (capsid) that encloses the nucleic acid.

nucleocytoplasmic   Relating to the cytoplasm and nucleus of cells.

nucleocytoplasmic ratio   The ratio of the volume of a cell's nucleus to the volume of its cytoplasm. Specific cell types have a fairly constant proportion; an increase suggests malignant neoplasms.

nucleolus, *pl.* nucleoli   The site of synthesis of ribosomal ribonucleic acid; it consists of a granular and a fibrillar portion and is situated within the cytoplasm of cells.

nucleoplasm   The protoplasm in the nucleus of a cell.

nucleus, *pl.* nuclei   **1.** The core of an object. **2.** The nucleus of a cell: a sphere within a cell that contains the genetic codes for maintaining and reproducing that cell. **3.** A group of central nervous system cells that support a common function, such as hearing or smell. **4.** In organic chemistry: the combination of atoms that form the framework of a molecule. **5.** The center of an atom around which electrons revolve.

nucleus pulposus   The pulpy, semifluid center of an intervertebral disk that loses some resiliency with age.

nuclide   A type of atom characterized by its atomic number, mass number, and energy content. It's capable of existing for a measurable time, usually greater than 10^{10} seconds.

null cell   A lymphocyte that lacks the surface marker for B or T cells; it develops in the bone marrow.

nullipara, *pl.* nulliparae   A woman who has not given birth to a viable infant. Designated on nursing charts as "para O."

numbness   A lack of sensation in any part of the body. The condition can result from any factor that interrupts the transmission of impulses from sensory nerves.

nummular dermatitis   A skin condition of unknown cause in which coin-shaped, scaling, eczema-like, or vesicular lesions appear on the forearms and front of the calves.

nurse practitioner   A nurse who has acquired expert knowledge in a specialized branch of practice by completing advanced training, such as a master's degree or certification, and clinical experience in a nursing specialty area.

nursing diagnosis   Descriptive interpretations of collected and categorized information indicating the problems or needs of a patient that nursing care can affect. According to the North American Nursing Diagnosis Association, "a clinical judgment about individual, community, or family responses to actual or potential health problems or to life processes. Nursing diagnoses provide the basis of selection of nursing interventions for which the nurse is accountable."

nursing process   An organizational framework for nursing practice that encompasses the five major steps a nurse must take when caring for a patient; assessment, diagnosis, planning, implementation, and evaluation.

nutrient   The nutritious component of food. Essential nutrients necessary for growth, normal functioning, and maintaining life include proteins, minerals, carbohydrates, fat, and vitamins.

nutrition   1. Nourishment. 2. The processes of taking in nutrients, assimilating them, and using them for growth, normal function, and maintenance of life.

nutritional anemia   A disorder in which there is an inadequate production of hemoglobin (red blood cells) because of a deficiency in iron, folic acid, or vitamin B^{12}.

nutritional care   The act of assuring the proper intake and assimilation of essential nutrients.

nyctalopia   Impaired vision in the dark, especially on entering a darkened room or while driving at night.

TIME LINE   Night blindness due to vitamin A deficiency usually occurs in elderly and disadvantaged patients. It's also a common side effect of the aging process.

nystagmus   Involuntary, rapid movements of the eyeball that may be horizontal, rotatory, vertical, or mixed.

TIME LINE   In children, pendular nystagmus may be idiopathic, or it may result from early-impaired vision associated with such disorders as optic atrophy, albinism, congenital cataracts, and severe astigmatism.

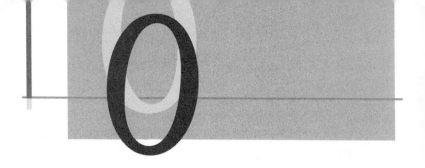

O Symbol for oxygen.

O₂ Symbol for molecular oxygen.

oat cell carcinoma A form of small cell cancer. The cells are shaped like oats, clump poorly, stain darkly, contain neurosecretory granules, and have little or no cytoplasm.

OB *abbr* 1. Obstetrics. 2. Obstetrician.

obesity A condition characterized by an excess of fat cells in the subcutaneous tissues of the body; weight is beyond physical requirements.

obligate To make necessary; only able to survive under special conditions. For example, an obligate parasite can survive only within a host organism.

oblique A diagonal direction; not horizontal or perpendicular; a 45-degree angle.

oblique bandage A bandage that is applied with spiral turns; it's usually used on an arm or leg.

oblique fissure of the lung 1. In the left lung: the groove marking the division between the upper and lower lobes. 2. In the right lung: the groove marking the division between the lower and middle lobes.

oblique fracture An angled or slanted break in a bone.

obliquus externus abdominis One of the thin, flat large muscles that form the outermost lateral walls of the abdomen.

obliquus internus abdominis One of the thin flat muscles, lying under the obliquus externus abdominis, that form the lateral wall of the abdomen.

obstetric anesthesia The anesthesia used for childbirth. Examples include a local anesthesia for episiotomy or episiotomy repair; paracervical block or pudendal block (regional anesthesia) for labor or delivery; and epidural, caudal, or saddle block (a wider block) for labor or delivery.

obstetric forceps Instrument designed to assist with the delivery of a fetus's head. The three parts of a forceps are the handle, shank, and blade.

obstetrician A physician who specializes in obstetrics, or pregnancy and childbirth.

obstetrics The branch of surgery involving pregnancy and childbirth. It includes care of the mother and fetus throughout pregnancy, childbirth, and the immediate postpartum period.

obstipation A condition of extreme constipation; usually caused by intestinal obstruction.

obstructive anuria A condition of almost total absence of urination; usually caused by urinary tract obstruction.

obtund 1. To dull or blunt. 2. To make less sensitive to pain or discomfort; to reduce the level of alertness, as by anesthesia.

obtundation The employment of an agent, such as preoperative general or local anesthesia, that clouds consciousness and reduces irritation or pain.

obturator A device or structure that closes or fills an opening. An example is a prosthesis used to close a cleft palate.

obturator externus A flat, triangular muscle on the external surface of the pelvic wall.

obturator foramen A large opening on the lower portion of the innominate bone. It's formed in the back by the ischium, on the top by the ilium, and in the front by the pubis.

obturator internus A muscle covering most of the lower portion of the lesser pelvis; it surrounds the obturator foramen.

obturator membrane A tough fibrous membrane covering the obturator foramen.

obturator muscle A muscle found in the pelvis and upper leg that helps the leg rotate outward.

occipital artery An external carotid artery that divides into six branches and supplies parts of the head and scalp.

occipital bone The bone in the lower back of the skull with an opening for the vertebral canal.

occipital lobe One of the five lobes of each cerebral hemisphere, located at the back of the cerebral hemisphere and shaped like a three-sided pyramid.

occipitofrontalis One of a pair of thin, broad muscles that cover the forehead.

occiput, *pl.* **occiputs, occipita** The back of the head. Also called *occiput cranii, occiput of cranium.*

occlusal Relating to the closing of an opening; relating to the surfaces of opposing teeth or masticating (biting) surface of molars.

occlusal trauma Progressive injury to a tooth and its supporting structures as the result of malocclusive, or abnormal, bite or poor biting habits.

occlusion The act of closing or closing off something; refers to bite or the relation between upper and lower teeth.

occlusion rim An artificial dental structure on which occluding surfaces are attached to temporary or permanent denture bases.

occlusive dressing A dressing that stops air or bacteria from contacting a wound or lesion.

occult Difficult to understand or see; hidden from view.

occult blood An amount of blood so small that it can be seen or detected only by a chemical test or microscopic examination.

occult carcinoma A minute carcinoma without obvious symptoms.

occult fracture A fracture that is initially undetectable by X-ray but is evident radiographically at a later time.

occupational asthma A respiratory condition caused by workplace exposure to allergenic or other irritating substances. Common workplace irritants include detergents, Western red cedar, cotton, flax, hemp, grain, flour, and stone.

occupational disability A condition that prevents a worker from performing a job; the condition is the result of a workplace disease or accident.

occupational disease A disease or condition caused by long-term workplace exposure to harmful substances or repetitive physical acts.

occupational lung disease Any one of several lung conditions resulting from inhaling dust, fumes, gases, or vapors while employed in a specific occupation.

occupational therapist A licensed, registered, or certified individual who evaluates the self-care, work, and play of disabled clients; the individual plans and implements restorative programs.

occupational therapy A therapy designed to promote recovery or rehabilitation in vocational skills and activities of daily life.

ochronosis A condition in which brown-black pigment is deposited in connective tissue and cartilage. Urine may darken on standing and blue macules may be seen on the sclera, fingers, ears, nose, genitalia, buccal mucosa, and axillae. The condition is often caused by phenol poisoning.

ocular Relating to the eye.

ocular hypertelorism An increase in the distance between two organs or body parts; for example, an extremely wide nose bridge and increased distance between the eyes.

ocular hypotelorism A decrease in distance between two organs or body parts; for example, an extremely narrow nose bridge and decreased distance between the eyes.

ocular myopathy A hereditary progressive weakness of ocular muscles of one or both eyes. Signs include decreased eye mobility and drooping of the upper lid. It can progress to complete paralysis of the muscles.

ocular spot An abnormal opacity in the eye. A shower of red and black dots may be seen in the eye after hemorrhage of a retinal vessel; opacities in the crystalline lens are characteristic in cataracts.

oculogyric crisis A condition in which the eyes become fixed in one position, usually upward, for minutes or hours. Usually seen in epidemic encephalitis or postencephalitic parkinsonism.

oculomotor nerve Cranial nerves originating in the brain stem that are essential for eye movements, supplying certain extrinsic and intrinsic eye muscles, including the pupil.

O.D. *abbr oculus dexter,* Latin for "right eye."

odontiasis The act of teething; cutting teeth.

odontitis The inflammation of a tooth.

odontogenic 1. Producing teeth. 2. Originating in tissues that form teeth.

odontogenic fibroma A rare, benign tumor of the jaw. Also called *central odontogenic fibroma.*

 ALERT Odontogenic fibroma occurs more frequently in women than in men.

odontogenic fibrosarcoma A malignant, or cancerous, tumor of the jaw that develops in a mesenchymal portion of a tooth or tooth germ.

odontogenic myxoma An uncommon, benign tumor of the jaw that develops in the mesenchyme of the tooth germ.

odontology Dentistry; the scientific study of teeth and of the structures of the mouth.

odynophagia An intense, squeezing pain when swallowing. It may be caused by a disorder of the esophagus or an irritation of the mucous membranes.

OH Symbol for hydroxyl.

ohm A unit of electrical resistance. One ohm is the electrical potential of 1 volt to produce a current of 1 ampere.

oil **1.** A greasy, combustible liquid that is insoluble in water and soluble in ether. Oils come from animal, vegetable, or mineral matter. **2.** A fat that is liquid at room temperature.

olecranon The projection of the ulna that forms the point of the elbow. When the forearm is fully extended, it fits into the olecranon fossa of the humerus.

olecranon bursa The bursa of the elbow.

olecranon fossa The hollow in the back of the humerus. The olecranon of the ulna fits into it when the forearm is extended.

oleic acid A colorless monounsaturated fatty acid found in almost all natural fats.

oleometer An instrument that measures the purity of oils.

olfactory Relating to the sense of smell.

olfactory center A group of neurons located near the junction of the temporal and parietal lobes that are responsible for detecting odors.

olfactory epithelium Organ of odor reception located in a small area of the nasal mucosa.

olfactory nerve One of two nerves involved with the sense of smell.

oligodactyly, oligodactylia A developmental anomaly in which one or more fingers or toes are missing.

oligodendroblastoma Tumor composed of young oligodendroglial cells. Also called oligodendro

oligodontia A genetic dental defect in which fewer than the normal number of teeth develop.

oligogenic Hereditary characteristics produced by a few genes.

oligohydramnios Presence of less than the normal amount of fluid.

oligomenorrhea Infrequent menstruation, usually occurring at intervals of more than 35 days to every 6 months.

 TIME LINE Teenage girls may experience oligomenorrhea associated with immune and hormonal function. However, prolonged oligomenorrhea, or the development of amenorrhea, may signal congenital adrenal hyperplasia or Turner's syndrome.

oligopepsia Lack of digestive tone.

oliguria A diminished flow of urine in relation to fluid intake, usually less than 400 ml in 24 hours. Also called *hypouresis.*

TIME LINE In elderly patients, oliguria may result from gradual progression of an underlying disorder; or from overall poor muscle tone secondary to inactivity, poor fluid intake, or infrequent attempts to void.

Ollier's dyschondroplasia An uncommon abnormal condition in which epiphyseal tissue spreads through the bones, causing irregular growth and deformity.

ombudsman A person who investigates complaints, reports findings, and helps to achieve equitable settlements.

omental bursa A peritoneal cavity located in back of the stomach, the lesser omentum, and the lower border of the liver and in front of the pancreas and duodenum. Also called *lesser peritoneal cavity.*

omentum, *pl.* **omenta** A fold in the peritoneum encompassing adjacent organs in the abdominal cavity.

omphalectomy Excision of the umbilicus or an attached tumor.

omphalocele A congenital condition in which part of the intestine protrudes through the abdominal wall near the naval. The protrusion is usually covered by a thin membrane.

omphalosite The underdeveloped of unequal conjoined twins. It's joined to the developed twin by umbilical cord vessels.

onchomycosis A disease of the nails in which they become opaque, white, thick, and brittle and crumble easily.

oncogenesis The production or beginning of a tumor or neoplasm.

oncogenic virus A virus able to cause a cancerous disease.

oncologist A physican who studies and treats tumors or neoplastic diseases, especially cancer.

oncology The study of tumors.

oncovirus A tumor-producing ribonucleic acid virus; associated with leukemia and sarcoma in animals.

Ondine's curse The loss of automatic control over breathing. Patients with the condition have a sensitivity to retained carbon dioxide.

one-and-a-half spica cast A cast used for immobilizing the trunk of the body for healing after surgical hip repair or for a fractured femur. Also used for correction and maintenance of correction of a hip deformity. It immobilizes the body from head to nipple line, one leg caudally to the toes, and the other leg caudally to the knee. For stability, a diagonal crossbar connects the parts of the cast encasing the legs.

ontogenetic, ontogenic   Acquired during the development of an individual organism.

ontogeny   Relating to the development of an individual organism from a single-celled ovum to birth.

onychia   Inflammation of the nail bed.

onycholysis   Distal nail separated from the bed.

oogamy   The fertilization of a large, non-motile, female gamete by a small, motile, male gamete, as seen in algae and the malarial parasite.

oogonium, *pl.* oogonia   Ovarian egg during fetal development; the primordial cell before it has developed completely.

ookinesis   The mitotic changes in the egg cell's nucleus as it matures and is fertilized.

oophorectomy   The surgical excision of an ovary. Oophorectomy is performed to remove an abcess, a cyst, or a tumor; to treat endometriosis; or to excise the source of estrogen in a patient with breast cancer.

oophoritis   The inflammation of an ovary; often occurs with salpingitis.

oophorocystectomy   Excision of an ovarian cyst.

oophoroplasty   Plastic repair of an ovary.

oophorosalpingectomy   The surgical removal of one or both ovaries and their oviducts, performed to excise an abcess, a cyst, or a tumor or to treat endometriosis.

oophorosalpingitis   Inflammation of an ovary and a fallopian tube.

oosperm   An ovum that has recently been fertilized; the resulting cell is a zygote.

ootid   A mature ovum at the end of the second meiotic division but before the fusion of the pronuclei to form the zygote.

opaque   Relating to a substance or surface that does not transmit or allow light to pass; not transparent or translucent.

open amputation   An amputation made with a straight, guillotine cut; there are no skin flaps. Also called *guillotine, flapless amputation.*

open-ended question   A question that requires an answer in sentence form, rather than a yes-or-no reply.

operating microscope   A special microscope used to perform delicate surgery, especially on the eye, ear, small blood vessels, or vocal cords.

operation   A surgical procedure performed with instruments or by a surgeon's hands.

operative cholangiography   In diagnostic radiology: a procedure done during surgery that outlines the major bile ducts; a

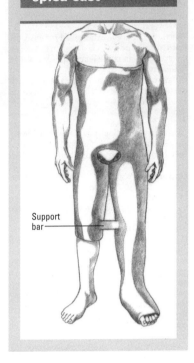

One-and-one-half spica cast

Support bar

radiopaque contrast material is injected directly into the ducts.

operator gene   In molecular genetics: a gene that is the starting point for reading genetic code. Also called *operator, operator locus.*

operculum, *pl.* opercula   A cover structure, such as the mucus plug over the cervix of the gravid uterus.

operon   In molecular biology: a portion of chromosome with an operator gene and one or more structural genes whose actions it controls.

ophthalmia   Severe inflammation of the eye, the conjunctiva, or deeper portions of the eye.

ophthalmic   Relating to the eye.

ophthalmitis   Inflammation of the deeper structures of the eye.

ophthalmologist   A physician who specializes in the medical care of the eye and its structures.

ophthalmology   The study of the physiology, anatomy, and pathology of the eye and the diagnosis and treatment of eye conditions.

ophthalmoplegia   Ocular paralysis.

ophthalmoscope   An instrument containing a light, a mirror with a single hole and several lenses for examining the interior structures of the eye. Also called *funduscope*.

ophthalmoscopy   The examination of the eye using an ophthalmoscope. Also called *funduscopy*.

opisthotonos   A severe muscle spasm causing the back to arch acutely, the head and heels to bend back, and the arms and hands to flex rigidly; the body is bowed forward.

Oppenheim's disease   An uncommon congenital disease in which the muscles are flabby and atonic, especially in the legs; deep reflexes are absent or very sluggish.

Oppenheim's reflex   A sign of pyramidal tract disease. The reflex is characterized by extension of the great toe and is elicited by stroking downward medial surface of the tibia.

opportunistic infection   1. An infection caused by an organism that does not ordinarily cause disease but that, under conditions of reduced immune resistance, will become pathogenic. Reduced immune response may be the result of such disorders as diabetes mellitus or cancer. 2. An unusual infection with a common pathogen, as cellulitis, meningitis, or otitis media.

opsonin   An antibody or complement split product that, on attaching to a foreign material, microorganism, or other antigen, enhances phagocytosis of that substance by leukocytes and other macrophages.

optic   Relating to the eyes or sight.

optic atrophy   Wasting of the optic disk caused by degeneration of nerve fibers in the optic nerve and optic tract.

optic disk   A small blind spot on the retina, located about 3 mm to the nasal side of the macula and insensitive to light; the retinal entrance of the optic nerve.

optician   An individual who fits, grinds, and dispenses prescription eyeglass lenses and contact lenses.

optic nerve   One of two cranial nerves made of coarse, myelinated fibers. They arise in the retinal ganglion, traverse the thalamus, and connect to the visual cortex.

optic neuritis   Inflammation of the optic nerve.

optics   1. In physiology: the study of vision and the functions of the eye; optics includes the relationship between the brain and the eye. 2. In physics: the study of electromagnetic radiation of wavelengths that are

shorter than radio waves but longer than X-rays.

optic stalk   One of two slender embryonic structures that become the optic nerve.

optometrist   One who tests the eyes for acuity, prescribes corrective lenses, and recommends eye exercises.

oral hygiene   The maintenance of teeth and other tissues and structures of the mouth. Oral hygiene includes brushing and flossing the teeth and cleaning dentures.

oral poliovirus vaccine (OPV)   An attenuated preparation of live poliovirus that confers immunity to poliomyelitis.

orbicularus ciliaris   One of the two zones of the ciliary body of the eye, extending from the ora serrata of the retina to the ciliary processes at the margin of the iris.

orbicularus oculi   The muscles of the eyelid that include the palpebral, orbital, and lacrimal muscles.

orbicularus oris   The muscle around the mouth; it includes fibers from other facial muscles, such as the buccinator, that are inserted into the lips, and fibers belonging to the lips.

orbital aperture   The opening in the skull to the eye orbit.

orbital fat   A semifluid layer of fat lining the bony eye orbit.

orbital pseudotumor   An inflammatory reaction, of unknown etiology, of the orbital tissues of the eye, characterized by protrusion of the eyeball (exophthalmos) and swelling (edematous congestion) of the eyelids.

orchiectomy   Excision of a testicle.

orchiopexy   Surgical intervention to bring an undescended testis into the scrotum, and to affix it so that it will not retract.

orchitis   Inflammation of the testes, usually caused by mumps, syphilis, or tuberculosis and characterized by swelling and pain.

orexigenic   Something that stimulates the appetite.

orf   A disease acquired from sheep that rarely occurs in humans. Symptoms include a painless vesicle, which may progress to a red, weeping nodule that crusts before healing.

organ   A part of the body that performs a specific function, such as the liver or kidney.

organelle, organella   1. Particles of living substance that include the nucleus, mitochondria, the lysosomes, and peroxisomes and centrioles. 2. Tiny organs of protozoa involved with locomotion, metabolism, and other processes.

organic   Any substance coming from living organisms; a chemical compound containing carbon.

organic chemistry A branch of chemistry dealing with the composition, properties, and reactions of chemical compounds that contain carbon.

organic dust Wind-borne, dried particles of plants, animals, fungi, or bacteria that may cause noninfectious respiratory disorders when inhaled.

organic evolution A theory about the origin and perpetuation of species that proposes that all forms of animal and plant life are descended from simpler forms, such as a single cell.

organism An individual living thing, animal or plant. It can be unicellular or multicellular and is able to carry on life functions.

organogenesis In embryology: the orgin and development of organs and organ systems during embryonic development.

orientation In molecular genetics: the insertion of a fragment of genetic material into a vector so that the placement of the fragment is in the same direction as the genetic map of the vector (the n orientation) or in the opposite direction (the u orientation).

orifice The opening or the outlet of any body cavity. Also called *ostium, orificium.*

ornithine carbamoyltransferase Liver enzyme that becomes elevated in liver disease.

oropharynx A division of the pharynx. It extends from the soft palate to the hyoid bone and contains the palatine tonsils and the lingual tonsils.

orthodontics The branch of dentistry concerned with the correction of malocclusion and dentofacial structures. Also called *dentofacial orthopedics.*

orthodromic conduction Relating to the conduction of nerve impulses in the normal direction.

orthogenesis The theory that evolution proceeds in a given direction and is fixed; evolution does not move in several directions as a result of natural selection and other environmental factors.

orthomyxovirus An influenza virus that belongs to the family Orthomyxoviridae.

orthopantogram An X-ray of the mouth showing a panoramic view of the alveolar bone, the complete dentition, and other contiguous structures.

orthopedic nurse A nurse whose main professional practice is in orthopedic (skeletal system) nursing.

orthopedics The study and treatment of the skeletal system, its joints, muscles, and associated structures.

orthopedic traction A procedure in which a pulling force is exerted on a body

part by means of ropes and pulleys attached to weights; countertraction is maintained.

orthoptic examination An ophthalmoscopic examination of the binocular function of the eyes. A stereoscopic instrument presents a slightly different picture to each eye. The examiner notes the degree to which the pictures are combined by the normal process of fusion.

orthosis An orthopedic apparatus used to support, align, prevent, or correct bone deformities; generally involves the use of braces or splints.

orthostatic hypotension Abnormally low blood pressure that occurs when a person stands up. Also called *postural hypotension.*

ALERT If you detect orthostatic hypotension, quickly check for tachycardia, altered level of consciousness, and pale, clammy skin; these signs suggest hypovolemic shock.

orthostatic proteinuria The presence of protein in the urine of an individual who is standing; the protein disappears when the individual lies down. The condition has no pathologic significance.

orthotonos A posture that is straight and rigid because of a tetanic spasm; commonly caused by a tetanus infection or strychnine poisoning.

Ortolani's test A test to evaluate the stability of a newborn's or infant's hip joints.

O.S. *abbr oculus sinister,* Latin for "left eye."

Os Symbol for osmium.

Osgood-Schlatter disease Inflammation or partial separation of the tibial tubercle; usually caused by chronic irritation from overuse of the quadriceps muscle. Also called *apophysitis tibialis adolescentium.*

Osler's nodes Raised, tender spots about the size of a pea that may be blue, red, or pink; found on the pads of the fingers or toes.

 CLINICAL TIP Osler's nodes are usually seen in subacute bacterial endocarditis and last 1 to 2 days.

osmium (Os) A hard, gray, pungent-smelling, toxic, metallic element. Its atomic number is 76; atomic weight, 190.2. It cannot be fused.

osmodysphoria Abnormal dislike of certain odors.

osmol, osmole The quantity of a substance in solution that forms one mole of active particles (an ideal nonelectrolyte); usually expressed in grams.

osmolality The concentration or osmotic pressure of a solution; expressed in osmols of solute per kilogram of solvent.

Osmosis

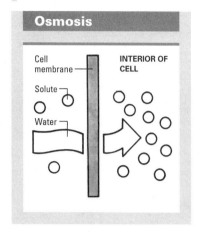

Cell membrane

INTERIOR OF CELL

Solute

Water

osmolar　Relating to the concentration of active particles in a solution; relating to the osmotic characteristics of a solution, expressed in osmols or milliosmols.

osmolarity　The osmotic pressure of a solution expressed in osmols or milliosmols per liter of the solution.

osmometry　The study of osmosis and the measurement of osmotic forces.

osmoreceptors　Special sensing cells in the hypothalamus that respond to changes in the blood's osmolality.

osmosis　The movement of a solvent such as water from a solution of lesser solute concentration to one of higher concentration through a semipermeable membrane that is permeable to the solvent, but not the solute. The rate of osmosis depends on the concentration, electrical charge, and temperature of the solute as well as the difference between the osmotic pressures of the solutions. Movement stops when the solute concentrations are equal.

osmotic diuresis　Increased passage of urine because of the presence of nonabsorbable or poorly absorbable substances, such as glucose, mannitol, or urea, in renal tubules.

osmotic fragility　The susceptibility of red blood cells to change in osmotic pressure. For example: When exposed to a strong (hypertonic) concentration of sodium in a solution, red cells give up their fluid, shrink, and break up. When exposed to a weak (hypotonic) concentration of sodium in a solution, red cells increase their intake of water, swell until the cell membrane's capacity is exceeded, then burst.

osmotic pressure　The pressure exerted on a semipermeable membrane separating solutions of different concentrations. Pressure varies with the concentration of the solution and with temperature.

osseous cell　Bone cell.

osseous labyrinth　The internal ear's bony portion, which has three cavities: cochlea, semicircular canal, and vestibule. It's responsible for transmitting sound vibrations from the middle ear to the acoustic nerve.

ossification　The development or formation of bone.

ossifying fibroma　A slow-growing, benign bone tumor that occurs mostly in the jaws, especially the mandible. It's composed of fibrous connective tissue.

ostearthrotomy　Excision of the articular end of a bone.

ostectomy　Excision of all or part of a bone.

osteitis　An inflammation of bone caused by infection, degeneration, or trauma and marked by tenderness and dull, aching pain.

osteitis fibrosa cystica　A degenerative bone condition in which normal tissue is replaced by cysts and fibrous tissue. It's usually associated with hyperparathyroidism. Also called *von Recklinghausen's disease.*

osteoanagenesis, osteanagenesis　The regeneration or development of bone.

osteoarthritis　A common form of arthritis, characterized by degenerative changes in one or many joints. Osteoarthritis includes loss of articular cartilage, proliferation of bone and cartilage in the joint, and subchondral bony sclerosis. It's characterized by pain and stiffness. Also called *degenerative arthritis, hypertrophic arthritis, degenerative joint disease.*

TIME LINE　Primary osteoarthritis is strongly associated with aging, and indeed, the aging process may predispose a person to the cartilage degeneration common in osteoarthritis.

osteoblast　A cell that is associated with bone production and that originates in the embryonic mesenchyme during the early development of the skeleton.

osteoblastoma　A benign, painful, fairly vascular bone tumor of fibrous tissue. It's found most commonly in the vertebra, femur, tibia, or upper extremity bones in children and young adults.

osteochondroma　A benign tumor consisting of bone and cartilage. Also called *chondrosteoma.*

osteochondrosis　A disease in children that affects the ossification centers. It may initially be characterized by degeneration and necrosis, followed by regeneration and recalcification. Also called *epiphyseal ischemic necrosis.*

osteoclasia   The absorption and destruction of bony tissue by osteoclasts.

osteoclasis   The surgical fracture or refracture of a bone to correct a deformity.

osteoclast   **1.** A large multinuclear bone cell that responds to parathyroid hormone and functions in the breakdown and absorption of bone. **2.** An instrument used in osteoclasis.

osteoclastic   **1.** Relating to osteoclasts. **2.** Something that destroys bone.

osteoclastoma   A giant cell bone tumor found most commonly at the end of a long bone. It usually appears as a mass surrounded by a thin shell of new bone.

osteocyte   A mature osteoblast embedded in bone matrix. It occupies a flat oval cavity and sends out protoplasmic projections that anastomose with those of other osteoblasts to create other small canals within the bone matrix.

osteodynia   Pain in a bone.

osteodystrophy   A defect in bone development. If associated with chronic kidney disease, it's called renal osteodystrophy and may result in dwarfism.

osteogenic, osteogenous   Derived from any structure involved in the development, growth, or repair of bone.

osteoid   Resembling a bone.

osteology   The study of bone.

osteolysis   The degeneration of bone from the loss of calcium; can result from disease, infection, or ischemia.

osteomalacia   Delayed or poor mineralization of bone; the adult equivalent of rickets.

 CLINICAL TIP Osteomalacia is associated with anorexia, fracture, pain, weakness, and weight loss.

osteomyelitis   Inflammation of bone that results from a local or general infection of bone and bone marrow. The bacterial infection is caused by trauma or surgery or by direct extension from a nearby infection, or can be introduced via the bloodstream.

osteon   The basic structural unit of compact bone that includes the haversian canal and its concentric rings of 4 to 20 lamellae, each 3 to 7 microns thick. The units are found along the long axis of bone.

osteopath, osteopathist   A physician of osteopathy.

osteopathy   A therapeutic approach to medicine that generally uses accepted forms of medical therapy and diagnosis, but that places greater emphasis on environmental conditions and adequate nutrition as well as the relationship of organs and the musculoskeletal system than is done in medicine.

osteopetrosis   A rare, inherited disease in which bone is abnormally dense, probably caused by faulty bone resorption from a deficiency of osteoclasts. The disease is most severe when it occurs in utero, infancy, or childhood. Fractures are common. Also called *ivory bones, marble bones.*

osteopoikilosis   An inherited condition (autosomal dominant trait) of the bones in which multiple areas of dense calcification appear throughout the osseous tissue, producing a mottled appearance. Can be diagnosed by X-ray examination and rarely produces symptoms.

osteoporosis   A disorder in which bone mass is reduced and fractures occur after minimal trauma. It occurs most commonly in postmenopausal women, in sedentary or immobilized individuals, and in persons on long-term steroid or heparin therapy.

osteorrhaphy   Suturing or wiring of a bone.

osteosarcoma   A primary, malignant bone tumor made up of anaplastic cells derived from mesenchyme. Also called *osteogenic sarcoma.*

osteosclerosis   Abnormally dense bone tissue. The condition is often associated with chronic infection, ischemia, and tumor formation and may result from faulty bone resorption involving the osteoclasts.

osteotomy   Cutting of a bone.

ostium primium   Opening in the lower portion of the membrane that divides the embryonic heart into right and left sides.

ostomate   An individual who has a surgically created ostomy.

ostomy   A term for a surgical procedure in which an artificial opening is created in a hollow organ. An ostomy is usually made in the bladder or intestines and allows for the passage of urine or intestinal contents through the abdominal wall. See illustration on page 220.

ostomy irrigation   The process of cleaning, stimulating, and regulating evacuation of an ostomy.

OTC   *abbr* over-the-counter, describing a drug available without a prescription.

otitis   Inflammation or infection of the ear. Kinds of otitis are otitis externa and otitis media. Otitis may be marked by pain, fever, poor hearing, tinnitus, and vertigo.

otitis externa   Inflammation or infection of the external auditory canal or auricle. Causes include allergy, bacteria, fungi, viruses, and trauma.

Permanent colostomy

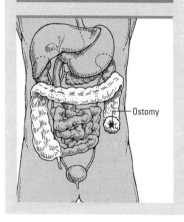

Ostomy

otitis media Inflammation or infection of the middle ear; tympanitis; a common affliction of childhood.

otocephaly A congenital malformation in which the lower jaw is missing, the mouth is defective, and the ears are united below the face.

otolith-righting reflex An involuntary tilting of the body in newborns that, when the infant is erect, causes the head to return to the upright position.

otoplasty Reconstructive plastic surgery that corrects ear deformities.

otorrhea A discharge from the ear. Otorrhea may be serous, sanguineous, or purulent if the external or middle ear is infected.

otosclerosis An inherited disorder characterized by irregular ossification, or formation of spongy bone, in the bony labyrinth of the inner ear, especially of the stapes. The disorder may cause tinnitus, hearing loss, and eventually deafness.

otoscope A device for examining the ear, including the external ear, eardrum, and ossicles (small bones in the middle ear). The instrument includes a device for insufflation, a light, and a magnifying lens.

ototoxic Something that is toxic, or harmful, to the eighth cranial nerve or the organs of balance and hearing.

ounce (oz) A measure of weight equal to $1/16$ of a pound in the avoirdupois system.

outcomes management A process of systematically tracking a patient's clinical treatment and responses. The system encourages caregivers to follow set guidelines (practice guidelines or critical paths) that research has shown to be the "one best way" to treat a specific medical condition.

outlet contracture An abnormally small pelvic outlet. It may be anteroposterior or transverse and, if small enough, may impede or prevent fetal passage through the birth canal during childbirth.

ovarian Relating to the ovary.

ovarian artery A thin branch of the abdominal aorta, arising caudal to the renal arteries, and supplying an ovary.

ovarian cancer A malignant tumor of the ovary that occurs infrequently in young adolescents and most commonly in women between ages 40 and 60.

ovarian cyst A sac that develops in or on an ovary. The cyst may be filled with fluid or semisolid material; it may be transient and physiologic or pathologic.

ovarian varicocele A varicose condition of the veins, or swelling, of the uterine broad ligament.

ovarian vein One of two veins (a left and a right) that emerge from plexuses of the broad ligament near the ovaries and the uterine tubes and drain into the vena cava.

ovariocentesis Puncture of an ovarian cyst or of an ovary.

ovariotomy Incision of an ovary, usually for biopsy.

ovary One of two female gonads located in the lower abdomen, next to the uterus, in a fold of the broad ligament.

overload 1. A burden beyond the capacity that a system was designed to handle. 2. In physiology: a factor that overstresses the body's abilities and that damages its health.

overoxygenation A condition in which the body's tissues, including blood, have more oxygen and less carbon dioxide than normal.

oviferous Able to produce ova.

oviparous Producing eggs that are hatched outside the body.

ovipositor An organ by which female insects deposit eggs on plants or in the soil.

ovomucin A glycoprotein coming from egg white.

ovomucoid Relating to a glycoprotein, similar to mucin, derived from egg white.

ovoviviparous Producing eggs that hatch within the body, as some fishes and reptiles.

ovulation Discharge of an ovum from the ovary upon rupture of a mature follicle. Discharge takes place as a result of cyclic ovarian and pituitary endocrine function and generally occurs on the 14th day after the 1st day of the last menstrual period. It may cause brief lower abdominal discomfort on the side of the ovulating ovary.

ovum, *pl.* **ova** **1.** An egg. **2.** A female germ cell expelled from the ovary during ovulation.

oxidation In chemistry: **1.** A process characterized by an increase in oxygen. **2.** A reaction whereby the positive valence of a compound or a radical increases through the loss of electrons.

oxidize To combine with oxygen, to remove hydrogen, or to lose electrons.

oxidizing agent A compound that gives up oxygen and attracts hydrogen. In chemical reactions, it accepts electrons and therefore increases the element's valence.

oxycephaly, oxycephalia A malformation characterized by a pointed or conical head shape. It's caused by premature closure of the coronal and sagittal sutures; a condition that results in accelerated upward growth of the head.

oxygen (O) A tasteless, odorless, colorless gas; its atomic number is 8; atomic weight, 15.999. Oxygen constitutes 20% of the atmospheric air and is essential for human and plant respiration. In respiratory therapy, oxygen is given to decrease the quantity of other circulating gases and increase the quantity of oxygen in the blood. In anesthesia, oxygen is a carrier gas for the anesthetic agents.

oxygen mask An instrument for administering oxygen. It fits snugly over the nose and mouth and may be held in place with the hand or secured with a strap. Oxygen flows at a prescribed rate and is humidified; inspiratory valves allow for inhalation while expiratory valves allow for exhalation.

oxygen tension The force with which oxygen molecules physically dissolved in blood are constantly trying to escape; expressed as partial pressure (Po_2).

oxygen therapy A procedure for relieving oxygen deficiency. Among the conditions for which it's administered are pulmonary edema, heart failure, and coronary thrombosis.

oxygen transport The process of absorbing oxygen from the lungs into hemoglobin and carrying it to peripheral tissues.

oxyhemoglobin Hemoglobin that contains oxygen. It's found in arterial blood and dissociates easily when there is a low concentration of oxygen.

oxyopia, oxyopy Acute vision; vision better than 20/20.

ozena Atrophic rhinitis with thick discharge and atrophy of the nasal chonchae and mucous membranes.

ozone (O_3) A form of oxygen that is a bluish, explosive gas; it's irritating and toxic to the pulmonary system and is characterized by molecules with three atoms. It forms when oxygen is electrically charged, as might happen during a lightning storm.

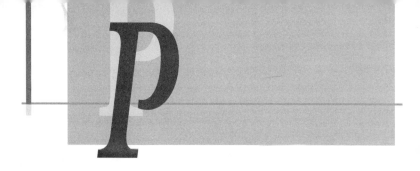

P 1. Symbol for gas partial pressure. See also *partial pressure.* 2. Symbol for phosphorus. 3. *abbr* position, posterior, postpartum, probability (in statistics), pulse, pupil.

P₁ In genetics: symbol for parental generation.

PA *abbr* physician's assistant.

PABA *abbr* para-aminobenzoic acid.

pabulum A food: a suspension of nutrients for easy absorption.

pacemaker 1. The natural rate at which something occurs. 2. A natural or artificial cardiac pacemaker; a device used for maintaining a normal sinus rhythm of the heart by electrically stimulating the heart muscle.

pachydactyly An abnormal thickening, or enlargement, of the fingers or the toes.

pachymeter A device for measuring the thickness of something thin such as a membrane.

pachynema A postsynaptic stage of mitosis, or cell division, in which the paired chromosomes contract as they become intertwined and spiral. At this stage the chromosomes are thicker than they were previously.

pachytene The third stage in meiotic prophase of gametogenesis. The paired chromosomes form tetrads, and the bivalent pairs become short, thick, and intertwined. Four chromatids are visible.

Pacini's corpuscles Special sensory organs that look like miniature white bulbs. The corpuscles are attached to nerve fibers in the subcutaneous, submucous, and subserous tissues of the body. They can be found in the palms of the hands, soles of the feet, genital organs, and joints.

packed cells The red blood cells that are left after plasma have been removed from whole blood. They may be given in blood transfusions administered to treat severe anemia.

 CLINICAL TIP Packed cells are administered to restore hemoglobin and red blood cells without taxing the vascular system with fluids.

packing 1. The act of filling a cavity or wound with absorbent material, such as a gauze, sponge, or pad. 2. The material used for packing a cavity or wound.

PAF *abbr* platelet-activating factor.

Paget's disease A common bone disease that usually affects middle-aged and elderly people. It's marked by inflammation of the bones, softening and thickening of the bones, excessive bone destruction, and unorganized bone repair; the result is bowing of the long bones; the cause is unknown.

pain receptor A free nerve ending that warns the body of possible harmful changes in the environment, such as extreme heat or cold; these endings are found throughout the body.

pain threshold The point at which a stimulus activates pain receptors. Persons with high thresholds experience pain much later than persons with low thresholds.

palatal 1. Relating to the roof of the mouth, or palate. 2. Relating to the lingual surface of a maxillary tooth.

palate The structure that separates the oral and nasal cavities and forms the roof of the mouth. The palate is divided into the soft (or fleshy) palate at the back of the mouth and the hard (or rigid) palate at the front of the mouth.

palatine Relating to the palate.

palatine arch The vault-shaped muscular structure that forms the soft palate and is located between the mouth and nasopharynx. An opening in it connects the mouth with the oropharynx; the uvula is suspended from the middle of the back edge of the arch.

palatine bone One of two bones of the skull that form the back of the hard palate, a portion of the nasal cavity, and the bottom of the eye orbit. The bone looks like a capital *L* and has three processes and horizontal and vertical parts.

palatine ridge One of the ridges on the front surface of the hard palate; there are four to six ridges all together.

palatine tonsil One of two small masses of lymphoid tissue located between the palatopharyngeal and palatoglossal arches on either side of the fauces.

paleogenetic A trait that is not newly acquired; a trait that originated in the past generation.

palindrome In molecular genetics: a segment of deoxyribonucleic acid or ribonucleic acid in which identical sequences run in both directions.

palliate To soothe or relieve the severity of something.

pallor A decrease, absence lack of color in the skin; pale, wane.

ALERT If generalized pallor suddenly develops, quickly look for signs of shock, such as tachycardia, hypotension, oliguria, and decreased level of consciousness. Keep emergency resuscitation equipment nearby.

palm The lower side, hollow or flexor surface, of the hand, between the wrist and the bases of the fingers.

palmar aponeurosis Ribbon-like fibrous tissue that runs from the tendon in the palm to the bases of the fingers. Also called *volar fascia*.

palmar crease One of several grooves that run across the palm of the hand to accommodate the hand's flexibility.

palmaris longus A long, slender, fusiform muscle in the forearm; It's located on the medial side of the flexor carpi radialis.

palmar metacarpal artery One of numerous arteries supplying the fingers; it originates in the deep palmar arch.

palmar reflex A grasping reflex seen in infants; the fingers curl when the palm of the hand is tickled. The reflex disappears at age 4 to 5 months.

palmature An abnormal condition marked by webbed fingers.

palmomental reflex A twitching of the chin elicited by scratching the palm of the hand. The reflex is an abnormal neurologic sign.

palpation The act of examining the body by applying slight pressure with the hands. The purpose is to feel the texture, size, and consistency of structures below the surface.

palpatory percussion The act of examining the body by applying percussion and light pressure. The vibrations produced by the percussion are evaluated by the examiner.

palpebral fissure The opening between the upper and lower eyelids.

palpebrate **1.** To wink or blink. **2.** Possessing eyelids.

palpitate To pulsate, or beat, rapidly. For example, the heart may beat unduly rapidly under conditions of stress, and some persons with heart problems may experience a racing heartbeat.

Palate

Hard palate — Soft palate

palpitation A pounding, rapid, or irregular heartbeat, usually associated with normal emotional responses or with some heart disorders.

ALERT If the patient complains of palpitations, ask him about dizziness and shortness of breath; inspect for pale, cool, clammy skin. Take the patient's vital signs noting hypotension and irregular or abnormal pulse. If these signs are present, suspect cardiac arrhythmia.

PAMP *abbr* pulmonary arterial mean pressure.

pampiniform Shaped like a tendril.

panacea **1.** A universal remedy. **2.** An old name for a healing herb or its liquid potion.

panacinar emphysema An obstructive emphysema that affects all lung areas. This form of the disease is characterized by dilation and atrophy of the alveoli and destruction of the lung's vascular bed.

panarthritis Inflammation of all the body joints or parts of a pancake kidney. A congenital condition in which the kidneys are fused together into one pelvic mass.

pancarditis An inflammation of the heart, including the endocardium, myocardium, and pericardium.

Pancoast's syndrome Several signs, including neuritic arm pain and atrophy of arm and hand muscles, that are associated with a tumor involving the brachial plexus in the apex of the lung.

pancreas   An elongated gland of three parts (a head, body, and tail) that stretches transversely behind the stomach between the spleen and the duodenum and secretes various substances, such as digestive enzymes, insulin, and glucagon.

pancreatectomy   A surgical procedure to remove the pancreas, or part of it, because of a tumor, cyst, pancreatitis, or trauma.

pancreatic cancer   A cancerous disease of the pancreas. Signs and symptoms include abdominal mass, anorexia, back pain, recent onset of diabetes, epigastric pain, flatulence, jaundice, pruritus, weakness, and weight loss; stools may be clay-colored if the pancreatic ducts are obstructed.

pancreatic diverticulum   One of two membranous pouches, deriving from the embryonic duodenum, that later form the pancreas and its ducts.

pancreatic duct   The primary duct of the pancreas that delivers pancreatic juice to the duodenum. Also called *duct of Wirsung.*

pancreatic enzyme   One of several enzymes secreted by the pancreas and needed for digestion of food. The most important enzymes are trypsin, chymotrypsin, steapsin, and amylopsin.

pancreatic hormone   One of several chemical compounds secreted by the pancreas and needed for proper cellular metabolism. Important pancreatic hormones include glucagon, insulin, and pancreatic polypeptide.

pancreaticoduodenal artery   The two arteries that distribute blood to the pancreas and duodenum.

pancreaticogastrostomy   Surgical procedure in which the pancreatic duct and the stomach are anastomosed.

pancreaticojejunostomy   Surgical procedure in which the pancreatic duct and the jejunum are anastomosed.

pancreatin   A mixture of pancreatic enzymes (mainly amylase, lipase, and protease), used to aid digestion.

pancreatitis   Inflammation, either acute or chronic, of the pancreas.

pancreatoduodenectomy   Surgical removal of the head of the pancreas and the loop of duodenum.

pancreatography   Visualization of the pancreas during surgery; a water-soluble contrast media is injected into the pancreatic ducts for viewing via X-rays while the abdomen is open. Viewing may also be via an endoscope or ultrasonography, computerized tomography, or radionuclide imaging.

pancreatolith   A pancreatic stone or calculus.

pancrelipase   A standardized preparation containing enzymes that is used as an aid to digestion when the pancreas is deficient.

pancytopenia   A deficiency of all cellular elements of the blood: red blood cells, white blood cells, and platelets.

pandemic   A widely spread epidemic occurring throughout a region, a country, or the world.

pandiastolic   Relating to complete diastole.

panencephalitis   Inflammation of both the gray and white matter of the brain. Usually caused by a virus, the onset of panencephalitis is insidious and the course, progressive with deterioration of mental and motor functions.

pangenesis   Darwin's theory that every particle of a parent reproduces itself in progeny.

panhypopituitarism   Low levels of pituitary hormones caused by deficiency of or damage to the pituitary gland.

panhysterectomy   Surgical removal of the cervix, fallopian tubes, ovaries, and uterus.

panniculus, *pl.* panniculi   A layer or sheet of membrane or tissue.

pannus   Minor vascularization of the eye's cornea; a thin layer of tissue overlaying the synovial cells inside a joint, usually seen in persons with inflammatory arthritis.

panophthalmitis   An inflammation all the structure of the eye; generally virulent pyogenic organisms, such as strains of meningococci, pneumococci, streptococci, anthrax bacilli, and clostridia.

panphobic melancholia   An unexplained fear of everything, an irrational dread; usually seen in persons with depression.

panthenol   An alcohol converted in the body to pantothenic acid, which is one of the B-complex vitamins. Also called *pantothenol, pantothenyl alcohol.*

Pao₂   Symbol for partial pressure of arterial oxygen.

Papanicolaou test   A common test that examines stained exfoliative cells; usually used to detect cancer of the cervix, but it may be used for tissue specimens from any organ. A smear of the cervix is obtained during a pelvic examination.

paper chromatography   The analysis of a substance by dissolving it in a solvent and filtering it through a strip of special paper.

papilla, *pl.* papillae   A small nipple-shaped elevation or projection. Examples of papilla include the conoid papillae of the tongue, the papillae of the corium, and the capillary blood vessels.

papilla of Vater   The duodenal end of the pancreatic and common bile duct drainage systems.

papillary   Relating to a papilla.

papillary adenocarcinoma   A malignant neoplasm characterized by small papillae of vascular connective tissue covered by neoplastic epithelium that projects into follicles, glands, or cysts.

papillary adenoma   A benign epithelial tumor characterized by papillary projections that grow into the alveoli or out of a cavity surface.

papillary carcinoma   A malignant neoplasm with numerous fingerlike projections; the most common thyroid tumor.

papillary duct   One of thousands of straight collecting renal tubules that descend through the medulla of the kidney and join with others to form the common ducts opening into the renal papillae.

papillary muscle   One of the muscular projections of the chordae tendineae in the ventricles of the heart.

papilledema   Inflammation and edema of the optic nerve; associated with increased intracranial pressure.

papillitis   The inflammation of a papilla, such as a lacrimal papilla or a renal papilla.

papilloma   A benign tumor that produces fingerlike projections from the epithelium. Also called *papillary tumor.*

papillomatosis   The abnormal development of many nipplelike or fingerlike growths.

papillomavirus   A virus that belongs to the papovavirus family and causes warts in humans and other animals. There are at least 58 viruses that produce warts in humans.

papovavirus   One of a group of deoxyribonucleic acid viruses, some of which may cause cancer in humans, originally isolated from the African green monkey.

Pap smear   *Informal.* A specimen of exfoliated genital epithelial cells and cervical mucus collected during a pelvic examination. Evaluation according to the Papanicolaou cytological classification is useful in detecting and diagnosing cancer of the vagina, cervix, and endometrium and also the human papillomavirus.

papulation   The production or development of papules.

papule   A small, solid, raised superficial skin lesion less than ³/₈″ (1 cm) in diameter.

PAR   *abbr* pulmonary arteriolar resistance.

para-aminobenzoic acid (PABA)   A crystalline substance used as a dietary supplement and a topical sunscreen.

para-aminosalicylic acid (PAS, PASA)   An antituberculosis drug.

paracentesis   Surgical puncture of a cavity for fluid aspiration.

paracervical block   Anesthesia of the plexus of nerves and ganglia in the uterine cervix produced by local injections of anesthetic into the area on each side of the uterine cervix.

paradidymis, *pl.* **paradidymides**   A structure composed of a few convoluted tubules situated on the spermatic cord of the epididymis in the male. Considered to be the vestigial remains of the caudal part of the embryonic mesonephric tubules.

paraffin bath   The application of heat to a specific area of the body through the use of heated liquid wax. It's an effective technique for heating traumatized or inflamed areas, especially the hands, feet, and wrists, and is used primarily for patients with joint conditions, such as arthritis and rheumatism.

paraganglion, *pl.* **paraganglia**   A collection of chromaffin cells situated outside the adrenal medulla, usually near the sympathetic ganglia along the aorta and its branches. Most paraganglia secrete epinephrine.

parageusia   Abnormal or perverted sense of taste.

paragonimiasis   Chronic infection with any of several flukes of the genus *Paragonimus.* Infestation with the lung fluke, *Paragonimus westermani*, occurs most commonly in Asia.

paragraphia   Disorder in which one word is written in place of another.

parainfluenza virus   A myxovirus with four serotypes that causes upper respiratory tract diseases of varying severity in infants and young children and, less commonly, in adults and animals.

paralysis, *pl.* **paralyses**   An abnormal condition characterized by the loss or impairment of motor function or the impairment of sensory function.

 ALERT If paralysis develops suddenly, suspect trauma or an acute vascular insult. After proper immobilization of the patient's spine, quickly determine level of consciousness and take vital signs. Elevated systolic blood pressure, widening pulse pressure, and bradycardia may signal increasing intracranial pressure.

paralytic ileus   A decrease in or absence of bowel motility that may occur following abdominal surgery or may be caused by numerous other conditions, most commonly by peritonitis.

paramesonephric duct   One of a pair of embryonic ducts that develops into the uterine tubes and the uterus in females and into a vestigial structure in males.

parameter A variable used to describe or measure a set of data representing a physiologic function or system that cannot itself be precisely determined by direct methods, as in the use of acid-base relationships of the blood as parameters for evaluating the function of a patient's respiratory system.

parametritis An inflammation of the tissue of the structures around the uterus.

paramyxovirus One of a genus of viruses that primarily cause respiratory infections in a number of vertebrate hosts. It includes viruses that cause parainfluenza, measles, mumps, and respiratory diseases in reptiles and birds.

paranasal Situated near or alongside the nasal cavity — for example, the paranasal sinuses.

paranasal sinuses The mucosa-lined air cavities in various cranial bones around the nose. They include the ethmoidal, frontal, maxillary, and sphenoidal sinuses, all of which communicate with the nasal cavity.

parapertussis An acute respiratory disease caused by the bacteria *Bordetella parapertussis.* The symptoms closely resemble those of pertussis but are usually milder.

paraphimosis A condition characterized by a retraction of the foreskin that causes a painful swelling of the glans penis. If the condition is severe and not treated it may result in dry gangrene.

paraplegia An abnormal condition characterized by the loss of sensation and motor function in the lower limbs, which may result in either complete or incomplete paralysis.

parapsoriasis A group of slowly evolving chronic skin diseases characterized by raised, red scaly eruptions which are commonly resistant to treatment.

paraquat poisoning A toxic condition resulting from ingesting paraquat dichloride, a highly poisonous contact herbicide. It's characterized by damage to the esophagus, and may result in kidney and liver failure several days after ingestion followed by progressive pulmonary insufficiency.

parasite A plant or animal living in or on and deriving nourishment from another organism. A facultative parasite may live on a host but is capable of independent existence.

parasitemia The presence of parasites, especially malarial parasites, in the blood.

parasitic fibroma A benign fibroid tumor of the uterus deriving part of its blood supply from the omentum.

parasitic thrombus An accumulation of the bodies and spores of malarial parasites formed in the capillaries of the brain causing a condition known as cerebral malaria.

parasympathetic Of or referring to the craniosacral division of the autonomic nervous system, consisting of the ocular, bulbar, and sacral divisions.

parasympathomimetic 1. Of or referring to a substance producing effects resembling those caused by stimulation of a parasympathetic nerve. 2. An agent that produces effects that mimic those produced by stimulation of parasympathetic nerves, especially the effects produced by acetylcholine.

parasystole A cardiac irregularity caused by the presence of two foci that independently initiate cardiac impulses at different rates. The two foci are usually the sinoatrial node, which is the normal pacemaker, and the ectopic focus usually found in the ventricle.

parathion poisoning A toxic condition caused by accidental inhalation or ingestion of the highly poisonous organophosphorus agricultural insecticide parathion. Can also be contracted by absorption through the skin or ingestion of contaminated food.

parathyroid gland One of several small bodies, usually four in number, attached to the posterior surface of the thyroid gland. Their main function is the secretion of parathyroid hormone, a major regulator of calcium and phosphorous metabolism.

parathyroid hormone (PTH) A hormone secreted by the parathyroid glands that controls the release of calcium from bones to the extracellular fluid, promotes renal reabsorption of calcium and increased renal excretion of phosphates, and indirectly promotes increased intestinal absorption of calcium. The maintenance of a constant concentration of calcium in the blood ensures normal neuromuscular irritability, blood clotting, and cell membrane permeability.

paratrooper fracture A fracture of the distal tibia, the internal or external malleolus, or both; results from subjecting the ankles to extreme force such as occurs when landing feet first following a jump from an elevated platform or parachuting from an airplane.

paratyphoid fever A bacterial infection, caused by any *Salmonella* species other than *Salmonella typhi,* characterized by symptoms similar to typhoid fever but usually less severe.

parenchyma The functional tissue of an organ as distinguished from its connective tissue or supporting framework.

parental generation (P$_1$) The initial generation with which a genetic study is begun; the parents of any individual, organism, or plant belonging to an F$_1$ generation.

parenteral   Not in or through the digestive system, but rather by injection through some other route such as subcutaneously, intravenously, intramuscularly, or intradermally.

parenteral absorption   The absorption of substances by body structures other than through the digestive tract.

parenteral nutrition   The I.V. administration of nutrients. Parenteral fluids usually consist of physiologic saline with amino acids, electrolytes, glucose, vitamins, and medications.

paresis   **1.** Slight or incomplete paralysis. **2.** A manifestation of neurosyphilis, characterized by progressive dementia resulting from degeneration of cortical neurons and generalized paralysis; generally occurs 10 to 20 years after initial syphilis infection.

paresthesia   Abnormal or heightened touch sensations, such as burning, numbness, prickling and tingling, that commonly occur without external stimulus.

parietal   **1.** Of or referring to the walls of a cavity. **2.** Of, referring to, or located near the parietal bone of the skull such as the parietal lobe of the brain.

parietal bone   One of a pair of bones that form part of the top and sides of the skull. Each parietal bone has two surfaces, four borders, and four angles and adjoins with five other bones: the opposite parietal, occipital, frontal, temporal, and sphenoid.

parietal lobe   The upper central lobe of each cerebral hemisphere that occupies the parts of the lateral and the medial surfaces that are covered by the parietal bones.

parietal lymph node   One of the small oval glands formed by the accumulation of lymph tissues that acts as a filter in the lymph vessels in either the walls of the thorax or the larger blood vessels of the abdomen and the pelvis.

parietal peritoneum   The serous membrane lining the abdominal and pelvic walls.

parietal pleura   The serous membrane lining the walls of the thoracic cavity.

parieto-occipital sulcus   A fissure on the medial surface of each cerebral hemisphere that divides the parietal and occipital lobes of the brain.

parity   In obstetrics: the classification of a woman by the number pregnancies carried to the point of viability (28 weeks' gestation) regardless of whether any of the children were living at birth. Usually denoted as P or para followed by the total number of pregnancies.

Parkinson's disease   A slowly progressing degenerative neurologic disorder characterized by a tremor of the resting muscles, a masklike or expressionless appearance of the

Parotid gland

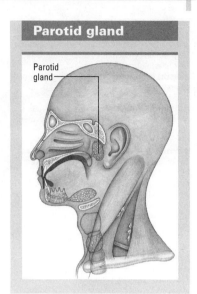

Parotid gland

face, shuffling gait, peculiar posture, and muscle rigidity and weakness.

paronychia   An inflammation of the fold of tissue at the margin of a nail.

CLINICAL TIP   Treatment may include soaking or hot compresses, antibiotics and, possibly, surgical incision and drainage.

parotid duct   A tubular canal, about 2³⁄₄" (7 cm) long, that drains the parotid gland and empties into the mouth.

parotidectomy   Surgical removal of the parotid gland.

parotid gland   The largest of the three main pairs of salivary glands situated at the side of the face in front of and below the external ear.

parotitis   Inflammation of one or both parotid glands, as in mumps.

parovarian cyst   Cyst located beside the ovary.

paroxysm   **1.** A sudden marked increase or recurrence of symptoms. **2.** A convulsion, seizure, or spasm.

paroxysmal cold hemoglobinuria   A rare autoimmune disorder in which the individual has episodes of hemolysis and hematuria after exposure to cold; caused by an immunoglobulin G antibody.

paroxysmal hemoglobinuria   Episodes of hemolysis and passage of hemoglobin in urine, occurring after infection, administration of vaccines, menstruation, or exposure to low temperatures.

paroxysmal nocturnal dyspnea   Sudden attacks of respiratory distress, usually occurring after several hours of sleep; caused by pulmonary edema resulting from congestive heart failure.

partial cleavage   Mitotic division of only the protoplasmic part of a fertilized ovum into blastomeres; restricted division.

partial placenta previa   Implantation of the placenta in the lower uterine segment so that it partially covers the internal os of the uterine cervix.

partial pressure   The pressure exerted by any single component in a mixture of gases, usually expressed in millimeters of mercury, or torr.

partial thromboplastin time (PTT)   A screening test for coagulation defects of the intrinsic system; activated partial thromboplastin is added to a sample of test plasma and to a control and the time in seconds it takes for each to clot is recorded and compared.

particle   1. A minute mass of material. 2. A submicroscopic component of matter and energy, such as the electron or proton.

particulate   Composed of particles.

PAS, PASA   *abbr* para-aminosalicylic acid.

passive euthanasia   The practice of allowing terminally ill individuals to die without taking heroic measures to prolong their lives, such as connecting their organic systems to artificial devices, when there is no hope for natural survival.

passive exercise   Movement of a body part using an externally applied force, such as a machine, another person, or voluntary movement of another part of the individual's body.

passive immunity   A form of acquired resistance to an infection resulting from transfer of antibodies either naturally through the placenta to a fetus or through the colostrum to an infant, or artificially by inoculation of antiserum.

passive movement   The moving of parts of the body by an outside force without voluntary action or resistance by the individual.

passive transport   The movement of small molecules across the cell membrane when the driving force is the concentration gradient; substances move from an area of high concentration to one of low concentration. Also called *passive diffusion.*

passive tremor   An involuntary trembling that occurs when the person is at rest; may diminish or stop during voluntary movement; a sign of Parkinson's disease.

Pasteurella   A genus of gram-negative, anaerobic ovoid or rod-shaped bacteria that are potentially pathogenic to man and domestic animals.

past health   A summary of a person's health to date, including past injuries, allergies, surgical procedures, immunizations, hospitalizations, and obstetric and psychiatric history; a component of the health history.

Patau's syndrome   Trisomy 13; a complex of birth defects in infants with an extra chromosome at position 13, occurring in approximately 1 in 5,000 births; usually fatal; characterized by mental retardation, deformed ears, cleft lip, cleft palate, microphthalmia, polydactyly, cardiac and renal anomalies, and malrotation of the intestines.

patella   A flat, triangular sesamoid bone at the front of the knee, within the tendon of the quadriceps muscle. Also called *knee cap.*

patellar ligament   The central portion of the tendon of the quadriceps muscle behind the knee; extends from the patella to the tibia.

patellar reflex   Knee jerk; a deep tendon reflex, elicited by a sharp tap on the patellar tendon with the leg hanging loosely at right angles to the thigh; normally characterized by contraction of the quadriceps muscle and extension of the leg at the knee.

patent ductus arteriosus (PDA)   Abnormal persistence of the fetal opening between the pulmonary artery and the aorta after birth; results in arterial blood recirculating through the lungs.

Paterson-Kelly syndrome   A condition associated with iron deficiency anemia, characterized by fissures at the side of the mouth, painful tongue, and the development of esophageal webs in the upper esophagus, resulting in dysphagia; also called *Plummer-Vinson syndrome.*

pathogen   Any microorganism that can produce disease.

pathogenesis   The development of an illness or abnormal condition, particularly the cellular changes and other pathologic events that occur during development of an illness.

pathognomonic   A sign or symptom that is specific to a disease or condition and on the basis of which a diagnosis can be made — for example, Koplik's spots, which are indicative of measles.

pathologic   1. Pertaining to the branch of medicine that studies the nature of disease, especially the changes in body tissue structure or function that cause or are caused by disease. 2. Indicative of or caused by disease.

pathologic absorption   The taking up into the bloodstream of any excremental or otherwise pathologic substance, such as pus, urine, or bile.

pathological anatomy   A subspecialty of pathology that deals with the study of organs and tissues of the body as related to disease; examination is done on tissues removed for biopsy or on postmortem specimens.

pathologic diagnosis   Determination of the nature of a disease by examining abnormal structural lesions by histologic techniques.

pathologic mitosis   Atypical, asymmetrical, or multipolar cell division that results in an unequal number of chromosomes in the nuclei of daughter cells; indicative of malignancy.

pathologic myopia   Progressive near-sightedness characterized by changes in the fundus of the eye, bulging of the posterior pole of the eye, and below-normal corrected acuity; also called *malignant myopia.*

pathologic retraction ring   One of the classic signs of threatened uterine rupture; a persistent ridge formed around the uterus at the junction of the upper and lower uterine segments during a prolonged or abnormal second stage of labor; obstructs delivery of the fetus.

pathologist   A physician who specializes in the study of the structural and functional manifestations of disease, usually in a hospital, school of medicine, or research center.

pathology   The branch of medicine that studies the characteristics of disease, as observed in the changes in structure and function of body tissues. Types include cellular pathology, which examines cellular changes in disease and holds that the cell is the starting point of disease, and clinical pathology, which applies the study of disease to the solution of clinical problems in medicine, using laboratory tests to aid clinical diagnosis.

pathophysiology   The study of the alterations in body or organ function seen in disease.

pathway   In neurology, the nerve structures that provide the route for transmission of nerve impulses from any part of the body to the spinal cord and cerebral cortex or from the central nervous system to the muscles and organs.

patient-controlled analgesia (PCA)   Treatment that allows the patient to control I.V. delivery of an analgesic (usually morphine) to maintain therapeutic serum levels. The specialized infusion device has a patient-controlled trigger and timing unit to deliver an analgesic dose at a controlled volume.

Patient's Bill of Rights   A list of patient's rights promulgated by the American Hospital Association that offers some guidance and protection to patients by stating the responsibilities of the hospital and its staff to patients and their families; not a legally binding document.

Pautrier's microabscess   A microscopic lesion of the epidermis, containing intensely staining mononuclear cells; seen in T-cell lymphoma and mycosis fungoides.

pavor   Excessive terror such as that seen in children with the sleep disorder night terrors.

PAWP   *abbr* pulmonary artery wedge pressure.

Payr's clamp   A clamp used in resection of the stomach or intestine.

Pb   Symbol for lead.

PBI   *abbr* protein-bound iodine.

p.c.   *abbr* Latin *post cibum,* after meals.

Pco_2   Symbol for partial pressure of carbon dioxide. See *partial pressure.*

PCP   *abbr* phencyclidine hydrochloride.

Pd   Symbol for palladium.

PDA   *abbr* patent ductus arteriosus.

PDR   abbr *Physician's Desk Reference.*

PE   *abbr* pulmonary embolism.

Péan's forceps   A type of curved or straight hemostatic clamp.

Pearson's correlation coefficient   In statistics, a test of the relationship between two variables; computed by dividing the covariance of the variables by the product of their standard deviations; designated by the symbol *r.*

peau d'orange   Orange-peel appearance of breast skin caused by edema; associated with breast cancer.

pectineus   A medial femoral muscle that arises from the iliopectineal line and inserts on the femur distal to the lesser trochanter; acts to flex and adduct the thigh.

pectoralis major   A large muscle of the upper chest wall that has subdivisions arising from the clavicle, sternum and upper ribs, and the aponeurosis of the external oblique muscle of the abdomen, respectively; inserts into the crest of the greater tubercle of the humerus; acts to flex, adduct, and medially rotate the arm.

pectoralis minor   A thin, triangular muscle of the upper chest wall beneath the pectoralis major; originates in the third, fourth, and fifth ribs and inserts at the coracoid process of the scapula; draws shoulder forward and down.

pectoriloquy   The transmission of vocal sounds through the chest wall, heard on auscultation, as in whispered pectoriloquy.

pediatrician, pediatrist   A physician who specializes in the branch of medicine that deals with the health and development of children and treatment of the diseases of children.

pediatric nurse practitioner (PNP)
A registered nurse who, by advanced study and clinical practice, is qualified to provide primary health care to infants and children.

pedicle clamp   Clamp forceps; a locking surgical instrument used to compress blood vessels or pedicles of tumors during surgery.

pediculosis   Infestation with lice, especially *Pediculus humanus.*

pedodontics   The field of dentistry that deals with the diagnosis and treatment of problems of the teeth and mouth in children.

pedogenesis   The production of offspring by larval forms, as in certain amphibians.

peduncle   **1.** A stalk or stem. **2.** A stalk-like structure in the brain such as the cerebral peduncle.

PEEP   *abbr* positive end-expiratory pressure.

Pelger-Huët nuclear anomaly   An inherited disorder that interferes with normal formation of nuclei in neutrophils and eosinophils; characterized by coarse, lumpy nuclear structure and dumbbell-shaped nuclei.

pellagra   A clinical syndrome that results from a deficiency of niacin or from a metabolic defect that interferes with the conversion of tryptophan to niacin; marked by dermatitis on body parts exposed to light or trauma, inflamed mucous membranes, diarrhea, and mental disturbances, including depression, irritability, disorientation, and hallucinations.

pelvic cellulitis   Parametritis; bacterial infection of the parametrium, the cellular tissue next to the uterus; can occur after childbirth or abortion.

pelvic classification   A grouping of the variations of the female pelvis; evaluation of the anatomic and spatial relationships of the bones of the pelvis; usually done to assess the adequacy of the pelvic structures for vaginal delivery.

pelvic congestion syndrome   A poorly understood gynecologic condition most commonly characterized by low back pain, dysuria, dysmenorrhea, vague lower abdominal pain, vaginal discharge, dyspareunia, leukorrhea, and discomfort when sitting or standing.

pelvic diaphragm   The caudal aspect of the body wall, made up of the levator ani and coccygeus muscles along with the fasciae above and below them.

pelvic inflammatory disease (PID)
Any ascending inflammatory condition of the upper female genital tract, especially one caused by bacterial infection.

pelvic inlet   The upper opening to the true pelvis, bounded by the sacral promonto-ry, the arcuate lines of the ilia, and the symphysis pubis and pubic crest.

pelvic minilaparotomy   A surgical technique in which the lower abdomen is entered through a small suprapubic incision, performed most commonly for sterilization by tubal ligation; also used for diagnosis and treatment of ovarian cysts, endometriosis, and infertility.

pelvic outlet   The lower opening to the true pelvis, bounded by the pubic arch, the sacrotuberous ligaments, part of the ischium, and the coccyx.

pelvic pole   The location of the breech of the fetus.

pelvic rotation   One of the five major determinants of gait; the alternate rotation of the pelvis to the right and the left of the central axis of the body, normally 4 degrees to each side of the central axis.

pelvic tilt   One of the five major determinants of gait; the lowering of the pelvis on the side of the swinging leg during the walking cycle.

pelvifemoral muscular dystrophy   A progressive muscular dystrophy that usually begins in the preadolescent period and most severely involves the pelvic girdle. Also called *Leyden-Möebius muscular dystrophy, limb-girdle muscular dystrophy.*

pelvimetry   The act of measuring the dimensions and capacity of the pelvis, especially the bony birth canal.

pelvis, *pl.* **pelves**   **1.** The lower portion of the trunk, bounded by the two hip bones laterally and anteriorly and the sacrum and coccyx posteriorly; the upper border is known as the pelvic inlet; the lower border, or pelvic outlet, is closed by the levator ani and coccygeus muscles. **2.** Any basin-like structure such as the renal pelvis.

pendular nystagmus   An undulating involuntary movement of the eyeball in which the oscillations of the eyes are equal in rate, amplitude, direction, and type of movement.

penetrance   In genetics, the regularity with which an inherited trait is manifest in the person who carries the gene. If a gene always produces its effect on the phenotype, it's fully and completely penetrant.

penile cancer   A rare malignancy of the penis occurring more commonly in uncircumcised men; associated with genital herpesvirus infection and poor personal hygiene.

penis   The male external reproductive organ, which also contains the urethra and serves as the organ of urinary excretion; consists of the root, the corpora cavernosa, the corpus spongiosum, and the glans penis.

pentosuria A rare benign error of metabolism that results in pentose being present in the urine.

Pepper syndrome A neuroblastoma of the adrenal gland that metastasizes to the liver.

pepsin Any of the enzymes secreted in the gastric juice that catalyze the hydrolysis of proteins.

peptic ulcer A lesion of the mucous membrane of the stomach, duodenum, or esophagus due to the action of gastric juices containing acid.

peptide Any compound composed of two or more amino acids joined by peptide bonds; constituents of proteins.

peracephalus A malformed fetus lacking a head and arms and having a defective thorax.

perceptual defect Any of a broad group of neurologic disorders that interfere with higher mental processes or with the conscious mental recognition of sensory stimuli.

percussion Striking a body part with sharp blows as part of physical examination; used usually in conjunction with auscultation to evaluate the size, borders, and condition of an internal organ.

percussor A small, hammerlike instrument used to tap the body lightly when performing percussion.

percutaneous Performed through the skin, as the aspiration of fluid or tissue from a space below the skin using a needle, catheter, and syringe.

percutaneous catheter placement The introduction of an intracatheter through the skin into an artery and its placement at the site to be studied, as in selective angiography and other diagnostic procedures.

percutaneous transhepatic cholangiography A radiologic procedure for examining the biliary system in which the radiopaque contrast material is introduced into the system through a catheter inserted through the skin into the liver or gallbladder.

percutaneous transluminal coronary angioplasty (PTCA) A technique to open stenosed atherosclerotic arteries in which a balloon catheter is inserted through the skin and into the vessel to the site of narrowing; the balloon is inflated, thus flattening the plaque against the arterial walls.

Perez's reflex The normal response of an infant, when held supported in the prone position, to cry, flex the limbs, and elevate the head and pelvis when a finger is run down the spine; persistence of the reflex after age 6 months may indicate brain damage.

perforate 1. To pierce or make a hole. 2. Riddled with holes.

perforating fracture A fracture caused by a projectile perforating the bone.

perianal abscess A purulent subcutaneous infection in the region around the anus; may be caused by a rectal fistula or sinus track.

periapical Pertaining to the tissues at or around the apex of a tooth.

periapical abscess An infection of the tissues around the root of a tooth, usually caused by a spread of the infection from dental caries or by trauma that causes necrosis of the pulp.

periapical infection Infection of the tissues surrounding the root of a tooth, usually resulting from spread of infection from the pulp of a tooth.

periarteritis Inflammation of the outer coat of an artery and of the tissue surrounding the artery.

periarteritis nodosa A progressive, systemic vasculitis characterized by the presence of numerous large, palpable nodules in clusters along small and middle-sized arteries; results from infarction and scarring of a related organ.

pericardectomy Surgical opening of the pericardial sac to remove accumulated fluid.

pericardiac artery One of several small branches of the thoracic aorta that supply the dorsal surface of the pericardium.

pericardiocentesis, pericardicentesis A surgical procedure in which the pericardial cavity is punctured for the aspiration of fluid from the pericardial space.

pericarditis Inflammation of the pericardium; may be caused by trauma, neoplasm, infection, uremia, myocardial infarction, or collagen disease.

 ALERT If the fluid accumulates rapidly, cardiac tamponade may occur, resulting in pallor, clammy skin, hypotension, pulsus paradoxus (a decrease in systolic blood pressure of 15 mm Hg or more during slow inspiration), neck vein distention, and, eventually, cardiovascular collapse and death.

pericardium The sac surrounding the heart and the roots of the great vessels; made up of an outer layer of fibrous tissue and an inner serous layer.

pericholangitis An inflammatory condition of the tissues surrounding the bile ducts.

perifolliculitis The presence of inflammation in the tissue surrounding a hair follicle.

perihepatitis Inflammation of the serous covering of the liver.

perilymph The clear fluid in the space between the osseous labyrinth and the membranous labyrinth in the inner ear.

perimeningitis Inflammation of the dura mater.

perimeter Line forming the boundary of a closed-plane figure.

perinatal Occurring within or pertaining to the time around birth; generally the period from the 20th week of gestation to the 28th day after birth.

perinatal death An inclusive term referring to the death of a fetus weighing more than 1,000 g at 28 or more weeks' gestation, stillbirth, and death of an infant within the neonatal period, up to 28 days after birth.

perinatal mortality The rate of fetal and infant death, from 28 weeks' gestation to the end of the neonatal period; includes stillbirths.

perinatal physiology The changes in physiology seen in the fetus and infant in the period surrounding birth; these changes in organ function must occur for the infant to adapt to extrauterine life.

perinatologist A physician who specializes in the treatment of the fetus and infant in the period surrounding birth.

perinatology The branch of medicine concerned with the diagnosis and treatment of disorders of the mother, fetus, and infant in the period surrounding childbirth.

perineal Of or pertaining to the perineum.

perineal care The procedure prescribed for cleaning of the perineum in the postpartum period.

perineorrhaphy Suture of the peritoneum; a surgical procedure to repair a tear or defect in the perineum.

perineotomy An incision into the perineum.

perinephritis Inflammation of the tissues surrounding the kidneys.

perineum 1. The pelvic floor and its associated structures; located between the symphysis pubis and the coccyx, and on the sides by the ischial tuberosities. 2. The body area between the thighs; bounded by the anus and scrotum in males and by the anus and vulva in females.

periodic Recurring at regular intervals.

periodontal Pertaining to the area around a tooth.

periodontal disease Any of a group of diseases of the tissues that surround and support a tooth; generally either inflammatory processes or conditions relating to diet.

periodontics, periodontia A branch of dentistry concerned with diseases of the periodontium, the tissues that enclose and support the teeth.

periodontist A dentist who specializes in the study of normal periodontal tissues and in treatment of diseases affecting these tissues.

periodontitis Inflammation of the periodontium, the tissues surrounding the tooth; usually represents an extension of gingivitis, or gum infection, into the deeper tissues.

perioophoritis Inflammation of the covering of the ovary.

periorbita The connective tissue covering the bones of the orbit of the eye.

periosteum The fibrous vascular connective tissue covering the bones, consisting of an inner layer of collagenous tissue and a layer of fine elastic fibers and an outer layer of dense vascular connective tissue; has bone-forming capability.

peripheral Of or pertaining to the edges of the body, an organ, or other structure.

peripheral acrocyanosis of the newborn A normal, transient condition of the newborn, characterized by cyanotic discoloration of the hands and feet.

peripherally inserted central catheter (PICC) Catheter inserted through a vein above the antecubital area; causes fewer and less severe adverse reactions than a traditional central venous catheter, and can be left in place for several months.

peripheral nervous system The portion of the nervous system made up of the motor and sensory nerves and ganglia outside the brain and spinal cord; consists of 12 pairs of cranial nerves, 31 pairs of spinal nerves, and their various branches.

peripheral parenteral nutrition (PPN) The delivery of nutrients through a short cannula inserted into a peripheral vein; generally provides fewer nonprotein calories than total parenteral nutrition because lower dextrose concentrations are used.

peripheral vascular disease Any disorder of the blood vessels of the extremities, especially those that interfere with blood flow.

peripheral vision The faculty of seeing objects that stimulate areas of the retina distant from the macula.

peristalsis The coordinated movement of smooth muscle in organs that moves their contents through them, as food is moved through the digestive tract and urine through the ureters.

peritoneal Of or pertaining to the peritoneum.

peritoneal cavity The potential space between the parietal and visceral peritoneum.

Permanent dentition

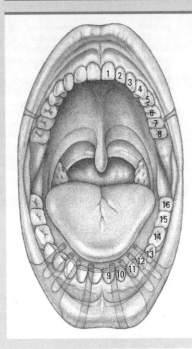

MAXILLARY

1. Central incisor: ages 7 to 8
2. Lateral incisor: ages 8 to 9
3. Canine: ages 11 to 12
4. First premolar: ages 9 to 11
5. Second premolar: ages 10 to 12
6. First molar: ages 6 to 7
7. Second molar: ages 12 to 13
8. Third molar: ages 17 to 25

MANDIBULAR

9. Central incisor: ages 6 to 7
10. Lateral incisor: ages 7 to 8
11. Canine: ages 11 to 12
12. First premolar: ages 9 to 12
13. Second premolar: ages 11 to 12
14. First molar: ages 6 to 7
15. Second molar: ages 12 to 13
16. Third molar: ages 17 to 25

peritoneal dialysis   A procedure performed to remove toxins, drugs, or other wastes normally excreted by the kidney; transfers these substances across the peritoneum by intermittently introducing and removing a dialysate from the peritoneal cavity.

peritoneal dialysis solution   A solution that mimics the electrolyte composition of interstitial fluid that is introduced across the peritoneum to remove toxic substances from the body and maintain electrolyte and acid-base balance in patients with compromised kidney function.

peritoneum   The extensive serous membrane that covers the abdominal wall and invests the viscera; divided into the parietal peritoneum and the visceral peritoneum.

peritonitis   An inflammation of the peritoneum; can be produced by bacteria or irritating substances introduced into the abdominal cavity by a penetrating wound or perforation of an organ.

peritonsillar abscess   An extension of acute tonsillitis to the tissue between the tonsil and pharynx, with formation of abscesses above and beyond the tonsils; also called *quinsy.*

periungual   Concerning the area around a fingernail or toenail.

perivascular goiter   An enlargement of the thyroid gland that surrounds a large blood vessel.

perivitelline   Located around the vitellus, or yolk.

permanent dentition   The eruption of the 32 permanent teeth, which begins with the appearance of the first permanent molars at about age 6 and is completed by age 12 or 13.

perochirus   A fetus with malformed hands.

perodactylus   A fetus with malformed fingers or toes, especially one in which one or more digits is absent.

perodactyly, perodactylia   A congenital anomaly characterized by deformed or absent fingers or toes.

peroneal   Pertaining to the outside of the leg, to the fibula, or to the muscles and nerves found there.

peroneal muscular atrophy   Charcot-Marie-Tooth disease; a progressive neuropathic condition characterized by the symmetrical weakening or atrophy of muscles of the lower legs and feet.

 CLINICAL TIP   Peroneal muscular atrophy is commonly first indicated by pes cavus.

perosplanchnia   A congenital anomaly in which the viscera is malformed.

PERRLA   Acronym for *p*upils *e*qual, *r*ound, *r*eactive to *l*ight, and *a*ccommodation; the qualities evaluated in assessment of the eyes.

persistent cloaca   A congenital anomaly caused by persistence of the common cavity into which the intestinal, urinary, and reproductive ducts empty; results from failure of the urorectal septum to form.

persistent vegetative state   A state of severe mental impairment in which only involuntary bodily functions are sustained.

Perthes' disease   Coxa plana; osteochondrosis of the head of the femur, characterized initially by epiphyseal necrosis followed by regeneration or recalcification; also called *Legg-Calvé-Perthes disease.*

pertussis   An acute, highly contagious respiratory disease usually caused by *Bordetella pertussi;* characterized by paroxysmal coughing that ends in a loud whooping inspiration produced by spasmodic closure of the glottis.

pertussis immune globulin   A sterile solution isolated from the plasma of immunized adults used to provide passive immunity against or to treat whooping cough.

pertussis vaccine   A component of the diphtheria and tetanus toxoids and pertussis inoculation; offers active immunity against whooping cough.

pes cavus   A deformity of the foot characterized by an excessively high arch; may be congenital or may develop later due to contractures.

pessary   A device placed in the vagina to support the uterus and rectum in patients with uterine prolapse, uterine retroversion, or cervical incompetence; also employed as a contraceptive device.

PET   *abbr* positron emission tomography.

petechiae, *sing.* **petechia**   Pinpoint purple or red spots on the skin that are caused by minute hemorrhages within the dermal or submucosal layers.

petechial fever   Any febrile illness accompanied by small petechiae on the skin, as seen in the late stage of typhoid fever.

petroleum   A semisolid mixture of hydrocarbons used as a base for ointments and alone as a topical protectant and emollient.

petroleum gauze   Absorbent cotton cloth of plain weave saturated with white petroleum; used as protective covering over wounds.

petroleum distillate poisoning   A toxic condition caused by the ingestion or inhalation of a petroleum distillate, such as gasoline, kerosene, glue, and various solvents.

petrosphenoidal fissure   A groove on the floor of the cranial fossa; located between the posterior edge of the wing of the sphenoid bone and the petrous part of the temporal bone.

Peutz-Jeghers syndrome   An autosomal dominant disorder, characterized by multiple intestinal polyps usually in the jejunum and abnormal pigmentation of the skin and mucous membranes, especially the lips and buccal mucosa.

Peyer's patches   Elevated areas of lymphoid tissue in the terminal ileum near its junction with the colon; made up of lymph nodules packed closely together.

peyote   1. Mescal; a cactus of the genus *Lophophora,* especially *L. williamsii,* from which the hallucinogenic drug mescaline is derived. 2. Mescaline.

Peyronie's disease   A disease of unknown cause characterized by plaques of fibrous tissue surrounding the corpora cavernosa of the penis, resulting in deformity and painful erections.

PFT   *abbr* pulmonary function test.

PG   *abbr* prostaglandin.

pH   A symbol representing the relative concentration of hydrogen ions in a solution compared to the hydrogen ion concentration of a standard solution; expressed on a scale, It's approximately equal to the negative logarithm of the hydrogen ion concentration; a value of 7 is neutral, below 7 is acid, and above 7 is alkaline.

phacomalacia   A softening of the lens of the eye, or a soft cataract.

phagomania   Another term for bulimia.

phagocyte   A scavenger cell; any cell that is able to engulf and digest microorganisms and cellular debris; classed as microphages, which are polymorphonuclear leukocytes that ingest bacteria, and macrophages, mononuclear cells that ingest dead tissue.

phagocytosis   The process by which cells engulf and digest solid substances, such as microorganisms and cell debris.

phakomatosis, phacomatosis, *pl.* **phakomatoses**   Any of a group of hereditary syndromes characterized by the development of benign tumorlike nodules of the eye, skin, and central nervous system.

phalanx, *pl.* **phalanges** 1. Any one of the tapering bones that make up the fingers and toes. 2. Any of the plates that make up the reticular membrane of the organ of Corti.

phantom limb syndrome The sensation that an amputated limb still exists; pain or discomfort may be experienced in the missing limb.

phantom tumor An accumulation of fluid in the interlobar spaces of the lung, resembling a tumor on radiologic examination; caused by heart failure.

pharmacist A specialist licensed to formulate and dispense medications and compounds and to fill prescriptions.

pharmacogenetics The study of the relationship between the genetic factors of a group or individual and the response of the group or individual to drugs.

pharmacokinetics The action of drugs within the body, including the routes and mechanisms of absorption and distribution, the biotransformation of the drug in the body, and the routes of excretion of the drug and its metabolites.

pharmacologist One who studies the actions of drugs.

pharmacology The science that studies the origin, nature, properties, uses, and actions of drugs.

PharmD *abbr* Doctor of Pharmacy. One trained to practice in a clinical setting, rather than dispensing medication.

pharyngeal aponeurosis A sheet of fibrous connective tissue in the wall of the pharynx; lined on inside with mucous membrane and partially covered by the constrictor muscle of the pharynx.

pharyngeal tonsil A collection of lymphoid tissue on the posterior wall of the nasopharynx; when swollen, results in the condition known as adenoiditis.

pharyngitis Inflammation or infection of the mucous membrane lining the pharynx and underlying tissues, usually producing a sore throat.

pharyngoconjunctival fever A febrile disease sometimes epidemic in schoolchildren characterized by fever, sore throat, and conjunctivitis that is caused by an adenovirus.

PhD *abbr* Doctor of Philosophy.

phenocopy A phenotypic trait induced by environmental factors that closely resembles one produced by a specific genotype.

phenol camphor An oily mixture of camphor and phenol, used as an antiseptic and toothache remedy.

phenol poisoning Poisoning caused by the ingestion or absorption of compounds containing phenol, such as carbolic acid, creosote, and naphthol; signs and symptoms include local corrosion, colic, and weakness.

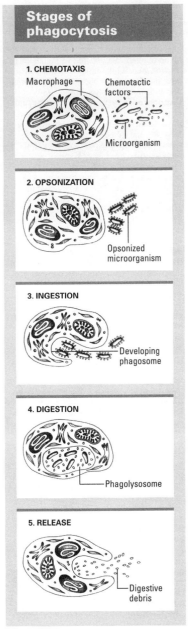

Stages of phagocytosis

1. CHEMOTAXIS
Macrophage — Chemotactic factors —
Microorganism

2. OPSONIZATION
Opsonized microorganism

3. INGESTION
Developing phagosome

4. DIGESTION
Phagolysosome

5. RELEASE
Digestive debris

phenylketonuria (PKU) An inborn metabolic disorder caused by absence or deficiency of phenylalanine hydroxylase, the enzyme responsible for the conversion of phenylalanine to tyrosine; results in accumulation of phenylalanine and its metabolites, causing mental retardation and other neurologic problems, light pigmentation, eczema, and a distinctive mousy odor.

pheochromocytoma A vascular tumor of chromaffin tissue derived from the adrenal medulla; characterized by secretion of epinephrine and norepinephrine, causing hypertension associated with attacks of palpitations, nausea, headache, dyspnea, anxiety, pallor, and profuse sweating.

pheromone A substance secreted to the exterior of the body by an individual that elicits, as through smell, a response from another individual of the same species.

Philadelphia chromosome Translocation of the long arm of chromosome 22, commonly seen in the abnormal marrow cells of patients with chronic myelocytic leukemia.

phimosis Constriction of the prepuce of the penis, preventing its retraction over the glans penis.

phlebectasia Swelling of a vein or a varicosity.

phlebemphraxis Obstruction of a vein by a clot or plug.

phlebogram 1. An X-ray of a vein that has been filled with contrast medium. 2. A graphic representation of the venous pulse, made with a phlebograph.

phlebograph An instrument used to produce a graphic record of the venous pulse.

phlebography 1. A technique for acquiring an X-ray image of veins by injecting a radiopaque contrast medium. 2. The technique of preparing a graphic recording of the venous pulse.

phlebophlebostomy Anastomosis of two veins.

phlebothrombosis A clot present within a vein not associated with an inflammatory condition of the vein wall; usually owing to hemostasis, hypercoagulability, or occlusion.

phlebotomus fever An acute, mild arbovirus infection occurring in five distinct forms in southern Europe, the Middle East, central Asia, and South and Central America, transmitted to man by the bite of an infected sandfly (genus *Phlebotomus);* characterized by rapidly developing fever, headache, conjunctivitis, and myalgia.

phlebotomy The incision of a vein for the purpose of drawing blood.

phlegm A thick mucous secretion such as that produced by the tissues lining the respiratory passages.

phlegmasia cerulea dolens A severe form of deep venous thrombosis, usually involving the femoral vein, with reactive arterial spasm and pronounced edema of the affected extremity.

phlegmonous gastritis A rare but severe form of stomach inflammation, in which there are abscesses in the stomach wall.

phlyctenular keratoconjunctivitis An inflammatory condition of the cornea and conjunctiva, characterized by tiny, ulcerating nodules of lymphoid cells in the conjunctiva.

phocomelia A developmental anomaly in which the upper portion of one or more of the limbs is absent so that the feet or hands are attached to the trunk of the body by short, irregularly shaped stumps.

phonocardiogram A graphic recording of heart sounds obtained from a phonocardiograph.

phonocardiograph A device that produces graphic recordings of heart sounds and murmurs.

phosphatase Any of the class of enzymes that act as catalysts in the release of inorganic phosphate in chemical reactions involving phosphorus.

phosphate A compound of phosphoric acid; important in the storage and utilization of energy and the transmission of genetic information.

phospholipid Any of a class of lipids, widely distributed in living cells, that contain phosphorus; the major form of lipids in cell membranes.

phosphomevalonate kinase An enzyme that catalyzes a reaction in the synthesis of cholesterol; transfers a phosphate group from adenosine triphosphate to produce adenosine diphosphate and 5-diphosphomevalonate.

phosphoric acid A strong mineral acid that is an important metabolite.

phosphorus (P) A nonmetallic element occurring in nature as a component of phosphate rock (atomic number, 15; atomic weight, 30.974); an essential element of the diet, It's abundant in all tissues and takes part in most metabolic processes; a major component of bone.

phosphorus poisoning A toxic condition caused by the ingestion or inhalation of white or yellow phosphorus.

 CLINICAL TIP Phosphorus poisoning is characterized by toothache, mandibular necrosis, anorexia, weakness, and anemia.

photoallergic   Of, pertaining to, or producing a delayed hypersensitivity reaction after exposure to light.

photoallergic contact dermatitis   A papulovesicular, eczematous, or exudative skin inflammation occurring after exposure to light in a previously sensitized person.

photochemotherapy   Treatment with a drug whose effect is enhanced by exposing the patient to light, such as the use of methoxsalen and ultraviolet light to treat psoriasis.

photophobia   Abnormal sensitivity of the eyes to light.

photosensitive   Having an increased reactivity to sunlight seen in skin as a result of exposure to certain drugs or from disorders, such as albinism or porphyria.

photosynthesis   The process by which green plants and blue-green algae formulate carbohydrates from atmospheric carbon dioxide and water in their chlorophyll tissues, using light for energy; the process releases oxygen.

phototherapy   The treatment of disease by the use of light, especially ultraviolet light or other concentrated rays; used to treat acne, psoriasis, and hyperbilirubinemia.

phototoxic   Characterized by or producing a rapidly developing, nonimmunologic reaction of the skin.

phreniclasia   Surgical crushing of the phrenic nerve.

phrenic nerve   One of a pair of branches of the cervical plexus, arising from the fourth cervical nerve; primarily acts as motor nerve for the diaphragm, but also provides sensory fibers to the pericardium.

phycomycosis   An infection caused by a species of fungi from the order Phycomycetes; usually characterized by inflammation and vascular thrombosis of the blood vessels of the affected organ.

physical chemistry   A natural science, a branch of chemistry that deals with the relationship between chemical and physical properties of matter.

physical examination   Evaluation of a patient to determine health status, using inspection, palpation, percussion, auscultation, and smell.

physical science   The study of the laws and properties of matter, as in chemistry and physics.

physical therapist   A person who is licensed to administer treatments under a physician's supervision to physically disabled people, including special exercises, application of heat or cold, and use of sonar waves.

physical therapy   A health profession that aims to promote health, prevent disability, and evaluate and rehabilitate injured or disabled people using physical measures, such as massage, manipulation, therapeutic exercises, cold, heat, hydrotherapy, electrical stimulation, and light.

physician   A health professional authorized to practice medicine, either one who has earned a degree of Doctor of Medicine (MD) after completion of a course of study at an approved medical school and satisfactory completion of National Board Examinations or one who has earned a degree of Doctor of Osteopathy (DO) by satisfactorily completing a course of study in an approved college of osteopathy.

physician's assistant (PA)   A person trained in certain aspects of the practice of medicine to provide assistance to a physician. A physician's assistant is trained by physicians and practices under the direction and supervision and within the legal license of a physician. Training programs vary in length from a few months to 2 years. Health care experience or academic preparation may be a prerequisite to admission to some programs. Most physician's assistants are prepared for the practice of primary care, but some practice subspecialties, including surgical assisting, dialysis, or radiology. National certification is available to qualified graduates of approved training programs. The national organization is the American Association of Physician's Assistants (AAPA). Also called *physician's associate.*

***Physician's Desk Reference* (PDR)**   An annual compendium containing information about drugs, primarily prescription drugs and diagnostics.

physics   The science of the laws, forces, and general properties of matter and energy.

physiologic contracture   A temporary condition in which a muscle tenses and shortens for a considerable period; can be produced by heat or drugs.

physiologic dead space   An area in the respiratory tract that includes the anatomical dead space plus the space in the alveoli occupied by air that doesn't contribute to the exchange of oxygen and carbon dioxide.

physiologic psychology   A branch of the science of the mind that studies the relationship between physiologic processes and behavior.

physiologic pump   A mechanism involved in the active transport of solutes; for example, the sodium-potassium pump, which moves sodium ions out of cells to the extracellular fluid, and potassium ions into cells from the extracellular fluid.

physiologic retraction ring   A ridge that forms at the junction of the thinned lower uterine segment and thickened upper segment during the second stage of normal labor; results from the progressive lengthening of the muscle fibers of the lower segment and concomitant shortening of those of the upper segment.

physiologic third heart sound A low-pitched extra heart sound that corresponds to rapid ventricular filling; heard early in diastole in a healthy child or young adult.

PI *abbr* In the patient record: present illness.

pia mater The innermost of the three meninges covering the brain and the spinal cord; firmly adhered to both structures and carries a rich supply of blood vessels, which nourish the brain tissue.

pica A craving to eat substances that aren't foods, such as dirt, clay, starch, or hair; may occur in pregnancy, in iron or zinc deficiencies, and in some forms of mental illness.

picornavirus A member of a family of small viruses (Picornaviridae) with a core of single-stranded ribonucleic acid; includes the enteroviruses, rhinoviruses, coxsackieviruses, and polioviruses.

PID *abbr* pelvic inflammatory disease.

piebald An autosomal dominant inherited condition marked by patchy areas of depigmentation of the hair and skin owing to an absence of functioning melanocytes and melanin in those areas.

Piedmont fracture An oblique fracture of the distal radius, with fragments of bone pulled into the ulna.

Pierre Robin syndrome An autosomal recessive condition marked by a complex of congenital anomalies, including abnormally small tongue and mandible, cleft palate, and defects of the eyes.

pigeon breast A structural defect of the chest; characterized by a prominent sternum and lengthening of the costal cartilages; may be caused by obstructed respiration in the infant or by rickets.

pigeon-breeder's lung A respiratory disorder caused by acquired hypersensitivity to bird droppings in those who come into close contact with birds; can result in pulmonary fibrosis.

pigment 1. Any organic normal or abnormal coloring material of the body such as melanin. 2. A paintlike medicinal preparation applied to the skin.

pilar cyst A common epidermal cyst, usually seen on the scalp, that is formed with an outer wall of stratified epithelium derived from the hair follicle.

pillion fracture A T-shaped fracture of the lower end of the femur with displacement of the condyles behind the femoral shaft;

caused when the knee of a person riding pillion on a motorcycle receives a sharp blow.

pilomotor reflex Goosebumps; contraction of the smooth muscle of the skin and erection of the hairs in response to a chilly environment, emotional stimulus, or gentle stroking.

pilonidal cyst A hair-containing dermoid cyst in the midline of the gluteal fold.

pilonidal fistula An abnormal sinus or pit that contains a tuft of hair which can lead to chronic inflammation and the production of pus; most commonly located close to the coccyx but also occurring in other regions of the body.

pilosebaceous Of or pertaining to the hair follicles and their oil, or sebaceous, glands.

pin 1. A slender metal rod used to secure and immobilize the fragments of a fractured bone. 2. A small metal peg used to fix an artificial crown to the root of a tooth.

pineal gland A small, flattened, cone-shaped structure suspended by a stalk in the epithalamus, situated between the superior colliculi and below the splenium of the corpus callosum; synthesizes and secretes melatonin in response to norepinephrine.

pinealoma A rare neoplasm of the pineal body made up of large epithelial cells; causes hydrocephalus, paralysis of upward gaze, gait disturbances, and precocious puberty.

pinhole test A test performed to distinguish a refractive error from organic disease in a person with diminished visual acuity.

pinocytosis The process by which cells imbibe extracellular fluid by developing saccular indentation, which close around the fluid and pinch off to form fluid-filled vesicles within the cell; thought to be a method of active transport.

pipette A calibrated, glass or transparent plastic open-ended tube used to measure or transfer small quantities of a liquid or gas.

piriformis A flat, pyramidal muscle that lies almost parallel with the gluteus medius; originates in the ilium and the second to fourth sacral vertebrae and inserts into the greater trochanter of the femur; acts to rotate the thigh.

Pirquet's test A tuberculin skin test , no longer in use, in which the tuberculin material was scratched onto the skin.

pisiform bone A small, pea-shaped bone in the proximal row of carpal bones; attached to the flexor retinaculum, the flexor carpi ulnaris, and the abductor digiti minimi.

pitch Sound frequency, measured as the number of sound waves per second.

pitting 1. Small, punctate indentations in fingernails or toenails, commonly a result of psoriasis. **2.** An indentation that remains for a short time after pressing edematous skin with a finger. **3.** Small, depressed scars in the skin or other organ of the body.

pityriasis alba A common idiopathic skin disorder, usually of children, characterized by round or oval, finely scaling patches of hypopigmentation, most commonly on the cheeks and the area around the mouth.

pityriasis rosea A self-limiting skin disease in which a solitary plaque is seen initially and then spreads over the trunk, arms, and thighs as a slightly scaling, pink, macular or papular rash.

pivot joint A uniaxial joint in which one bone rotates within a bony or ligamentous ring, as in the atlantoaxial joint.

PK *abbr* psychokinesis.

PKU *abbr* phenylketonuria.

placebo An inactive substance prescribed as if it were an effective dose of a needed medication; used in controlled clinical trials to determine the efficacy of an experimental treatment.

placenta A highly vascular organ present in mammals during pregnancy joining mother and fetus, through which the fetus absorbs oxygen, nutrients, and other blood-borne substances and excretes carbon dioxide and other wastes.

placenta accreta Abnormal adherence of the placenta to the uterine wall.

placenta bipartita Bilobate placenta.

placenta circumvallata Cup-shaped placenta.

placental hormone Any one of the hormones produced by the placenta, including human placental lactogen, chorionic gonadotropin, and other hormones with estrogenic, progesteronic, or adrenocorticoid activity.

placental insufficiency An abnormal condition of pregnancy in which the placenta fails to perform its function properly, retarding fetal growth and jeopardizing fetal survival.

placenta previa Implantation of the placenta so that it adjoins or covers the internal os of the uterine cervix.

 CLINICAL TIP The most common symptom of placenta previa is painless hemorrhage in the last trimester.

plagiocephaly, plagiocephalism A congenital malformation of the skull caused by irregular closure of the coronal or lambdoidal sutures; results in an asymmetrical, twisted appearance.

plague An infectious disease transmitted to humans by fleas infected with the bacillus *Yersinia pestis* or by contact with infected rats, the primary host.

plague vaccine An agent prepared with cultures of killed *Yersinia pestis*, the causative organism of plague, that provides active immunity against the disease.

planar xanthoma A tumor composed of foam cells that manifests itself as yellowish, orange or red flat macules or slightly raised plaques occurring in either localized clusters or widely distributed over the body.

plane **1.** A flat surface determined by three points in space. **2.** An imaginary surface formed by extension of a longitudinal section through an axis, as the coronal, horizontal, and sagittal planes that are used to identify the position of body parts.

plantar aponeurosis The tough bands of fibrous tissue that surround the soles of the feet, radiating from the heel to the base of the toes.

plantar neuroma A tumor involving nerve cells on the sole of the foot.

plantar reflex Flexion of the toes in response to stroking the outer surface of the sole from heel to toes.

plantar wart A painful lesion on the sole of the foot, caused by a human papillomavirus.

plantigrade Characterizing a gait in which the full sole of the foot touches the ground such as that of humans.

plaque **1.** Any flat patch on the skin or any body surface. **2.** A thin film made up of mucin and colloidal material that adheres to the teeth.

plasma The colorless fluid of the lymph and the blood in which the leukocytes, erythrocytes, and platelets are suspended.

plasma cell An oval cell found in the bone marrow, connective tissue, and blood that is characterized by a round nucleus with a cartwheel heterochromatin pattern; derived from B lymphocytes, It's active in antibody formation.

plasma cell leukemia An unusual disease of the blood-forming tissues in which the predominant cells in peripheral blood are plasma cells.

plasmacytoma, *pl.* **plasmacytomas, plasmacytomata** **1.** A malignant tumor of plasma cells. **2.** A focal neoplasm that contains plasma cells.

plasmapheresis Removal of plasma from blood that has been withdrawn from a donor, and retransfusion of the formed elements into the donor.

plasma protein Any one of the various proteins, including albumin, fibrinogen, and the gamma globulins, dissolved in the blood; holds fluid in vessels by osmosis, and has a role in coagulation and immune responses.

Plasmodium

TROPHOZOITES	GAMETOCYTES

plasma thromboplastin antecedent (PTA)   Factor XI; a stable blood factor essential in the intrinsic pathway of coagulation.

plasmocyte   Plasma cell.

Plasmodium   A genus of protozoa, several species of which cause malaria, transmitted to humans by the bite of an infected mosquito.

plate   A flat structure such as a thin layer of bone.

platelet   A disk-shaped cell found in the blood that is important in blood coagulation.

platinum (Pt)   A silvery white, soft metallic element (atomic number, 78; atomic weight, 195.09).

platypelloid pelvis   A rare type of pelvis with a flattened inlet, in which the anteroposterior diameter is shorter and the transverse diameter is wider than normal; usually makes vaginal delivery impossible.

platysma   One of a pair of muscles that originate from the neck and insert in the lower jaw and the skin around the mouth; acts to open the jaw and wrinkle the skin on the neck.

pledget   A small, flat compress or a tuft of cotton, wool, or lint; used to wipe the skin and absorb drainage.

pleiotropy   Production of a variable factor that modifies basic patterns of inheritance such as a gene.

plethora   Edema and blood vessel distention.

plethysmogram   A tracing representing variations in volume or blood flow in a body part or organ produced by a plethysmograph.

plethysmograph   An instrument that measures and records variations in the volumes of body parts and organs and in the amount of blood passing through them.

pleura, *pl.* pleurae   A delicate serous membrane enclosing the lung and lining the thoracic cavity, creating a potential space known as the pleural cavity.

pleural cavity   The potential space that lies between the visceral and parietal pleurae; contains small amounts of fluid that acts as a lubricant.

pleural effusion   Accumulation of fluid in the interstitial and air spaces of the lung.

pleural space   The potential space between the visceral and parietal layers of the pleurae. The space contains a small amount of fluid that acts as a lubricant, allowing the pleurae to slide smoothly over each other as the lungs expand and contract with respiration.

pleurisy   Inflammation of the pleura, characterized by dyspnea and stabbing pain, leading to restriction of breathing.

pleurodynia   Acute pain in the intercostal muscles and the diaphragm's muscular attachment to the chest wall; caused by fibrositis or irritation of pleural surfaces.

pleuropericardial rub   A coarse friction sound heard on auscultation of the lungs; a sign of inflammation of the pleurae (pleurisy) or of pericarditis with pleural involvement.

pleurothotonos   A tetanic, prolonged contraction of the muscles of one side of the body, resulting in bending of the body to that side.

plexiform neuroma   A neoplasm composed of twisted nerve trunks.

pleximeter   A device, such as a percussor or finger, used to receive light taps in mediate percussion.

plexus, *pl.* plexuses   A network of intersecting nerves, blood vessels, or lymphatic vessels.

plica, *pl.* plicae   A ridge or fold of tissue within the body.

plicae transversales recti   Transverse folds of the rectum; transverse folds in the rectum that support the weight of feces.

plica semilunaris   The semilunar fold of the conjunctiva; a fold of mucous membrane at the inner corner of the eye.

Plimmer's bodies Encapsulated bodies of different shapes and sizes found in the cytoplasm of cancerous cells; once thought to be the causative parasites, but now thought to be products of cell necrosis.

ploidy The status of a cell nucleus regarding the number of chromosome sets in the karyotype; as a suffix, denotes the degree of multiplication of chromosome sets, such as haploidy and diploidy.

plumbism Form of poisoning caused by the absorption of lead or a lead salt.

Plummer's disease Hyperthyroidism caused by a toxic nodular goiter.

Plummer-Vinson syndrome A disorder seen in middle-aged women with chronic iron-deficiency anemia, characterized by dysphagia caused by esophageal webs at the level of the cricoid cartilage.

Pm Symbol for promethium.

PMI *abbr* point of maximum impulse.

PND *abbr* **1.** postnasal drip. **2.** paroxysmal nocturnal dyspnea.

pneumococcal Of, pertaining to, or caused by pneumococci.

pneumococcal vaccine A solution containing purified antigens of the 23 types of *Streptococcus pneumoniae;* provides active immunity against pneumococcal disease, including pneumococcal pneumonia.

pneumococcus, *pl.* pneumococci A gram-positive diplococci of the species *Streptococcus pneumoniae;* the most common cause of bacterial pneumonia

pneumocystosis Infection with the parasite *Pneumocystis carinii,* which produces an interstitial plasma cell pneumonia.

CLINICAL TIP Pneumocystosis is usually seen in infants or debilitated or immunosuppressed people.

pneumoencephalogram A radiograph of the fluid-containing structures of the brain made after withdrawing some cerebrospinal fluid and replacing it with air, oxygen, or helium.

pneumoencephalography A procedure for radiographic visualization of the ventricular space, basal cisterns, and the subarachnoid space overlying the cerebral hemispheres; requires intermittently withdrawing cerebrospinal fluid and replacing it with a gas.

pneumomediastinum The presence of air or gas in the mediastinal tissues, which may interfere with breathing or circulation and can lead to pneumothorax or pneumopericardium; can be caused by trauma or another pathologic process, or may be induced for diagnostic test.

pneumonitis Inflammation of the lung.

pneumothorax A collection of air in the pleural space; may result from an open chest wound that permits the entrance of air or from the rupture of a vesicle on the surface of the lung. Common types of pneumothorax are open, closed, and tension. See the illustration on page 242.

PNH *abbr* paroxysmal nocturnal hemoglobinuria.

PNP *abbr* pediatric nurse practitioner.

P.O. *abbr* by mouth.

Po Symbol for polonium.

Po₂ Symbol for partial pressure of oxygen.

podiatrist A health professional, with the degree Doctor of Podiatric Medicine (DPM) trained to diagnose and treat disorders of the feet.

podiatry The study of the anatomy, physiology, and pathology of the foot and of diagnosis and treatment of diseases of the foot.

poikilocytosis Presence in the blood of erythrocytes exhibiting an abnormal degree of variation in shape.

poikiloderma atrophicans vasculare A chronic patchy dermatitis characterized by hyperpigmentation or hypopigmentation, telangiectasia, atrophy of the epidermis, and symmetrical redness on the breasts and buttocks.

poikiloderma of Civatte A common skin condition among middle-aged women; characterized by blotchy areas of hyperpigmentation and telangiectasia interspersed with dry, scaly, pale punctate areas on the face, neck, and upper chest; believed to be associated with photosensitivity.

point of maximal impulse (PMI) The place on the chest where the left ventricular pulse is felt most strongly, usually in the fifth intercostal space just medial to the left midclavicular line.

poison Any substance that impairs function, damages tissue structure, or destroys life when introduced into the body in relatively small amounts.

poison control center One of a network of facilities that provide information regarding all aspects of poisoning; also maintains records of occurrence of poisonings and refers patients to treatment centers.

poisoning The morbid condition or physical state produced by ingestion or exposure to a poisonous substance.

poison sumac A shrub of the genus *Rhus,* common in North America, containing the highly allergic resin urushiol; skin contact produces severe dermatitis in many people.

polar body **1.** One of the small abortive cells with haploid chromosomes produced during unequal division of the primary and

Tension pneumothorax

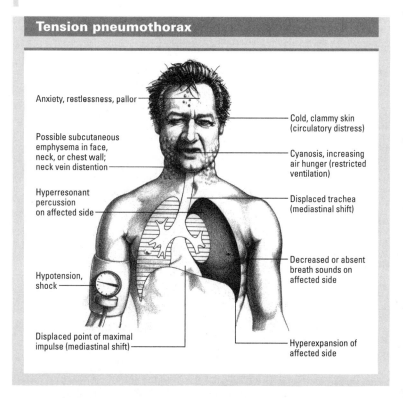

Anxiety, restlessness, pallor

Possible subcutaneous emphysema in face, neck, or chest wall; neck vein distention

Hyperresonant percussion on affected side

Hypotension, shock

Displaced point of maximal impulse (mediastinal shift)

Cold, clammy skin (circulatory distress)

Cyanosis, increasing air hunger (restricted ventilation)

Displaced trachea (mediastinal shift)

Decreased or absent breath sounds on affected side

Hyperexpansion of affected side

secondary oocyte. **2.** The metachromatic granules located at ends of bacterial cells.

polarity   In physics: the distinction between a negative and a positive electrical charge.

pole   **1.** Either extremity of an imaginary axis drawn through a cell, organ, ovum, or nucleus. **2.** The point of origination of a dendrite on a nerve cell.

polioencephalitis   An inflammatory disease of the gray matter of the brain caused by poliovirus infection.

polioencephalomyelitis   An inflammatory disease of the gray matter of the brain and the spinal cord caused by poliovirus infection.

poliomyelitis   An acute viral disease caused by one of the three polioviruses; mild form characterized by fever, sore throat, headache, vomiting, stiff neck and body; may progress to severe form, which includes central nervous system involvement, pleocytosis, and paralysis.

poliosis   The absence or loss of melanin in patches or strands of hair, most commonly on the scalp, eyebrows, or eyelashes. Also called *trichopoliosis.*

poliovirus hominis   The virus that causes poliomyelitis in humans.

poliovirus vaccine   A vaccine derived the poliovirus hominis organism that provides immunity to the virus.

pollakiuria   Abnormally frequent urination.

pollen coryza   Acute rhinitis caused by exposure to plant pollen. Also called *allergic coryza.*

polonium (Po)   A radioactive metallic element, with the atomic number 84 and an approximate atomic weight of 210, which is isolated from pitchblende. One isotope of polonium is radium.

polus, *pl.* **poli**   Either of the two points at the extreme ends of the axis of any organ.

polyarteritis   The inflammation of a number of arteries at the same time.

polyarteritis nodosa   A disease characterized by inflammation and necrosis of segments of medium-sized arteries in muscle tissue, accompanied by secondary ischemia of the tissue supplied by those arteries. Also called *Kussmaul's disease.*

 CLINICAL TIP The cause of polyarteritis nodosa is unknown, but the condition may involve hypersensitivity.

polychromatophile A cell that stains easily with acid, basic, and neutral dyes.

polychromatophilia **1.** The tendency of certain cells (such as the erythrocytes in individuals with pernicious anemia) to stain with both acid and basic dyes. **2.** A condition characterized by the presence of polychromatophiles.

polyclonal Of or relating to proteins from more than one clone of cells or designating a group of identical cells or organisms derived from several identical cells.

polycystic kidney disease A disease characterized by the formation of multiple cysts located throughout both kidneys, and usually associated with hypertension, hematuria, and uremia.

polycystic ovary A disorder characterized by tissue changes and symptoms including anovulation, abnormal menstruation, obesity, and virilization (such as hirsutism and clitoromegaly); commonly associated with infertility.

polycythemia An abnormal increase in the number of circulating red blood cells.

polydactyly, polydactylia, polydactylism A congenital malformation characterized by the formation of more than five digits on either the hands or feet.

polydipsia Chronic, excessive thirst.

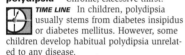 *TIME LINE* In children, polydipsia usually stems from diabetes insipidus or diabetes mellitus. However, some children develop habitual polydipsia unrelated to any disease.

polyhybrid In genetics: pertaining to or describing an individual, organism, or strain that is heterozygous for more than three specific traits, that is the offspring of parents differing in more than three specific gene pairs, or that is heterozygous for more than three particular characteristics or gene loci being followed.

polyhybrid cross In genetics: the mating of two individuals, organisms, or strains that have different gene pairs that determine more than three specific traits or in which more than three particular characteristics or gene loci are being followed.

polyleptic Of or relating to a disease characterized by multiple remissions and exacerbations, such as malaria and epilepsy.

polyleptic fever A fever that occurs in two or more paroxysms, such as smallpox.

polymenorrhea Menstrual cycle of less than eighteen days.

polymorphic Type of ventricular tachycardia in which the QRS complexes change beat to beat.

polymorphism **1.** Occurrence in more than one form. **2.** The existence of more than one morphologic type in a species or other group.

polymorphocytic leukemia A type of leukemia characterized by the predominance of mature, segmented granulocytes. Also called *granulocytic leukemia.*

polymorphonuclear Describing cells having nuclei with a variety of forms.

polymorphonuclear leukocytes A white blood cell having nuclei with a variety of forms, including eosinophils, basophils, and especially neutrophils. Also called *granulocyte.*

polymorphous Occurring in more than one form.

polymyalgia rheumatica A collagen disease, which occurs more commonly in women, characterized by an elevated sedimentation rate and muscle pain at more than one anatomic site.

polymyositis The simultaneous inflammation of a number of voluntary muscles.

polypeptide A peptide formed by a number of amino acids with peptide bonds.

polyphagia Excessive food ingestion.

polyradiculitis Inflammation of several or many nerve roots.

polysome In genetics: a group of ribosomes joined together by a molecule of messenger ribonucleic acid containing the genetic code.

polysomy The presence of a chromosome in at least triplicate in an otherwise diploid somatic cell as the result of chromosomal nondisjunction during meiotic division in the maturation of gametes.

polyuria The excessive excretion of urine from the kidneys.

Pompe's disease A type of glycogen storage disease that is due to a deficiency of acid maltase (lysosomal alpha-1,4-glucosidase). Also called *type 2 glycogenosis.*

pons, *pl.* pontes **1.** The part on the ventral surface of the brain between the medulla oblongata and the mesencephalon. **2.** A formation of tissue resembling a bridge that connects two parts of the same organ or structure.

popliteal artery A continuation of the femoral artery, which passes through the popliteal space behind the knee, then subdivides into the anterior and posterior tibial arteries.

popliteal node One of the surface lymph nodes that drain the skin on the back of the leg and part of the foot or the deeper lymph nodes that drain the knee joint, the structures deeper within the leg, and the surface lymph nodes.

popliteal pulse   The pulse that can be felt over the popliteal artery (behind the knee) when an individual is lying down with the leg slightly flexed.

pork tapeworm infection   An intestinal or tissue infestation with the species of tapeworm found in swine, *Taenia solium.*

porphobilinogen   A chemical substance that is generated in the body and is excreted in large quantities in the urine of individuals with the metabolic disease porphyria.

porphyria   A group of disorders, either hereditary or acquired as a result of exposure to certain environmental toxins, characterized by an abnormal increase in the production and excretion of porphyrins and associated with any of a variety of clinical manifestations, including photosensitivity and hemolytic anemia.

portacaval shunt   A surgically created shunt either between the portal and systemic venous systems or between the portal vein and the vena cava.

portal fissure   A fissure on the liver's visceral surface, between the caudate and quadrate lobes, through which several nerves and vessels pass, including the portal vein, the hepatic artery, the hepatic nerve plexus, and lymphatic vessels.

portal hypertension   Increased blood pressure in the portal circulation caused by obstruction of the portal vein (as may occur in cirrhosis of the liver, for example).

portal vein   A vein formed by the superior mesenteric vein and splenic vein behind the pancreas that ascends anterior to the inferior vena cava and forms right and left branches in the liver and, within the liver, splits into branches resembling an artery and conveys blood through the hepatic veins. Also called *hepatic portal vein.*

Porter-Silber reaction   The chemical reaction to the presence of 17-hydroxycorticosteroids. The 17-hydroxycorticosteroid test is performed to assess the function of the adrenal glands.

positive   1. The presence of a substance or the occurrence of a particular reaction demonstrated in a laboratory test. 2. The presence or demonstration of a sign on physical examination, usually an indication of a disease or disorder. 3. Relating to the positive chemical charge of an element or compound.

positive end-expiratory pressure (PEEP)   A technique used in respiratory therapy in which expiration is impeded mechanically, so that the pressure in the airway is greater than the pressure in the atmosphere.

positive feedback   An increase in function in response to signal that is returned to the organ or structure (for example, the increase in urinary flow that occurs once urination has started).

positive pressure   1. Pressure that is higher than the ambient atmospheric pressure. 2. Any technique used in respiratory therapy that involves the delivery of compressed air or gas at a pressure higher than the pressure in the atmosphere.

positive relationship   The expression of a direct relationship between two variables tested in an experimental study, such that an increase or decrease in one can be expected to increase or decrease correspondingly in the other.

positive signs of pregnancy   Three signs that indicate that conception has occurred: the detection of fetal heart sounds on auscultation, the presence of an X-ray or ultrasound image of a fetal skeleton, and the presence of fetal parts detected on palpation.

positron emission tomography (PET)   A computerized diagnostic technique that involves the use of radioactive substances to create sectional images of metabolic and physiologic function in tissue.

postcommissurotomy syndrome   A condition that may occur following surgery on a cardiac valve, characterized by fever, chest pain, pericardial or pleural rub, and pericardial or pleural effusion. Its cause is unknown.

postconcussion syndrome   A condition caused by an injury to the head, characterized by headache, dizziness, hypersensitivity to stimulation of the nerves, and impaired ability to concentrate. Also called *posttraumatic syndrome, traumatic neurasthenia.*

posterior   Of or relating to the back (or dorsal) surface of an organ, structure, or body.

posterior atlanto-occipital membrane   One of a two broad, fibrous membranes located between the arch of the atlas and the occipital bone, which forms part of the atlanto-occipital joint and through which pass the vertebral artery and the suboccipital nerve.

posterior costotransverse ligament   One of the short, quadrangle-shaped ligaments that pass behind the costotransverse joint from the tip of each vertebral transverse process to the posterior surface of the neck of each rib below. Also called *lateral costotransverse ligament.*

posterior longitudinal ligament   A thick, fibrous band that runs vertically along the entire length of the spine and connects the posterior surfaces of the vertebral bodies.

posterior mediastinal node One of the lymph nodes located along the thoracic aorta that drains lymph from the esophagus, diaphragm, liver, and pericardium and sends lymph to the thoracic duct and inferior tracheobronchial nodes.

posterior mediastinum The portion of the mediastinum that lies between pericardium and the spine, containing the descending aorta, thoracic duct, esophagus, azygos veins, and vagus nerves.

posterior nares The two openings inside the nose that allow the passage of air between the nose and the nasopharynx. Also called *choanae.*

posterior tibial artery A division of the popliteal artery, which begins just below the popliteal space, passes behind the tibia, and serves the muscles of the lower leg and foot.

posterior tibialis pulse The pulse of the posterior tibial artery, which can be felt on the medial aspect of the ankle, just behind the prominence of the ankle bone.

posterior vein of the left ventricle One of the branches of the coronary sinus that serve the myocardium.

postinfectious glomerulonephritis Glomerulonephritis that may occur as a late complication of pharyngitis, particularly when due to streptococcal infection ("strep throat"). Also called *acute glomerulonephritis, acute poststreptococcal glomerulonephritis.*

postmature infant An infant who remains in the uterus until after the end of the normal 42 weeks of pregnancy.

postmenopausal Of or relating to the phase of life following the cessation of menses (menopause), or to a woman who is in this phase of life.

postpericardiotomy syndrome A condition characterized by the symptoms of pericarditis, which may include fever, that may occur repeatedly for weeks or months after pericardiotomy.

postpill amenorrhea The absence of normal menstrual cycles beyond 3 months after a woman discontinues the use of oral contraceptives.

postpolycythemic myeloid metaplasia A condition characterized by anemia, enlargement of the spleen, and hematopoiesis in the liver and spleen, which occurs commonly in individuals with polycythemia rubra vera.

postprandial (pp) After a meal.

postpuberty, postpubescence The period of development ranging from 1 to 2 years after puberty, characterized by a slowing in the growth of the bones and the establishment of physiologic functions of the reproductive years.

postural drainage The use of body positioning to promote drainage of secretions from the lungs and bronchi into the trachea.

posture The position of the body as a whole or of the limbs.

potassium (K) An alkaline metallic element with an atomic weight of 39.102 and the atomic number 19. This extremely abundant element always occurs in combination with other elements. The salts of potassium are commonly used medicinally.

potential trauma The existence of malocclusion of the teeth or a similar problem that presents a risk for tissue injury.

potentiation The interaction between two or more drugs given simultaneously in which the combined effect is greater than would occur if the agents had been given alone.

Pott's fracture A fracture of the lower part of the fibula and the malleolus of the tibia, resulting in the outward displacement of the foot.

poultice A pulpy, mushy preparation of powders or other absorbent substances, which may or may not be medicated, wet with watery or oily fluids and spread between layers of gauze or cloth.

 CLINICAL TIP A poultice is usually applied hot to the body surface to provide emollient, relaxing, stimulant, or counterirritant effects.

power of attorney An instrument authorizing another person to act as one's agent or attorney; an "attorney-in-fact." Power of attorney operates only with the continued consent of the person who granted it. If the grantor of the power should become incompetent or die, power of attorney is automatically revoked. Compare *durable power of attorney.*

poxvirus A member of the Poxviridae family of viruses, including the viruses that cause smallpox and molluscum contagiosum.

PPD *abbr* Purified protein derivative, the material used in testing for tuberculin sensitivity.

PPLO *abbr* pleuropneumonia-like organism.

PPV *abbr* positive pressure ventilation

p.r. *abbr* by rectum.

Pr Symbol for praseodymium.

Prader-Willi syndrome A congenital disorder characterized by short stature, mental retardation, excessive eating and severe obesity, and impaired maturity of the secondary sex characteristics.

praseodymium (Pr)   A metallic element in the rare earth group, with an atomic weight of 140.907 and the atomic number 59.

preagonal ascites   Ascites that forms just before death.

precipitate   1. To cause a substance in solution to separate from or settle out as a solid. 2. A solid, previously in solution, that has separated from or settled out.

precipitin   An antibody that can form with its specific, soluble antigen to create a complex that precipitates in solution. Also called *precipitating antibody.*

precordial   Of or relating to the precordium (plural: precordia) — the epigastrium and the anterior surface of the lower part of the thorax.

precordial movement   Any motion in the precordial area.

predictive hypothesis   A hypothesis formulated in an attempt to predict the effects of the interactions of certain variables.

predictive validity   An index of how well a test or measurement tool can be expected to measure future performance in a real-life task.

preeclampsia   An abnormal condition characterized by the development of hypertension during pregnancy, accompanied by edema or proteinuria, usually after the 20th week of gestation.

preferential anosmia   The loss of ability or inborn inability to perceive certain odors.

preferred provider organizations (PPO)   Entities through which employer health benefit plans and insurance carriers purchase health care service for members from a select group of providers.

pregnancy   The process and period of time from conception through birth.

pregnancy rate   The statistical expression of the ratio of pregnancies per 100 woman-years in a given population over a certain period of time. The rate is derived by multiplying the number of pregnancies by 1,200 months, dividing that product by the number of women observed, and multiplying this product by the number of months in the observation period.

preload   Stretching force exerted on the ventricular muscle by the blood it contains at the end of diastole.

premature   1. Immature; not completely developed. 2. An event or episode that occurs before the expected, usual, or appropriate time. 3. Of or relating to a premature infant.

premature atrial contraction (PAC)   An abnormal heart rhythm characterized by the occurrence of an atrial beat before the expected excitation. On an electrocardiogram,

PACs are demonstrated by the presence of an early P wave followed by a normal QRS complex.

premature infant   Any infant born before the end of the 37th week of pregnancy.

premature ventricular contraction (PVC)   A commonly occurring abnormal heart rhythm, usually not clinically significant, characterized by the occurrence of a ventricular beat before the expected electrical impulse. On an electrocardiogram, PVCs are demonstrated by the absence of a P wave and the presence of an early and wide QRS complex.

premenopausal   1. Of or relating to the period of time before the cessation of menstruation. 2. A woman who is premenopausal.

premenstrual syndrome (PMS)   A syndrome that occurs just prior to the onset of menstruation, characterized by any one or more of the following signs and symptoms: nervous tension, irritability, weight gain, edema, headache, breast tenderness, mastalgia, dysphoria, and lack of coordination occurring during the last few days of the menstrual cycle preceding the onset of menstruation.

premolar   One of the eight bicuspid teeth.

prenatal   Of or relating to the period of time before birth.

prenatal development   The development of an embryo and fetus from the moment of conception through birth.

prepatellar bursa   A bursa located in the knee joint, between the quadriceps tendon and the lower portion of the femur.

preprandial   Before a meal.

prepuberty   The 2 years (approximately) just before puberty during which the physical changes occur that lead, ultimately, to sexual maturity. These changes include increased skeletal growth and the appearance of secondary sex characteristics.

prepuce   The loose, retractable fold of skin that covers the glans penis. Also called *foreskin.*

presbycusis   Progressive, symmetrical, bilateral sensorineural hearing loss, usually of high frequency tones, caused by loss of hair cells in the organ of Corti.

presbyopia   A loss of visual acuity for distant objects, commonly occurring with advancing age.

prescreen   To evaluate patients to determine which should receive a particular treatment or diagnostic procedure, according to predetermined criteria.

prescription   A written order for medication, diagnostic testing, treatment, or therapeutic or prosthetic device given by a duly licensed health care professional and filled by a pharmacist or another person who is so authorized.

prescription drug   A medication that is available to the public only as prescribed by a duly licensed health care professional, as designated by the U.S. Food and Drug Administration.

presentation   The fetus' position in the uterus, especially referring to the portion of the fetus that will first enter the birth canal.

presomite embryo   The embryo before the appearance of somites, which usually occurs around 19 to 21 days postfertilization of the ovum in humans.

pressure   A force, usually measured in units of mass per unit of area (for example, pounds per square inch, or psi), that is applied to a surface by a fluid or an object.

pressure bandage   A strip or roll of gauze used to apply pressure, most commonly used to prevent edema, aid in blood clotting, or support varicose veins.

pressure dressing   A dressing in which pressure is exerted on the covered area to prevent fluids collecting in the underlying tissues, most commonly used for hemostasis.

pressure point   The area over any artery in which one can feel a pulse. Applying pressure to this point can help stop blood flowing from a wound.

presumed consent   A legal principle based upon the belief that a rational, prudent person would consent in the same situation, if able. Applies primarily to emergency care of unconscious patients, but may be expanded to cadaver organ donors.

presynaptic   1. Located before or proximate to a synapse. 2. Occurring prior to crossing a synapse.

presynaptic element   Any neurological structure (such as a neuron) that is located near a synapse.

presystolic   Pertaining to the beginning of systole.

pretibial fever   An acute infection marked by a rash on the pretibial region, and accompanied by headache, fever, chills, enlarged spleen, myalgia, and low white blood cell count. Caused by *Leptospira autumnalis*, the infection is transmitted to man through contact with the urine of infected animals or by water, soil, or vegetation contaminated by this urine.

prevalence   In epidemiology: the number of cases of a disease that are present in a population during a period in time. Prevalence is expressed as a ratio in which the number of events is the numerator and the population at risk is the denominator.

preventive   Serving to avert the occurrence of a disease or lessen its incidence.

preventive care   A method of nursing in which the goal is to maintain health and prevent disease. This care emphasizes early detection of disease, identifying those at risk, and counseling.

preventive treatment   Any course of action designed to either prevent the occurrence of a disease or prevent a mild disease from becoming worse.

priapism   Persistent abnormal erection of the penis, without sexual desire; It's commonly accompanied by pain and tenderness, and occurs in diseases and injuries of the spinal cord.

ALERT   If the patient has priapism, apply an ice pack to the penis, administer analgesics, and insert an indwelling urinary catheter to relieve bladder distention.

primary afferent fiber   A nerve fiber that conveys sensory impulses from the intrafusal fibers of the muscle spindle to the central nervous system.

primary amputation   The removal of a limb or other appendage after severe trauma; It's performed as soon as the patient recovers from shock and before the occurrence of infection.

primary apnea   Absence of breathing, which may be caused by a head injury. A self-limited condition, It's common immediately after birth; the newborn then breathes when carbon dioxide reaches a certain level.

primary atelectasis   A condition in which the lungs do not expand fully at birth, affecting premature infants and those under the effects of maternal anesthesia.

primary biliary cirrhosis   Chronic inflammation of the liver.

primary bronchus   One of two main air passages of the lungs. Branching from the trachea and conveying air to the lungs, the right and left primary bronchi are shaped differently (the right primary bronchus is wider and shorter, about 1″ [2.5 cm] long), so that most foreign objects in the trachea usually enter the right bronchus. See illustration on page 248.

primary carcinoma   A malignant new growth at the location of its origin.

primary dental caries   Dental caries appearing in previously healthy tooth enamel.

primary tuberculosis   The form of the disease occurring in childhood, usually affecting the lungs, the posterior pharynx and, less commonly, the skin.

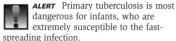 *ALERT*   Primary tuberculosis is most dangerous for infants, who are extremely susceptible to the fast-spreading infection.

Primary bronchus

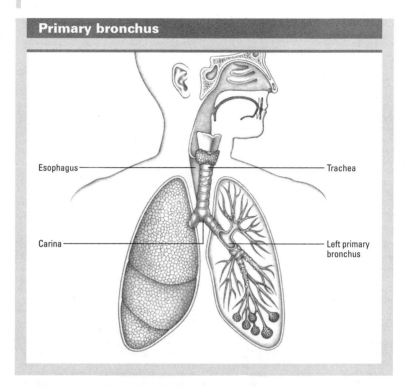

Esophagus — — Trachea

Carina — — Left primary bronchus

prime mover A muscle that directly brings about a specific movement.

primigravida A woman in her first pregnancy.

primitive groove A shallow linear depression, running lengthwise down the middle of the caudal end of the embryonic disc. Clearly visible during the third week in human embryos, it indicates the cephalocaudal axis resulting from the active involution of cells forming the primitive streak.

primitive node A small mass of tissue forming a knot or protuberance at the cephalic end of the primitive streak, occurring in the early stages of the development of human embryos and those of higher animals.

primitive reflex Any reflex that is normally present in an infant or fetus that later disappears; when an adult exhibits signs of reflexes common only in infants, It's usually an indication of serious neurological disease.

primitive ridge A ridge that borders the primitive groove in the early embryo.

primordial dwarf An abnormally undersized person with perfectly proportioned

head and extremities as well as normal intellectual and sexual development.

primordial germ cell A large round diploid cell, found in the early embryo, from which the oogonia and spermatogonia are later formed.

primordium, *pl.* primordia The earliest discernible indication during embryonic development of an organ, tissue, or part; anlage; rudiment.

PR interval The portion of an electrocardiogram between the onset of the P wave (atrial depolarization) and the onset of the QRS complex (ventricular depolarization); It's illustrated by an inverted U-shaped curve (beginning of P wave) that flattens out abruptly (Q wave) and then peaks sharply (R wave).

Prinzmetal's angina A variant of angina pectoris, a form of unstable angina, in which the attacks occur during rest. Attacks are indicated by an ST-segment elevation on an electrocardiogram.

PRL *abbr* prolactin.

p.r.n. *abbr pro re nata*, which means "as needed" in Latin. In other words, the patient's needs determine the schedule of administration.

proarrhythmia   Rhythm disturbance caused or made worse by drugs or other therapies.

procaryotae   In bacteriology: a kingdom of plants with two divisions, Cyanobacteria and Bacteria, including all cellular organisms in which the nucleoplasm has no basic protein and lacks a true nucleus.

proctitis   Condition in which rectum and anus become inflamed as a result of trauma, infection, drugs, allergy, or radiation injury.

proctologist   A physician who specializes in the branch of medicine called proctology.

proctology   The branch of medicine concerned with the colon, rectum, and anus.

proctoscope   A speculum or tubular instrument containing a light and a magnifying lens for inspecting the rectum and the distal portion of the colon.

prodromal labor   The early stage of labor prior to the strong and frequent contractions that result in progressive dilation of the uterine cervix.

prodrome   1. A symptom indicating the onset of a disease. 2. The earliest stage of a disease.

professional liability   A legal concept describing the obligation of a professional person to pay a patient or client for damages caused by the professional's act of omission, commission, or negligence, after a court determines that the professional was negligent. Professional liability better describes the responsibility of all professionals to their clients than does the concept of malpractice, but the idea of professional liability is central to malpractice.

progenitive   Capable of producing offspring or descendants; reproductive.

progenitor   1. A parent or ancestor. 2. Precursor; a person or thing that precedes.

progeny   1. Offspring; the result of a specific mating, whether of individuals or organisms. 2. The descendants of a known or common ancestor.

progeria   A congenital syndrome in which there is extreme premature aging in childhood; symptoms include gray hair, wrinkled skin, lack of pubic and facial hair, small stature, and the posture and physique of an aged person. Death from coronary artery disease commonly occurs before age 10.

prognathism   Projection of the jaw.

prognosis   A forecast as to the expected outcome of a disease, depending upon the characteristics of the patient and taking into consideration the outcome of the disease in previous patients with similar characteristics.

progressive systemic sclerosis   The most common form of scleroderma, which is characterized by induration and thickening of the skin and by fibrotic degenerative changes in various body organs, including the heart, lungs, kidneys, and GI tract.

prokaryote   Cellular organisms lacking a true nucleus and a nuclear membrane; therefore, nuclear material occurs throughout the cytoplasm. Examples of prokaryocytes include viruses, bacteria, chlamydiae, rickettsiae, actinomycetes, mycoplasmas, and some algae.

prolactin (PRL)   A hormone secreted by special cells of the anterior pituitary gland, which in conjunction with other hormones (estrogen, progesterone, thyroxine, insulin, growth hormone, glucocorticoids, and human placental lactogen), is responsible for stimulating the development and growth of the mammary glands in postpartum mammals.

prolapse   The falling down or sinking of a part from its normal position in the body, as in prolapse of the uterus, rectum, or anus.

promethium (Pm)   A radioactive, rare-earth, metallic chemical element; atomic number, 61; atomic weight, 147.

promyelocyte   A large, single nucleus blood cell whose presence in the circulating blood is abnormal.

pronation   1. The act of assuming the prone position, in which the ventral surface of the body is downward. 2. The act of turning the forearm so the palm is downward and backward. 3. The act of lowering the medial margin of the foot during an outward rotation.

pronator reflex   A reaction to tapping the distal end of the radius or ulna while holding the hand vertically; the result is pronation of the patient's forearm.

pronator teres   A forearm muscle which arises from a humeral and an ulnar head.

prone   1. Lying face downward. 2. Referring to a hand whose palm is facing downward.

proneness profile   A screening process during prenatal care that examines the possibility of problems occurring in development for the newborn. The process should begin as early as possible and continue after the newborn's delivery.

pronephric duct   One of a pair of ducts present in the early stages of vertebrate embryonic development connecting the pronephric tubules with the cloaca.

prophase   The initial stage in cell reduplication in mitosis as well as in the two meiotic divisions.

prophylaxis Prevention of disease, in which chemical or mechanical agents may be used to prevent infection.

propionic fermentation The creation of propionic acid as a result of using bacteria to ferment sugars or lactic acid.

proprioceptive reflex Any involuntary reaction to stimulation of proprioceptive receptors (such as when the respiratory rate increases during exercise).

proprioceptor Sensory nerve terminals (such as those found in muscles, tendons, joints, and the vestibular apparatus), that respond to stimuli to provide information about movements and position of the body.

proptosis Abnormal protrusion of an organ or area of the body.

prosopothoracopagus Equal conjoined twins who are united laterally in the frontal plane, the fusion extending from the oral region through the thorax.

prostaglandin (PG) Any of a group of components derived from extremely potent unsaturated fatty acids that act like hormones in the cells in which they are synthesized and surrounding cells.

prostate A male gland that contributes a secretion to the seminal fluid causing the liquefaction of the coagulated semen. The prostate surrounds the neck of the bladder and the urethra.

prostatectomy Surgical procedure in which the entire prostate gland or a portion of It's removed, as a result of either a benign or malignant growth.

prostatic catheter A long instrument for male catheterization (about 16″ [40.5 cm]) with a short angular tip for passing an enlarged prostate obstructing the urethra.

prostatic ductule One of many small excretory tubes carrying the secretion of the prostate gland and opening into the prostatic portion of the urethra.

prostatitis Chronic condition in which the prostate gland becomes inflamed, usually from infection.

prosthesis, *pl.* prostheses 1. An artificial substitute for a missing body part, such as a limb or eye. 2. A device used for functional reasons, as in a hearing aid.

prostrate Lying face down on a surface.

prostration Extreme exhaustion.

protactinium (Pa) A radioactive metallic chemical element; atomic number, 91; atomic weight, 231.

protease Any enzyme that catalyzes the breakdown of protein.

protein Any of a group of complex organic compounds containing carbon, hydrogen, nitrogen, oxygen, and usually sulfur. Some compounds contain phosphorus, iron, iodine, or other essential elements. Proteins consist essentially of combinations of amino acids; each protein has a unique, genetically defined sequence of amino acids that determines its shape and function.

protein-calorie malnutrition Spectrum of disorders resulting from either prolonged or chronic inadequate protein or calorie intake, or from high metabolic requirements for protein and energy.

protein-energy malnutrition A deficiency of protein and energy (calories); spectrum of disorders resulting from prolonged, chronic or inadequate protein or caloric intake, or high metabolic protein and energy requirements. Disorders that commonly lead to PEM include cancer, GI disorders, chronic heart failure, alcoholism, and conditions with high metabolic needs, such as burns.

proteolipid A form of lipoprotein that is mostly composed of lipid material (more than half of the molecule).

proteolysis The splitting of proteins by the addition of water to the peptide bonds.

Proteus A genus of motile, gram-negative, rod-shaped bacteria normally found in fecal material, water, and soil.

CLINICAL TIP Commonly found in patients treated with oral antibiotics, the infections are associated with urinary tract infections, pyelonephritis, abdominal and wound infections, diarrhea, bacteremia, and endotoxic shock.

prothrombin The precursor of thrombin, this plasma protein forms thrombin when exposed to thromboplastin and calcium; thrombin is the initial stage for formation of blood clots.

prothrombin time (PT) A one-stage test that identifies abnormalities in plasma coagulation as a result of a deficiency of factors V, VII, or X.

protocol A description of specific steps in patient care for a particular condition or circumstance; may also describe how to administer a medication.

protoporphyria A disorder characterized by excessive levels of protoporphyrin in the feces and a wide variety of photosensitive skin changes.

protoporphyrin A kind of porphyrin that, in combination with ferrous iron and protein, forms hemoglobin, catalase, and myoglobin. The only naturally occurring isomer, It's an intermediate in heme biosynthesis.

protozoa, *sing.* protozoon The simplest organisms of the animal kingdom, Protozoa have more complex structures than bacteria. These unicellular organisms range in size from submicroscopic to macroscopic;

as self-contained units with organelles, they are responsible for complex functions, such as nutrition, excretion, and respiration, and can attach to other organisms.

protozoal infection   An illness caused by unicellular microorganisms of the class Protozoa.

provitamin   A precursor of a vitamin; a substance present in some foods that may be converted into a vitamin by the body.

proximal   Nearest to.

proximal radioulnar articulation   The pivot joint between the radial head, the ulna, and the annular ligament, which is responsible for the motion of the head of the radius in pronation and supination.

proximal renal tubular acidosis (proximal RTA)   A disorder in which there is an abnormal amount of acid accumulation and excessive secretion of bicarbonate.

prurigo   Any of several types of skin eruptions in which there is an encrusted, dome-shaped papule, characterized by chronic inflammation and itching.

pruritus   Itching; an unpleasant sensation that leads to rubbing or scratching the skin in an effort to obtain relief. Scratching the skin may lead to secondary infection.

pruritus ani   Intense chronic itching in the anal area.

PSA   *abbr* prostate-specific antigen.

psammoma body   A round mass of chalky material found in benign and malignant tissue neoplasms as well as in some tissue that is chronically inflamed.

pseudesthesia   A feeling or sensation not linked to an external stimulus or one not corresponding appropriately to the stimulus causing it (such as phantom limb pain).

pseudocyst   An abnormal cavity resembling a cyst that contains fluid but is not lined with epithelium.

pseudogene   In molecular genetics: a deoxyribonucleic acid sequence that is similar to a gene and may be derived from one, but does not function as one.

pseudojaundice   A condition in which the skin has a yellowish color that is caused by blood changes rather than by hyperbilirubinemia.

pseudomembranous stomatitis   A condition in which the mouth becomes extremely inflamed and produces a membrane-like exudate.

pseudomonad   A bacterium of the genus *Pseudomonas.*

Pseudomonas   A genus of gram-negative bacteria known for their fluorescent pigments and strength with which they resist antibiotics. The genus comprises several hundred species, including several found in soil and water and some pathogens (such as *Pseudomonas aeruginosa)* that cause severe and commonly fatal infections involving the urinary tract, wounds, abscesses, and the bloodstream.

psittacosis   A chronic respiratory and systemic disease caused by the bacterium *Chlamydia psittaci,* which can be transmitted to humans and other animals by infected birds, especially parrots. This disease may be asymptomatic or marked by mild influenza-type symptoms or by a severe, fatal pneumonia.

psoas major   An abdominal muscle that flexes the thigh or trunk, originating from the lumbar vertebrae and the fibrocartilages and the lower thoracic vertebrae and the lumbar vertebrae.

 ALERT If you elicit a positive psoas sign in a patient with abdominal pain, suspect appendicitis.

psoriasis   A common, chronic dermatologic condition with polygenic inheritance. Marked by rounded red lesions covered by grayish or silvery white dry scales, psoriasis is caused by an overabundance of epithelial cells. Affected areas include nails, scalp, genitalia, and the lumbosacral region.

psoriatic arthritis   A type of rheumatoid arthritis in which patches of psoriasis affect the skin and nails, especially the joints of the fingers and toes. This chronic systemic disease is shown as a "pencil in cup" deformity on an X-ray.

PSVT   *abbr* paroxysmal supraventricular tachycardia.

psychiatric nurse practitioner   A nurse practitioner with special training in the treatment of mental disorders.

psychiatric nursing   The branch of nursing specializing in the treatment of mental disorders. Theories of human behavior and the use of the self are essential to this type of nursing practice.

psychiatry   The branch of medicine that concerns itself with the causes, treatment, and prevention of mental disorders.

psychoanalyst   One who specializes in psychoanalysis (usually a psychiatrist) and uses psychoanalytic theory to treat patients.

psychobiology   1. The study of how the body and mind interact to affect personality development. 2. A theory introduced by Adolf Meyer that views an individual as an integrated unit, emphasizing the biological, emotional, and sociocultural factors that determine a human being's psychological makeup or mental status.

psychologist   One who specializes in the study of psychology.

psychology 1. The branch of science that studies the mind and its processes, particularly how It's affected by environment. 2. A profession that applies theories and techniques to understand and treat an individual's problems, particularly the relationship between the person and his environment. 3. The thought processes, behavior, and attitudes of a human being.

psychomotor development A child's gradual achievement of tasks requiring cognitive skills and muscular strength (e.g., the infant's ability to turn over, sit, and crawl; the toddler's ability to walk, talk, control excretory functions, and begin solving cognitive problems).

psychophysics The science that deals with the relationship between patterns of physical stimuli and sensory responses.

Pt Symbol for platinum.

PT *abbr* prothrombin time.

PTA *abbr* plasma thromboplastin antecedent.

PTCA *abbr* percutaneous transluminal coronary angioplasty.

pterygium An abnormal, thick, triangular fold of membrane extending medially from the nasal border of the cornea to the inner canthus of the eye.

pterygoideus lateralis One of the muscles responsible for mastication.

pterygoid plexus A network of veins, located between the temporalis and the pterygoideus lateralis, that drains into the facial vein and extends between structures in the infratemporal fossa.

PTH *abbr* parathyroid hormone.

ptosis An abnormality in which the upper eyelid droops, either congenitally, as a result of a weak levator muscle, or due to paralysis of the third cranial nerve.

TIME LINE Astigmatism and myopia may be associated with childhood ptosis. Congenital ptosis is typically discovered by an infant's parents; this ptosis is unilateral, constant, and accompanied by lagophthalmos, which causes the infant to sleep with open eyes.

PTT *abbr* partial thromboplastin time.

ptyalism Excessive flow of saliva; sometimes occurring in early pregnancy.

Pu Symbol for plutonium.

pubarche The beginning of puberty, in which secondary sexual characteristics begin to develop (such as beginning of growth of pubic hair).

pubic symphysis The pelvic joint, which consists of two pubic bones divided by a fibrocartilage disk and connected by two ligaments.

pubis, *pl.* **pubes** One of two pubic bones that, in conjunction with the ischium and the ilium, form the hip bone; these bones connect the pubic bone from the opposite side at the symphysis pubis.

pubococcygeus exercises Isometric exercises intended to help the vaginal introitus contract or to avoid leakage of urine by voluntarily contracting the muscles of the pelvic diaphragm and perineum.

pudendal block A type of local anesthesia that dulls the pain during the expulsive second stage of labor.

pudendal nerve A branch of the pudendal plexus that arises from the second, third, and fourth sacral nerves. Passing between the piriformis and coccygeus, the pudendal nerve leaves the pelvis through the greater sciatic foramen.

pudendum, *pl.* **pudenda** The external genitalia of humans, especially of women. The female pudendum consists of the mons veneris, the labia majora, the labia minora, the vestibule of the vagina, the urinary meatus, and the vestibular glands. The male pudendum consists of the penis, scrotum, and testes.

puerperal 1. Of or pertaining to the period from the end of childbirth until involution of the uterus is complete (usually 3 to 6 weeks). 2. Of or pertaining to a woman (puerpera) who has just given birth to an infant.

puerperal fever A condition, marked by systemic bacterial infection and septicemia, affecting puerperal women as a result of unsterile obstetric practices.

puerperium The period of time beginning immediately after childbirth and ending when the involution of the uterus is complete (approximately 6 weeks) during which a woman adjusts to the changing needs of her body.

pulmonary, pulmonic Of or pertaining to the lungs or the respiratory system.

pulmonary alveolus A terminal air sac of the lung in which the exchange of oxygen and carbon dioxide takes place.

pulmonary arteriolar resistance (PAR) The loss of pressure per unit of blood flow from the pulmonary artery to a pulmonary vein.

pulmonary artery wedge pressure (PAWP) The force in the capillary end of the pulmonary artery, measured by catheterizing a branch of the pulmonary artery and inflating a balloon at its tip. This force is an indication of mean left atrial pressure and left ventricular end-diastolic pressure. Also called *pulmonary wedge pressure.*

pulmonary atrium   One of many spaces at the end of an alveolar duct into which alveoli open.
pulmonary edema   An abnormal condition in which extravascular fluid is accumulated in lung tissues and alveoli.
pulmonary embolism (PE)   Foreign matter that forms a blockage in a pulmonary artery; this blockage could be caused by fat, air, tumor tissue, or a thrombus that usually arises from a peripheral vein.
pulmonary function test (PFT)   A method of examining the lung's capacity to make an efficient exchange of oxygen and carbon dioxide.
pulmonic stenosis   A cardiac disorder in which the right ventricle of the heart has concentric hypertrophy with a small increase in diastolic volume.
pulp   Any soft, spongy animal or vegetable tissue (such as pulp present within the spleen, the pulp chamber of the tooth, or the distal phalanges of the fingers and the toes).
pulpitis   Inflammation of the dental pulp, usually the result of bacterial infection.
pulse   1. A rhythmic beating or vibrating movement. 2. A brief electromagnetic wave. 3. The expansion and contraction of an artery in a regular, rhythmic pattern; this happens when the left ventricle of the heart ejects blood as it contracts, thus causing waves of pressure.
pulse deficit   The difference between the ventricular rate measured at the heart's apex and the arterial rate of the radial pulse.
pulse point   One of many sites on the body's surface in which arterial pulsations can be easily palpated; one of the most common sites is the point over the wrist's radial artery.
pulse pressure   The numerical difference between the systolic and diastolic pressures, usually 30 to 40 mm Hg.
pulsus alternans   A pulse in which the weak and strong beats alternate regularly without changing the cycle length.
pulsus paradoxus   An pulse in which there is a large decrease in systolic pressure and pulse-wave amplitude during inspiration, as commonly happens in constrictive pericarditis.

ALERT   A paradoxical pulse may signal cardiac tamponade — a life-threatening complication of pericardial effusion occuring when sufficient blood or fluid accumulates and compresses the heart.
punch biopsy   The surgical removal and microscopic examination of tissue for purposes of diagnosis; this tissue is obtained by a punch, an instrument used for indenting,

perforating, or excising a segment of tissue. For example, a punch is used to extract bone marrow from the sternum.
punch forceps   An instrument used in surgery to excise a portion of tissue (such as bone or cartilage).
punctum lacrimale, *pl.* **puncta lacrimalia**   A small opening on the lacrimal papilla of an eyelid into which tears drain to enter the lacrimal canaliculi.
puncture wound   An injury in which the skin is penetrated by a sharp object (such as a knife or glass fragment).
punitive damages   Punitive damages are compensation in excess of actual damages as a form of punishment to the wrongdoer, and reparation to the injured; awarded only in rare instances of malicious and willful misconduct. Also called *exemplary damages.* Compare *general damages, special damages.*
Punnett square   A diagram in the form of a checkerboard that shows how many different combinations of male and female gametes are possible when one or more pairs of independent alleles are crossed.
pupil   The round opening at the center of the iris that allows light to enter the eye.
purified protein derivative (PPD)   A form of tuberculin that is introduced into the skin to test for tubercle bacilli infection; if a past or present infection exists, there may be a positive reaction within 48 to 72 hours.
purine   One of many colorless crystalline nitrogenous compounds, which are end products in the digestion of certain proteins; some purines are synthesized in the body.
Purkinje's fibers   Muscle fibers that spread through the heart in a complex network to convey the impulses necessary for the near-simultaneous contraction of the right and left ventricles.
purpura   A group of hemorrhagic diseases, characterized by lesions, ecchymoses or petechiae, and a tendency to bruise easily.

CLINICAL TIP   Purpura may be caused by a change in the number of platelets, vascular defects, or reactions to certain drugs.
pus   A creamy, viscous, liquid inflammation product, usually yellow or yellow-green, caused by liquefaction necrosis.
P value   In research: the statistical probability that a given finding will occur by chance alone compared with the known distribution of possible findings.
PVC   *abbr* 1. polyvinyl chloride. 2. premature ventricular contraction.
PVR   *abbr* pulmonary vascular resistance.
P wave   The portion of the cardiac cycle that is represented as an inverted U-shaped curve on an electrocardiogram. Following the

end of the T wave and preceding the spike of the QRS complex, the P wave shows atrial depolarization, in which the atria pump blood into the ventricles.

PWP *abbr* pulmonary wedge pressure.

pyelogram A radiograph of the kidneys and ureters, especially showing the pelvis of the kidney. An I.V. pyelogram uses a radiopaque dye to show the size and location of the kidneys, any cysts that might exist there, the outline of the ureters and bladder, the filling of the renal pelvises, and the patency of the urinary tract.

pyelonephritis Inflammation of the kidney and its pelvis.

pygoamorphus Unequal conjoined twins in which the parasite is an amorphous mass attached to the sacral region of the more developed twin.

pyloric orifice The opening of the stomach into the duodenum positioned at the level of the cranial border of the first lumbar vertebra.

pyloric sphincter A muscular ring that separates the pylorus from the duodenum in the stomach.

pyloric stenosis A condition in which the pyloric sphincter becomes thinner at the outlet at the stomach, which causes a blockage in the small intestine preventing the flow of food.

pyloroplasty An operation in which incision of the pylorus and reconstruction of the pyloric channel is performed to eliminate an obstruction or accelerate gastric emptying to treat a gastric ulcer.

pylorospasm A spasm of the pylorus (for example, as in pyloric stenosis).

pylorus, *pl.* pylori, pyloruses The portion of the stomach surrounded by a strong band of circular muscle; stomach contents travel through the pylorus and are emptied into the duodenum.

pyorrhea 1. A pus discharge. 2. An inflammation of the tissues surrounding the teeth, as occurring in periodontitis.

pyosalpinx A condition in which pus collects in a fallopian tube.

pyramidal tract Two groups of fibers in the spinal cord in which motor impulses are conveyed to the anterior horn cells from the opposite side of the brain.

pyridoxine One of the B complex vitamins, derived from pyridine. This water-soluble vitamin is converted in the body to pyridoxal and pyridamin for synthesis.

pyrogen A fever-producing substance (such as some bacterial toxins).

pyrosis A burning sensation, commonly as a result of the reflux of highly acidic stomach contents; possibly a symptom of esophagitis.

pyrrole A type of organic compound; its derivatives are used in the manufacture of pharmaceuticals and may be added to whole blood or to plasma as a preservative.

pyruvic acid The end product of glucose metabolism.

pyuria The presence of pus in the urine, commonly a sign of urinary tract infection.

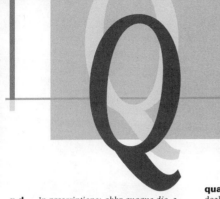

q.d.   In prescriptions: *abbr quaque die,* a Latin phrase meaning "every day."

Q fever   An acute febrile illness, usually respiratory, caused by *Coxiella burnetii.*

q.h.   In prescriptions: *abbr quaque hora,* a Latin phrase meaning "every hour."

qi   Pronounced "chee," this vital energy or "life force" flows through the body along invisible channels and influences bodily functions, according to traditional Chinese medicine. An obstruction or imbalance of *qi* results in illness.

Qigong   Pronounced "chee goong," this ancient Chinese health discipline consists of breathing exercises, deep concentration, and physical exercises aimed at balancing *qi* to maintain health and prevent disease.

q.i.d.   In prescriptions: *abbr quater in die,* a Latin phrase meaning "four times a day."

QRS complex   Part of the cardiac cycle that appears on an electrocardiogram as a sharp positive or negative deflection following the less acute curve of the P wave and preceding the ST segment. It represents ventricular depolarization, in which the electrical impulse is conducted over the bundle of His and the Purkinje fibers, causing ventricular contraction.

q.s.   In prescriptions: *abbr quantum satis,* a Latin phrase meaning "quantity required."

quadriceps femoris   The great extensor muscle of the anterior thigh that forms a large dense mass covering the front and sides of the femur and is composed of the rectus femoris, the vastus lateralis, the vastus medialis, and the vastus intermedius.

quadrigeminal pulse   A pulse in which a pause occurs after every fourth beat.

quadriplegia   Paralysis of the arms, legs, and trunk of the body below the level of an associated injury to the spinal cord.

qualitative   Of or referring to the quality, value, or nature of something.

quality of life   A legal and ethical standard that's determined by relative suffering or pain, not by the degree of disability.

quantum theory   In physics: theory that deals with the interaction of matter and electromagnetic radiation according to which radiation consists of small units of energy called *quanta.*

quarantine   **1.** Isolation of people with communicable disease or those exposed to communicable disease during the contagious period to prevent spread of the illness. **2.** A period (usually 40 days) of detaining travelers or vessels originating from an infected area to allow for inspection or disinfection.

quartan   Referring to the 4th day or recurring at 72-hour intervals.

quartan malaria   Malaria caused by *Plasmodium malariae* that's characterized by febrile paroxysms occurring every 72 hours.

Queckenstedt's test   A test in which the jugular vein on each side of the neck is compressed alternately to detect a spinal canal obstruction. The pressure of the spinal fluid is measured by a manometer that's connected to a lumbar puncture needle or catheter.

Queensland tick typhus   A tick-borne infection caused by *Rickettsia australis* that occurs in Australia and resembles mild Rocky Mountain spotted fever.

quellung reaction   The swelling of the capsule of a bacterium, usually observed when the organism is exposed to specific antisera.

quickening   The first notable fetal movement in utero, usually occurring at 16 to 20 weeks' gestation.

Quincke's pulse   An alternate blanching and reddening of the skin, such as by pressing the front edge of the fingernail and watching the blood in the nail bed recede and return.

Quincke's sign   Alternate blanching and flushing of the skin.

quinidine   Antiarrhythmic drug used to treat atrial flutter, atrial fibrillation, premature ventricular contractions, and tachycardia.

quinine   White, bitter crystalline alkaloid made from cinchona bark that's used in antimalarial medications.

quinolones Class of synthetic broad-spectrum antibacterial drugs displaying bactericidal action.

quinone Term used for a group of aromatic compounds that bear two oxygens instead of two hydrogens.

quintuplet One of five children born at one birth.

Q wave Part of the cardiac cycle that appears on the electrocardiogram as a short abrupt downward line from the end of the tail of the P wave. It represents the first part of the QRS complex, but usually isn't prominent; its absence may be without clinical significance.

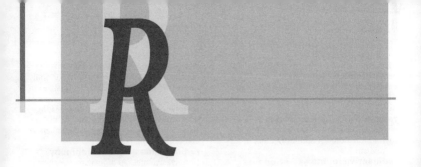

rabies An acute, usually fatal, infectious disease of the central nervous system spread by animals to people through contaminated saliva, blood, or tissue. Animal reservoirs include skunks, bats, foxes, dogs, raccoons, and cats, but almost never rodents.

rabies immune globulin (RIG) Antirabies immune globulin.

rabies vaccine A sterile suspension of killed rabies virus prepared from human diploid cells. Also called *HDCV.*

race A class of genetically related individuals who share specific physical characteristics.

racemose Similar in appearance to a bunch of grapes, used in describing structures in which many branches terminate in nodular, cystlike forms.

racemose aneurysm A significant dilation of long, tortuous blood vessels; some may be up to 20 times their normal size.

rachicentesis Lumbar puncture.

rachitic **1.** Of or related to rickets. **2.** Similar to a rickets-afflicted individual.

rachitis **1.** Rickets. **2.** An inflammatory disease of the vertebral column.

racial immunity Natural immunity commonly occurring in most members of a race.

rad *abbr* radiation absorbed dose; basic unit of absorbed dose of ionizing radiation. One rad is equivalent to the absorption of 100 ergs of radiation energy per gram of matter.

radial artery An artery in the forearm, beginning at the bifurcation of the brachial artery, passing in 12 branches to the forearm, wrist, and hand.

radial keratotomy A surgical procedure for treating myopia in which several tiny incisions are made on the cornea.

radial nerve The largest branch of the brachial plexus, beginning on each side as a continuation of the posterior cord.

radial pulse The pulse of the radial artery palpated at the wrist over the radius. The radial pulse is commonly taken because of the ease with which it's palpated.

radial recurrent artery Part of the radial artery, arising distal to the elbow, ascend-

ing between the branches of the radial nerve, and supplying several muscles of the arm and elbow.

radial reflex Flexion of the forearm when the distal radius is tapped.

radiant energy Energy released by electromagnetic radiation, such as radio waves, light, X-rays, and gamma rays.

radiation **1.** The release of energy, rays, or waves. **2.** In medicine: the use of a radioactive substance for diagnosing or treating a disease.

radical A group of atoms that acts together and forms a component of a compound; it can't exist in a free state.

radical mastectomy Surgical removal of an entire breast, pectoral muscles, axillary lymph nodes, and all fat, fascia, and adjacent tissues, usually in the treatment of breast cancer.

radical neck dissection Surgical dissection and removal of lymph nodes and removable tissues under the skin of the neck, performed to prevent the spread of malignant tumors of the head and neck that may be controlled.

radicotomy, radiculectomy Sectioning of nerve roots of the spine to relieve pain or spastic paralysis.

radiculomeningomyelitis Inflammation of the nerve roots, the spinal cord, and its covering.

radioactive Emitting radiation due to disintegration of the nucleus of an atom.

radioactive contamination The undesirable addition of radioactive material to the skin or environment.

radioactive contrast media A solution or colloid containing materials of high atomic number that's used in diagnostic radiology to observe soft-tissue structures.

radioactive decay Disintegration of the nucleus of an unstable nuclide by the spontaneous release of charged particles or photons, or both.

radioactive element An element capable of spontaneous degeneration of its nucle-

257

us, accompanied by the release of alpha or beta particles or gamma rays.

radioactive iodine (RAI, sodium iodide) (^{131}I)   A thyroid hormone antagonist.

radioactive iodine excretion   The elimination of radioactive iodine given in a thyroid function test and for treating hyperthyroidism.

radioactive iodine excretion test   A technique for determining thyroid function by measuring the quantity of radioactive iodine in urine after a patient is given an oral tracer dose of the radioisotope ^{131}I.

radioactive iodine uptake (RAIU)   The absorption of radioactive iodine by the thyroid, given orally as a tracer dose in a thyroid function test and in larger doses for treating hyperthyroidism.

 ALERT Below normal iodine uptake may be caused by renal failure, diuresis, severe diarrhea, X-ray contrast media studies, or ingestion of such iodine preparations as iodized salt, cough syrups, and some multivitamins.

radioallergosorbent test (RAST)   A test in which radioimmunoassay is used to identify and measure immunoglobulin E antibodies in serum.

radiobiology   Branch of science focused on the cellular and tissue response to radiation.

radiocarpal articulation   The condyloid joint at the wrist connecting the radius and distal surface of an articular disk with the scaphoid, lunate, and triangular bones.

radiochemistry   Branch of chemistry that deals with the study of radioactive materials and their use in treating diseases.

radiographic magnification   Observation by magnification achieved with a small X-ray tube; a common diagnostic tool in orthopedics.

radiography   The production of shadow images on photographic emulsion by ionizing radiation.

radioimmunoassay (RIA)   A radiologic technique that may be used to measure the serum level of an antigen, antibody, or other proteins.

radioiodine   A radioactive iodine isotope used in the treatment of certain thyroid disorders and in scanning techniques in diagnostic radiology.

radioisotope   A radioactive isotope of an element, used in diagnosis and treatment of diseases.

radioisotope scan   A two-dimensional image of the gamma rays released by a radioisotope, showing its occurrence in a spe-

cific body site. In diagnostic scanning, the radioactive isotope may be given I.V. or orally.

radiologist   A doctor who specializes in radiology.

radiology   Branch of medicine dealing with radioactive substances and the diagnosis and treatment of disease using ionizing and nonionizing radiation.

radionuclide angiocardiography   Noninvasive method of imaging the chest in which a radionuclide, such as thallium or technetium, is circulated through the heart and major vessels to assess ventricular function.

radiopaque   A material that doesn't allow X-rays or other radiant energy to pass through. Because bones are relatively radiopaque, they appear as white areas on an exposed X-ray film.

radiopaque dye   A chemical substance that doesn't let X-rays pass through it. Radiopaque iodine compounds are commonly used to delineate the inside of hollow organs, such as heart chambers and blood vessels.

radiopharmaceutical   A drug that demonstrates spontaneous disintegration of unstable nuclei with the release of nuclear particles or photons.

radiopharmacist   A person specialized in the clinical aspects of radiopharmacy, who prepares and dispenses prescribed radioactive tracers.

radiopharmacy   A facility where radioactive drugs are prepared and dispensed and where radioactive and other related materials are stored.

radioreceptor assay (RRA)   Sensitive, reliable blood test to detect human chorionic gonadotropin by means of a gamma counter to reveal radioactivity; can detect pregnancy as early as 1 week after conception.

radioresistance   The resistance of cells, tissues, organs, organisms, or any substances to the adverse effects of radiation.

radioresistant   Unaffected by or protected against damage by radioactive emissions, such as X-rays, alpha particles, or gamma rays.

radiosensitive   Sensitive to radioactive emissions, such as X-rays, alpha particles, or gamma rays.

radiosensitivity   Susceptibility of cells, tissues, organs, organisms, or other substances to the effects of radiation.

radiotherapy   The treatment of neoplastic disease by ionizing radiation.

radium (Ra)   A radioactive metallic element of the alkaline-earth group with atomic number 88 and atomic weight 226.

Passive range of motion exercises

ABDUCTION

ADDUCTION

DORSIFLEXION

PLANTAR FLEXION

EXTENSION

FLEXION

EXTERNAL ROTATION

INTERNAL ROTATION

EVERSION

INVERSION

SUPINATION

PRONATION

radon (Rn)   A radioactive, inert, gaseous, nonmetallic element with atomic number 86 and atomic weight 222.

RAI   *abbr* radioactive iodine.

RAIU   *abbr* radioactive iodine uptake.

RA latex test   *abbr* rheumatoid arthritis latex test.

rale   An abnormal respiratory sound heard in auscultation during inspiration, characterized by discontinuous bubbling noises, indicating a pathologic condition.

CLINICAL TIP Fine rales have a crackling sound, and medium rales are medium-pitched bubbling or gurgling sounds, whereas coarse rales have a lower pitch.

Ramsay Hunt syndrome   A neurologic disorder caused by a varicella-zoster virus in-fection that's characterized by severe ear pain, facial nerve paralysis, vertigo, hearing loss, and generalized encephalitis.

ramus, *pl.* rami   A small, branchlike structure extending from a larger one or dividing into two parts, such as a branch of a nerve or artery.

range of motion (ROM) exercise   Range through which a muscle or joint can be extended and flexed.

ranula   A cyst lying under the tongue because of obstruction by a salivary duct or mucous gland.

raptus haemorrhagicus   An unexpected, massive hemorrhage.

RAS   *abbr* reticular activating system.

ray   A beam of radiation moving in a direction away from the source.

Raynaud's phenomenon Intermittent bilateral ischemic attacks of the fingers or toes and, sometimes, the ears or nose, that are characterized by severe pallor and usually accompanied by paresthesia and pain.

Rb Symbol for rubidium.

RBC *abbr* red blood cell.

RBE *abbr* relative biological effectiveness.

RCP *abbr* Royal College of Physicians.

RCPSC *abbr* Royal College of Physicians and Surgeons of Canada.

RCS *abbr* Royal College of Surgeons.

RDA *abbr* recommended daily allowance; dietary needs as outlined by the Food and Nutritional Board, National Academy of Sciences Research Council.

RDS *abbr* respiratory distress syndrome.

reabsorption Act or process of absorbing again.

Reach to Recovery A national volunteer organization that offers counseling and support to women who have breast cancer and to their families. Many of the members have had mastectomies themselves.

reaction A response to a substance, treatment, or other stimulus.

reagent A substance involved in a chemical reaction.

reapproximate To rejoin tissues separated by surgery or trauma and restore their anatomic relationship.

rebound 1. Recovery from illness. 2. A sudden contraction of muscle following relaxation, usually observed when inhibitory reflexes are lost.

rebound tenderness Inflammation of the peritoneum indicated by pain that occurs by the sudden release of a hand pressing on the abdomen.

 ALERT Rebound tenderness is a reliable sign of peritonitis. If you discover rebound tenderness in a patient who's experiencing constant, severe abdominal pain; quickly take his vital signs and monitor continuously for signs of shock, such as hypotension and tachycardia.

rebreathing bag In anesthesia: a flexible bag attached to a mask that acts as a reservoir for anesthetic gases during surgery or for oxygen during resuscitation. The bag may be squeezed to pump gas or air into the lungs.

receiver In communication theory: the person to whom a message is sent.

recess A small hollow cavity such as the epitympanic recess in the tympanic cavity of the inner ear.

recessive gene 1. Of, related to, or describing a gene, the effect of which isn't evident or hidden if a dominant gene exists at the same locus. If both genes are recessive

and produce the same trait, it's expressed in the individual. 2.The member of a pair of genes that can't express itself when a more dominant allele is present; it can only be expressed in the homozygous state.

Recklinghausen's tumor A benign tumor, originating from smooth muscle containing connective tissue and epithelial cells, that occurs in the oviduct wall or posterior uterine wall.

reclining Leaning backward.

recombinant A cell or organism that's the consequence of the recombination of genes within the deoxyribonucleic acid molecule, regardless of whether it was naturally or artificially induced.

recombination In genetics: the formation of a new combination and arrangement of genes within the chromosome because of independent assortment of unlinked genes, crossing over of linked genes, or intracistronic crossing over of nucleotides.

recon In molecular genetics: the smallest unit in genetics capable of recombination.

recovery room (RR, R.R.) An area near the operating room where patients are taken following surgery. It has equipment and staff trained in monitoring vital signs and adequacy of ventilation as the patient recovers consciousness.

recrudescent hepatitis Acute viral hepatitis characterized by a relapse during recovery.

rectal reflex The normal response to evacuate (defecate) feces accumulated in the rectum.

rectocele A hernial protrusion of part of the rectum into the vagina. It occurs after the muscles of the vagina and pelvic floor have been weakened by childbearing, old age, or surgery and may reflect a congenital weakness in the wall and, if severe, result in dyspareunia and difficulty in evacuating the bowel.

rectosigmoid Refers to the lower sigmoid colon and upper rectum.

rectouterine pouch A deep pouch between the rectum and uterus.

rectum The distal portion of the large intestine, beginning as a continuation of the sigmoid colon from the level of the third sacral vertebra and ending in the anal canal.

rectus abdominis A pair of anterolateral abdominal muscles that extend the length of the ventral aspect of the abdomen and are separated by the linea alba.

rectus muscle A muscle with a relatively straight form.

recumbent Lying down or leaning backward.

Rectum

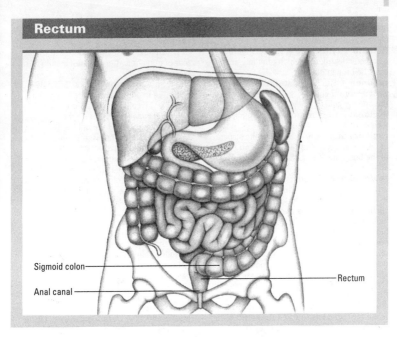

Sigmoid colon

Rectum

Anal canal

recurrent bandage   A bandage that's wrapped several times around itself.

recurvatum   Backward thrust of the knee occurring as a result of weakness of the quadriceps.

red cell indices   Characterization of red cell population regarding size, hemoglobin content, and hemoglobin concentration.

 ALERT Hemoconcentration due to prolonged tourniquet constriction can interfere with accurate test results.

red marrow   The red vascular substance, made up of connective tissue and blood vessels, that's found in the many bone cavities.

reduce   In surgery: return a part to its original position after displacement, such as the reduction of a hernia by returning the bowel to its normal position.

reduction   **1.** Addition of hydrogen to a substance. Also called *hydrogenation.* **2.** Removal of oxygen from a substance. **3.** Decrease in the valence of the electronegative part of a compound. **4.** Addition of one or more electrons to a molecule or atom. **5.** Correction of a fracture or hernia. **6.** Reduction of data such as in converting interval data to an ordinal or nominal scale of measurement.

Reed-Sternberg cell   A large, multinucleated reticuloendothelial cells in the lymphatic system in Hodgkin's disease.

reentry mechanism   Failure of a cardiac impulse to follow the normal conduction pathway; instead, it follows a circular path.

referred pain   Pain occurring at a site other than that of an injured or diseased part of the body.

refined birth rate   Ratio of total births to the total female population during a period of 1 year.

reflex action   The immediate, involuntary action or movement of an organ or part of the body in response to a stimulus.

reflex apnea   Involuntary halting of respiration because of irritating, noxious vapors or gases.

reflex dyspepsia   Impaired digestion associated with the disease of an organ that isn't directly involved with digestion.

reflexology   Form of body work involving application of pressure to specific points on the feet or hands. These points are believed to be connected to, and have a therapeutic effect on, specific body parts or organs.

reflux   A backward or return flow of a fluid.

refraction   **1.** Change of direction of light as it passes from one medium to another of different density. **2.** A test to measure and correct refractive errors of the eye.

refractory period   Period of relaxation following the excitation of a neuron or the contraction of a muscle.

Refsum's syndrome   A rare, inherited metabolic disorder in which phytanic acid can't be broken down.

regimen   Strict, regulated scheme of diet, exercise, or other activity designed to achieve therapeutic goals.

regional   Of or referring to a geographical area or part of the body.

regional anatomy   Study of the structural relationships within the organs and parts of the body, such as surface or cross-sectional anatomy.

regional anesthesia   Anesthesia of an area of the body by injecting a local anesthetic to block a group of sensory nerve fibers, such as brachial plexus anesthesia, epidural anesthesia, paracervical block, pudendal block, and spinal.

registered nurse (RN)   A professional nurse who has graduated from a school of nursing accredited by the National League for Nursing and who has taken and passed the National Council Licensure Examination for Registered Nurses (NCLEX-RN).

Registered Therapist (RT)   An X-ray technician who has satisfied the certification requirements of the American Registry of Radiologic Technicians.

regulative development   Embryonic development in which a fertilized ovum produces blastomeres that share similar developmental goals and are each capable of giving rise to a single embryo.

regulatory gene   In molecular genetics: a genetic unit that regulates or suppresses the action of genes.

regulatory sequence   In molecular genetics: a group of deoxyribonucleic acid nucleotides regulating gene expression.

regurgitation   1. Return of swallowed food into the mouth. 2. Backward flow of blood through a defective heart valve, named for the affected valve such as aortic regurgitation.

rehabilitation   The process of treatment and education of a person or part to return to normal or near-normal function after disease, injury, or addiction.

rehabilitation center   A facility that provides various therapies, such as occupational, physical, vocational, or speech, and training for rehabilitation.

Rehfuss stomach tube   A special gastric tube with a graduated syringe, used for removing specimens of the stomach contents for study following a test meal.

Reifenstein's syndrome   Male hypogonadism characterized by azoospermia, undescended testes, gynecomastia, testosterone deficiency, and elevated gonadotropin levels.

reinforcement   In psychology: a process in which a response is strengthened by the fear of punishment or the anticipation of reward.

Reiter's syndrome   An arthritic disorder, occurring in adult men, caused by a myxovirus or Mycoplasma infection.

CLINICAL TIP Reiter's syndrome commonly affects the ankles, feet, and sacroiliac joints and is usually associated with conjunctivitis and urethritis.

rejection   In medicine: an immunologic response to materials regarded as foreign, such as grafts or transplants.

relapse   1. The appearance of symptoms after a patient has recovered from disease or illness. 2. The recurrence of a disease after apparent recovery.

relapsing fever   An acute infectious disease, characterized by recurrent febrile episodes, that's caused by *Borrelia* strains.

relapsing polychondritis   A rare disease marked by inflammation and destruction of cartilage and replacement by fibrous tissue; its cause is unknown.

relative growth   Comparison of the increases in size of similar organisms, tissues, or structures at various time intervals.

relative risk   An evaluation of the incidence of adverse effects that may occur when a specific factor or event exists compared with the expected adverse effects when the factor or event is absent.

releasing hormone (RH)   A hormone, produced by the hypothalamus, secreted into the anterior pituitary by a portal system.

reliability   In research: the extent to which a test or device produces the same results when it's repeated over time by different investigators under identical conditions.

rem   Acronym for roentgen equivalent man. One dose of ionizing radiation that has the same effect as one roentgen of X-radiation or gamma radiation.

REM   *abbr* rapid eye movement.

remission   The elimination or reduction of the clinical symptoms of a chronic or malignant disease.

remittent fever   A fever that abates and exacerbates but doesn't return to normal.

remote afterloading   In radiotherapy: a technique in which an applicator is placed in or on the patient and is then loaded from a safe source with a high-activity radioisotope.

renal artery   A pair of large, visceral branches of the abdominal aorta that arises caudally to the superior mesenteric artery between the first and second lumbar vertebrae.

renal biopsy   Surgical removal of kidney tissue for microscopic observation to diagnose a renal disorder, help stage disease, and suggest the appropriate therapy and prognosis.

renal calculus   A calculus formed in the kidney.

renal calyx   The first unit within the renal system carrying urine from the kidney cortex to the ureters and into the pelvis for excretion.

renal cell carcinoma   A malignant tumor in the kidney, primarily made up of large cells with clear cytoplasm.

renal colic   Sharp, severe pain occurring in the lower back, radiating forward into the area of the groin.

renal cortex   The outer layer of the kidney that contains about 1.25 million renal tubules, which remove bodily wastes as urine.

renal failure   Failure of the kidneys to perform its essential functions of excreting wastes, concentrating urine, and conserving electrolytes.

renal hypertension   Hypertension occurring as a consequence of kidney disease.

renal infarction   Ischemia of the kidney due to thrombosis or embolus.

renal rickets   Caused by acute nephritis, this condition is marked by rachitic changes in the skeleton.

renal tubular acidosis (RTA)   Abnormal condition associated with persistent dehydration, metabolic acidosis, hypokalemia, hyperchloremia, and nephrocalcinosis.

renin   An enzyme that's produced by and stored by the kidneys.

rennin   A milk-curdling enzyme occurring in gastric juices of infants; it also occurs in the rennet produced in the stomach of calves and other ruminants.

reovirus   A ubiquitous, double-stranded ribonucleic acid virus found in the respiratory and alimentary tracts.

replacement   Substitution of a missing part or substance with a similar structure or substance.

replication   1. The act of reproducing, duplicating, or copying. 2. In research: the repetition of an experiment under identical conditions to confirm initial findings. 3. In genetics: the duplication of the deoxyribonucleic acid (DNA) strands or DNA synthesis.

replicator   In genetics: the part of the deoxyribonucleic acid molecule that initiates and controls the replication of the polynucleotide strands.

replicon   In genetics: a replication unit; part of the deoxyribonucleic acid molecule which undergoes replication. It's regulated by the regulator, which controls replication and coordinates it with cell division.

repolarization   Recovery of the myocardial cells after depolarization during which the cell membrane returns to its resting potential.

repressor gene   In molecular genetics: a unit of genetic information that inhibits another gene's activity.

reproduction   The production of offspring by animals and plants; procreation; the transmission of life from one organism to successive generations similar to the parents, to maintain the continuity of a species.

repulsion   1. The act of repelling, disjoining; a force that separates two bodies or elements. 2. In genetics: in linked inheritance where the alleles of two or more mutant genes are located on homologous chromosomes so that each chromosome of the pair carries one or more mutant and wild-type genes, which are located close enough to be inherited together.

RES   *abbr* reticuloendothelial system.

research instrument   A testing instrument for measuring a specific object such as a questionnaire.

research measurement   An assessment of the amount or incidence of a defined variable obtained with a research instrument.

resect   The surgical removal of part or all of an organ or structure.

resection   The removal of a significant portion of an organ or structure.

reserve   A potential supply that may be used to maintain the body's vital functions during an emergency.

reservoir bag   Part of the anesthesia equipment that allows gas to accumulate, forming a reserve supply of gas that may be used when flow is inadequate.

resident   1. A doctor in one of his postgraduate years of clinical training, the duration of which depends on the specialty. 2. A person who resides in a long-term care facility.

residual volume   The volume of gas remaining in the lungs after a maximum expiration.

resonance   An echo or sound that's produced by percussion of an organ during a physical examination.

resorption   Loss of a substance through physiologic or pathologic means, such as loss of dentin and cementum of a tooth.

respiration   1. External respiration is the act of breathing (inhalation and exhalation). 2. Internal respiration is the molecular exchange of oxygen and carbon dioxide in the body tissues.

respirator   An instrument that's used to modify air for inspiration or to artificially improve pulmonary ventilation.

respiratory acidosis   Caused by reduced alveolar ventilation, this condition is marked by increased partial pressure of arterial carbon dioxide, excess carbonic acid, and increased plasma hydrogen-ion concentration. Hypoventilation inhibits the excretion of carbon dioxide, which consequently produces excessive carbonic acid and thus lowers blood pH.

respiratory alkalosis   Caused by both respiratory and nonrespiratory factors, this condition is marked by decreased partial pressure of arterial carbon dioxide, decreased hydrogen-ion concentration, and increased blood pH. Extreme anxiety can precipitate hyperventilation associated with respiratory alkalosis.

respiratory center   A region in the brain that controls breathing.

respiratory distress syndrome of the newborn (RDS)   An acute lung disease of premature infants and infants of diabetic mothers.

respiratory exchange ratio (R)   The ratio of the net expiration of carbon dioxide to the net inspiration of oxygen, as defined by carbon dioxide uptake and oxygen uptake.

respiratory failure   Failure of the cardiac and pulmonary systems to adequately exchange oxygen and carbon dioxide in the lungs. Respiratory failure may be hypoxemic or ventilatory.

respiratory rate   The rate of breathing at rest that's controlled by the hydrogen ion concentration in the cerebrospinal fluid.

respiratory rhythm   Recurrent cycle of inspiration and expiration that's controlled by muscles in the chest and the respiratory centers in the brain.

respiratory syncytial virus (RSV)   A group of myxoviruses that causes giant cells or syncytia to form in tissue culture.

respiratory tract   The complex arrangement of organs and structures through which pulmonary ventilation and exchange of oxygen and carbon dioxide between the ambient air and blood is accomplished.

respiratory tract infection   An infectious disease of the upper or lower respiratory tract.

respiratory volume   Measurements used to assess lung functioning, including tidal volume, inspiratory reserve volume, expiratory reserve volume, residual volume, and vital capacity.

resting cell   A cell not undergoing division.

restless legs syndrome   A treatable condition marked by uneasiness, tiredness, and itching within the lower leg muscles that may be accompanied by twitching and pain.

restriction endonuclease   In molecular genetics: an enzyme that cleaves deoxyribonucleic acid at a specific site.

resuscitator   An instrument that fits over the mouth and nose that's designed to pump air into the lungs.

retarded dentition   Delayed eruption of the deciduous or permanent teeth due to malnutrition, hereditary causes, malposition of the teeth, or a metabolic imbalance.

rete   An arterial or venous network.

retention of urine   An involuntary accumulation of urine in the bladder because of an inability to urinate; may be caused by urethral obstruction or muscle tone loss, neurologic dysfunction, or trauma to the bladder.

reticular   Having a netlike pattern or structure of veins.

reticular activating system (RAS)   A functional system in the brain that controls the overall degree of the central nervous system, including wakefulness, attention, concentration, and introspection.

reticular formation   A dense group of neurons located in the brain stem that controls vital bodily functions, such as breathing and heart rate.

reticulocyte   An immature erythrocyte that has a netlike pattern of particles at the former nuclear site; they comprise less than 1% of circulating erythrocytes.

reticuloendothelial system (RES)   A functional system responsible for defending the body against infection and disposing of cellular breakdown products.

retina   A 10-layered, delicate, nervous tissue membrane of the eye that receives images and transmits impulses through the optic nerve to the brain.

retinaculum extensorum manus   Thickened band of antebrachial fascia covering the tendons of the forearm extensor muscles at the distal ends of the radius and ulna.

retinaculum flexorum manus   Thick, fibrous band of antebrachial fascia that envelops the carpal canal around the forearm flexor muscle tendons at the distal ends of the radius and ulna. Also called *flexor retinaculum of the hand, volar ligament.*

retinal   An aldehyde preform of vitamin A that's necessary for night, day, and color vision.

retinal detachment   Separation of the retina from the choroid, occurring as a consequence to a hole in the retina that enables vitreous humor to leak.

retinene One of two carotenoid pigments occurring in the rods of the retina that are preforms of vitamin A and light-activated.

retinitis Inflammation of the retina.

retinitis pigmentosa Group of retinal diseases that may be inherited, characterized by retinal atrophy, weakening of the retinal vascular system, clumping of pigment, and narrowing of the visual field.

retinoblastoma, *pl.* **retinoblastomas, retinoblastomata** A common childhood hereditary neoplasm arising from retinal germ cells.

retraction of the chest The visible depression of soft tissues of the chest between and around the cartilaginous and bony ribs, occurring with increased inspiratory effort.

TIME LINE If you detect retractions in a child, check quickly for other signs of respiratory distress, such as cyanosis, tachypnea, and tachycardia.

retractor An instrument used during surgery for holding back the edges of tissues and organs to expose underlying anatomy.

retroaortic node A node in one of three pairs of lumbar lymph nodes serving structures in the abdomen and pelvis.

retroflexion The flexing backward of an organ such as the bending backward of the uterus at an angle with the cervix.

retrograde Moving backward; movement in an opposite direction to that considered to be normal.

retrograde depolarization Depolarization that occurs backward toward the atrium instead of downward toward the ventricles; results in an inverted P wave.

retrograde pyelography A radiologic technique used to examine the structures within the kidney's collecting system; especially to locate a urinary tract obstruction.

ALERT Be especially attentive to catheter output if ureteral catheters have been left in place, as inadequate output may reflect catheter obstruction and require irrigation. Protect ureteral catheters from dislodgment.

retroperitoneal Of or related to structures attached to the abdominal wall and partially covered by peritoneum.

retroperitoneal fibrosis An inflammatory disorder in which fibrous tissue covers large blood vessels in the lower lumbar area.

retropharyngeal abscess Pus present in the tissues behind the pharynx; difficulty swallowing, fever, and pain may occur.

retroplacental Behind the placenta.

retroversion The tipping backward of an organ, commonly without flexion.

retrovirus A virus that belongs to the oncoviruses.

Reverdin's needle A surgical needle that has an eye that can be opened and closed with a slide.

reverse Barton's fracture Fracture of the volar articular surface of the radius with displacement of the carpal bones and radius.

reversed bandage A roller bandage that lies smoothly and conforms to the contour of the extremity.

review of systems (ROS) In health history: a system-by-system review of the bodily functions. Initially begun during the patient interview, the ROS is completed during the physical examination.

Reye's syndrome Acute encephalopathy and fatty infiltration of the internal organs following acute viral infections, such as influenza B, chickenpox (varicella), the enteroviruses, and the Epstein-Barr virus. The syndrome has also been associated in children with administration of aspirin and other salicylates.

R factor A genetic factor in bacteria that controls resistance to certain drugs and may be transmitted to progeny and other bacterial cells. The portion of the episome involved in replication and transmission is called *resistance transfer factor.*

Rh Symbol for rhodium.

rhabdomyoblastoma Benign tumor arising from striated muscle.

rhabdomyolysis Disorder in which skeletal muscle is destroyed, causing intracellular contents to spill into extracellular fluid.

rhabdomyoma, *pl.* **rhabdomyomas, rhabdomyomata** A striated muscle tumor occurring in the uterus, vagina, pharynx, tongue, and heart.

rhabdomyosarcoma, *pl.* **rhabdomyosarcomas, rhabdomyosarcomata** A highly malignant tumor, originating from striated muscle cells, that commonly occurs in the head and neck and also in the genitourinary tract, extremities, body wall, and retroperitoneum.

rhabdovirus A member of the ribonucleic acid viruses, including the causative organism of rabies.

rhagades Fine linear scars or cracks in the skin, especially around the mouth.

Rh$_0$(D) immune globulin An immunizing agent administered after abortion, miscarriage, ectopic pregnancy, or delivery to prevent Rh sensitization.

rhenium (Re) A hard, brittle, metal with atomic number 7 and atomic weight 186.2.

rheumatic aortitis Inflammation of the aorta, which may occur with rheumatic fever, that's marked by disseminated focal lesions leading to fibrosis.

rheumatic arteritis A complication of rheumatic fever in which arteries and arterioles become inflamed.

rheumatic fever An inflammatory disease sometimes occurring if group A beta-hemolytic streptococcal infection is inadequately treated.

rheumatic heart disease Damage caused to heart muscle and valves by rheumatic fever.

rheumatoid arthritis A chronic, systemic collagen disease marked by inflammation, stiffness, and pain in the joints and related structures that result in crippling deformities.

rheumatoid factor (RF) An immunoglobulin occurring in the serum of most patients with rheumatoid arthritis.

rheumatologist A doctor specializing in rheumatology.

rheumatology The study of the causes and treatment of rheumatic disorders (inflammation, degeneration, or metabolic derangement of connective tissue).

Rh factor, Rh₀(D) antigen An antigenic substance found in erythrocytes of most people. The presence of the factor indicates that a person is Rh + (Rh positive); its absence makes a person Rh– (Rh negative).

RHIA *abbr* registered health information administrator.

Rh incompatibility In hematology: two blood groups that are antigenically different and, therefore, aren't compatible because one group lacks the Rh factor.

rhinitis Inflammation of the mucous membranes in the nose, commonly accompanied by a mucous discharge and swelling of the membranes.

rhinodynia Pain of the nose.

rhinolaryngitis Inflammation of the mucous membranes of the nose and larynx.

rhinopathy A disease (including malformation) of the nose.

rhinophyma A severe form of rosacea characterized by prominent blood vessels, redness, sebaceous overgrowth, and swelling.

CLINICAL TIP The skin of the nose and cheeks may appear distorted.

rhinoplasty Plastic surgery in which the shape of the nose is changed. The surgery may be reconstructive, restorative, or cosmetic; and bone or cartilage may be removed, tissue grafted from another part of the body, or synthetic material implanted to alter the shape.

rhinoscope A speculum used for examining the interior of the nose through the anterior nares or through the nasopharynx.

rhinoscopy An examination of the interior of the nose performed to view the mucous membranes. The purpose of the examination is to detect inflammation, deformities, or asymmetry such as a deviated septum.

rhinotomy An incision made along one side of the nose to drain pus from an abscess or a sinus infection.

rhinovirus Any of about 100 serologically distinct, ribonucleic acid viruses that infect the upper respiratory tract and cause the common cold.

RHIT *abbr* registered health information technician.

rhitidosis, rhytidosis Wrinkling of the cornea of the eye.

rhizotomy Sectioning of the nerve roots of the spine to relieve pain or spastic paralysis; also called *radicotomy, radiculectomy.*

Rh neg, Rh– *abbr* Rhesus factor negative.

rhodium (Rh) A gray-white metal of the platinum group. Its atomic number is 45; atomic weight, 102.905.

rhodopsin A photosensitive purple-red compound found in the retinal rods. Protein, opsin, and a derivative of vitamin A, retinal, make up the compound.

rhomboideus major A muscle located in the upper back. Rhomboideus major is below and parallel to rhomboideus minor.

rhomboideus minor A muscle located in the upper back. Rhomboideus minor is above and parallel to rhomboideus major.

rhonchi, *sing.* rhonchus A dry rattling sound heard on auscultation of the upper respiratory airway (throat or bronchial tubes); usually caused by an obstruction, thick secretions, muscular spasm, neoplasm, or external pressure.

TIME LINE Because a respiratory tract disorder may begin abruptly and progress rapidly in an infant or child, observe closely for signs of airway obstruction.

rhotacism A speech disorder in which the letter *r* is overused or mispronounced.

Rh pos, Rh+ *abbr* Rhesus factor positive.

rhus dermatitis A skin rash, or dermatitis, caused by contact with poison ivy, poison oak, or poison sumac, all plants of the genus *Rhus.*

rhytidoplasty, rhitidoplasty Plastic surgery to remove facial wrinkles by tightening the skin.

RIA *abbr* radioimmunoassay.

rib Any of 12 pairs of elastic arches of bone (12 on each side of the body) that form a large part of the thoracic skeleton.

riboflavin A vitamin that's part of the B complex group. It's water-soluble, heat-stable, yellow, and crystalline and is found in milk, eggs, leafy green vegetables, whole grains, and enriched cereals. It's an essential nutrient for humans.

ribonucleic acid (RNA)   A nucleic acid that plays a role in the flow, or transmission, of genetic instructions. RNA is located in the nucleus and cytoplasm of cells, and it carries the genetic material for RNA viruses.

ribonucleic acid (RNA) polymerase In molecular genetics: a general term for an enzyme that catalyzes the assembly of ribonucleoside triphosphates into RNA. Single-stranded deoxyribonucleic acid serves as the template.

ribonucleic acid (RNA) splicing   In molecular genetics: the process by which base pairs that interrupt the continuity of genetic information in deoxyribonucleic acid are removed from the precursors of messenger RNA.

ribosome   A molecular structure that contains ribonucleic acid, receives genetic information, and is responsible for protein synthesis.

rice diet   A diet used in the treatment of chronic renal disease, hypertension, and obesity. The diet includes rice, fruit, fruit juices, and sugar and is supplemented with vitamins and iron. Salt is forbidden.

rickets   A condition of abnormal bone growth caused by insufficient vitamin D, calcium and, commonly, phosphorus. Rickets occurs in infancy and childhood; in adults, the condition is osteomalacia.

rickettsia, *pl.* rickettsiae   A bacteria of the genus *Rickettsia*. Rickettsiae are small, rod-shaped, or oval organisms that occur intracellularly as parasites in fleas, lice, mites, and ticks. The bacteria cause disease in man, and sometimes other animals.

rickettsiosis, *pl.* rickettsioses   The infectious diseases caused by bacteria of the genus *Rickettsia*.

rider's bone   A bony deposit, or formation, found on the lower portion of the tendon of the thigh's adductor muscle. The formation may develop in persons who ride horseback extensively.

ridge   A projecting structure, such as the bony ridge of the mandible that contains the alveoli.

Rieder's cell leukemia   A form of acute leukemia in which malignant neoplasms of blood-forming tissues are present. The blood cells have immature cytoplasm and indented, lobulated fairly mature nuclei.

rifampin   An antibiotic used in the United States to treat tuberculosis.

RIG   *abbr* rabies immune globulin.

right bundle-branch block   A cardiac condition in which an impaired electrical sig-

nal is sent from the atrioventricular bundle to the right ventricle.

right common carotid artery   The shorter of the two common carotid arteries, arising from the brachiocephalic trunk, passing obliquely from the level of the sternoclavicular articulation to the cranial border of the thyroid cartilage, and dividing into the right internal and the right external carotid arteries; supplies blood to the head and neck.

right coronary artery   One of two branches of the ascending aorta, arising in the right posterior aortic sinus, passing along the right side of the coronary sulcus, dividing into the right interventricular artery and a large marginal branch, supplying both ventricles, the right atrium, and the sinoatrial node.

right hepatic duct   The duct that drains bile from the right lobe of the liver into the common bile duct.

righting reflex   The ability of an animal to return to its optimal, or normal, body position after it has been moved from that position.

right pulmonary artery   The larger and longer of two arteries carrying blood from the heart to the lungs. It originates in the pulmonary trunk, bends to the right behind the aorta, and divides into two branches at the base of the right lung.

right-sided heart failure   A cardiac condition in which the right ventricle of the heart becomes impaired and there's congestion and elevated pressure in the veins and capillaries. Left-sided heart failure may occur at the same time.

right subclavian artery   A large artery that originates in the brachiocephalic artery. Arising from the right subclavian artery are several branches: the axillary, vertebral thoracic, and internal thoracic arteries and the cervical and costocervical trunks that pass blood to the right side of the upper body.

rigor   **1.** A stiffening, or rigid, condition of a dead body (rigor mortis). **2.** A stiffening of the muscles that's caused by heat. **3.** A violent shivering that may accompany a high fever.

rigor mortis   The stiffening of muscles that occurs shortly after death.

RIND   *abbr* reversible/resolving ischemic neurologic deficit.

ring chromosome   A circular chromosome formed after both ends have been lost and the two broken ends joined to create a ring. It's common type of chromosome in bacteria.

Ringer's injection   A fluid and electrolyte replacement solution that consists of sodium chloride, potassium chloride, and calcium chloride in water.

Ringer's injection, lactated   A fluid and electrolyte replacement solution consisting of calcium chloride, potassium chloride, sodium chloride, and sodium lactate in water. It closely approximates the electrolyte concentration in blood plasma.

Rinne's tuning fork test   A hearing test that's helpful in determining the type of hearing loss: conductive or sensorineural.

risk management   The identification, analysis, evaluation, and elimination or reduction, to the extent possible, of risks to hospital patients, visitors, or employees. Risk management programs are involved with both loss prevention and loss control; they also handle all incidents, claims, and other insurance- and litigation-related tasks.

risorius   One of 12 muscles of the mouth. Originating in the fascia over the masseter and inserting into the skin at the corner of the mouth, it's activated by mandibular and buccal branches of the facial nerve and retracts the angle of the mouth to produce a smile.

Risser cast   Used to treat scoliosis, a Risser cast extends from the chin to the cervical area to the chin. In rare cases, it extends over the hips to the knees and may include one arm as far as the elbow. Also called *Risser jacket.*

risus sardonicus   A grinning, masklike expression caused by a spasm of the facial muscles. It's commonly seen in tetanus.

Ritter's disease   An uncommon staphylococcal infection that occurs in newborns. It starts with red spots around the mouth and on the chin, and gradually spreads over the entire body.

RIU   *abbr* radioactive iodine uptake.

RMSF   *abbr* Rocky Mountain spotted fever.

Rn   Symbol for radon.

RN   *abbr* registered nurse.

RNA   *abbr* ribonucleic acid.

RN,C   *abbr* registered nurse, certified.

Robertsonian translocation   The exchange of entire chromosome arms, with the break occurring at the centromere, usually between two nonhomologous acrocentric chromosomes, to form one large metacentric chromosome and one small chromosome that carries little genetic material and may be lost through successive cell divisions, leading to a reduction in total chromosome number.

Rocky Mountain spotted fever (RMSF)   An infectious disease occurring in the temperate zones of North and South America, caused by *Rickettsia rickettsii*, and carried by wood ticks. Chills, fever, severe

headache, myalgia, mental confusion, and rash are signs and symptoms of the disease.

rod   **1.** A straight cylindrical mass. **2.** A slender cylindrical sensory element in the retina.

rodenticide poisoning   Poisoning caused by the ingestion of an agent created for killing rats, or rodents.

rodent ulcer   A slow growing cancer that destroys soft tissues and bones. It's usually found at the outer edges of the eye and on the tip of the nose.

roentgen   An international unit for measuring X-rays or gamma rays. In radiotherapy or radiodiagnosis, it's the unit of the emitted dose. (The quantity of X-rays or gamma rays that creates 1 electrostatic unit of ions in 1 cc of air [0.001293 g] at 32° F [0° C] and 760 mm Hg of pressure.)

roentgen fetometry   Radiographic techniques for measuring a fetus in utero.

roentgenology   The study of diagnostic and therapeutic uses of X-rays.

Rolando's fracture   A fracture at the base of the first metacarpal.

rolfing   A type of deep-tissue massage designed to release kinks in the connective tissues to improve body alignment and functions; formally known as Structural Integration.

roller bandage   A commercially prepared bandage of varying widths. It's tightly rolled and usually applied as a circular bandage.

rolling effleurage   A type of circular, rubbing massage that promotes circulation and relaxation of muscles and is especially effect on the shoulders and buttocks.

ROM   *abbr* **1.** range of motion. **2.** rupture of membranes. **3.** right otitis media.

Romberg's sign   A swaying (or falling) when a person stands with feet together and eyes closed. It's an indication that the person has lost a sense of position. Also called *rombergism.*

TIME LINE Romberg's sign can't be tested in children until they can stand without support and follow commands. A positive sign in children commonly results from spinal cord disease.

rooting reflex   A response in newborns to the cheek being touched or stroked. The infant turns the head toward the stimulated side and begins to suck. The reflex usually disappears by 3 to 4 months of age.

ROP   *abbr* retinopathy of prematurity.

Rorschach test   A personality assessment test developed by Hermann Rorschach, a Swiss psychiatrist.

ROS   *abbr* review of systems.

rosacea   Chronic skin disease that produces flushing and dilation of small blood vessels in the face, especially the nose and cheeks.

rose fever   A type of seasonal hay fever to grass pollens, which are released at the same time roses and other late spring and early summer flowers are blooming.

roseola   A rose-colored rash seen in diseases such as measles.

roseola infantum   A noninfectious illness, seen in infants and young children, in which there's a high (sustained or spiking) fever, mild pharyngitis, and lymph node enlargement. The rash usually appears after the fever subsides.

rose spots   A common symptom of typhoid and paratyphoid fevers, rose spots are small red (erythematous) macules that appear on the upper abdomen and chest and last for 2 to 3 days.

rotameter   An instrument for measuring the flow of gases during the administration of an anesthetic.

rotary joints   Joints in which one bone pivots around a stationary bone. Also called *pivot joints.*

rotation   1. Movement around an axis. 2. The turning of the fetal head during labor. 3. The motion of a bone around its central axis, which may lie in a separate bone. 4. A procedure to turn a tooth into its proper position.

Rotor syndrome   An inherited liver condition; the trait is recessive.

rouleaux, *sing.* rouleau   A roll or stack of red blood cells.

Rovsing's sign   In acute appendicitis: Pressure on the left lower quadrant of the abdomen (corresponding to McBurney's point) will cause pain in the right lower quadrant.

Royal College of Physicians (RCP)   A professional organization of physicians in the United Kingdom.

Royal College of Physicians and Surgeons of Canada (RCPSC)   A national Canadian organization that recognizes and confers membership on certain qualified physicians and surgeons.

Royal College of Surgeons (RCS)   A professional organization of surgeons in the United Kingdom.

RPF   *abbr* renal plasma flow.

RR   *abbr* recovery room.

RRA   *abbr* radioreceptor assay.

R-R interval   In an electrocardiogram: The interval from the peak of one QRS complex to the peak of the next.

RRT   *abbr* registered respiratory therapist.

RSV   *abbr* respiratory syncytial virus.

RT   *abbr* 1. respiratory therapy. 2. radiotherapy.

RTA   *abbr* renal tubular acidosis.

rtc   *abbr* return to clinic. It's noted on the chart, usually followed by a date on which a subsequent appointment has been made for the patient.

ru   *abbr* radiation unit.

Ru   1. *abbr* roentgen unit. 2. Symbol for ruthenium.

rubella   An acute contagious viral disease that usually occurs in children and has these signs: arthralgia, fever, lymph node enlargement, mild upper respiratory infection, and a generalized fine pink rash.

rubella and mumps virus vaccine   A standardized suspension containing live attenuated mumps and rubella viruses; used to immunize against rubella and mumps.

rubella embryopathy   A congenital abnormality that results from the mother having had rubella during the early stages of pregnancy.

rubella syndrome   Exposure of a nonimmune mother to rubella during the first trimester of pregnancy.

rubella virus vaccine   A standardized suspension containing live attenuated rubella virus; used to immunized against rubella.

rubescent   Reddening.

rubidium (Rb)   A soft, rare, slightly radioactive metallic element of the alkali metals group. Its atomic number is 37; atomic weight, 85.47. It's used in radioisotope scanning.

Rubin's test   A test to evaluate the cause of infertility by assessing patency of the fallopian tubes. A cannula inserted into the cervix is used to introduce pressurized carbon dioxide gas (CO_2) into the fallopian tubes. The test may cause discomfort in the patient's shoulders.

rubor   Redness, a sign of inflammation.

rudiment   An organ or tissue that's incompletely developed or nonfunctional.

Ruffini's corpuscles   A variety of oval-shaped nerve endings in the dermis that adapts to sensations of pressure. Also called *Ruffini's endings.*

ruga, *pl.* rugae   A wrinkle or fold such as the rugae of stomach: large folds of mucous membrane that are seen when the organ is empty.

rule of nines   A method for calculating the amount of an adult's body surface that has been burned, with 9% assigned the head and each arm, twice 9% to each leg and to the front and back of the trunk, and 1% to the perineum.

rumination   Regurgitation, or spitting up, of small amounts of food after most feedings, a condition common in infants. It may be caused by overfeeding, eating too fast, or swallowing air.

rupture   A forcible tear or break in the skin or another body organ such as a hernia.

Russell dwarf   A person who has Russell's syndrome, a congenital disorder characterized by short stature as well as incurved fifth fingers, triangular-shaped face, downturned corners of the mouth, other skeleton abnormalities and varying degrees of mental retardation. Also called *Russell-Silver syndrome.*

Russell's bodies   The mucoprotein inclusions found in cancerous growths and simple inflammatory growths.

Russell traction   An orthopedic device that combines suspension and traction to align and immobilize the legs, used to treat diseases of the hip and knee and to treat fractured femurs as well as hip and knee contractures.

ruthenium (Ru)   A rare, very hard metallic element. Its atomic number is 44; atomic weight, 101.07.

rutin   A bioflavonoid obtained from buckwheat and other plants and used to treat fragile capillaries.

RV   *abbr* residual volume.

RVC   *abbr* responds to verbal commands.

R wave   The first upward part of the QRS wave in a normal electrocardiogram. It's a straight, upward line and represents the middle part of the QRS complex.

Rx   *abbr* prescription.

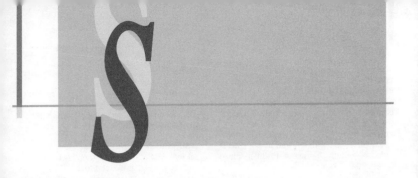

S Symbol for: **1.** sulfur. **2.** saturation of hemoglobin.

S₁ The first heart sound in the cardiac cycle, heard during closure of mitral and tricuspid valves. The sound is dull, prolonged, "lubbed."

S₂ The second heart sound, heard during closure of the semilunar valves just before ventricular diastole. The sound is a "dub" sound.

S₃ The third heart sound, heard during rapid ventricular filling in diastole. It's generally detected only in children and physically active young adults.

S₄ The fourth heart sound, heard during atrial contraction. It's rarely audible. When heard, it indicates abnormally increased resistance to ventricular filling.

SA *abbr* **1.** surgeon's assistant. **2.** sinoatrial. **3.** surface area.

Sabin-Feldman dye test A test for diagnosing toxoplasmosis. The results depend on the presence of antibodies that block the uptake of methylene blue dye by the cytoplasm of the *Toxoplasma* organisms.

sac A pouch, or sacklike structure; for example, the abdominal sac in the embryo eventually develops into the abdominal cavity.

saccharide One of the carbohydrates. Saccharides include monosaccharides, oligosaccharides, and polysaccharides; that is, all sugars and starches. Almost all carbohydrates are saccharides.

saccharin, saccharine A white, crystalline compound that's much sweeter than table sugar (sucrose). Saccharin is often used as a sugar substitute and as a sweetener in pharmaceutical preparations.

saccule A small bag or pouch, as the laryngeal saccule.

sacral Relating to the sacrum.

sacral foramen One of several openings between the fused segments of the sacral vertebrae in the sacrum through which the sacral nerves pass.

sacral node A node, located in the sacrum, that's in one of the parietal lymph nodes of the abdomen and pelvis.

sacral plexus A network of motor and sensory nerves formed by the lumbosacral trunk from the fourth and fifth lumbar and the first, second, and third sacral nerves.

sacroiliac articulation A joint in the pelvis formed by the joining of the sacrum and the ilium. Movement of the joint is limited.

sacrospinalis A large muscle that runs along the spine from the sacrum to the head.

saddle block anesthesia A regional nerve block that affects the buttocks, perineum, and inner thighs. It's introduced into the dural sac or fourth lumbar interspace.

saddle joint A joint that has two saddle shaped surfaces, which are at right angles to each other. This type of joint allows no axial rotation but flexion, extension, adduction, and abduction are possible. The carpometacarpal joint of the thumb is an example of such a joint.

sagittal In anatomy: relating to an imaginary straight line that extends from the front to the back through the median of the body (or a part of the body).

sagittal plane An imaginary plane that divides the body vertically into right and left sides. Also call a median or midsagittal plane.

sagittal suture A fibrous joint in which the opposed surfaces of the skull are closely jointed. It runs down the midline from the coronal suture to the upper part of the lambdoid suture.

SaH, SAH *abbr* subarachnoid hemorrhage.

salicylate poisoning A toxic condition resulting from an overdose of a salicylate, such as aspirin or oil of wintergreen.

ALERT Symptoms include rapid breathing, headache, irritability, ketosis, hypoglycemia, and vomiting. In extreme cases, seizures and respiratory failure may occur.

saline cathartic A purgative, such as Epsom salts, given to achieve quick, complete evacuation of the bowel.

saline infusion A saline solution administered therapeutically into a vein or under the skin.

saline irrigation The washing of a body cavity or wound with an isotonic aqueous solution of sodium chloride or a similar salt solution.

saline solution A solution containing sodium chloride, or common salt. Depending on the therapeutic use, the solution may be hypotonic, isotonic, or hypertonic.

saliva A clear, somewhat viscous fluid that moistens and softens food and keeps the mouth moist. It's secreted by the salivary and mucous glands in the mouth and is composed of water, mucin, organic salts, and the digestive enzyme ptyalin.

salivary duct A duct that secretes saliva.

salivary fistula An abnormal opening between a salivary gland or duct to the mouth or skin of the face or neck.

salivary gland One of the six glands that secrete saliva and aid digestion.

Salmonella A rod-shaped, gram-negative bacteria that includes species causing typhoid fever, paratyphoid fever, and some forms of gastroenteritis or food poisoning.

salmonellosis A disease caused by a *Salmonella* infection, often caused by eating food contaminated with the *Salmonella* bacteria. Symptoms usually include sudden, crampy abdominal pain; fever; and bloody, watery diarrhea. Incubation period is 6 to 48 hours.

salpingectomy Removal of one or both fallopian tubes by surgery; also to remove a cyst, a tumor, or an abscess on a fallopian tube.

salpingitis An inflammation or infection of a fallopian tube.

salpingo-oophorectomy Removal of a tube and an ovary. Also called *oophorosalpingectomy.*

salpingopexy Surgical fixation of a fallopian tube.

salpingostomy Creation, by surgery, of an artificial opening in a fallopian tube. The purpose is to restore patency in a tube that has been closed by infection or chronic inflammation or to drain an abscess or accumulated fluid.

saltation In genetics: an abrupt change or mutation in a species. Also the jerk motions that may occur in persons with chorea.

samarium (Sm) A rare metallic element. Its atomic number is 62; atomic weight, 150.35.

sand bath The application of warm, dry or damp sand to the body.

Sandhoff's disease A disease similar to Tay-Sachs that's characterized by defects in the enzymes hexosaminidase A and B. Severity decreases with increasing age of onset.

SA *abbr* sinoatrial.

saphenous nerve A large, long branch of the femoral nerve that supplies the medial side of the leg, ankle, and foot.

saponin A soapy material found in some plants. It forms a durable foam when shaken in watery solutions; saponin can dissolve red blood cells in high dilutions. Soapwort and certain lilies contain saponin.

sarcoidosis cordis A form of sarcoidosis, a disease in which granulomatous lesions affect organs and tissues of the body. In sarcoidosis cordis, lesions develop in the myocardium.

sarcoma, *pl.* **sarcomas, sarcomata** A tumor, usually malignant, of soft and connective tissue. Sarcomas usually originate in fibrous, fatty, muscular, synovial, vascular, or neural tissue.

sarcoma botryoides A tumor derived from embryonal muscle cells. It forms an edematous, polypoid, grapelike mass and is usually found in the upper vagina, on the uterine cervix, or on the neck of the urinary bladder. It's seen most often in infants and young children.

sarcoplasmic reticulum Tubules and sacs in skeletal muscles that aid muscle contraction and relaxation by releasing and storing calcium ions.

Sarcoptes scabiei The genus and species of acarids; a mite that causes scabies and itching in humans.

sartorius The long, ribbonlike muscle of the thigh. It extends from the pelvis to the calf of the leg and allows the thigh to rotate extend and rotate laterally and the leg to rotate medially.

saturated In chemistry: **1.** A solution that contains the maximum amount of solute. **2.** A hydrocarbon that has all carbon bonds filled and no double or triple bonds; it can't unite directly with another compound.

saturated fatty acid A fatty acid lacking double bonds. It's found mostly in animal fats and tropical oils and can be produced by hydrogenation of unsaturated fatty acids, which are found in vegetable oils. Saturated fatty acids seem to contribute to a high serum cholesterol level and, therefore, seem to be associated with coronary heart disease.

saturated solution A solution that contains the maximum amount of solute.

sauna bath A bath of high temperature and humidity (steam) that induces sweating.

It's often followed by a cold shower. It isn't advised for persons with a fever or those who are dehydrated. Prolonged exposure to a sauna can produce dehydration.

Sayre's jacket   A plaster cast that supports and immobilizes the spine. Used to treat vertebral abnormalities.

Sb   Symbol for antimony.

SBE   *abbr* **1.** self–breast examination. **2.** subacute bacterial endocarditis.

Sc   Symbol for scandium.

SC   *abbr* subcutaneous.

scabies   A contagious skin disease caused by the itch mite, *Sarcoptes scabiei*.

scale   **1.** A thin flake of dried horny epidermis. **2.** A thin layer of tartar on the teeth. **3.** To remove tartar from the teeth. **4.** A measuring device with predetermined units.

scalp   Skin covering the head, that's covered by hair; excludes the face and ears.

scamping speech   Speech characterized by the lack of consonants or whole syllables. Both are left out because the person can't form the sounds.

scandium (Sc)   A rare gray metallic element. Its atomic number is 21; atomic weight, 44.956.

scanning   Careful visual examination of an area, organ, or system of the body. In a scan, an image is created and recorded on a photographic plate after the area to be examined has been injected with a radioactive substance. The liver, brain, and thyroid can be examined by various scanning techniques.

scanning electron microscope (SEM)   A device similar to an electron microscope that displays an image on a television screen; the image appears to be three-dimensional. SEM can examine a sample of any convenient size or shape.

scanning electron microscopy   The technique using a scanning electron microscope in which a beam of electrons is accelerated and focused on an electrically conducting sample. The beam is moved in a point-to-point manner over the surface of the specimen. The number of electrons emerging from the sample is proportionate to the shape, density, and other properties of the sample.

scanning speech   A speech pattern characterized by words that are broken because of pauses between syllables. Speech is slow and hesitant and often found in persons with advanced multiple sclerosis.

scaphocephaly, scaphocephalis, scaphocephalism   A condition in which one has a misshapen head that resembles the keel of a boat. The condition is congenital and results from premature closure of the sagittal suture.

Scabies: Cause and effect

Infestation with *Sarcoptes scabiei*, the itch mite, causes scabies. This mite has a hard shell and measures a microscopic 0.1 mm.

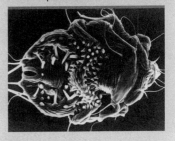

The bottom illustration shows the erythematous nodules with excoriation that appear in patients with scabies.

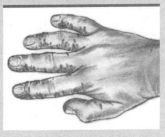

scapula   The shoulder blade; a flat, triangular bone on the back of the shoulder. It has two surfaces, three borders, three angles, and a prominent dorsal spine. See illustration on page 274.

scapulohumeral muscular dystrophy   A limb-girdle muscular dystrophy that begins in the shoulder girdle.

scapulohumeral reflex   A normal response in which the upper arm rotates outward when the vertebral border of the scapula is tapped, or percussed. Absence of the reflex may indicate a lesion in the fifth cervical segment of the spinal cord.

scarification   Many small scratches in the skin, such as are made when a vaccine is administered.

scarlet fever   An acute contagious childhood disease that's caused by group A ß-hemolytic streptococci. Symptoms include a sore throat, fever, enlarged lymph nodes in

Scapula

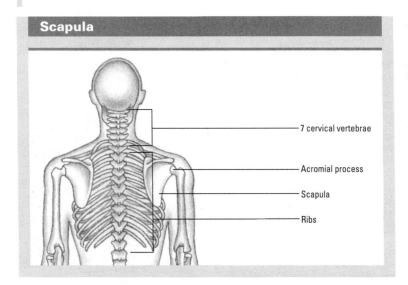

7 cervical vertebrae

Acromial process

Scapula

Ribs

the neck, flushed face, red or white strawberry tongue, bright red rash, and lines of hyperpigmentation. Also called *scarlatina*.

scattergram   A plot, or graph, showing the distribution of two variables in a sample population. Variables are plotted on vertical (x) and horizontal (y) axes. The values are indicated by a symbol, usually dots, and aren't connected. Also called *scatterplot*.

scattering   In radiology: a change in direction of a photon (a subatomic particle) resulting from a collision.

Schick test   A skin test to determine immunity to diphtheria. A positive reaction is marked by redness for 24 to 36 hours at the test site. Redness lasts 4 to 5 days and leaves a brown mark. A negative reaction is marked by absence of redness or swelling, especially after 48 hours.

Schilder's disease   One of several severe, neurologic diseases beginning in childhood. Symptoms include blindness, deafness, spasticity, adrenal insufficiency, and mental deterioration. White matter in the brain is destroyed. Also *called Schilder's encephalitis.*

Schiller's test   A test for cancer of the vagina or cervix; used as a guide in selecting biopsy sites.

Schilling test   A test to determine disorders of vitamin B_{12} metabolism including pernicious anemia. In the test, B_{12} labeled with radioactive cobalt is administered orally, then GI absorption is determined by the amount of radioactivity in urine samples collected over 24 hours.

Schiøtz tonometer   A device for measuring intraocular pressure by gauging the depth of corneal indentation. The measure is translated into millimeters of mercury by using a conversion table.

schneiderian carcinoma   A malignant tumor of the nasal mucosa and paranasal sinuses.

School Nurse Practitioner (SNP)   A registered nurse who's qualified by postgraduate study to perform the duties of a nurse practitioner in a school.

Schultz-Charlton phenomenon   A skin reaction to the injection of scarlet fever antitoxin or scarlet fever convalescent serum. If the skin has a bright red rash, it will blanch.

Schwabach's test   A hearing test, using these tuning forks: 256, 512, 1024, or 2048 Hz. The tester, who has normal hearing, and the patient each occlude one ear. The tester then alternates the fork between the mastoid process of the patient's open ear and the tester's ear. The process continues until one of them no longer hears the tone. It's used to determine conductive and sensorineural hearing impairment.

Schwann's cells   Large nucleated cells found outside the central nervous system that form the neurilemma and a thin layer of myelin around nerve fibers.

sciatica   A condition characterized by severe pain coursing down the sciatic nerve from the back and buttocks and along the posterior or lateral aspect of the leg, commonly caused by compression or swelling of the sciatic nerve, which may result from a ruptured intervertebral disk in the lower back.

SCID *abbr* severe combined immunodeficiency disease.

science The systematic observation of natural phenomena for the purpose of determining the laws that govern the observed phenomena. Pure science is concerned with gathering facts solely for the purpose of obtaining new knowledge.

scientific method A systematic method of research involving data gathering and problem solving. The basic process involves the statement of the problem, the collection of relevant data to formulate a hypothesis, the development of an experimental method to help prove or disprove the hypothesis, and the drawing of conclusions from the observed experimental results.

scintillation A particle emitted from the disintegration of a radioactive element.

scintiphotography A diagnostic procedure involving the photography of radioactive scintillations given off from body tissues following the introduction of a radioactive substance into the body.

scintiscan A two-dimensional graphic representation of the scintillations produced when a radioactive substance is introduced into the body for diagnostic purposes. The intensity of the record indicates the concentration of the substance in specific organs or tissues.

scirrhous carcinoma A hard, fibrous tumor composed of dense connective tissue.

sclera The tough, white outer coating of the eyeball, extending from the optic nerve to the cornea.

sclerectomy Excision of part of the sclera.

scleredema A disease of unknown cause characterized by nonpitting hardening of the skin beginning on the face or neck and spreading downward to the shoulder, arms, and thorax. The condition is usually preceded by one of a variety of infectious processes, especially a staphylococcal infection, and often occurs in association with diabetes mellitus.

sclerema neonatorum A severe, sometimes fatal condition occurring mainly in preterm or seriously debilitated infants and characterized by a rapidly progressing, generalized hardening of the skin and subcutaneous tissue.

sclerodactyly A localized form of scleroderma affecting the fingers and, less frequently, the toes. May be one of several presenting systems of systemic scleroderma.

scleroderma A relatively rare autoimmune disease characterized by a chronic hardening and thickening of the skin and degeneration of the connective tissue of the skin, lungs, and internal organs. Occurs in a localized form and as a systemic disease.

sclerokeratitis Inflammation of the sclera and cornea.

scleromalacia perforans A condition of the eyes characterized by degeneration and thinning of the sclera, occurring as a complication of rheumatoid arthritis.

sclerosis A hardening of a tissue or part as a result of inflammation or from increased formation of connective tissue.

sclerotome **1.** An instrument used to make an incision in the sclera. **2.** In embryology: the paired segmented masses of mesenchymal tissue in the developing embryo that originate from somites and develop into the vertebrae and ribs.

scolex, *pl.* **scolices** The headlike segment of an adult tapeworm by which it attaches itself to the wall of the intestine; may possess hooks, grooves, or suckers for this purpose.

scoliosis An appreciable lateral curvature of the spine resulting from numerous causes, including congenital malformations of the spine, muscle paralysis, poliomyelitis, sciatica, and unequal leg length.

scorbutic pose The characteristic position of advanced infantile scurvy in which the child lies flat, with thighs and legs semiflexed and hips rotated outward.

scratch test A skin test to determine the allergic reaction to a substance, performed by applying a small amount of the suspected allergen on a superficial scratch.

 CLINICAL TIP A positive reaction is indicated by the formation of a wheal in 15 minutes.

screening **1.** A preliminary test or examination to detect the most common symptoms of a disorder that may require further investigation. **2.** The examination or testing of a large group of individuals or a population to detect a specific disease or disorder or to determine who may be at a higher risk for developing a specific condition.

Scribner shunt A type of arteriovenous bypass, used in hemodialysis, consisting of an external U-shaped tube inserted between the radial artery and the cephalic vein. Also called *Quinton-Scribner shunt.*

scrofula Former name for tuberculous cervical lymphadenitis, a tuberculosis of the cervical lymph nodes occurring either as a primary infection or spread through the lymph system or the blood from another primary site.

scrotoplasty   Repair of the scrotum.

scrotum   The pouch of skin that contains the testes and their accessory organs.

scrub typhus   An acute, typhuslike infectious disease caused by several strains of the genus *Rickettsia* that's transmitted from rats to humans through the bite of an infected larval mite. It occurs primarily in Asia, India, northern Australia, and the western Pacific islands.

scruple (scr.)   A unit of mass or weight of the apothecaries' system, equal to 20 grains or 1.296 g.

scultetus binder   A many-tailed bandage with an attached central piece that's applied with the tails overlapping and held in place by pinning or tying the last two tails.

scurvy   A condition caused by a lack of ascorbic acid (vitamin C) in the diet.

Se   Symbol for selenium.

sebaceous cyst   An incorrect term for an epidermal cyst or pilar cyst.

sebaceous gland   One of the many small glands in the skin that secrete an oily substance, sebum.

seborrhea   Any of several common skin conditions caused by an oversecretion of sebum and characterized by excessive oiliness and dry scales.

seborrheic blepharitis   An inflammation of the eyelids associated with seborrhea of the scalp, eyebrow, and the skin behind the ears and characterized by greasy scaling of the margins of the lids.

seborrheic dermatitis   A chronic, inflammatory skin disease of unknown cause characterized by dry or moist greasy scales and yellow crusted patches on the various parts of the body including the scalp, ears, face, and genitalia.

seborrheic keratosis   Benign tumor of the epidermis with many yellow or brown raised lesions on the skin.

sebum   A substance composed of keratin, fat, and cellular debris secreted by the sebaceous glands of the skin. Combined with sweat, sebum forms a moist, oily, acidic film that protects the skin against drying and bacterial and fungal infections.

secondary areola   A second pigmented ring appearing around the areola of the breast during pregnancy.

secondary biliary cirrhosis   A cirrhosis of the liver caused by chronic bile duct obstruction with or without infection.

secondary bronchus   A lobar or segmental bronchus, a subdivision of the primary bronchus.

secondary dental caries   Dental cavities that develop at the edges of or under an existing dental restoration.

secondary fissure   A fissure between the uvula of the cerebellum and the pyramid. Also referred to as the *postpyramidal fissure.*

secondary host   An animal or plant in which one or more of the asexual larval or intermediate stages of a parasite develop. Humans are secondary hosts for malaria parasites.

secondary nutrient   A substance that stimulates the flora of the intestinal tract to synthesize other nutrients.

secondary sequestrum   A piece of dead bone that becomes partially detached from the sound bone during the process of necrosis but may be pushed into place.

secondary sex characteristic   Any of the physical characteristics of sexual maturity specific to the male or female but not directly involved in reproduction.

secondary shock   A delayed or deferred shock, developing an hour or more following the injury or burn that causes it.

secrete   To generate, separate or discharge a substance into a cavity, a vessel, or an organ or onto the skin surface.

secretin   A digestive hormone produced by the mucosal lining of the duodenum and jejunum when acidic, partially digested food enters the intestine from the stomach.

secretin test   A test of pancreatic function that measures the pancreatic secretion produced as a response to an intravenous injection of secretin.

secretory duct   A smaller duct that has a secretory function and joins with an excretory duct of a gland.

secretory phase   The phase of the menstrual cycle following ovulation. During this phase, also referred to as the luteal phase, the corpus luteum develops and secretes progesterone.

secundigravida   A woman pregnant for the second time; also referred to as gravida II.

sedation   Inducing a state of quiet, calmness, or sleep, especially by means of a sedative or hypnotic medication.

segment   A portion or section of a body, organ, or object, set apart by naturally occurring or artificially established borders.

segmental bronchus   An air passage branching from a lobar bronchus and further dividing into smaller passages called *bronchioles.*

segmental fracture   The fracture of a bone in two places; also referred to as a double fracture. The resulting bone fragments may either pierce the skin, as in an open fracture, or may be contained within the skin, as in a closed fracture.

Secondary bronchus

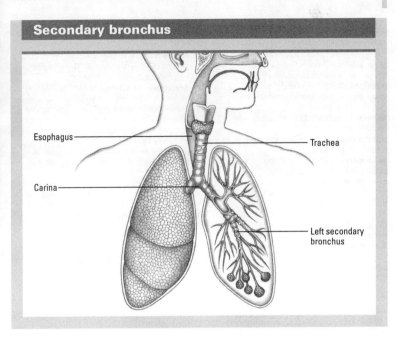

Esophagus

Trachea

Carina

Left secondary bronchus

segmentation   1. The process of dividing into segments or similar parts, as the formation of somites or metameres. **2.** The division of a fertilized egg into blastomeres; cleavage.

segmentation nucleus   The nucleus of the zygote formed by the fusion of the male and female pronuclei in the fertilized ovum.

segmented hyalinizing vasculitis   A chronic, relapsing inflammation of the blood vessels of the lower legs usually affecting middle-aged people with circulatory problems. It's characterized by nodular or purpuric skin lesions that may become ulcerated, resulting in scars.

seizure threshold   The minimum amount of stimulus required to produce a convulsive seizure; also called *convulsant threshold.*

selenium (Se)   A nonmetallic element resembling sulfur, with an atomic number of 34 and an atomic weight of 78.96.

self-differentiation   Specialization and diversification of a tissue or part resulting solely from intrinsic factors and independent of outside influences.

self-limited   Of a disease or condition: tending to run a definite limited course and ending without treatment.

self-retaining catheter   An indwelling urinary catheter constructed to be retained in the bladder and urethra. One of the double

channels allows urine to drain from the bladder; the other channel has a balloon at the bladder end and a diaphragm at the external end to inflate the balloon, which holds the catheter in place.

sella turcica   A saddle-shaped depression crossing the midline of the superior surface of the body of the sphenoid bone; it contains the pituitary gland.

semen   The thick, whitish secretion of the male reproductive organs that's discharged during ejaculation. It's composed of spermatozoa in their nutrient plasma, secretions from the prostate, seminal vesicles, and various other glands.

semicircular duct   One of three long ducts of the membranous labyrinth of the inner ear.

semi-Fowler's position   A position in which the patient is inclined with the upper half of the body raised by elevating the head of the bed. The head isn't raised the full 18″ to 20″ (46 to 51 cm) above level as with the full Fowler's position. The knees are also raised.

semilunar cartilage   Interarticular cartilage of the knee joint.

semilunar valve   A valve with half-moon–shaped cusps, as the aortic valve and the pulmonic valve. The term is sometimes applied to any one of the cusps composing such a valve.

semimembranosus   One of three posterior femoral muscles located at the back and inner side of the thigh that flexes and rotates the leg and extends the thigh.

seminal duct   Any duct, such as the deferent duct or the ejaculatory duct, through which semen passes.

seminal vesiculitis   Inflammation of a seminal vesicle.

seminiferous   Producing, carrying, or transferring semen.

seminuria   Discharge of semen in the urine; also called *spermaturia.*

semitendinosus   One of three posterior femoral muscles located at the back and inner part of the thigh that flexes and rotates the leg and extends the thigh; remarkable for the great length of its tendon of insertion.

senescent   Aging.

Sengstaken-Blakemore tube   A triple-lumen catheter used to stop hemorrhaging from esophageal varices. Two lumens end in two balloons; one is inflated in the stomach to hold the catheter in place and compress the vessels around the cardia and the other is inflated in the esophagus to exert pressure against the varices in the wall of the esophagus. The third lumen is used to aspirate stomach contents.

senile cataract   The most common form of cataract, associated solely with aging, in which a hard opacity forms most often in the cortical area of the lens or, less frequently, in either the nucleus of the lens or the subcapsular area.

senile delirium   A syndrome associated with extreme age, usually of acute onset and characterized by disorientation, mental feebleness, restlessness, insomnia, aimless wandering, and hallucinations.

senile involution   The progressive degeneration that occurs with advancing age and results in the progressive shrinking of tissues and organs.

sensible perspiration   Fluid loss from the body through the sweat glands that forms an observable moisture on the surface of the skin.

sensitivity   1. The ability to feel or respond to a stimulus. 2. Heightened or abnormal susceptibility to a substance, such as a drug or an antigen.

sensitization   1. Administration of an antigen to induce the production of specific antibodies; immunization. 2. Exposure to an antigen resulting in the development of a hypersensitivity.

sensorineural hearing loss   Hearing loss caused by a defect or lesion of the inner ear or the acoustic nerve resulting in a distortion of sound that makes discrimination difficult.

sensorium   1. The center in the brain that processes all sensations. 2. The complete sensory apparatus of the body.

sensory   1. Relating to the senses or sensation. 2. Referring to a structure, such as a nerve, that receives and transmits impulses from sense organs to the reflex and higher centers of the brain.

sensory nerve   A peripheral afferent nerve that conducts sensory impulses from the sense organ receptors of the body to the brain or spinal cord.

septic abortion   Spontaneous or induced termination of a pregnancy associated with a serious pathogenic infection of the uterus and leading to a generalized infection that's life-threatening. To prevent death, treatment requires immediate and intensive care, systemic antibiotic therapy, evacuation of the uterus and, often, emergency hysterectomy.

septic arthritis   An acute infectious arthritis, characterized by tissue and joint inflammation, caused by bacteria that spreads through the blood from a primary site of infection or by joint contamination during trauma or surgery.

septicemia   A systemic infection caused by the presence of pathogenic microorganisms or their toxins in the blood. It's diagnosed by blood culture and treated aggressively with antibiotics.

septic fever   An elevation of body temperature associated with septicemia.

septic shock   A form of shock associated with septicemia thought to result from the action of bacterial endotoxins on the vascular system causing large volumes of blood to be isolated in the capillaries and veins.

ALERT Watch closely for signs of disseminated intravascular coagulation (abnormal bleeding), renal failure (oliguria, increased specific gravity), heart failure (dyspnea, edema, tachycardia, distended neck veins), GI ulcers (hematemesis and melena), and hepatic abnormality (jaundice, hypoprothrombinemia, and hypoalbuminemia).

sequestered antigens theory   A theory of autoimmunity, maintaining that tissues that are anatomically sequestered from the lymphoreticular system during embryonic development may not be recognized as belonging to the body. Such tissues would cause an autoimmune response if exposed to the lymphoreticular system in adult life.

sequestrum, *pl.* sequestra   A piece of dead bone partially or entirely separated from the surrounding or adjacent healthy bone during the process of necrosis.

sequestrum forceps Forceps with small, powerful, serrated jaws used for removing bone fragments that form a sequestrum.

sequoiosis A type of hypersensitivity pneumonitis that occurs in logging and sawmill workers. It's caused by the inhalation of *Graphium* and *Aureobasidium* fungal spores found in moldy redwood sawdust.

serologic diagnosis A diagnosis made through laboratory examination of blood serum reactions to antigens.

serology The study of blood serum for evidence of infection by evaluating in vitro antigen-antibody reactions.

serosa Any serous membrane that lines the external walls of body cavities and secretes a watery exudate; the tunica serosa, for example.

serosanguineous Of a discharge containing both serum and blood.

serositis Inflammation of a serous membrane.

serotonin A naturally occurring derivative of tryptophan found in platelets and in cells of the intestine, pineal body, and central nervous system. It has many physiologic functions including inhibiting gastric secretion, stimulating smooth muscle, and serving as a central neurotransmitter.

Serratia A genus of motile, gram-negative bacteria, many of which are opportunistic pathogens that can cause infections in humans. Infections with *Serratia* organisms are often contracted in hospitals.

serratus anterior A thin muscle of the chest wall extending from the ribs under the arm to the scapula. It serves to draw the scapula forward and also to rotate the scapula to raise the shoulder.

serum The clear, thin, sticky portion of any body fluid; the clear liquid that separates from blood during clotting. Like plasma, it contains no blood cells or platelets; unlike plasma, it contains no fibrinogen.

serum albumin The major plasma protein, which helps to maintain the blood's oncotic pressure.

serum sickness A hypersensitivity reaction that occurs 2 to 3 weeks after antiserum administration. It's characterized by fever, rash, joint pain, edema, and lymphadenopathy.

sesamoid bone Any one of numerous small, round, bony masses embedded within a tendon or joint capsule, found primarily in the hands, feet, and knees.

severe combined immunodeficiency disease (SCID) A group of rare congenital diseases characterized by extreme impairment of both cell-mediated and humoral immunity resulting from a marked deficiency of B cells and T cells.

sex A classification of male or female based on criteria such as the type of gametes produced by the individual, and various anatomic and chromosomal characteristics.

sex chromatin A densely staining mass within the nucleus of female interphase cells of most mammalian species. According to the Lyon hypothesis, it's a single, condensed, inactive X chromosome.

sex chromosome A chromosome associated with the determination of the sex of an offspring. In mammals, an unequal pair of chromosomes, the X and the Y, carry the genes that transmit sex-linked traits and conditions.

sex-influenced Of or pertaining to a genetic trait or condition, as patterned baldness, that's fully expressed in one sex only.

sex-linked disorder Any disease or abnormal condition that's determined by a gene carried on a sex chromosome.

sex-linked ichthyosis A chronic skin disorder affecting only males and transmitted as an X-linked recessive trait from the female. *CLINICAL TIP* The disorder may be present at birth or appear in early infancy and is characterized by large, thick, dry scales that are dark and that cover the neck, extremities, trunk, and buttocks.

sexual generation Production of a new organism by the union of male and female gametes.

SG *abbr* specific gravity.

SGA *abbr* small for gestational age.

sheath A tubular structure that encloses or surrounds an organ or body part, as the sheath of the rectus abdominis muscle.

sheep cell test A method that mixes human blood cells with the red blood cells of sheep to determine the absence or the deficiency of human T-lymphocytes. The sheep cell test is used to diagnose several diseases, such as DiGeorge syndrome.

shield In radiation technology: a material used to prevent or reduce the passage of charged particles or radiation; for example, a lead shield.

shift to the left In hematology: an increase in the number of band cells, the immature stage of neutrophil development in which the cells have only one or a few lobes.

shift to the right In hematology: an increase in the percentage of polymorphonuclear neutrophils having three or more lobes, indicating cell maturity.

Shigella A genus of gram-negative, facultatively anaerobic, pathogenic bacteria that cause gastroenteritis and bacterial dysentery such as *Shigella dysenteriae.*

shigellosis　An acute infectious disease of the bowel caused by bacteria of the pathogenic genus *Shigella;* characterized by fever, intestinal pain, diarrhea with mucus and blood in the stools. Also called *bacillary dysentery.*

shin splints　Strain of the long flexor muscle of the toes caused by strenuous athletic activity and characterized by pain along the shin in the lower leg.

Shirodkar's operation　A surgical procedure performed to correct an incompetent cervix in which the cervical canal is closed with a surrounding purse-string suture, called a *cerclage.*

shock　An abnormal physiologic state characterized by reduced cardiac output, circulatory insufficiency, tachycardia, hypotension, restlessness, pallor, and diminished urinary output. Shock may be caused by a variety of conditions including trauma, infection, hemorrhage, poisoning, myocardial infarction, and dehydration.

shock lung　A sudden, severe pulmonary edema resulting from increased permeability of the alveolar capillary membrane resulting in acute respiratory failure. Also called *adult respiratory distress syndrome (ARDS).*

shoulder girdle　Area formed by the clavicle and the scapula.

shoulder joint　The ball-and-socket articulation formed by the head of the humerus and the cavity of the scapula.

shreds　Slender strands of mucous filaments in the urine that indicate an inflammation of the urinary tract.

shunt　1. To divert the flow of a body fluid from one cavity or vessel to another. 2. A tube or device surgically implanted in the body to divert the flow of body fluid.

Shy-Drager syndrome　A rare, progressive disorder, characterized by orthostatic hypotension, impotence in males, constipation, urinary retention or urgency, anhidrosis, general neurologic dysfunction, tremor, rigidity, incoordination, ataxia, and muscle wasting.

Si　Symbol for silicon.

sialoadenotomy　Incision and drainage of a salivary gland.

sialogogue　An agent that stimulates the flow of saliva.

sialography　A radiographic technique in which a salivary gland is filmed following the injection of an X-ray opaque substance into its duct.

Siamese twins　Conjoined twin fetuses produced from the same ovum. The severity of the condition ranges from two well-developed individuals joined by a superficial connection to that in which the heads or complete torsos are united and several internal organs are shared, or a small, incompletely developed twin is attached to a much larger and more fully developed twin.

sibilant crackles　Abnormal, shrill hissing or whistling sounds produced by the presence of a viscid secretion in the bronchial tubes in respiratory diseases, such as asthma or bronchitis.

sickle cell　A crescent-shaped erythrocyte that contains hemoglobin S, an abnormal form of hemoglobin.

sickle cell anemia　A chronic and incurable hereditary disorder occurring in people homozygous for hemoglobin S (Hb S). The presence of Hb S results in distortion and fragility of erythrocytes.

sickle cell thalassemia　A heterozygous hemolytic disorder in which the genes for sickle cell and thalassemia are inherited.

sickle cell trait　A heterozygous form of sickle cell anemia in which hemoglobin S and hemoglobin A occur in erythrocytes.

sideroblastic anemia　A heterogenous, chronic blood disorder marked by normocytic or macrocytic anemia, hypochromic and normochromic erythrocytes, and decreased erythropoiesis and hemoglobin synthesis.

siderosis　1. A form of pneumoconiosis due to the presence of iron dust or particles. 2. Discoloration of tissue because of excess iron. 3. An excess of iron in circulating blood.

SIDS　*abbr* sudden infant death syndrome.

Sigma Theta Tau　A national honor society for nurses.

sigmoid　1. Resembling an S shape. 2. The sigmoid colon.

sigmoid colon　Part of the colon describing an S-shaped curve between the pelvis and rectum.

sigmoidectomy　Excision of the sigmoid colon.

sigmoid mesocolon　A peritoneal fold that joins the sigmoid colon with the pelvic wall, forming a curved line of attachment.

sigmoidopexy　Attachment of the sigmoid colon to another structure.

sigmoidoscope　An endoscope that enables observation of the membrane lining of the colon; it's used to study the lumen of the sigmoid colon.

sigmoidotomy　Incision into the sigmoid colon.

sign　An objective finding indicating disease, such as a fever or rash; they're often accompanied by symptoms of disease.

silicon (Si)　A common nonmetallic element with atomic number 14 and atomic weight 28.086.

Inheritance patterns in sickle cell anemia

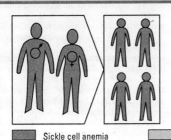
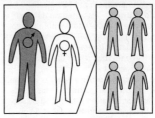

When both parents have sickle cell anemia, childbearing, if possible at all, is dangerous for the mother, and all offspring will have sickle cell anemia.

When one parent has sickle cell anemia and one is normal, all offspring will be carriers of sickle cell anemia.

silicosis   A pulmonary condition caused by prolonged exposure and continual inhalation of silicon dioxide dust.

silk suture   A nonabsorbable, braided, black suture material that's used to close incisions, wounds, and cuts; it's removed after about 7 days.

silo filler's disease   A rare pulmonary disorder affecting workers in closed, poorly ventilated spaces, such as silos, who inhale nitrogen oxide from fermented fodder.

silver (Ag)   A soft, white, precious metal with atomic number 47 and atomic weight 107.88.

simian crease   A crease that crosses the palm from the fusion of the proximal and distal palmar creases; it's usually seen in congenital disorders such as Down syndrome.

simple angioma   A tumor composed of a network of small vessels or distended capillaries bound together by connective tissue.

simple fracture   An uncomplicated, closed bone fracture in which the skin isn't broken.

simple mastectomy   A surgical procedure in which only the breast is removed and the underlying muscles and lymph nodes are left intact.

simple protein   A protein that yields only amino acids on hydrolysis, including albumins, globulins, alcohol-soluble proteins, albuminoids, histones, and protamines.

Sims' position   A semiprone position in which the patient lies on the left side with

the right knee and thigh drawn toward the chest.

sinew   A tendon of a muscle.

sinoatrial (SA) block   A cardiac conduction disorder during which an SA nodal impulse is blocked from activating the atrial myocardium.

sinoatrial (SA) node   A group of several cells in the right atrial wall near the opening of the superior vena cava.

sirenomelia   A congenital condition in which the lower extremities are fused and feet are lacking.

Sister Kenny's treatment   Treatment of poliomyelitis in which the patient's limbs and back are wrapped in warm, moist cloths; after the pain is relieved, the patient exercises the affected muscles.

situs   The normal site or position.

sitz bath   A bath commonly used for patients who have undergone rectal or perineal surgery in which only the hips and buttocks are immersed in water or saline solution.

Sjögren-Larsson syndrome   An autosomal recessive disorder that's marked by ichthyosis, mental deficiency, and spastic paralysis.

skeletal fixation   A method of firmly attaching fractured bone fragments with wires, screws, plates, or nails.

skeletal traction   Type of orthopedic traction used to treat fractures and correct orthopedic abnormalities.

skeleton The supporting framework of the body that protects delicate structures, provides attachments for muscles, allows body movement, serves as major reservoirs of blood, and produces red blood cells.

Skene's glands Paraurethral ducts of the female urethra that open just within the urethral orifice.

skew Deviating from a straight line or symmetrical pattern, such as data that don't follow the expected statistical curve.

skilled nursing facility (SNF) An institution or part of an institution that meets criteria for accreditation established by sections of the Social Security Act that determine the basis for Medicaid and Medicare reimbursement for skilled nursing care, including rehabilitation and various medical and nursing procedures.

Skillern's fracture A complete fracture of the distal radius with a greenstick fracture of the distal ulna.

skin The membranous protective covering of the body; also the largest organ.

skin cancer Abnormal, cutaneous tissue growth as a result of ionizing radiation, genetic defects, chemical carcinogens, or overexposure to the sun.

CLINICAL TIP A common and curable malignancy, it's also the most frequent secondary lesion in patients with other cancers.

skinfold calipers An instrument that measures the breadth of a skinfold, commonly on the posterior aspect of the upper arm or over the lower ribs.

skinfold thickness The thickness of a skinfold gripped by calipers; it estimates the amount of subcutaneous fat for use in determining nutritional needs.

skin graft Part of the skin implanted to cover areas where it has been lost through burns, injury, or excised tissue.

skin prep The cleaning of skin with an antiseptic before surgery or venipuncture; usually done to eliminate bacteria and pathologic organisms and reduce the risk of infection.

skin test The intradermal injection or topical application of a test substance to determine the body's reaction to it.

skin traction A basic type of orthopedic traction used in the treatment of fractured bones and correction of orthopedic abnormalities.

skull The bony structure of the head, consisting of the cranium and facial skeleton. The cranium contains and protects the brain.

SL *abbr* 1. soda lime. 2. sublingual.

SLE *abbr* systemic lupus erythematosus.

sling A bandage designed to support an injured body part.

sling restraint A therapeutic device that's used to assist in immobilizing patients, especially in orthopedic traction.

slit lamp An ophthalmic instrument used to examine the conjunctiva, lens, vitreous humor, iris, and cornea.

slit lamp microscope A microscope for ophthalmic visualization of the posterior surface of the corneal endothelium.

slough The shedding or elimination of dead tissue cells of the endometrium, which are shed during menstruation.

slow virus A virus that remains dormant in the body for a long time before symptoms occur.

Sm Symbol for samarium.

SMA 6 *abbr* sequential multiple analysis, 6 serum test.

SMA 12 *abbr* sequential multiple analysis, 12 channel biochemical profile.

SMA 20 *abbr* sequential multiple analysis, 20 chemical constituents.

SMA 60 *abbr* sequential multiple analysis, 60 chemical constituents.

SMAC *abbr* sequential multiple analyzer computer.

small-for-gestational-age (SGA) infant An infant whose weight and size at birth is below the 10th percentile of appropriate-for-gestational-age infants.

small intestine Part of the digestive system from the stomach to the iliocecal junction, extending for about 23′ (7 m); it's divided into the duodenum, jejunum, and ileum.

smallpox An acute, infectious, viral disease marked by fever, prostration, and a vesicular, pustular rash.

smear A thin specimen for microscopic study prepared by spreading a film of tissue onto a glass slide.

smegma A foul-smelling secretion of sebaceous glands occurring in the genital area.

Smith fracture A reverse Colles' fracture of the wrist, involving displacement of the bone fragment toward the volar aspect.

Smith-Petersen nail A three-flanged stainless steel nail used to secure a fracture of the femur neck.

Sn Symbol for tin.

SN *abbr* student nurse.

snare A device for removing small projections from a surface; a wire noose is placed around the growth and gradually tightened.

sneeze A sudden, forceful, involuntary expulsion of air through the nose and mouth; a reflex caused by an irritation to mucous membranes of the upper respiratory tract.

Snellen chart A visual acuity testing chart in which letters, numbers, or symbols are arranged in decreasing size from top to bottom.

Snellen test A visual acuity test using the Snellen chart. The person being tested stands 20′ (6 m) from the chart and reads as much of the chart as possible.

SNF *abbr* skilled nursing facility.

snout reflex A sign marked by facial grimace, usually indicating bilateral corticopontine lesions, elicited by tapping the nose.

snuffles A nasal discharge in infants that may be due to congenital syphilis.

soap A compound of fatty acids and an alkali that's used in detergents, liniments, enemas, and other products.

SOB *abbr* shortness of breath.

socket A hollow into which a correspondingly shaped bone or organ fits.

soda A compound of sodium, especially sodium bicarbonate, sodium carbonate, or sodium hydroxide.

soda lime (SL) A compound used as an absorbent of carbon dioxide, such as in an anesthesia rebreathing system.

sodium (Na) A soft, gray alkaline metal with atomic number 11 and atomic weight 22.99.

sodium arsenate poisoning Toxicity due to the ingestion of sodium arsenate; the symptoms and treatment are similar to those for arsenic poisoning.

sodium chloride Common table salt with several uses, including as a fluid and electrolyte replenisher, isotonic vehicle, irrigating solution, and enema.

sodium glutamate A glutamic acid salt used in the treatment of hepatic coma and for improving food flavor.

sodium pump A hypothetical mechanism that transports sodium ions across cellular membranes against an opposing concentration gradient.

soft diet Liquid or semisolid food that's soft, easily digested, low in residue, and well tolerated and provides essential nutrients.

soft palate Located in the posterior part of the palate, this structure is composed of mucous membrane, muscular fibers, and mucous glands and forms the roof of the mouth.

soft radiation Low energy and low penetrating power radiation.

solar plexus A complex network of nervous tissue surrounding the celiac roots and the superior mesenteric arteries around the first lumbar vertebra.

solar radiation The emission and diffusion of radiant energy from the sun, overexposure to which may cause sunburn, keratosis, skin cancer, or photosensitivity reactions.

soleus A broad, flat posterior muscle of the leg lying under the gastrocnemius and arising by tendinous fibers from the head of the fibula, from the popliteal line, and from the medial border of the tibia.

solution A homogeneous mixture of two or more substances dispersed molecularly in another dissolving substance. The molecules of each substance don't undergo chemical reaction.

solvent A liquid in which another substance can be dissolved.

somatic With reference to the body.

somatic cell An undifferentiated body cell having the diploid number of chromosomes.

somatic delusion A false belief regarding body image or function.

somatist A psychotherapist or psychiatrist who believes all neuroses and psychoses are caused by diseases of the body.

somatomegaly An abnormally large body due to excessive somatotropin or inadequate somatostatin.

somatoplasm The nonreproductive protoplasm of body cells, excluding germ cells.

somatopleure The body wall layer of an early developing embryo.

somatostatin A hormone made in the hypothalamus that inhibits the release of somatotropin from the anterior pituitary gland.

somite In vertebrates: a pair of mesodermal tissue masses arranged segmentally along the length of the neural tube during early embryonic development.

somnambulism Sleepwalking; a condition occurring during the first third of sleep marked by complex motor activity and no recall on awakening.

sonorous crackle A snoring sound caused by the vibration of thick secretions lodged in a bronchus.

souffle A soft sound heard through a stethoscope, commonly over the pregnant uterus, caused by circulating blood in the large uterine arteries.

sparganosis An infection caused by fish tapeworm larvae, marked by painful eye or subcutaneous inflammation.

spasmodic torticollis Torticollis marked by transient neck muscle spasmotic episodes. Examination rarely reveals a physical cause.

spastic aphonia Spasmodic contraction of the throat abductor muscles resulting in an inability to speak.

spastic bladder Neurogenic bladder due to a spinal cord lesion located above the voiding reflex center.

spastic paralysis The involuntary contraction of a muscle with associated loss of muscular function.

SPE *abbr* sucrose polyester.

spec *abbr* 1. specimen. 2. speculum.

specialist A healthcare professional with advanced postgraduate or clinical training in a specialty.

special sense One of the five senses of sight, smell, touch, taste, or hearing.

species (Sp) In taxonomic classification: the subcategory below genus; includes individuals of the same genus who have similar structure and chemical composition and, thus, can interbreed.

species immunity A type of natural immunity shared by members of a species.

specific activity In nuclear medicine: the radioactivity of a radioisotope per unit mass of the element or compound, expressed in microcuries per millimol or disintegrations per second per milligram.

specific gravity Ratio of the density of one substance to the density of another approved as a standard. Water is the accepted standard for liquids and solids; hydrogen is the accepted standard for gases.

specimen A sample of a substance, the purpose of which is to show the characteristics of the whole.

SPECT *abbr* single photon emission computed tomography.

spectrometer An instrument for measuring wavelengths of rays of a spectrum, the index of refraction, and the angles between faces of a prism.

spectrometry The measurement of wavelengths of light and other electromagnetic waves.

spectrophotometry An instrument that measures color in a solution by determining the amount of light absorbed; it's used to calculate the concentration of substances in solution.

spectrum, *pl.* spectra 1. A range of properties occurring in increasing or decreasing magnitude. The arrangement of radiant or electromagnetic energy is based on wavelength and frequency. 2. The range of effectiveness of an antibiotic. A broad-spectrum antibiotic works well against a wide range of microorganisms.

speculum A retractor that enlarges the opening of a cavity for inspection.

speech 1. The expression of thoughts in verbal sounds. 2. The act of communicating verbally, requiring the coordination of larynx, mouth, lips, tongue, lungs, throat, and abdomen.

speech dysfunction Any defect or abnormality of speech, including aphasia, alexia, stammering, stuttering, aphonia, and slurring.

speech pathology 1. The study of the speech organs and related defects and disorders. 2. The diagnosis and treatment of speech disorders by a speech pathologist or therapist.

speech therapist A professionally trained person skilled in speech pathology who treats people with speech disorders.

speed shock Shock caused by too-rapid direct injection of a drug; most drugs must be directly injected over a specific time period to avoid speed shock. No drug should be injected in less than 1 minute unless the patient is in cardiac or respiratory arrest, or the order specifies so.

spermatic cord A cord extending from the deep inguinal ring through the scrotum and into the testis.

spermatic fistula An abnormal passage that communicates with the testis or seminal ducts.

spermatid A male germ cell that originates from a spermatocyte and becomes a mature spermatozoon in the final phase of spermatogenesis.

spermatocele A cyst of the epididymis or rete testis that contains spermatozoa.

spermatocide A chemical substance that destroys spermatozoa either by reducing their surface tension or by creating an acidic environment.

spermatocyte A male germ cell that originates from a spermatogonium.

spermatogenesis The process of forming spermatozoa that includes spermatocytogenesis, in which spermatogonia become spermatocytes that develop into spermatids, and spermiogenesis, in which the spermatids become spermatozoa.

spermatozoon, *pl.* spermatozoa A mature male germ cell formed in the seminiferous tubules of the testes; each spermatozoon is about 50 micrometers ($1/500''$) in length and consists of a head (with a nucleus), neck, and tail.

spermaturia Sperm in the urine.

sphenoidal fissure A cleft between the great and small wings of the sphenoid bone.

sphenoidal sinus One of a pair of paranasal cavities lined with mucous membrane. A large sphenoidal sinus may extend into the roots of the pterygoid processes, the great wings, or occipital bone.

sphenoid bone The bone located at the skull base, anterior to the temporal bones and the basilar part of the occipital bone; it resembles a bat with extended wings.

sphenomandibular ligament A pair of flat, thin ligaments making up part of the temporomandibular joint between the mandible and the temporal bone.

spherocyte   A spherical erythrocyte containing more than the usual amount of hemoglobin.

spherocytic anemia   A hematologic disorder caused by the presence of spherocytes.

sphincter   A muscle that surrounds a tube, duct, or orifice such that its contraction alters the size of the lumen or orifice.

sphincteroplasty   Repair of a sphincter.

sphincter pupillae   A muscle that expands the iris and narrows the pupillary diameter.

sphygmogram   Related to a tracing produced by a sphygmograph; a curve occurring on the tracing represents an atrial pulse.

sphygmograph   An instrument designed to record the atrial pulse.

sphygmomanometer   An instrument, consisting of an inflatable cuff, inflatable bulb, and a gauge, designed to measure arterial blood pressure.

spica bandage   A figure-eight bandage in which each turn overlaps the next, forming a succession of V-like designs. This bandage is used to provide support, apply pressure, or hold a dressing securely.

spica cast   An orthopedic cast that immobilizes part or all of the trunk or extremity.

spina bifida   A common neural tube defect caused by one or more vertebral arches failing to fuse.

spina bifida anterior   Incomplete fusion of the anterior surface of the vertebral column.

spina bifida occulta   A defective closure of the vertebral column in the lumbosacral region without hernial protrusion of the spinal cord or meninges.

spinal aperture   large opening formed by the vertebral body and its arch.

spinal canal   The cavity inside the vertebral column.

spinal cord   A long, almost cylindrical structure lodged in the vertebral canal and extending from the base of the skull to the upper lumbar region.

spinal cord compression   A serious complication due to pressure on the spinal cord.

spinal cord injury   A traumatic disruption of the spinal cord, usually accompanied by extensive musculoskeletal involvement.

spinal cord tumor   A spinal cord neoplasm of which more than 50% are extramedullary, about 25% intramedullary, and the remainder extradural.

spinal curvature   A persistent deviation of the vertebral column from its usual position.

spinal fusion   The fastening of an unstable part of the spine, usually by surgery or less commonly by skeletal traction or immobilization of the patient in a body cast.

spinal headache   Occurring after spinal anesthesia or lumbar puncture, it's caused by a loss of cerebrospinal spinal fluid from the subarachnoid space through the puncture site.

spinal manipulation   The forceful passive movement of vertebral segments beyond their active limit of movement.

spinal nerves   The nerves emerging from the spinal cord; there are 31 pairs (8 cervical, 12 thoracic, 5 lumbar, 5 sacral, and 1 coccygeal).

spinal tract   An ascending or descending pathway for nerve impulses occurring in the white matter of the spinal cord.

spindle   1. The fusiform appearance of achromatin during the late prophase and metaphase stages of mitosis. 2. A burst of electrical activity (14 waves per second) usually seen on electroencephalographic examination. 3. A sensory organ consisting of neurotendinous and neuromuscular spindles.

spindle cell carcinoma   A mass of rapidly growing fusiform squamous cells that may be difficult to differentiate from a sarcoma.

spinnbarkeit   The clear, slippery, elastic characteristic of cervical mucus during ovulation; it's also a useful indicator of peak fertility during a menstrual cycle.

spinocerebellar disorder   A genetic disorder in which the spinal cord, cerebellum, and other nervous system tissue undergo gradual degeneration.

spiral fracture   A disruption of bone tissue that's spiral, oblique, or transverse to the long axis of the fractured bone. See illustration on page 286.

spiral reverse bandage   A bandage that's turned and folded back on itself to fit body shape.

spirochete   A motile and spiral-shaped bacterium.

spirogram   A recording made by a spirometer of respiratory movements.

spirograph   An instrument that records respiratory movements.

spirometer   A device used to determine pulmonary function; it measures and records the amount of respiratory gases.

spirometry   Measurement of pulmonary function by a spirometer.

splanchnopleure   An early embryonic layer formed by association of endoderm and splanchnic mesoderm.

S-plasty   A technique used in plastic surgery in which an S-shaped incision is

Spiral fracture

The fracture line crosses the bone at an oblique angle, creating a spiral pattern. This type of break usually occurs in a long bone.

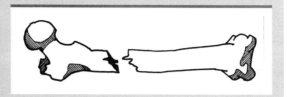

made in loose skin to reduce tension and improve healing.

spleen   A soft, highly vascular, lymphatic organ located between the stomach and diaphragm on the left side.

 ALERT If the patient has a history of abdominal or thoracic trauma, don't palpate the abdomen as this may aggravate internal bleeding. Instead, examine for left-upper-quadrant pain and signs of shock, such as tachycardia and tachypnea. If you detect these signs, suspect splenic rupture.

splenectomy   The surgical removal of the spleen.

splenic flexure syndrome   Recurrent pain and abdominal distention in the upper left abdomen caused by gas trapped in the large intestine below the spleen, at the splenic flexure.

splenius capitis   One of a pair of deep muscles of the back.

splenomegaly   An enlargement of the spleen that may occur with portal hypertension, hemolytic anemia, Niemann-Pick disease, or malaria.

splenopexy   Fixation of a movable spleen.

splenorrhaphy   Repair of the spleen.

splint   **1.** An orthopedic appliance used to immobilize, restrain, or support part of the body. **2.** In dentistry: something used to anchor the teeth or modify the bite.

splinter fracture   A comminuted fracture with long and sharp-pointed bone fragments.

splinter hemorrhage   Bleeding under a fingernail or toenail that looks like a splinter and is usually observed in trauma patients or in those with bacterial endocarditis.

split gene   In molecular genetics: a genetic unit whose gene sequence is broken.

split Russell traction   A device that's used to immobilize, position, and align the lower extremities in congenital hip disloca-tion and hip and knee contractures and for correcting orthopedic deformities.

spondylitis   Inflammation of the spinal vertebrae, causing stiffness and pain.

spondylolisthesis   The forward movement of one vertebra over the one lying below it.

spondylosis   Fixation or stiffness of a vertebral joint.

spongioblastoma, *pl.* spongioblas-tomas, spongioblastomata   Tissue growth consisting of spongioblasts, embryonic epithelial cells occurring around the neural tube that infiltrate nerve cells or the lining of ventricles and the spinal cord canal.

spongiosis   Edematous swelling within the cells of the epidermis.

spontaneous   Occurring naturally and without external restraint.

spontaneous abortion   Expulsion of the fetus from the uterus before the 20th week of gestation, caused by fetal abnormalities or maternal environment.

spontaneous delivery   A vaginal birth occurring without any mechanical assistance, such as an obstetric forceps or a vacuum aspirator.

spontaneous evolution   The unaided delivery of a fetus lying in the transverse position.

spontaneous generation   The hypothesis that living organisms can arise from inanimate matter; abiogenesis.

spontaneous labor   Labor that starts and progresses without mechanical or pharmacologic stimulation.

spore   **1.** The reproductive unit of some fungi or protozoa. **2.** A form that can resist external conditions, such as heat and drought, and chemicals.

sporicide   An agent that can kill spores.

sporiferous   Capable of producing or bearing spores.

sporogenesis   The formation or reproduction by spores; sporogeny.

sporogenous   Relating to an animal or plant that can reproduce by spores.

sporogeny   The formation and development of spores.

sporogony   Reproduction by spores, particularly the formation of sporozoites in a sporozoan protozoan, such as *Plasmodium.*

sporophore   The spore-producing part of an organism or plant.

sporophyte   The asexual, spore-bearing stage in a plant that demonstrates alternation of generations.

sporotrichosis   A chronic fungal infection resulting in skin ulcers and subcutaneous nodules along lymphatic channels that's caused by *Sporothrix schenckii.*

sprain   A joint injury involving the tendons, muscles, or ligaments, accompanied by pain, swelling, and skin discoloration.

sprain fracture   A fracture caused by the separation of a tendon or ligament at the point of insertion, together with a piece of bone.

spring forceps   An instrument with a spring mechanism that's used for grasping an artery to stop or prevent bleeding. Also called *bulldog forceps.*

spring lancet   A surgical knife with a spring-triggered blade that's used in the collection of small blood specimens.

sprinter's fracture   A break in the anterior superior or inferior ilium spine that may occur during a muscular spasm, such as at the start of a sprint.

sprue   A condition caused by intestinal malabsorption of nutrients.

sputum   Expectorated material coughed up from the lungs and through the mouth.

squamous cell carcinoma   A malignant neoplasm composed of squamous epithelial cells, commonly occurring in the lungs, skin, larynx, nose, and bladder.

squeeze dynamometer   An instrument that measures the muscular strength of a hand grip.

squinting eye   Strabismus that can't be focused with the rigid eye.

Sr   Symbol for strontium.

SR   *abbr* **1.** sedimentation rate **2.** sinus rhythm.

SRS-A   *abbr* slow-reacting substance of anaphylaxis.

ss   *abbr* steady state.

SSSS   *abbr* staphylococcal scalded skin syndrome.

stable element   A nonradioactive element, such as calcium, iron, lead, potassium, and sodium, that can't undergo spontaneous nuclear degeneration.

staccato speech   Speech in which pauses between words break the flow in a phrase or sentence.

stadium, *pl.* **stadia**   A stage in the course of a disease.

staging   **1.** The determination and classification of a disease, organism, or process into distinct developmental periods or phases. **2.** The process of classifying tumors based on size, nodal involvement, and metastatic progress.

stain   A dye, pigment, or agent that discolors microscopic objects or tissues, thus aiding study and identification.

stance phase of gait   The first part of the gait cycle starting with the strike of the heel on the ground and ending with the lift of the toe at the beginning of the swing phase; it's the brief period when both feet are on the ground.

stapedectomy   The replacement of the stapes of the middle ear with a graft and prosthesis to restore hearing.

stapes   An ossicle in the middle ear, resembling a stirrup, whose function is to transmit sound vibrations from the incus to the internal ear.

staphylococcal infection   An infection caused by *Staphylococcus,* commonly resulting in abscesses of the skin and other organs.

staphylococcal scalded skin syndrome (SSSS)   Epidermal erythema, peeling, and necrosis that make the skin appear scalded.

staphylokinase   An enzyme, produced by some staphylococci strains, that rapidly converts plasminogen to plasmin in several animal hosts.

starch   **1.** A polysaccharide composed of long chains of glucose subunits; the chief molecule used to store food in plants. In animals, excess glucose is stored as glycogen, which shares a similar molecular structure. **2.** A demulcent.

Starr-Edwards prosthesis   An artificial cardiac valve that prevents the backward flow of blood by obstructing the valve opening.

start point   In molecular genetics: the first nucleotide transcribed from the deoxyribonucleic acid template during the formation of messenger ribonucleic acid.

starvation   Prolonged food deprivation resulting in body dysfunction.

stasis   **1.** The standing still of blood or other fluids in a body vessel. **2.** Stillness.

stasis ulcer   A necrotic, craterlike skin lesion caused by severe venous congestion, usually affecting the lower leg.

stat, STAT   *abbr* at once, immediately.

static Stationary, lacking motion, at rest, in equilibrium.

static imaging In nuclear medicine: a diagnostic method of observation of internal body structures by giving a radioactive material to a patient.

station The degree of descent of the presenting part of the fetus through the maternal pelvis, relative to the maternal ischial spines.

status 1. A state or condition, such as emotional status. 2. An unrelenting state or condition, such as status asthmaticus.

status asthmaticus A severe and prolonged asthma attack in which bronchospasm fails to respond to oral medication, sometimes resulting in hypoxia, cyanosis, and unconsciousness.

STD *abbr* sexually transmitted disease.

steady state (SS) A physiologic idea that all life's forces and processes are in homeostasis. Living organisms are in dynamic equilibrium, working to balance the internal and external environments to avoid a deficiency or excess that may cause illness.

Stearns' alcoholic amentia Alcohol-induced insanity marked by an emotional disturbance that lasts longer but is less severe than delirium tremens and includes increased mental clouding and amnesia.

steatorrhea Excessive fat in the feces that floats, is frothy and foul-smelling, and occurs in celiac disease and malabsorption syndromes.

Steele-Richardson-Olszewski syndrome A rare but progressive neurologic disorder that usually affects middle-aged men.

stellate fracture A bone fracture with a central point of injury from which several fissures radiate.

stem cell leukemia A type of leukemia that's difficult to classify because the predominant cell is too immature to classify.

stent 1. A material compound used to make dental impressions or medical molds. 2. A device used in anchoring skin grafts or for supporting tubular structures in the body, such as vessels and cavities, during surgical anastomosis.

stereognosis 1. The ability to perceive and understand the form and nature of objects by touching. 2. Perception by the senses of the solidity of objects.

stereognostic perception The recognition of objects by touching.

stereoscopic microscope A microscope that enables an object to be observed three-dimensionally through a double optical system with independent light paths.

sterile 1. Barren; inability to reproduce due to an abnormality, such as the absence of spermatogenesis in a man or fallopian tube blockage in a woman. 2. Aseptic; free from living microorganisms.

sterilization 1. A process or action that results in an inability to produce offspring. 2. The destruction of microorganisms by heat, water, chemicals, radiation, or gases.

sternoclavicular articulation The double-gliding connection of the sternum and clavicle.

sternocostal articulation The gliding joint of each rib cartilage and the sternum, excluding the first rib joint, in which the cartilage is directly connected with the sternum to form a synchondrosis.

sternum A long, flattened bone forming the middle part of the thorax. It supports the clavicles, articulates with the first seven pairs of ribs, and is made up of the manubrium, gladiolus, and xiphoid process.

stertorous Laborious breathing that produces a snoring sound.

stethoscope An instrument used to mediate auscultation; it consists of two earpieces connected by flexible tubing to a diaphragm, which is placed against the patient's chest or back.

Stevens-Johnson syndrome An inflammatory disease that initially presents with fever followed by skin bullae and ulcers on the mucous membranes of the lips, eyes, mouth, nasal passage, and genitalia.

stillbirth 1. The birth of a fetus that has died before or during delivery. 2. A fetus, born dead, weighing over 1,000 g (2 lb, 3 oz) that would have been expected to live.

stillborn 1. An infant that was born dead. 2. Related to an infant dead on birth.

Still's disease Rheumatoid arthritis affecting the larger joints of children below age 16.

Stokes-Adams attack Sudden episode of light-headedness or loss of consciousness caused by an abrupt slowdown or stoppage of the heart beat.

stoma, *pl.* **stomas, stomata** 1. A minute pore, orifice, or surface opening. 2. An artificial, surgically created opening of an internal organ on the body surface, such as for a colostomy or tracheostomy. 3. A new opening surgically created between two structures, such as for a gastroenterostomy or pancreaticogastrostomy.

stomach A saclike organ of digestion that's located in the upper left abdomen and divided into the fundus, body, and pylorus.

stomach pump A pump, connected to a tube passed through the mouth or nose into the stomach, that's used to withdraw the stomach contents.

Sternoclavicular and sternocostal articulations

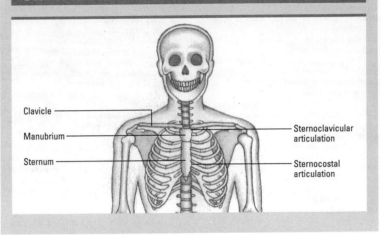

Clavicle

Manubrium

Sternum

Sternoclavicular articulation

Sternocostal articulation

stomatitis   An inflammation of the mouth that may result from bacterial, viral, or fungal infection; exposure to chemicals or drugs; vitamin deficiency; or a systemic inflammatory disease.

STPD   *abbr* standard temperature, standard pressure, dry.

strain   **1.** To use physical force to an extreme, resulting in damage. **2.** To filter solids or particles from liquid. **3.** The injury, usually muscular, resulting from using excessive physical force. **4.** A classification of a subgroup of a species. **5.** An emotional state reflecting mental pressure or fatigue.

strapping   The bandaging of adhesive tape strips to a body area to place pressure and hold a structure in place, such as in the treatment of strains, sprains, dislocations, and fractures.

stratified epithelium   Squamous or columnar cells arranged in three or more layers.

stratiform fibrocartilage   A fibrocartilage structure that forms a thin layer of osseous grooves through which certain muscles glide.

stratum, *pl.* strata   A uniform, thick sheet or layer, usually occurring with other layers, such as the layers of the epidermis.

stratum basale   The basal layer of the epidermis composed of a single layer of columnar cells.

stratum granulosum   The granular layer of the epidermis in which cells contain visible cytoplasmic granules that die, become keratinized, move to the surface, and flake away; it's absent in the palms and soles.

stratum lucidum   A layer of the epidermis that occurs only in the thick skin of the palms and soles.

stratum spinosum   A layer of the epidermis that's composed of several layers of polygonal cells.

strawberry gallbladder   Indicative of cholesterolosis; a small, yellow gallbladder flecked with deposits on the red mucous membranes, resulting in a strawberry-like appearance.

Streptobacillus   A genus of nonmotile, gram-negative, necklace-shaped bacteria.

streptococcal infection   An infection caused by pathogenic bacteria belonging to the genus *Streptococcus* or their toxins.

Streptococcus   A genus of nonmotile, gram-positive bacteria whose classification is based on serologic types, hemolytic action when grown on blood agar, and reaction to bacterial viruses. Most species can cause disease in humans.

streptokinase   An enzyme produced by streptococci that's capable of converting plasminogen to plasmin in animal hosts.

streptolysin   A substance, produced by some streptococci, that yields hemoglobin from red blood cells.

stress fracture   A bone fracture involving one or more metatarsals that's caused by repeated, prolonged, or abnormal stress.

stress test   A test measuring the efficiency of a body system under monitored stress conditions.

stria, *pl.* **striae**　A streak or line, such as that seen on the abdomen after pregnancy, usually due to rapidly developing skin tension. Purplish striae are indicative of hyperadrenocorticism.

striated muscle　A type of muscle, such as the skeletal muscles.

stridor　A high-pitched respiratory sound, usually heard during inspiration, caused by an obstruction of the trachea or larynx.

 ALERT If you detect stridor, quickly check the patient's vital signs and examine him for other signs of partial airway obstruction, including choking or gagging, tachypnea, dyspnea, shallow respirations, intercostal retractions, nasal flaring, tachycardia, cyanosis, and diaphoresis.

string carcinoma　A malignancy of the large intestine that appears to be tied in segments, similar to a string of beads, on radiologic observation.

stroke volume　Amount of blood pumped out of the heart in a single contraction.

strontium (Sr)　A metallic element with atomic number 38 and atomic weight 87.62.

structural chemistry　The study of the molecular structure of chemical substances.

structural gene　In molecular genetics: a unit of genetic information containing the code of amino acid sequence of a polypeptide.

Stryker wedge frame　An orthopedic bed that can rotate the patient to the supine or prone position.

ST segment　Part of the cardiac cycle that appears as a short, upward curve following the spiked QRS complex before the rise of the T wave on an electrocardiogram.

stump　Part of a limb left after amputation.

stump hallucination　The sensation that an amputated limb is still present.

stupor　A state of lethargy and unresponsiveness during which a person appears unaware of his surroundings.

Sturge-Weber syndrome　A congenital condition consisting of a port wine–colored capillary hemangioma over a sensory dermatome of a facial nerve branch.

sty, stye　A purulent infection of a meibomian or sebaceous gland of the eyelid, usually due to a staphylococcus.

stylet, stilet, stilette　A slender, metal probe used for inserting in or passing through a needle, tube, or catheter to remove debris from its lumen or for inserting in a catheter to stiffen it as it's placed in a vein or through an orifice.

stylohyoideus　One of four muscles of the styloid process and hyoid bone that lie anterior and superior to the posterior belly of the digastricus.

stylohyoid ligament　Attachment of the tip of the styloid process of the temporal bone to the hyoid bone.

styptic　**1.** A substance with astringent qualities that's used to control bleeding. A chemical styptic induces blood coagulation. A cotton pledget used as a compressor to control bleeding is a mechanical styptic. **2.** Acting as an astringent or agent to control bleeding.

subacromial bursa　The saclike, fluid-filled cavity separating the acromion and deltoid muscle from the point of insertion of the supraspinatus muscle and the greater tubercle of the humerus.

subacute bacterial endocarditis (SBE)　A chronic bacterial infection of the heart valves, presenting initially with a fever and followed by heart murmur, splenomegaly, and the development of tissue clumps (vegetations) around an intracardiac prosthesis or on the valve flaps.

subacute glomerulonephritis　A rare, noninfectious disease marked by inflammation of the kidney and the capillary loops in the glomeruli of the kidney. Symptoms include decreased urine production, hematuria, proteinuria, and edema. This persistent condition may develop into the lobular or malignant forms.

subacute sclerosing panencephalitis　A rare and severe form of leukoencephalitis that generally affects children and adolescents. Caused by the measles virus, it's a progressive disease that produces cerebral dysfunction within several weeks or months, leading to seizures, blindness, dementia, and death within a year.

subarachnoid　Located between the arachnoid and the pia mater.

subarachnoid block anesthesia　Anesthesia in which a local anesthetic is injected into the subarachnoid space around the spinal cord.

subarachnoid cisterns　Subarachnoid reservoirs containing cerebrospinal fluid.

subarachnoid hemorrhage (SAH)　An intracranial hemorrhage into the subarachnoid space.

subcapital fracture　Break or rupture of a bone just below its head, especially an intracapsular fracture of the neck of the femur.

subclavian artery　An artery situated inferior to the clavicle that has six branches connecting the vertebral column, spinal cord, ear, and brain.

subclavian steal syndrome　A disease in which there's a cerebral or brain stem ischemia as a result of an obstruction in the subclavian artery.

subclavian vein   An extension of the axillary vein, which, together with the internal jugular, forms the brachiocephalic vein.

subcutaneous   Under the skin.

subcutaneous emphysema   Crackling beneath the skin on palpation.

subcutaneous fascia   A band of fibrous tissue that continues over the entire body between the skin or forms an investment for muscles and other organs.

subcutaneous mastectomy   An operation in which the breast tissue is removed but the skin, nipple, and areola are preserved so that later reconstructive surgery is possible.

subcutaneous nodule   A small, solid node that can be felt under the skin.

subdural   Located between the dura mater and the arachnoid.

subinvolution   Incomplete involution, as when the uterus fails to return to its normal size and condition after delivery. This can be the result of infection, uterine fibromyomas, or incomplete delivery of the placenta.

subjective   Pertaining to or perceived only by the individual, such as pain.

sublimate   To divert consciously unacceptable instinctual drives into more socially or morally acceptable channels.

sublingual   Under the tongue.

sublingual gland   The smallest of the salivary glands, located under the tongue.

subluxation   Incomplete or partial dislocation.

submandibular duct   A passage for the secretion of saliva from the submandibular gland.

submandibular gland   One of three chief, paired salivary glands in the submandibular triangle that extend from the diagastricus to the stylomandibular ligament.

submetacentric   A chromosome in which the centromere is equidistant from the center of the chromosome and one end so that the arms are unequal.

subperiosteal fracture   A crack in a bone that doesn't alter its alignment or contour so that the periosteum isn't broken.

subserous fascia   One type of fascia, located beneath the serous membranes.

substance P   A peptide present in nerve cells scattered throughout the body that causes vasodilation and stimulates contraction of GI smooth muscle. It acts as a neurotransmitter controlling pain, touch, and temperature.

substantia spongiosa ossium   Inner spongy layer of bone.

substernal goiter   A swelling in the front part of the neck, in which a portion of

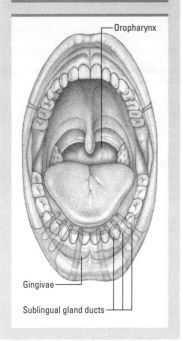

Sublingual gland

— Oropharynx

Gingivae —

Sublingual gland ducts —

the enlarged thyroid gland is located beneath the sternum.

subthalamus   A large mass in the diencephalon that sends optic and vestibular impulses to the globus pallidus.

subungual hematoma   An accumulation of blood under the nail, usually as a result of injury.

succussion splash   A procedure in which a person's body is shaken, which makes a splashing sound, indicating there's free fluid and air or gas in a body cavity.

sucking blisters   Soft pads that form on an infant's lips when he begins to suck. Although they look like blisters, they are not.

sucrose   Sugar obtained from sugar cane, sugar beets, and sorghum. It's composed of fructose and glucose and is used extensively as a sweetener.

sucrose polyester (SPE)   An artificial fat that increases the excretion of cholesterol in the feces, thereby reducing plasma cholesterol levels in the diet.

suction curettage   A procedure in which growths or other material are removed from the wall of a cavity (for example, specimen of the endometrium or the products of conception) by application of a vacuum.

sudden infant death syndrome (SIDS) The sudden, unexpected, and inexplicable death of an infant who appears to be healthy. It occurs during sleep, typically in infants between the ages of 3 weeks and 5 months. Also called *crib death.*

sudoriferous duct A passage that leads from a sudoriferous or sweat gland to the skin's surface.

sudoriferous gland A gland that secretes sweat and that's located in the subcutaneous tissue.

suffocative goiter An enlargement of the thyroid gland that causes dyspnea as a result of pressure on the trachea.

sugar Several sweet, water-soluble carbohydrates that can be crystallized; they can be divided into two main categories — monosaccharides and disaccharides. They are the chief source of energy in animals.

sulcus, *pl.* sulci A shallow trench or depression, especially one of those on the brain's surface.

sulfhemoglobin A greenish substance formed by treating blood with hydrogen sulfide so that normal oxygen binding doesn't occur.

sulfur, sulphur (S) A nonmetallic element that commonly occurs in yellow crystalline form or in masses, especially in volcanic areas. An odorless, tasteless, multivalent element occurring in protein, sulfur is a laxative and is used to treat skin diseases; atomic number, 16; atomic weight, 32.06.

Sulkowitch's test An examination in which urine is checked to see if calcium is present.

sundowning A condition in which institutionalized geriatric patients experience confusion and disorientation at day's end.

superficial reflex Any neural reflex elicited by tactile stimulation of the skin, cornea, or mucous membranes.

superficial spreading melanoma The most common type of malignant tumor, characterized by a period of radial growth atypical of melanocytes in the skin.

CLINICAL TIP It occurs most often as a small, pigmented macule on the lower leg or back.

superficial temporal artery An artery that's easily felt and is therefore used to take a patient's pulse. It's located on either side of the head in front of the ear.

superinfection A new infection occurring during antimicrobial therapy for an existing infection; it may occur at the site of the original infection or at a new one.

superior Situated above or directed upward; for example, the head is superior to the torso.

superior aperture of the minor pelvis An orifice bordered by the crest and pecten of the pubic bones, the arch-shaped lines of the ilia, and the anterior margin of the base of the sacrum.

superior aperture of the thorax An elliptical orifice at the top of the thorax bounded by the first thoracic vertebra, the first ribs and cartilage, and the upper margin of the manubrium sterni.

superior costotransverse ligament A strong band of fibers rising from the crest of the neck of a rib to the transverse process of the vertebra above, except that of the first rib.

superior mediastinum The division of the mediastinum that extends from the pericardium to the root of the neck. It contains the trachea, the aortic arch, the esophagus, and the origins of the sternohyoidei and the sternothyroidei.

superior mesenteric artery A vessel through which blood passes from the heart to the small intestine and proximal half of the colon. It's divided into the following branches: inferior pancreaticoduodenal, jejunal, ileal, ileocolic, right colic, and middle colic arteries.

superior sagittal sinus One of the sinuses of the dura mater, this cavity drains blood into the internal jugular vein from the brain.

superior thyroid artery A vessel through which blood passes from the heart to the thyroid gland and several head muscles. It originates from the external carotid artery, one of the arteries in the neck.

superior vena cava The vein that drains blood from the head, neck, upper extremities, and chest. The second largest vein in the body, it empties deoxygenated blood into the right atrium of the heart.

supination 1. Assuming a supine position, horizontally on the back. 2. The act of turning certain joints, as in rotation of the elbow and wrist, to allow the palm of the hand to turn up.

supine Lying on the back with face upward.

supplemental inheritance The interaction of two independent pairs of nonallelic genes that supplement each other so a genetic trait can be expressed.

suppression amblyopia Impairment of vision as a result of cortical inhibition of central vision to avoid diplopia or double vision.

suppressor gene In molecular genetics: a genetic unit that changes the result of a specific gene mutation.

suppressor mutation In molecular genetics: a mutation in which a function lost by a preceding mutation is completely or partially restored in a different genetic site.

supraclavicular nerve The common trunk, which is a branch of the cervical plexus, arising from the third and mostly the fourth cervical nerve.

suprainfection A secondary infection resulting from an opportunistic pathogen; for example, when treating one infection with antibiotics leads to a fungal infection.

suprapubic Situated above the pubic arch.

suprarenal Located superior to the kidney.

supraspinal ligament A single, long, fibrous band attached to the tips of the spinous processes of the vertebrae.

supraspinatus muscle Muscle that abducts the arm.

surface area (SA) The total surface area exposed to the external environment. As the object's linear dimensions increase, there's a proportional increase in the surface area and volume. Therefore, if two objects are similarly shaped, the larger one will have less surface area per unit volume than the smaller one.

surface biopsy A procedure in which living tissue is scraped from the surface of a lesion and examined under a microscope.

surface tension The contraction of a surface of a liquid to minimize its surface area.

surface thermometer An instrument that measures the surface temperature of any body part.

surfactant An agent, such as soap or detergent, that reduces surface tension by dissolving in water.

surfer's nodules A small boss or node occurring over body prominences of surfer's feet and legs as a result of repeated trauma from contact with a rough surfboard.

surgical anesthesia The depth of anesthesia at which it's considered safe to perform surgery.

surgical pathology Tissue specimens obtained and examined during surgery by a surgical pathologist to determine how the operation should proceed.

surgical scrub 1. An antibacterial agent that's used by anyone performing or assisting with surgery to prevent infection. 2. The act of using an antibacterial solution to wash hands, forearms, and fingernails.

suspension A liquid that contains solid particles that aren't dissolved; stirring or shaking the liquid maintains the dispersal.

sutura, *pl.* suturae A type of fibrous joint in which certain bones are so tightly connected by a thin layer of fibrous tissue that they are immovable; found only in the skull.

sutura dentata A type of immovable fibrous joint in which toothlike forms connect along the margins of connecting skull bones.

sutura limbosa A type of immovable fibrous joint in which there are overlapping and interlocking of the beveled and serrated surfaces of some of the connecting skull bones, such as the parietal and temporal bones.

sutura serrata A type of immovable fibrous joint in which there's interlocking of connecting bones along edges resembling the teeth of a fine-toothed saw.

suture 1. A joint, as between the cranial bones. 2. To use suture material to connect the cut or torn edges of a surgical or accidental wound.

SV *abbr* stroke volume.

S⊽o₂ *abbr* mixed venous oxygen saturation.

swab A wire or clamp used to hold absorbent cotton; its many uses include applying medication, removing material for examination, and cleaning or drying an area.

Swan-Ganz catheter A flexible surgical instrument with a balloon at the tip for measuring pulmonary arterial pressures.

swan-neck deformity A condition, associated with rickets, in which the kidney tubules are abnormally formed.

S wave The final phase of the QRS complex, which shows the cardiac cycle on an electrocardiogram as a sharply slanting downward line. It goes from the peak of the R wave to the beginning of the upward curve of the T wave.

sweat duct One of the tubes for the passage of sweat secretions to the surface of the skin from the many sweat glands throughout the body.

sweat test Often performed as an initial test to diagnose cystic fibrosis, this procedure examines the excretion of sodium and chloride from the sweat glands.

 ALERT The presence of pure salt depletion, common in hot weather, may cause a false positive test result.

swimmer's itch A dermatologic condition common in swimmers, caused by an allergic reaction to schistosome cercarias. They die under the skin, causing a rash of short duration, erythema, and urticaria.

Synapse

Labels: Presynaptic terminal, Synaptic cleft, Neurotransmitter substance, Axon cytoplasm, Synaptic vesicles, Postsynaptic membrane, Postsynaptic receptor

sycosis barbae   A bacterial inflammation involving the bearded region. If neglected, crust will form and it may become chronic.

Sydenham's chorea   An acute disorder usually affecting children and adolescents. Closely linked with rheumatic fever, it affects motor activities and speech.

symbiosis   In biology: organisms of different species living in close association with each other for their mutual benefit.

symmetric tonic neck reflex   The reflexive extension of the arms and bending of the knees when the head and neck are extended, a normal response in infants.

sympathectomy   An operation in which part of the sympathetic nerve pathways are interrupted to relieve chronic pain in such vascular diseases as arteriosclerosis.

sympathetic ophthalmia   A condition in which both eyes suffer inflammation of the uveal tract as a result of a uveal tract injury to one eye.

sympathetic trunk   One of two long nerve strands, one on each side of the vertebral column, extending from the base of the skull to the coccyx.

sympathizing eye   In sympathetic ophthalmia: a healthy eye that acquires an infection by lymphatic or blood-borne metastasis.

sympatholytic   Opposing the effects of impulses conveyed by adrenergic postganglionic fibers of the sympathetic nervous system.

sympathomimetic   Mimicking the effects of impulses conveyed by adrenergic postganglionic fibers of the sympathetic nervous system.

symptom   A change in condition or characteristic of a disease that's perceived by the patient.

synapse   The area between two neurons or between a neuron and an effector organ; nerve impulses are transmitted through the action of a chemical neurotransmitter, such as acetylcholine or norepinephrine. The impulse causes the release of the neurotransmitter after it reaches the end of one neuron, which then binds with receptors in the other neuron, muscle, or gland. Electrical charges are then triggered that either inhibit or continue to transmit the impulse.

synapsis, pl. synapses   The formation of double or bivalent chromosomes from pairing homologous chromosomes during the early prophase of meiosis.

synaptic cleft   A narrow, elongated opening between the presynaptic and postsynaptic membranes.

synaptic junction   The plate where the membranes of the presynaptic neuron and the postsynaptic receptor cell meet the synaptic cleft.

synaptic transmission   Use of a neurotransmitter to pass an impulse across a synapse from one nerve fiber to another.

syncope   A temporary state of unconsciousness, usually preceded by a light-headed feeling. Caused by transient cerebral hypoxia, it may be prevented by either lying down or placing the head between the knees.

ALERT If you see a patient faint, ensure a patent airway and take vital signs. Then place the patient in a supine position, elevate his legs, and loosen any tight clothing. Be alert for tachycardia, bradycardia, or an irregular pulse.

syndrome of inappropriate antidiuretic hormone   A condition that causes excessive release of antidiuretic hormone, resulting in extreme water retention and sodium excretion.

synotia   A birth deformity in which the ears are in front of the neck; development of the lower jaw is commonly defective as well.

synovectomy   Removal of destructive, proliferating synovium; typically in the wrists, knees, and fingers.

synovia   A clear and viscous fluid that lubricates joints, bursae, and tendons. Resembling a raw egg white, it's secreted by synovial membranes.

synovial bursa   A closed sac in the connective tissue between the muscles, tendons, ligaments, and bones that's filled with synovial fluid.

synovial chondroma   A rare, cartilaginous body formed in the connective tissue below the synovial membrane of the joints.

synovial chondromatosis   A rare disorder in which multiple nodules form in the synovial membranes, resulting from changes in the synovial linings of joints.

synovial fluid   A clear, viscid fluid that lubricates the joints. Secreted in the bursae and tendon sheaths, it contains fat, albumin, mucin, and mineral salts.

synovial joint   Connected by ligaments lined with synovial membrane, articular cartilage covers the contiguous bony surfaces of this movable joint.

synovial sarcoma   A growth that begins as a soft swelling and often metastasizes through the bloodstream to the lung before it's discovered to be malignant; composed of synovioblasts.

synovial sheath   A tubular structure around the tendon of a muscle that helps the tendon glide through a fibrous or bony tunnel, such as under the flexor retinaculum of the wrist.

synovitis   A condition in which the synovial membrane of a joint becomes inflamed either from an aseptic wound or injury.

synthetic   Of or pertaining to a substance produced artificially.

synthetic chemistry   The science involving building an artificial chemical compound from its elements or other starting materials.

syphilis   An infectious disease, usually transmitted by sexual contact or acquired in utero, that's caused by the spirochete *Treponema pallidum.*

CLINICAL TIP   There are three clinical stages of syphilis, with the duration of each stage varying; the last stage is characterized by destructive lesions involving many organs and tissues.

syringe pump   A type of pump, especially useful for giving intermittent I.V. medications to pediatric patients, because it gives the greatest control over small-volume infusions; used with syringe sizes from 1 to 60 ml and low-volume tubing.

systemic lupus erythematosus (SLE)   A chronic inflammatory multisystemic disorder of connective tissue, characterized principally by involvement of the skin, joints, kidneys, and serosal membranes.

systole   The normal action of the heart, in which the ventricles contract to drive blood into the aorta and pulmonary artery.

systolic click   Short, dry, clicking heart sounds occurring in midsystole or in late systole. Usually insignificant, the sounds sometimes indicate a disorder of the mitral or aortic valves; the timing of the click may indicate the nature of the disorder.

systolic gradient   The pressure difference between two communicating cardiac chambers, such as the left atrium and left ventricle, during systole.

systolic murmur   An auscultatory sound, either benign or pathologic, that occurs during systole. Usually less significant than diastolic murmurs, systolic murmurs are generally caused by mitral or tricuspid regurgitation or pulmonary obstruction.

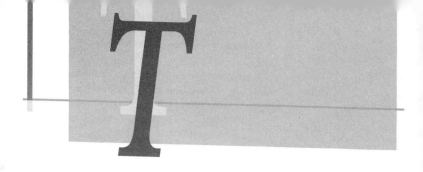

T 1. *abbr* tumor in the TNM system for staging malignant neoplastic disease. 2. Symbol for temperature.

T₃ Symbol for triiodothyronine.

T₄ Symbol for thyroxine.

Ta Symbol for tantalum.

TA *abbr* transactional analysis.

tabes dorsalis A disorder in which all or part of the body degenerates and loses peripheral reflexes, occurring 15 to 20 years after an initial infection of syphilis.

tablet A solid dosage form that contains a medicinal substance in pure or diluted form.

tachycardia A condition characterized by a regular but accelerated action of the heart, usually l00 to 150 beats per minute.

ALERT After detecting tachycardia, first perform an electrocardiogram to examine for reduced cardiac output, which may initiate or result from tachycardia. Take the patient's other vital signs; if the patient has increased or decreased blood pressure and is drowsy or confused, administer oxygen, begin cardiac monitoring, and determine his level of consciousness.

tachyphylaxis 1. In pharmacology: rapidly decreasing effectiveness of a drug after repeated use. 2. In immunology: rapid immunization against the effect of toxic doses as a result of previous exposure, such as by injection.

tachypnea An excessive rate of respiration, marked by quick, shallow breaths, as in hyperpyrexia.

TIME LINE When assessing a child for tachypnea, be aware that the normal respiratory rate varies with age. Pediatric tachypnea may result from congenital heart defects, metabolic acidosis, meningitis, or cystic fibrosis. Bear in mind that hunger and anxiety may also cause tachypnea.

tactile Of or pertaining to touch.

tactile anesthesia The loss of the sense of touch in the fingers, possibly caused by disease or trauma.

tactile fremitus A vibration in the chest wall that may be felt when a hand is applied to the thorax while the patient is speaking. It's most commonly due to consolidation of a lung or a part of a lung or may be caused by congestion, inflammation, or infection.

tactile image A picture or conception of an object sensed through the fingers rather than perceived through the sense of sight.

Taenia A genus of tapeworm of the family Taeniidae, class Cestoda. Among the most common of human parasites, these large intestinal tapeworms have an armed scolex and a series of segments in a chain.

taeniasis Infection with any of the tapeworms of the genus *Taenia*.

tai chi chuan Ancient Chinese exercise program based on Taoist teachings and the theory and practice of traditional Chinese medicine. Although originally a martial art, *tai chi* is practiced today to promote health and longevity; includes movement, meditation, and breathing exercises.

tail fold A tail bud present in the early stages of fetal development, which later forms the hindgut. This same tail bud forms a caudal appendage in animals.

tail of Spence An extension of breast tissue that projects from the upper outer quadrant of the breast toward the axilla.

Takayasu's arteritis A progressive occlusion of the brachiocephalic trunk and the left subclavian and left common carotid arteries above their origin in the aortic arch, leading to loss of pulse in both arms and carotids as well as many symptoms associated with brain ischemia.

talipes A congenital malformation of the foot, which remains twisted in an abnormal position. Also called *clubfoot*.

talus, *pl.* **tali** The highest of the tarsal bones, which helps to form the ankle joint.

tamponade Application of pressure, or compression of a blood vessel (such as a tampon, a pressure dressing applied to a hemorrhage, or cardiac tamponade) to stop the flow of blood to an organ or body part.

Tangier disease An autosomal recessive disorder characterized by a deficiency of high-density lipoproteins.

CLINICAL TIP Symptoms include enlargement and orange coloring of the tonsils and pharynx and a low blood cholesterol level.

tantalum (Ta)   A rare, metallic element, atomic number, 73; atomic weight, 180.95. It has been used for plates or disks to replace cranial defects, for prosthetic appliances, and for wire sutures.

tapeworm   A worm whose segmented, ribbon-shaped body has a scolex. Belonging to the class Cestoda, this intestinal parasite infects man when the eggs of tapeworms make their way into the tissues and produce larvae, which develop within the alimentary canal.

tapeworm infection   An infection resulting from eating food that has been infested with a parasitic worm or its larvae. Raw or undercooked meat can be infected with several species of parasitic worms, and can cause this intestinal infection.

tapotement   A short, rapid tapping motion of the fingertips or sides of the hands in massage.

tardive dyskinesia   A disorder associated with parkinsonism and extended use of the phenothiazine drugs used to treat this condition. Most commonly affecting the aged, symptoms include repeated involuntary facial, limb, and trunk movements.

tardy peroneal nerve palsy   A disorder affecting a single nerve, in which there's excessive compression of the peroneal nerve where it crosses the head of the fibula.

tardy ulnar nerve palsy   A disorder in which the first dorsal interosseous muscle atrophies. Possibly caused by trauma to the ulnar nerve at the elbow, this condition makes fine manipulations difficult to perform.

target cell   An abnormal red blood cell that shows, when stained, a dark center and a peripheral ring of hemoglobin, separated by a pale, unstained ring containing less hemoglobin; seen in certain types of anemia, jaundice, and other disorders.

target organ   **1.** In radiotherapy: an organ that's chosen to receive irradiation for therapeutic purposes. **2.** In nuclear medicine: an organ that's chosen to receive the highest concentration of a radioactive tracer for diagnostic purposes. **3.** In endocrinology: an organ that's most affected by a specific hormone.

tarsal   Pertaining to the tarsus or any bones of the tarsus, such as the ankle bone.

tarsal bone   One of the seven bones of the tarsus (ankle), which includes the talus, calcaneus, cuboid, navicular, and the three cuneiforms.

tarsal gland   One of many sebaceous follicles between the tarsi and the conjunctiva of the eyelids.

tarsal tunnel syndrome   A disorder in which the posterior tibial nerve is compressed, resulting in pain, numbness, and tingling in the sole of the foot.

tarsometatarsal   Pertaining to the tarsus and the metatarsus, especially at the instep of the foot, where the metatarsal bones meet the cuneiform and cuboid bones.

tarsus, *pl.* tarsi   **1.** The region of the junction between the foot and the leg. **2.** One of the plates of connective tissue, approximately 1" (2.5 cm) long, that form the framework of an eyelid.

tartar   A hard substance that collects on teeth and gums; it's made up of organic matter, phosphates, and carbonates.

tartaric acid   A powder, either white or colorless, that's prepared commercially from maleic anhydride and hydrogen peroxide. Found in many plants, its salts are used in food preparation (cream of tartar) and have been used as cathartics.

taste   The sense, effected by receptors in the tongue, that can distinguish sweet, salty, sour, and bitter qualities as a result of the transmission of nerve impulses to the thalamus and cortex of the brain.

taste bud   One of the small organs of the gustatory nerve located throughout the tongue and the roof of the mouth.

TAT   *abbr* tetanus antitoxin.

Taylor brace   A steel brace that's padded and used for spinal support. Also called *Taylor splint.*

Tay-Sachs disease   A disease in which sphingolipids are accumulated in the brain. This neurodegenerative disorder is caused by an enzyme deficiency of hexosaminidase A, an inherited condition occurring chiefly among northeast European Jews. It's specifically characterized by infantile onset (3 to 6 months); affected children die between the ages of 2 and 5 years.

Tb   Symbol for terbium.

TB   *abbr* tuberculosis.

T binder   A T-shaped girdle or bandage, used for the perineum after childbirth and sometimes for the head.

TBP   *abbr* **1.** bithionol. **2.** total bypass.

Tc   Symbol for technetium.

T cell   A small lymphocyte found in the blood, lymph, and lymphoid tissues. Acting as the body's helper, cytotoxic, and suppressor cells, T cells originate in the bone marrow and mature in the thymus.

TD   *abbr* toxic dose.

TD50   *abbr* median toxic dose.

tDNA   *abbr* transfer DNA.

Te   Symbol for tellurium.

teardrop fracture   A tear-shaped indirect break of one of the short bones, such as a vertebra.

tear duct   Any duct that carries tears secreted by the lacrimal glands.

tearing   Increase in the amount of tear production as a result of infection, irritation, or emotion.

technetium (Tc)   A radioactive, metallic element, atomic number, 43; atomic weight, 99.

teething   The periodic eruption of deciduous teeth through the gums. The entire process is usually finished at about 30 months when a complete set of 20 teeth has erupted.

T effector cells   T cells that are produced as stem cells in red bone marrow, matured in the thymus, and stored in the lymph nodes; they produce proteins called lymphokines, which stimulate inflammation and phagocytosis.

telangiectasia   Permanent dilation of groups of superficial capillaries and venules.

telangiectasis   A small, red lesion, usually on the skin or mucous membranes, produced by permanent dilation of preexisting blood vessels.

telangiectatic epulis   A benign mass of the gingiva in which blood vessels are prominent, making the tumor appear red.

telangiectatic glioma   A bright pink tumor made up of a network of blood vessels and glial cells.

telangiectatic nevus   A common neonatal dermatologic condition in which flat, bright pink areas of capillary dilation appear on the face (especially lower occiput, upper eyelids, upper lip, bridge of the nose, and the back of the neck).

telangiectatic sarcoma   A malignant tumor of mesodermal cells that develops a rich vascular network.

tellurium (Te)   A nonmetallic or metaloid element; atomic number, 52; atomic weight, 127.60.

telophase   The last of four stages of nuclear division in mitosis and of the two divisions in meiosis.

temperate phage   A bacteriophage in which the host bacterium contains its complete gene complement.

temperature   1. The degree of sensible heat or cold. 2. In physiology: a measure of sensible heat of the metabolism of the human body, normally constant at 98.6° F (37° C); temperature is balanced by the thermotaxic nerve mechanism.

template   In genetics: the strand of deoxyribonucleic acid that molds to synthesize messenger ribonucleic acid.

temporal arteritis   A progressive disease chiefly occurring in women over age 70 in which the cranial blood vessels (especially the temporal artery) become inflamed.

temporal artery   One of three cerebral arteries: the superficial temporal artery, the middle temporal artery, and the deep temporal artery.

temporal bone   One of two large bones containing the hearing organs, forming part of the lateral surfaces and base of the skull.

temporal bone fracture   A crack of the temporal bone; as a result, the ear may bleed.

temporalis   The muscle that closes the jaws and retracts the mandible, necessary for chewing.

temporal lobe   The cerebral region below the lateral fissure.

temporal veins   Veins that drain the temporal region of the head.

temporomandibular joint   Formed by parts of the mandibular fossae of the temporal bone, the articular tubercles, the mandibular condyles, and five ligaments, this combined hinge and gliding joint connects the mandible to the temporal bone.

temporomandibular joint pain dysfunction syndrome   A disorder in which a defective or dislocated temporomandibular joint causes pain in the face and dysfunction in the mandible.

temporoparietalis   One of two muscles of the scalp that appear over the temporal fascia and are inserted into the galea aponeurotica; the muscles are broad and thin, and are divided into three parts.

TEN   *abbr* toxic epidermal necrolysis.

tenaculum, *pl.* tenacula   An instrument with a clamp and long handles for holding or immobilizing an organ or a piece of tissue.

tenalgia   Pain in a tendon. Also called *tenodynia.*

tendinitis, tendonitis   An inflamed tendon, which is usually caused by strain.

TIME LINE A common form of tendinitis in adolescents of both sexes is patellar tendinitis associated with inflammation of the tibial epiphysis in Osgood-Schlatter disease.

tendo calcaneus   A powerful tendon at the back of the heel; the common tendon of the soleus and gastrocnemius.

tendon   A fibrous cord, generally covered in delicate fibroelastic connective tissue except at points of attachment, by which a muscle is attached to bone.

tenesmus   Repeated, ineffectual straining during defecation or urination.

tenodesis Suturing of a tendon to a muscle.

tenodynia Pain in a tendon. Also called *tenalgia*.

tenomyotomy Surgical procedure that involves cutting of tendon and muscle.

tenosynovitis Condition in which a tendon sheath is inflamed as a result of repeated strain or trauma, high levels of blood cholesterol, calcium deposits, gout, gonorrhea, or rheumatoid arthritis.

tenotomy A procedure in which a tendon is severed, either totally or partially, in order to treat muscular imbalance, such as in strabismus of the eye or clubfoot.

TENS *abbr* transcutaneous electrical nerve stimulation.

tensor fasciae latae A muscle that arises from the iliac crest, the iliac spine, and the deep fascia lata, one of 10 in the gluteal region.

tentorial herniation A condition in which brain tissue protrudes into the tentorial notch as a result of tumor, hemorrhage, or tumor.

ALERT Tentorial herniation causes drowsiness, confusion, dilation of one or both pupils, hyperventilation, nuchal rigidity, bradycardia, and decorticate or decerebrate posturing. Irreversible brain damage can occur rapidly.

tentorium, *pl.* **tentoria** An anatomic part that resembles a tent or covering, such as the tentorium of the cerebellum.

tentorium cerebelli An extension of the dura mater that supports the occipital lobe and covers the cerebellum. Its internal border is free, but its external border is attached to the skull.

teratism Any anomaly of formation or development, resulting from either inheritance, environment, or both; a condition that produces a severely deformed fetus.

teratogen Any substance or process that causes malformation of a fetus by affecting normal prenatal development.

teratologist A person who practices teratology.

teratology The study of congenital and developmental malformations, their causes, and effects.

teratoma, *pl.* **teratomas, teratomata** A tumor consisting of various kinds of unrelated tissue; this type of tumor is most commonly found in the ovaries or testes.

terbium (Tb) A rare-earth metallic element; atomic number, 65; atomic weight, 158.294.

teres, *pl.* **teretes** Long and round, as a muscle or ligament.

teres major A muscle of the shoulder that's flat and broad.

teres minor A muscle of the shoulder that's long and rounded.

terminal Of a structure or process: pertaining to its end, such as terminal cancer or terminal bronchiole.

terminal nerve A small nerve that begins in the cerebral hemisphere in the olfactory trigone and considered by many to be part of the olfactory nerve.

terminal sulcus of the right atrium Occurring between the superior and inferior venae cavae, this shallow groove on the right atrium's external surface corresponds to a ridge on the internal surface (crista terminalis).

termination codon In molecular genetics: a unit in the genetic code that causes termination in the synthesis of a growing polypeptide chain.

termination sequence In molecular genetics: an ending segment of deoxyribonucleic acid (DNA) that's converted to messenger ribonucleic acid from the DNA template.

term infant Any infant born between the 37th- and 43rd-week gestational period, usually measuring between 19″ and 21″ (48 and 53 cm) from head to heel and weighing between 6 and 9 lb (2,700 and 4,000 g).

tertian malaria A disease in which febrile paroxysms occur every third day (counting the day of occurrence as the first day of the cycle) because of a synchronized infection with a single brood of *Plasmodium vivax* or *Plasmodium ovale*. Vivax malaria, caused by *P. vivax*, is the most common form of malaria and the one that's most likely to recur because of latent forms that persist in the liver.

tertiary 1. Third in order. 2. Belonging to the third level of development.

testcross In genetics: crossing a dominant with a recessive phenotype to ascertain whether the resulting phenotype is homozygous or heterozygous, or the degree of genetic linkage.

testicular artery One of two branches of the abdominal aorta that supplies the testis.

testicular cancer A neoplastic disease most commonly affecting men between ages 20 and 35 in which there's a progressive, malignant tumor on the testis.

testicular vein One of two veins that form the greater mass of the spermatic cords, coming from the convoluted venous plexuses.

testis, *pl.* **testes** One of two male gonads that are responsible for production of semen. Although they're located in the scro-

Thalamus of the brain

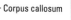

- Corpus callosum
- Thalamus
- Hypothalamus
- Midbrain

tum in adult males, they're located in the abdominal cavity behind the peritoneum in the fetus.

testosterone The major androgenic hormone; it regulates gonadotropic secretion, stimulates skeletal muscle, and is responsible for other male characteristics and spermatogenesis. Production of testosterone occurs in the interstitial cells of the testes in response to stimulation by the luteinizing hormone of the anterior pituitary gland.

tetanus An acute, often fatal, infectious disease caused by tetanospasmin, a potent neurotoxin elaborated by an anaerobic bacillus, *Clostridium tetani.*

 ALERT Generally entering the body through a contaminated puncture wound, tetanus can have mild to severe symptoms, ranging from localized muscular spasms to trismus (lockjaw), seizures, and paralysis.

tetanus and diphtheria toxoids An active form of detoxified tetanus and diphtheria toxoids for the purpose of producing a slow immunization to the two diseases.

tetanus immune globulin (TIG) A specific immune globulin derived from the blood of human donors that can be injected for the prevention and treatment of tetanus.

tetanus toxoid An active agent containing detoxified tetanus toxin that permanently immunizes the body to tetanus infection.

tetany Hyperexcitability of nerves and muscles as a result of a lessened concentration of extracellular ionized calcium; symptoms include seizures, muscle twitching and cramps, and sharp flexion of the wrist and ankle joints.

tetrad In genetics: a group of four chromosomal elements formed in the pachytene state of the first meiotic prophase stage of gametogenesis.

tetrahydrocannabinol (THC) The active principle in the plant *Cannabis sativa,* which is used to prepare hashish, marijuana, ganja, and bhang. It occurs in two isomeric forms, both considered psychotomimetically active.

tetralogy of Fallot A combination of congenital cardiac defects consisting of pulmonic stenosis, interventricular septal defect, dextroposition of the aorta so that it overrides the interventricular septum and receives venous as well as arterial blood, and right ventricular hypertrophy.

tetraploidy A condition in which four complete sets of chromosomes are present.

T fracture A break situated between two condyles in which the fracture lines are shaped like a T.

TGF *abbr* transforming growth factor.

Th Symbol for thorium.

thalamus, *pl.* thalami One of two large organs that form part of the diencephalon and most of the lateral walls of the third ventricle of the brain.

thalassemia A group of hereditary hemolytic anemias in which a decreased rate of synthesis of one or more hemoglobin peptide chains produces microcytic, hypochromic, and short-lived red blood cells.

thallium (Tl)   A heavy, soft, bluish-white metal that also has some nonmetallic properties; atomic number, 81; atomic weight, 204.37. Its salts are active poisons.

thallium imaging   A procedure used to diagnose myocardial infarction and coronary artery disease by giving a patient a thallium isotope I.V. either while at rest or after a treadmill stress test. The isotope doesn't collect in areas of poor blood flow and damaged cells, so they show up as "cold spots" on a scanner; as a result, it's sometimes called *cold spot myocardial imaging* or *thallium scintigraphy.*

thallium poisoning   A condition in which thallium salts, especially thallium sulfate, are eaten or absorbed into the skin, causing toxicity.

THC   *abbr* tetrahydrocannabinol.

theca, *pl.* thecae   An enclosing case or sheath (for example, an ovarian follicle or the theca cordis).

theca cell tumor   A rare ovarian fibroid tumor that's benign and contains theca cells and, usually, granulosa (follicular) cells.

Theden's bandage   A strip or roll of gauze or other material used to facilitate blood clotting by continuing upward over a compress and below the injury.

thelarche   The beginning of development of the breasts, which begins before puberty, normally occurring between ages 9 and 13.

T helper cells   Cells that increase the immune response of T effector cells and B cells.

therapeutic equivalent   A drug that has an equal measure of effectiveness in treating one condition as another drug and can be substituted for it.

therapeutic index   The ratio, used to evaluate dosage safety, of a drug's toxic dose to its effective dose.

therapeutic plasma exchange (TPE)   Processing and reinfusing plasma from the patient's blood for therapeutic purposes.

therapeutic radiopharmaceutical   A drug used to irradiate body tissues internally (iodine 131), to ablate thyroid tissue in hyperthyroid patients (cesium 137, iridium 192, radium 226), or to treat malignant tumors by implanting in a sealed source (strontium 90).

Therapeutic Touch   A method of energetic healing in which the practitioner passes her hands over the patient's body in an attempt to transmit her own energy to the patient. Like a number of alternative therapies originating in the East, Therapeutic Touch is based on the theory that vital energy flows through all human beings.

thermal burn   Trauma to the tissues caused by contact with fire or extreme heat exposure (for example, to the skin).

thermistor   An instrument that's able to measure extremely small changes in temperature.

thermocautery   Cauterization by means of a hot wire or needle.

thermogenesis   Heat production, especially within the human body.

thermography   Use of an infrared detector to indicate different temperatures of the body on film, sometimes used to diagnose breast tumors.

thermometer   A sealed glass tube that contains liquid (usually mercury) that's an instrument for measuring temperature. It's marked in degrees of Celsius or Fahrenheit.

thermopenetration   The process of warming the body tissues by using diathermic techniques for purposes of therapy.

thermoradiotherapy   A procedure in which ionizing radiation is applied to an anatomic site in which there has been an artificial increase in temperature.

thermostable   Able to withstand changes in temperature without undergoing change.

thermotherapy   Use of heat for the treatment of disease, which can be either dry heat (heat lamps, diathermy machines, electric pads, or hot water bottles) or moist heat (warm compresses or immersion in warm water).

theta wave   A type of brain wave with a low frequency (4 to 7 hertz) and a low amplitude (10 microvolts).

thiamine, thiamin   A crystalline compound of the B complex vitamin group, which is necessary for normal metabolism and function of the nervous system. This water-soluble compound occurs chiefly in pork, organ meats, legumes, nuts, and whole grain cereals and breads.

third-party reimbursement   Reimbursement for services rendered to a person, in which an entity other than the giver or receiver of the service is responsible for payment. Third-party reimbursement for the cost of a subscriber's health care is commonly paid by insurance plans.

third-space fluid shift   Movement of fluid out of the intravascular space into another body space, such as the abdominal cavity.

Thiry's fistula   A passage created surgically in an experimental animal's abdomen to study internal secretions.

Thomas splint   1. A support, used in the treatment of chronic joint diseases, that's made of a curved steel bar and held on the limb by a cast or bandage. 2. A rigid splint, made out of metal, that's used to immobilize and position a patient's fractured femur. The

Thoracentesis

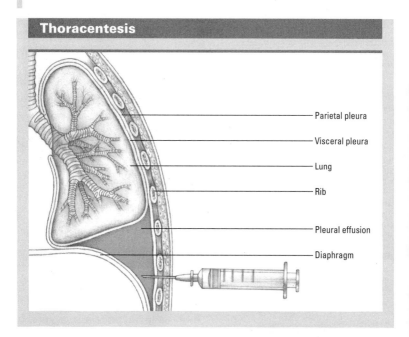

- Parietal pleura
- Visceral pleura
- Lung
- Rib
- Pleural effusion
- Diaphragm

splint extends from a ring at the hip to be-yond the foot.

thoracentesis, thoracocentesis Sur-gical puncture and drainage of the thoracic cavity for diagnostic or therapeutic purposes.

thoracic aorta The upper portion of the aorta, which supplies the heart, ribs, chest muscles, and stomach; it begins at the caudal border of the fourth thoracic vertebra and di-vides into seven branches.

thoracic arteries The three arteries (lat-eral, superior, and internal) that distribute blood to the pectoral muscles, mammary glands, axillary area of the chest wall, the di-aphragm, and the structures of the medi-astinum and the anterior thoracic wall.

thoracic duct The canal that ascends from the cisterna chyli to the junction of the left subclavian and left internal jugular vein.

thoracic medicine The study of medi-cine that diagnoses and treats disorders in-volving chest structures and organs, especial-ly the lungs.

thoracic nerves The nerves on each side of the thorax, which include 11 inter-costal nerves and 1 subcostal nerve.

thoracic outlet compression syn-drome A disorder in which the fingers suffer from paresthesia, possibly caused by compression of the nerve root by a cervical disk or by carpal tunnel syndrome.

thoracic parietal node One of the lymph glands that's divided into sternal nodes, intercostal nodes, and diaphragmatic nodes, and associated with many lymphatic vessels.

thoracic vertebra Bony segments of the spine, designated T1 to T12. T1 is located be-low the seventh cervical vertebra (C7), and T12 is located above the first lumbar vertebra (L1).

thoracic visceral node One of the three groups of lymph nodes that serves the thymus, pericardium, esophagus, trachea, lungs, and bronchi.

thoracodorsal nerve A branch of the brachial plexus, usually occurring between two subscapular nerves.

thorax The part of the body between the neck and the thoracic diaphragm, encased by the ribs. It's responsible for respiration and circulation and covers part of the abdominal organs.

thorium (Th) A rare, heavy, gray, radio-active metal; atomic number, 90; atomic weight, 232.04.

thready pulse Common in hypovolemia, a weak pulse rate that's often fairly rapid and difficult to count.

threatened abortion A condition in which bleeding of the uterus and severe cramping before the 20th week of gestation indicates the threat of a miscarriage.

threshold   The point, or minimum level, at which a stimulus produces an effect.

thrill   A sensation, or feeling, of vibration felt by an examiner's hand at the site of an aneurysm or over the heart if a harsh murmur occurs.

throb   A deep, pulsating discomfort or pain; a pulsating movement.

thrombasthenia   A rare hemorrhagic disease in which hemostasis occurs because of an abnormality in the membrane surface of the platelet.

thrombectomy   The surgical removal of a thrombus from a blood vessel.

thrombin   An enzyme formed in plasma during clotting from calcium, prothrombin, and thromboplastin.

thromboangiitis obliterans   An inflammatory condition that includes thrombus of the blood vessels mostly of the legs and feet. It occurs most often in young men and can lead to gangrene. Also called *Buerger's disease.*

thrombocytopathy   A general term for a disorder of blood coagulation that results from abnormal platelet function.

thrombocytopenia   A reduction in the number of blood platelets, usually caused by destruction of erythroid tissue in bone marrow. The condition may be a result of neoplastic disease or an immune response to a drug.

TIME LINE In older adults, platelet characteristics change; granular constituents decrease and platelet-release factors increase. These changes may reflect diminished bone marrow and increased fibrinogen levels.

thrombocytopenic purpura   A bleeding disorder in which there's a noticeable decrease in platelets. As a result, the patient may have multiple bruises and petechiae and may hemorrhage into tissues.

thrombocytosis   A marked increase in the number of platelets.

thromboembolism   The blocking of a blood vessel with an embolus that has been carried in the blood from a clot origin site.

thrombogenic   A device or process that may cause, or lead to thrombosis formation.

thrombophlebitis   Inflammation of a vein, often involving clot formation. Common causes include chemical irritation, blood hypercoagulability, immobilization, infection, postoperative venous stasis, prolonged sitting or standing, trauma to the vessel wall, or a long period of I.V. catheterization.

thrombophlebitis purulenta   Inflammation of a vein along with the formation of a soft thrombus that infiltrates the vessel wall.

thromboplastin   A substance found in blood and tissues. A complex substance that initiates the clotting process by converting prothrombin to thrombin, it's also present in red blood cells; initiation occurs in the presence of calcium ions.

thrombosis, *pl.* thromboses   The development of a thrombus within a blood vessel.

thrombotic thrombocytopenic purpura (TTP)   A disorder characterized by thrombocytopenia, hemolytic anemia, and neurologic abnormalities.

thrombus, *pl.* thrombi   A blood clot.

thulium (Tm)   A rare metallic element. Its atomic number is 69; atomic weight, 168.93.

thymoma   A tumor on the thymus gland.

thymosin   A hormone that's secreted by the thymus gland and helps maintain immune functions. Children have the most thymosin; older adults have the least.

thymus, *pl.* thymuses, thymi   A symmetric lymphoid organ located in the mediastinum. It extends superiorly into the neck to the lower edge of the thyroid gland and inferiorly as far as the fourth costal cartilage. The thymus reaches maximum development at puberty and goes into decline throughout adulthood.

thymusectomy   Surgical removal of the thymus.

thyrocervical trunk   A short, thick, arterial branch, deriving from the first portion of the subclavian arteries, close to the medial border of the scalenus anterior. It supplies blood to muscles and bones in the back, head, and neck.

thyroid acropathy   A condition in which the extremities swell and the digits club.

thyroid cancer   A neoplasm of the thyroid gland. Thyroid cancer is usually slow growing and has a prolonged clinical course.

thyroid cartilage   It forms the Adam's apple and is the largest cartilage of the larynx with two laminae fused at an acute angle in the middle line of the neck.

thyroid dermoid cyst   A tumor originating from embryonal tissues. It's believed to have developed in the thyrolingual duct or thyroid gland.

thyroidectomy   Surgical removal of the thyroid gland. The procedure is performed to treat colloid goiter, tumors, or hyperthyroidism that hasn't responded to antithyroid drugs or iodine therapy.

thyroid function test   A laboratory test for evaluating increased or decreased function of the thyroid gland.

thyroid gland   A vascular organ located at the base of the neck front. It weighs about 30 g (a little more than 1 ounce), has two lobes that are connected in the center by a narrow isthmus, and contains active substances such as thyroxine.

thyroid hormone   A compound containing iodine and secreted by the thyroid gland. Thyroid hormone consists mostly of thyroxine (T_4) and has small amounts of triiodothyronine (T_3), a substance that's four times more potent than T_4.

thyroiditis   Inflammation of the thyroid gland. Acute thyroiditis is caused by infections, such as staphylococcal or streptococcal infections; it's very painful and symptoms include abscesses. Acute thyroiditis may progress to a subacute, diffuse disease of the gland.

thyroid-stimulating hormone (TSH) A hormone, or substance, secreted by the front lobe of the pituitary gland, that controls the release of thyroid hormone and is necessary for proper thyroid function and growth.

thyrotropin-releasing factor (TRF)   A hormone, secreted by the median eminence of the hypothalamus, that regulates the secretion of thyroid-stimulating hormone. It's also involved in the release of prolactin. Also called *protirelin*.

thyroxine (T_4)   A hormone of the thyroid gland, formed from thyroglobulin and transported in the blood. It influences metabolic rate and is used to treat hypothyroidism.

ALERT Free-fatty acids, heparin, iodides, lithium, phenytoin, phenylbutazone, and high doses of salicylates, sulfonamides, and sulfonylureas may decrease thyroxine levels.

thyroxine-binding globulin   A plasma protein that binds with and transports thyroxine in the blood.

Ti   Symbol for titanium.

TI   *abbr* therapeutic index.

tibia   The shin bone. It's located below the knee and is the second longest bone of the body.

tibial torsion   A twisting, either lateral or medial, of the tibia, causing a rotation of the foot.

tibiotarsal joint   The joint between the tibia and the tarsal bones.

tick bite   A puncture wound or bite from a blood-sucking tick, which is a small, toughskinned, parasitic arachnid.

tick paralysis   An uncommon, progressive, reversible disorder caused by certain ticks that release a neurotoxin. The disorder is seen mostly in children.

tidal volume (VT)   The quantity of air inspired and expired during one cycle of normal breathing.

tide   The rise and fall in volume of a certain component of body fluids.

Tietze's syndrome   A painful nonsuppurative swelling of one or more costal cartilages. The condition causes pain that may radiate to the neck, shoulder, or arm and often mimics the chest pain of coronary artery disease. Also called *costal chondritis*.

TIG   *abbr* tetanus immune globulin.

tinea   A term that describes a group of fungal skin diseases caused by dermatophytes. The diseases are named by site and are characterized by itching, scaling and, occasionally, painful lesions. Also called *ringworm*.

tinea capitis   A contagious fungal disease of the scalp. The symptoms include circular, bald patches ranging in size from $1/2''$ to $2\ 1/2''$ (1 to 6 cm) in diameter with slight erythema, scaling, and crusting and hair loss at the site of infection. Also called *tinea tonsurans*.

tinea cruris   An acute or chronic fungal infection of the groin, caused by *Trichophyton* or *Epidermophyton floccosum*. The infection is generally superficial and is most common in the tropics and among males. Also called *jock itch, ringworm of the groin*.

tinea pedis   A chronic, superficial fungal infection of the foot. The infection generally involves the skin between the toes and on the soles and is characterized by severe itching, scaling, and pustular lesions. It's common worldwide and is usually caused by *Trichophyton mentagrophytes, T. rubrum*, and *Epidermophyton floccosum*. Also called *athlete's foot, ringworm of the feet*.

tinea unguium   A fungal infection of the nail that starts on the surface or distal edges of the nail and migrates to under the nail plate. Tinea unguium is caused by *Trichophyton* and, occasionally, by *Candida albicans* and is more common on the toes than the fingers. It can cause complete crumbling and destruction of the nails.

tinea versicolor   A common, noninflammatory fungal infection of the skin in which there are finely desquamating, pale or tan patches on the upper trunk and upper arms. The patches often itch and don't tan.

Tinel's sign   A distal tingling sensation upon percussion of a damaged nerve. It indicates a divided nerve or the beginning of regeneration. Also called *distal tingling on percussion*.

Tine test   A skin test with tuberculin. A small disk with multiple tines bearing tuberculin antigen is used to puncture the skin.

The site is checked 48 to 72 hours later for redness and swelling, which if present is considered positive.

tinnitus   A ringing, buzzing, roaring or clicking in one or both ears. It may be a sign of acoustic trauma.

TIME LINE An expectant mother's use of ototoxic drugs during the third month of pregnancy can cause labyrinthine damage in the fetus, resulting in tinnitus.

tin (Sn)   A white metallic element. Its atomic number is 50; atomic weight, 118.69.

tissue dose   In radiotherapy: the amount of radiation absorbed by tissue in the region of interest, expressed in rads.

tissue fixation   A process for preserving the cells of a tissue specimen.

tissue fixative   The fluid used to preserve cells for later identification and examination.

tissue response   A reaction or change in cells after they have received stimulus or been acted upon by a disease or toxin.

tissue typing   A series of tests for evaluating the compatibility of tissues between a donor and a recipient. Tissue typing is done before an organ transplant.

titanium (Ti)   A dark-gray, brittle, metallic element. Its atomic number is 22; atomic weight, 47.90; specific gravity, 4.5.

titubation   Posture characterized by a staggering or stumbling gait and a swaying head or trunk while sitting.

Tl   Symbol for thallium.

TLC   *abbr* **1.** total lung capacity. **2.** *Informal.* Tender loving care.

Tm   Symbol for thulium.

TMJ   *abbr* temporomandibular joint.

TNM   A system for staging malignant neoplastic disease.

tntc   *abbr* too-numerous-to-count. Usually applied to organisms or cells viewed on a slide under a microscope.

Tobruk plaster   A plaster cast splint with tapes for skin traction coming through openings in the plaster and connected with a Thomas splint.

tocodynamometer, tokodynamometer   An electronic instrument that's used to monitor and record contractions during labor.

tocopherol   A group of fat-soluble, oily, pale-yellow liquids possessing some biological vitamin E activity.

togavirus   A family of ribonucleic acid viruses that includes the organisms responsible for dengue, encephalitis, yellow fever, and rubella.

tolerance dose   In radiotherapy: the quantity of radiation that a body structure,

tissue, or organ can receive before irreversible damage occurs.

tomography   An X-ray technique that records detailed internal body images at a predetermined depth or plane.

tonicity   The quality of tissue tone, or tonus.

tonic neck reflex   A normal response in infants. A supine infant will extend the arm and leg on the side of the body to which the head is quickly turned. At the same time, the infant will flex the limbs of the opposite side.

ALERT The absence or persistence of the tonic neck reflex may indicate central nervous system damage.

tonometer   A device used during an eye examination for measuring intraocular tension or pressure.

tonometry   A means for measuring intraocular tension or pressure. Usually used for detecting glaucoma.

tonsil   A small, rounded mass of lymphoid tissue. The term is often used to designate the palatine tonsil.

tonsillectomy   The surgical removal of the palatine tonsils.

tonsillitis   An infection or inflammation of the palatine tonsil or tonsils.

tonus, tone   A normal state of slight contraction of the body tissues and muscles.

tooth, *pl.* **teeth**   Any of the hard calcified structures that develop in the jaws. Teeth have three parts: the crown, neck, and root, and are part of the digestive system, being used to cut, grind, and process food in the mouth.

tophi   Accumulations of urate salts; in gout, occurs throughout the body.

topical anesthesia   A gel, ointment, or solution applied to the skin, mucous membrane, or cornea as a topical anesthetic.

TOPV   *abbr* trivalent oral poliovirus vaccine.

TORCH   An acronym for a group of infections that may cross the placental barrier and cause symptoms in babies but be silent in the mother. The group of infections include toxoplasmosis, other agents, rubella, cytomegalovirus, and herpes simplex viruses.

TORCH syndrome   Infection of the fetus or newborn by one of the TORCH agents. The outcome of a pregnancy complicated by a TORCH agent may be abortion or stillbirth, intrauterine growth retardation, or premature delivery.

torpid idiocy   Severe mental retardation marked by dullness and inactivity.

torpor   Absence of response to normal stimuli.

torque   A force that produces rotation, or torsion; for example the forces produced by contraction of the medial femoral muscles tend to rotate the thigh medially.

torr   A unit of pressure, commonly meaning 1 mm Hg, the amount of pressure required to raise a column of mercury 1 mm.

torsion   The act of twisting or turning away from the normal position or rotating about an axis.

torsion fracture   A spiral fracture, usually caused by a twisting or forceful rotating of a limb from the normal position.

torsion of the testis   Rotation or twisting of the spermatic cord that cuts off the blood supply to the testicle, epididymis, and other structures. If the blood supply is reduced for any length of time, the result is atrophy of the testis; if the supply is completely cut off for 6 hours, gangrene of the testis may set in.

torticollis   A condition in which the cervical muscles are contracted so that the head is inclined or twisted to one side.

torulopsosis   A yeast infection caused by *Torulopsis glabrata,* a normal inhabitant of the oropharynx, GI tract, and skin. The disease is found mostly in severely debilitated patients, in people with impaired immune function and, sometimes, in patients who have had prolonged urinary catheterization.

total anomalous venous return   A rare congenital cardiac anomaly in which the pulmonary veins attach directly to the right atrium or to various veins draining into the right atrium rather than directing flow to the left atrium.

total cleavage   Mitotic division of the fertilized ovum into blastomeres.

total lung capacity (TLC)   The volume of air in the lungs after breathing in.

total nutrient admixture (TNA)   Daily allotment of total parenteral nutrition solution, including lipids and other solution components; commonly given in a single, 3-L bag. Also called *3:1 solution.*

total parenteral nutrition (TPN)   The administration of total caloric needs in a nutritionally adequate solution of glucose, protein hydrolysates, minerals, and vitamins through a catheter inserted into the superior vena cava.

total renal blood flow (TRBF)   A measure of the total volume of blood flowing into the renal arteries. The average TRBF for a normal adult is 1,200 ml/minute.

Tourette syndrome   Condition characterized by facial and vocal tics, uncontrollable use of obscenities, and generalized lack of coordination.

tourniquet test   A test to determine the ability of capillaries to withstand pressure. During the test, a blood pressure cuff is applied to a person's arm and is inflated to a pressure between the diastolic and systolic blood pressure for 5 minutes.

toxic amblyopia   Loss of some vision from poisoning with quinine, lead, wood alcohol, arsenic, tobacco, or other poisons.

toxic dementia   Impaired memory, judgment, and abstract thinking from excessive use of or exposure to a poison.

toxic dose (TD)   In toxicology: the amount of a substance, or agent, that will produce toxic effects.

toxic epidermal necrolysis (TEN)   A rare skin disease, afflicting mostly adults, in which skin erosions, skin redness, and superficial necrosis are present. The condition makes the skin appear scalded and it often leaves scars.

toxic goiter   An enlarged thyroid gland, which causes swelling in the front of the neck, from exophthalmia and systemic disease.

toxicity   1. The quality or amount to which something is poisonous. 2. A condition caused by exposure to a toxin or to toxic amounts of a substance.

toxic nodular goiter   An enlarged thyroid gland with numerous nodules; usually of long standing and occurring most frequently in elderly individuals.

toxicologist   A specialist in toxicology.

toxicology   The study of poisons and their detection and effects as well as methods of treating the conditions that poisons produce.

toxic shock syndrome (TSS)   A severe illness caused by infection with *Staphylococcus aureus* that produces a unique toxin, enterotoxin F. It's characterized by a sudden high fever, vomiting, diarrhea, and myalgia. A sunburnlike rash may be present and skin may peel from the palms and soles. During the acute stage, hypotension (and shock) may occur.

CLINICAL TIP TSS is most common in menstruating women using high-absorbency tampons but has been observed in newborns, children, and men.

toxocariasis   Infection with the roundworm *Toxocara canis,* a common worm larvae found in cats and dogs.

toxoid   A modified toxin (a toxin that has been treated with chemicals or heat) that has lost its toxic effect. It still retains its properties for stimulating the formation of an antitoxin.

Toxoplasma   A genus of protozoa of which the species *T. gondii* is an intracellular parasite of cats and other hosts that causes toxoplasmosis in humans.

toxoplasmosis   An infection with the protozoan intracellular parasite *Toxoplasma gondii*. If toxoplasmosis crosses the placental barrier, it involves the liver and brain and causes cerebral calcification, seizures, blindness, microcephaly or hydrocephaly, and mental retardation in the newborn.

TPN   *abbr* total parenteral nutrition.

trabecula carnea, *pl.* **trabeculae carneae**
Irregular bands or bundles of muscle projecting from the inner walls of the ventricles. There are three types: simple muscular ridges, bundles, and papillary muscles.

trace element   A nutritional element occurring in extremely small amounts in food and body tissues. Examples include aluminum, bromine, chromium, cobalt, copper, fluorine, iron, iodine, manganese, nickel, silicon, zinc.

trace gas   A vapor that escapes into the air, or atmosphere, during an anesthetic procedure.

tracer   A radioactive isotope that allows a structure to be identified or a process to be followed.

tracer depot method   In nuclear medicine: a technique for determining local skin or muscle blood flow, based on the rate at which a radioactive tracer deposited in a tissue is removed by diffusion into the capillaries and washed out by the local blood supply.

trachea   A cylindrical structure or tube in the neck that's composed of cartilage and membrane. It extends from the larynx to the right and left bronchi and is commonly called the windpipe.

 ALERT Tracheal deviation is the hallmark of life-threatening pneumothorax. If you detect tracheal deviation, be alert for these signs of respiratory distress: tachypnea, dyspnea, decreased or absent breath sounds, stridor, nasal flaring, accessory muscle use, asymmetrical chest expansion, restlessness, and anxiety.

tracheal breath sound   The breath sound heard in trachea auscultation.

tracheitis   An inflammation of the trachea.

tracheobronchial tree (TBT)   The primary structure for breathing and for carrying air to and from the lungs, the tracheobronchial tree consists of the trachea, the bronchi, and the bronchial tubes.

tracheobronchitis   An inflammation of the trachea and bronchi.

tracheostomy   The surgical creation of an opening through the neck into the trachea; used to relieve upper airway obstruction and aid breathing.

trachoma   A chronic infection of the eye conjunctiva and cornea. Trachoma is caused by *Chlamydia trachomatis*, a bacterium; symptoms of the infection include inflammation, pain, sensitivity to light, and tearing.

tract   A group of tissues and structures, usually of some length, that function together such as the digestive tract.

traction   1. The action of pulling a part of the body along the long axis. 2. In orthopedics: the act of exerting force through a system of weights and pulleys to align, immobilize, or relieve pressure in a limb, bone, or group of muscles.

traction frame   An orthopedic mechanism that supports the pulleys, ropes, and weights from which traction is applied or parts of the body are suspended.

tragus, *pl.* **tragi**   The cartilage projection at the front opening of the ear.

transaminase   An enzyme that catalyzes the transfer of an amino group from a donor to an acceptor.

transcellular fluids   A form of extracellular fluid that includes cerebrospinal fluid, lymph, and fluids in such spaces as the pleural and abdominal cavities.

transcondylar fracture   A fracture of the humerus that occurs transversally and at the level of the condyles. Also called *diacondylar fracture.*

transcription   In molecular genetics: the process by which single-stranded ribonucleic acid is formed from a double-stranded deoxyribonucleic acid.

transcutaneous electrical nerve stimulation (TENS) unit   An instrument, usually portable, that transmits painless electrical impulses to peripheral nerves or a painful area.

transduction   In molecular genetics: a method of genetic recombination in bacteria by which deoxyribonucleic acid is transferred from one cell to another, thereby changing the genetic makeup of the second.

transfection   In molecular genetics: the process by which an animal cell or bacteria is artificially infected with the deoxyribonucleic acid or ribonucleic acid of a virus to produce a mature virus.

transfer DNA (tDNA)   In molecular genetics: deoxyribonucleic acid (DNA) transferred from its original source and present in transformed cells.

transfer factor   A leukocyte extract that transfers hypersensitivity to an antigen from one person to another.

transferrin   A trace protein in the blood that binds and transports iron.

transfer RNA (tRNA)   In molecular genetics: a kind of ribonucleic acid (RNA) that transfers the genetic code from messenger RNA for the production of a specific amino acid.

transformation **1.** A change from one form to another. **2.** In oncology: the change that a cell undergoes as it becomes malignant, or cancerous. **3.** In molecular genetics: the process by which genes are integrated into chromosomes in a form that's recognized by the apparatus of the host cell.

transforming growth factor A protein or group of proteins, created by tumor cells, that cause a disorderly and abnormal increase in cells in a culture that was once normal.

transfusion Introduction of blood or its components directly into the bloodstream. Components of a transfusion include any of the following: whole blood, plasma, platelets, or packed red blood cells.

transfusion reaction Adverse reaction to transfusion therapy; the most severe form being a hemolytic reaction, which destroys red blood cells and may become life-threatening. Signs of a transfusion reaction include: fever, chills, rigors, headache, and nausea.

transposition **1.** Displacement of a viscus to the opposite side. **2.** The process of carrying a tissue flap from one situation to another without severing its connection entirely until it's united at the new location. **3.** The exchange of position of two atoms within the molecule.

Trendelenburg's position Position in which the head is low and the body and legs are on an inclined plane; used in central venous catheter insertion to distend neck and thoracic veins for optimum visibility and accessibility.

trisomy Presence of an extra chromosome.

Trousseau's sign Carpal (wrist) spasm elicited by applying a blood pressure cuff to the upper arm and inflating it to a pressure 20 mm Hg above the patient's systolic blood pressure; indicates the presence of hypocalcemia.

truss Elastic, canvas, or metallic device for retaining a reduced hernia within the abdominal cavity.

TSH *abbr* thyroid-stimulating hormone.

T suppressor cells Cells that suppress or limit the immune response of T effector cells and B cells.

tumor resistance The ability of a tumor to withstand the effects of chemotherapeutic drugs, either during the initial treatment or developed over successive treatments.

tunica A coat or covering of a blood vessel, organ, or body part.

tunica adventitia The fibrous elastic covering of blood vessels.

tunica intima The inner coat of a blood vessel.

tympany Musical, drumlike sound heard on percussion over a hollow organ, such as the stomach; a normal sound.

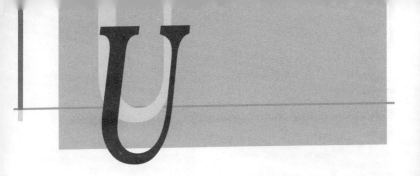

u Symbol sometimes used for micron (properly μ), as in u/ml, representing μ/ml.

U 1. Symbol for uranium. 2. *abbr* unit.

ulcer An open sore or defect of the surface of an organ or tissue caused by the sloughing of necrotic tissue that's caused by inflammation, infection, or malignancy.

ulcerative blepharitis A condition in which inflammation of the eyelids is accompanied by formation of sticky crusts on the lid margins, caused by a staphylococcal infection of eyelash follicles and eyelid glands.

ulcerative colitis A chronic, recurrent ulceration of the colon of unknown cause in which there's abdominal cramping, rectal bleeding, and diarrhea containing blood, pus, and mucus.

ulna The inner and larger bone of the forearm that lies parallel with the radius; it's on the side opposite that of the thumb.

ulnar artery A brachial artery arising near the elbow, it distributes blood to the forearm, wrist, and hand. This artery passes obliquely in a distal direction to become the superficial palmar arch.

ulnar nerve Originating in the medial and lateral cords of the brachial plexus, this nerve distributes to the muscles and the skin on the medial part of the hand and ulnar side of the forearm.

ulocarcinoma, *pl.* **ulocarcinomas, ulocarcinomata** Carcinoma of the gums.

ultracentrifuge A centrifuge with an extremely high rate of rotation that's used to separate and sediment the molecules of a substance; it can produce sedimentation of viruses in blood plasma.

ultrafilter 1. An apparatus for performing laboratory ultrafiltration. 2. A semipermeable membrane.

ultrafiltrate The liquid or minute particles that have passed through an ultrafilter.

ultrafiltration Filtration through an ultrafilter to separate extremely minute particles. It occurs both naturally (filtration of plasma at the capillary membrane) and in the laboratory (separation of a substance in colloid solution from its dispersion medium).

ultrasonography The visualization of deep structures of the body by measuring and recording the reflection of pulses of ultrasonic waves directed into the tissues.

ultrasound Mechanical radiant energy with a frequency greater than 20,000 vibrations per second. These high-frequency sound waves have been used in fetal monitoring, imaging internal organs, and cleaning dental and surgical instruments.

ultraviolet Light at the violet (short) end of the spectrum, which occurs naturally in sunlight. Beyond the visible spectrum, ultraviolet light has powerful chemical properties, which include producing vitamin D by their action on ergosterol in the skin and inducing sunburn and tanning of the skin.

ultraviolet radiation A range of electromagnetic waves that extends from the short or violet end of the spectrum to the beginning of the X-ray spectrum.

umbilical 1. Of or pertaining to the umbilicus. 2. Of or pertaining to the umbilical cord.

umbilical catheterization The passage of a catheter through an umbilical artery or vein; this procedure can be used to provide a neonate with parenteral fluid, to obtain blood samples, to perform an exchange transfusion, or to administer fluids in an emergency.

umbilical cord An elastic structure that connects the umbilicus and the placenta in the gravid uterus; it gives passage to the umbilical arteries and vein and transmits nourishment from the mother to the fetus.

umbilical fissure A groove on the visceral surface of the liver that separates the right and left lobes of the liver; it holds the ligamentum teres.

umbilical fistula An abnormal passage from the umbilicus to the intestine or, more commonly, to the urachus.

umbilical hernia Protrusion of part of the intestine at the umbilicus due to a defect in the abdominal wall; it's covered with skin and subcutaneous tissue.

umbilical vein Either of the paired veins that carry blood from the placenta in the early embryo; they later fuse to form a single vessel.

unconscious   Without awareness, sensation, or cognition; insensible; unable to respond to sensory stimuli or to have subjective experiences.

unconsciousness   A state in which there's no response to sensory stimuli or to environment; it may be caused by illness, shock, or injury.

undifferentiated malignant lymphoma   A neoplastic disease of the lymphoid tissue characterized by many large stem cells with undefined borders, pale cytoplasm, and large nuclei.

undisplaced fracture   A break or rupture in a bone characterized by fissures in the osseous tissue that radiate in several directions but don't displace the fragmented sections.

unengaged head   A floating head of a fetus.

unequal cleavage   The process by which fertilized ovum are divided into unequal blastomeres in mitosis; the blastomeres are larger near the yolk and smaller near the nucleus portions of the protoplasm.

unequal twins   One of two separate, nonjoined offspring produced in the same pregnancy in which one is fully formed and the other has developmental abnormalities.

unicellular reproduction   A form of reproduction in which a new organism is formed without fertilizing a female egg; parthenogenesis.

uniovular   Developing from one ovum (for example, monozygotic twins).

unipolar lead   An electrocardiographic conductor with exploring and indifferent electrodes; the exploring electrode is placed on the precordium or a limb as the indifferent electrode is in the central terminal.

unit   1. A single thing. 2. A quantity recognized as a standard of measurement.

unit dose   An individual labeled packet prepared by a pharmacist containing one dose of medication that the nurse is to give the patient on the ordered schedule.

United States Pharmacopeia (USP)
A legally recognized compendium of standards for drugs. Periodically revised, it includes tests for determining strength, quality, and purity.

United States Public Health Service (USPHS)   A federal agency that regulates the arrival of people, goods, or substances from other countries to protect the health of U.S. citizens.

univalent   Monovalent; the ability of one atom in a chemical element to attract or displace one atom of hydrogen.

universal antidote   A remedy once given when the exact poison wasn't known; it consisted of 50% activated charcoal, 25% magnesium oxide, and 25% tannic acid. This mixture is no longer recommended by most authorities; activated charcoal alone is now preferred.

universal donor   A person with O blood type, which lacks both A and B antigens and can be transfused in limited amounts to any patient in an emergency, with little risk of adverse reaction, regardless of the recipient's blood type.

universal recipient   A person with AB blood type, which has neither anti-A nor anti-B antibodies; AB individuals may receive A, B, AB, or O blood.

Unna's boot   A method of treating varicose ulcers in which a layer of a gelatin–glycerin–zinc oxide paste is applied to the leg; a spiral bandage covered with several layers of paste then goes over the dressing to produce an inflexible boot.

unsaturated alcohol   An alcohol that's derived from unsaturated hydrocarbons (for example, an alkene or olefin).

unsaturated fatty acid   One of many glyceryl esters of certain organic acids; during chemical reactions double or triple valence bonds joining some atoms commonly split and recombine with other substances.

upper extremity suspension   An orthopedic procedure used to correct bone fractures and upper limb defects.

upper motor neuron paralysis   A loss or impairment of motor function to the area of the brain or spinal cord that controls the upper motor neurons, which extend from the centers in the brain to the spinal column.

upper respiratory tract   The upper portion of the respiratory system, containing the nose, nasal cavity, ethmoidal air cells, frontal sinuses, sphenoidal sinuses, maxillary sinus, and the larynx.

uranium (U)   A hard, heavy, radioactive metallic element; atomic number, 92; atomic weight, 238.03.

urea   A crystalline solid, $CO(NH_2)_2$, the diamide of carbonic acid. Odorless and colorless, urea is produced in the liver from carbon dioxide and ammonia. Urea is the natural end product of protein metabolism and is present in blood, lymph, and urine.

Ureaplasma urealyticum   A microorganism that inhabits the urogenital systems of men and women; it's a sexually transmitted infection that's asymptomatic.

uremia   1. An excess in the blood of urea and other nitrogenous end products of protein and amino acid metabolism. 2. A disorder in which excessive amount of these substances are present in the blood (for example, in renal failure).

uremic frost A crystal deposit on the skin resembling that of dew or vapor, caused by kidney failure and uremia.

ureter The fibromuscular tube, about 12″ (30.5 cm) long, that conveys the urine from the kidney to the bladder.

ureteral dysfunction A condition in which the usual peristaltic flow of urine through a ureter is disturbed due to a malfunction of ureteral motor nerves.

ureteritis Inflammation of a ureter as a result of irritation of a stone or infection.

ureterocele Sacculation of the terminal portion of the ureter into the bladder, which may cause a urine flow obstruction, hydronephrosis, and loss of renal function.

ureterolithotomy Surgical incision made to remove a calculus from the ureter.

urethra The membranous canal conveying urine from the bladder to the exterior of the body. About 1″ (2.5 cm) long in women, it's located behind the symphysis pubis, anterior to the vagina. Much longer in men (about 8″ [20.5 cm]), it begins at the bladder and passes through the prostate gland, tissue connecting the pubic bones, and the urinary meatus of the penis.

urethral Of or pertaining to the urethra.

urethritis Inflammation of the urethra in which dysuria occurs, usually caused by a bladder or kidney infection.

urethrocele In women: a prolapse of the female urethra, in which a segment of the urethra and the surrounding connective tissue protrudes into the anterior wall of the vagina.

urethrorrhea Abnormal urethral discharge.

urethrostaxis Urethral oozing of blood.

URI *abbr* upper respiratory infection.

uric acid A substance present in the blood and eliminated in the urine that's an end-product of protein metabolism.

uricaciduria A condition in which urine contains an excessive amount of uric acid; this commonly occurs with urinary calculi or gout.

urinalysis A urine examination in which the urine is tested for color, turbidity, specific gravity, and pH.

urinary Of or pertaining to urine or the formation of urine.

urinary bladder The musculomembranous sac, located in the anterior part of the pelvic cavity, that serves as a reservoir for urine; it then discharges it through the urethra.

urinary calculus A small or large stone formed in any part of the urinary tract. Some

calculi can pass through the urine; larger ones may obstruct the flow of urine.

urinary hesitancy A difficulty in beginning urination, with decreased flow throughout, and usually caused by an obstruction between the bladder and the urethral opening.

TIME LINE The most common cause of urinary obstruction in male infants is posterior structures. Infants with this problem may have a less forceful urinary stream, and may also present with failure to thrive, a palpable bladder, or fever due to urinary tract infection.

CLINICAL TIP Urinary hesitancy symptom of a prostate gland enlargement in men and stenosis of the urethral opening in women.

urinary incontinence Loss of control over bladder and urethral sphincters, resulting in involuntary leakage of urine.

TIME LINE Causes of incontinence in children include infrequent and incomplete voiding that may also lead to urinary tract infection. Ectopic ureteral origin is an uncommon congenital anomaly associated with incontinence.

urinary tract infection (UTI) A bacterial infection, most commonly caused by *Escherichia coli* or a species of *Klebsiella*, *Proteus*, *Pseudomonas*, or *Enterobacter*, affecting one or more parts of the urinary tract.

TIME LINE Diagnosing a UTI in elderly patients can be problematic because many present only with urinary incontinence, changes in mental status, anorexia, or malaise. In addition, many elderly patients without UTIs present with dysuria, frequency, urgency, or incontinence.

urination The elimination of urine.

urine A clear, amber-colored fluid secreted by the kidneys, passed through the ureters, stored in the bladder, and discharged through the urethra. Healthy urine has a slight acid reaction, the characteristic odor of urea, and a specific gravity between 1.005 and 1.030.

urine output The daily volume of urine excreted, usually from 24 to 68 oz (710 to 2,010 ml).

urinoma, *pl.* **urinoma, urinomatas** A collection of urine encapsulated by fibrous tissue.

urinometer Any instrument, such as a gravitometer or hydrometer, that measures the specific gravity of urine. See illustration on page 312.

urobilin An amorphous, brownish pigment normally present in feces and, in lesser amounts, in urine. It's an oxidized form of urobilinogen.

Urinometer

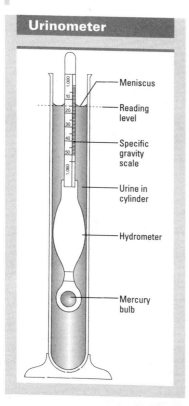

- Meniscus
- Reading level
- Specific gravity scale
- Urine in cylinder
- Hydrometer
- Mercury bulb

urobilinogen   A substance formed in the intestine as a result of the bacterial breakdown of bilirubin. This colorless compound is partially excreted in feces, the rest is resorbed, then excreted again in bile or urine.

urogenital sinus   An elongated sac into which open the ureter, mesonephric and paramesonephric ducts, and bladder; it's formed by division of the cloaca in the early embryo.

urogenital system   The organs and structures that form the kidneys, ureters, bladder, urethra, and the male and female genital structures. The female genital structure contains the ovaries, uterine tubes, uterus, clitoris, and vagina; the male genital structure contains the testes, seminal vesicles, seminal ducts, prostate, and penis.

urogram   A radiograph of part of the urinary tract, obtained by urography.

urography   Radiography of a part of the urinary tract, involving injecting an opaque substance, which then shows up on an X-ray when the passes through or is ex-

creted from the portion being studied. There are several kinds of urography, including cystoscopic urography, retrograde pyelography, and I.V. pyelography.

urokinase   An enzyme that's a powerful activator of the fibrinolytic system. Produced in the kidney and present in urine, pharmaceutical preparations of urokinase are used to treat pulmonary embolism.

urologist   A doctor who specializes in urology.

urology   The branch of medicine that deals with the urinary tract in both male and female and with the male genital tract.

uroporphyria   A rare congenital disorder in which the urine secretes an excessive amount of uroporphyrin in the urine. Signs and symptoms include blistering dermatitis, hemolytic anemia, splenomegaly, and photosensitivity.

uroporphyrin   A porphyrin normally excreted in the urine in small amounts.

urorectal septum   A caudally and outwardly growing wedge of endoderm-covered mesoderm that divides the cloaca into the urogenital sinus and rectum in the embryo.

urticaria   A vascular reaction caused by dilation and increased permeability of the capillaries. Symptoms include the development of transient wheals with pale centers and well-defined erythematous margins.

ALERT In acute cases of urticaria, quickly evaluate respiratory status and take vital signs. If you note any respiratory difficulty or signs of impending anaphylactic shock, begin cardiopulmonary resuscitation.

urticaria pigmentosa   A rare form of mastocytosis in which pigmented skin lesions become urticarial as a result of irritation, either by mechanical or chemical means.

urushiol   A poison found in some of the plants of the genus *Rhus* and their sap (for example, poison ivy, poison oak, and poison sumac).

use effectiveness   Of a contraceptive method: the success rate of a method or device in preventing pregnancy. Various factors, such as human error and improper and inconsistent use, will lower the success rate of any contraceptive method.

use test   The careful and systematic elimination and subsequent addition of certain substances in the diet or environment for the purpose of identifying the item to which the patient is allergic.

USPHS   *abbr* United States Public Health Service.

uta   A form of American leishmaniasis that occurs in the Andes of Peru and Argentina. Caused by *Leishmania viannia peruviana*, it's characterized by a single or a few ulcer-like, self-limited lesions.

uterine anteflexion   A condition marked by the forward curvature of the uterus at the juncture of the isthmus of the uterine cervix and the lower uterine segment.

uterine anteversion   The forward tipping or tilting of the uterus. It isn't clinically significant if anteversion is mild; in the most common position of the uterus there's slight anteversion.

uterine cancer   Any neoplasm of the uterus (for example, cervical cancer, which affects the cervix; endometrial cancer, which affects the lining of the body of the uterus).

uterine retroflexion   A position of the uterus in which the body of the uterus is bent backward on itself at the isthmus of the cervix and the lower uterine segment.

uterine retroversion   A tipping of the uterus in a posterior direction. It's neither unusual nor clinically significant to have mild degrees of retroversion; however, severe retroversion is commonly associated with dyspareunia, chronic pelvic discomfort, and an inability to use a contraceptive diaphragm.

utero-ovarian varicocele   A varicose condition of the veins of the pampiniform plexus of the female.

uterus   The hollow muscular reproductive organ in female mammals in which the fertilized ovum is implanted. The fetus is then nourished and develops in this pear-shaped organ; where no fertilization occurs, the decidua of menses flows from the uterus.

UTI   *abbr* urinary tract infection.

uvea   The vascular middle coat of the eye, consisting of the iris, the ciliary body, and the choroid.

uveitis   An inflammatory condition of the uvea, including the iris, ciliary body, and choroid. Signs and symptoms include inflammation around the cornea, pus in the anterior chamber, a pupil that has an irregular shape, opaque deposits on the cornea, pain, and lacrimation.

uvula, *pl.* uvulae   A pendent, fleshy mass hanging from the soft palate above the root of the tongue from the posterior border of the soft palate.

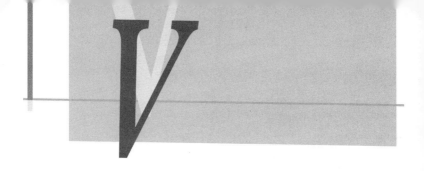

v Symbol for: **1.** venous blood. **2.** vein. **3.** volt.

V Symbol for: **1.** vanadium. **2.** rate of gas flow.

VT *abbr* tidal volume.

vaccination Any inoculation with vaccine as a preventive measure to induce immunity or to lessen the symptoms of associated infectious diseases. Although vaccines originally were inoculations against smallpox only, there are now vaccines to induce immunity against various other diseases.

vaccine A suspension containing killed or attenuated microorganisms or antigenic proteins derived from them, used for preventive inoculation or in treatment of infectious diseases. Depending on the type of vaccine, this suspension may be an intradermal, intramuscular, or subcutaneous injection; there are also vaccines that are taken orally.

vaccinia A disease that may infect humans as a result of either direct contact with cattle infected with a poxvirus or the smallpox vaccine intended to induce immunity.

vacuole **1.** Any small space or cavity formed in the protoplasm of a cell. **2.** A small space in the body, often consisting of secretions, fat, or cellular debris, that's surrounded by a membrane.

vacuum aspiration A procedure in which the fetus and placenta are removed from the uterus by suction; it's possible to terminate a pregnancy with this type of abortion up to the 14th week of pregnancy.

vagal Of or pertaining to the vagus nerve.

vagina The canal in the female that extends from the vulva to the cervix uteri. This portion of the female genitalia is located in front of the rectum and behind the bladder.

vaginal bleeding The passage of blood from the vagina, unrelated to the normal flow of blood during the menses.

TIME LINE Eighty percent of postmenopausal vaginal bleeding is benign; endometrial atrophy is the predominant cause. Malignancy should be ruled out.

vaginal cancer A neoplastic disease of the vagina that rarely occurs alone and is often secondary to cervical, endometrial, vulvar, or ovarian cancer.

vaginal discharge A discharge from the vagina, which normally produces a clear or pearly-white discharge.

TIME LINE Female newborns who have been exposed to maternal estrogens in utero may have a white mucus vaginal discharge for the first month after birth; a yellow mucus discharge indicates a pathologic condition.

vaginal instillation of medication The use of a suppository, gel or medicated cream, instilled into the vagina, to treat a vaginal infection or an infection of the uterine cervix.

vaginal jelly A translucent substance that usually contains a spermicide and is used in conjunction with a cervical cap or a contraceptive diaphragm to prevent contraception. There are also antimicrobial medications that take the form of a vaginal jelly.

vagotomy Interruption of the impulses carried by the vagus nerve, by cutting certain branches of this nerve; this gastric surgery is performed to lessen the secretions of gastric acid, thereby preventing a gastric ulcer.

vagotonus Increased activity and stimulation of the vagus nerve, which results in bradycardia with faintness, decreased cardiac output, and syncope.

vagovagal reflex A reflexive stimulation of the vagus nerve in which laryngeal or tracheal irritation produces a slower pulse rate.

vagus nerve One of the nerves of the cranium that makes speech, swallowing, and many other bodily functions possible.

valence In chemistry: a number, either positive or negative, indicating the combining power of an element in a chemical compound. A positive valence refers to how many hydrogen atoms one atom of a chemical element can displace; a negative valence refers to how many hydrogen atoms can be bonded with one atom of a chemical element.

valgus   A deformity in which a part of a limb is bent outward or twisted (for example, in talipes valgus, the heel of the foot is twisted away from the midline of the body).

valine   An amino acid that's essential for optimal growth in infants and for nitrogen equilibrium in adults. It's produced by the digestion or hydrolytic decomposition of proteins.

vallecula   In anatomy: any depression or furrow on an organ's surface or structure.

vallecula epiglottica   A depression between the lateral and median glossoepiglottic folds on each side of the posterior oropharynx.

vallecular dysphagia   A condition in which swallowing is painful or difficult, due to the lodgment of food in the valleculae, which in turn causes the vallecula epiglottica to become inflamed.

Valsalva's maneuver   Forcible exhalation effort against a closed air passage; for example, a person trying to exert force would hold his breath and contract his muscles.

Valsalva's test   An exercise to determine whether eustachian tubes are obstructed. After deep inhalation, the mouth and nose are held tightly closed, and a strong attempt at exhalation is made. A popping sound indicates that the air has entered the middle ear cavities, proving the eustachian tubes are open.

valve   A membranous fold in a canal that ensures that fluid contents flow in proper direction and there's no return flow.

valve of lymphatics   Any of the small, usually doubled, cusps in the lymphatic system that control lymph flow and ensure that there's no reflux of venous blood.

valvotomy   A surgical procedure in which a defect is corrected by incision of a valve (for example, incision of a valve of the heart to allow it to open and close properly).

valvular heart disease   A disorder characterized by stenosis of a cardiac valve, resulting in obstruction of the flow of blood, or degeneration of the valve, which leads to a reflux of blood. The disorder may be the result of a congenital defect or an acquired disease.

valvular stenosis   An acquired or congenital disorder in which any of the cardiac valves becomes narrow or constricted.

valvulitis   A disorder in which a valve, especially one in the heart, becomes inflamed, generally as a result of bacterial endocarditis, syphilis, or rheumatic fever.

vanadium (V)   A rare, gray metallic element; atomic number, 23; atomic weight, 50.942.

van den Bergh's test   A way to determine the amount of bilirubin present in the blood serum; the normal range is from 0.2 to 1.4 mg per 100 ml of serum. A small percentage (about 15%) should be direct, or conjugated, bilirubin.

vanillylmandelic acid (VMA)   A substance produced by the metabolic process of epinephrine and norepinephrine, which is excreted in the urine; a high level of VMA indicates a pheochromocytoma.

 ALERT   Epinephrine, norepinephrine, lithium, chlorpromazine, reserpine, monoamine oxidase inhibitors, levodopa, and salicylates may cause abnormal test results.

vapor bath   Application of steam to the body.

varicella-zoster virus (VZV)   A virus causing chickenpox (varicella) and shingles (herpes zoster), a member of the herpesvirus family.

varicelliform   Resembling the rash occurring with chickenpox.

varicocele   A varicose condition of the veins of the pampiniform plexus, marked by a bluish, painful swelling of the scrotum.

varicose   1. Of a vein: exhibiting varicosis, or a varicosity. 2. Unnaturally and permanently enlarged (for example, bulging veins sometimes seen in limbs).

varicose vein   A vein with inadequate valves that's twisted and dilated.

varicosis   A varicose condition of the veins of any part, most commonly affecting the veins in the lower extremities of individuals between the ages of 30 and 60.

varicosity   A condition in which something is twisted and swollen; usually refers to a vein.

variegate   Having different and varying features, especially variations in color.

variegate porphyria   An autosomal dominant hepatic porphyria, caused by partial deficiency of protoporphyrinogen oxidase activity. Symptoms include skin lesions and photosensitivity.

varioloid   1. Resembling smallpox. 2. A situation in which a vaccinated person or one who has previously had smallpox contracts a mild form of the disease.

varix, *pl.* varices   1. A twisting, enlarged vein. 2. A dilated, twisting artery or an enlarged, tortuous lymphatic.

varus   A disorder in which a portion of a limb is abnormally twisted toward the midline (for example, the heel and foot in talipes varus).

vas, *pl.* vasa   Any of the vessels in the body, especially the vessels carrying blood or lymph.

vascular Of or pertaining to a blood vessel.

vascular access port (VAP) A long-term central venous catheter implanted in a pocket under the skin; uses an attached indwelling catheter tunneled through subcutaneous tissue to position the tip in a central vein; accessed with a specially designed, noncoring needle; usually delivers intermittent infusions. VAP is often chosen when an external catheter isn't suitable; for arterial access; or implantation into the epidural space, peritoneum, or pericardial or pleural cavity.

vascular insufficiency A condition in which insufficient peripheral blood flow occurs as a result of the following: occlusion of vessels with atherosclerotic plaques, thrombi, or emboli; arteriovenous fistulas; hematologic hypercoagulability; heavy smoking; or vascular walls weakened by disease.

vasculitis A disorder in which the blood vessels are inflamed, either from an allergic reaction or as a result of disease.

vas deferens, *pl.* **vasa deferentia** The excretory duct of the testis, which unites with the excretory duct of the seminal vesicle to form the ejaculatory duct.

vasectomy A surgical procedure in which a portion of the vas deferens is removed for purposes of male sterilization.

vasoconstriction A stricture of the caliber of vessels, especially constriction of the arterioles and veins in the skin and abdominal viscera, leading to decreased blood flow.

vasoconstrictor 1. Of or pertaining to anything that constricts blood vessels. 2. An agent that causes vasoconstriction; for example, common exogenous vasoconstrictors include stress, fear, changes in temperature, and narcotic drugs.

vasodilation, vasodilation Increased caliber or distention of blood vessels, particularly arterioles, often caused by nerve impulses or medications that encourage smooth muscles of the vascular system to relax.

vasodilator 1. An agent that promotes dilation of blood vessels. 2. Pertaining to the relaxation of the smooth muscle in the walls of the blood vessels. 3. Producing dilation of blood vessels.

vasovagal reaction Sudden collapse of a vein during venipuncture, possibly caused by vasospasm due to pain or anxiety.

vasotomy Incision into the vas deferens.

vasovasostomy The surgical restoration of the ends of the severed vas deferens in which function is restored after vasectomy.

vastus intermedius A muscle in the center of the thigh, one of four of the quadriceps femoris.

vastus lateralis The largest of the four muscles that make up the quadriceps femoris; located on the outside of the thigh, extending from the hip joint to the common quadriceps tendon, inserted in the patella; extends the leg.

vastus medialis One of the four muscles that make up the quadriceps femoris; located on the inside of the thigh, inserting into the patella by the common quadriceps tendon; extends leg.

VC *abbr* vital capacity

VD *abbr* venereal disease.

VDRL test *abbr* Venereal Disease Research Laboratory test, a serologic flocculation test for syphilis; positive results also occur in presence of other treponemal diseases such as yaws.

Ve Symbol for expired volume.

VE Symbol for volume expired in one minute.

vector 1. A carrier, especially one that transmits disease; classified as either a biological vector, an animal (usually an arthropod) in which the infecting organism completes part of its life cycle, or a mechanical vector, which transmits the infecting organism from one host to another but isn't essential to its life cycle. 2. A quantity having direction and magnitude, usually represented by a line resembling an arrow.

veganism Adherence to a strict vegetarian diet that excludes all protein foods of animal origin.

vegetable albumin Any albumin produced in plants.

vegetal pole, vegetative pole The relatively inactive part of the egg where the yolk is situated; usually opposite the animal pole.

vegetarianism The practice of restricting the diet to vegetables, fruits, grains, and nuts; diet may include eggs and milk products, but no animal flesh.

vegetation Any abnormal plantlike growth of tissue, especially a funguslike growth of pathologic tissue, as in the bacterial vegetation sometimes seen around the cardiac valves.

vegetative 1. Pertaining to nutrition and growth. 2. Of or pertaining to plants. 3. Functioning involuntarily; used to denote a state of impaired consciousness in which the individual is incapable of performing voluntary actions. 4. Inactive; denoting the stage of the cell cycle in which the cell isn't replicating.

vehicle 1. An inert substance with which a medication is mixed to facilitate measurement and administration. 2. Any body fluid or structure that passively conveys a stimulus or infectious agent.

Veillonella   A genus of gram-negative anaerobic cocci occurring in pairs; found in the digestive tract of humans and animals, especially in the mouth.

Veillon tube   A glass tube with a rubber stopper at one end and a cotton plug at the other, used for the laboratory growth of bacteriologic cultures.

vein   One of the many vessels that convey blood from organs or body parts to the heart.

vein ligation and stripping   A surgical procedure consisting of the ligation and removal of the saphenous vein from groin to ankle, performed to treat recurrent thrombophlebitis or severe varicosities or to obtain a blood vessel to graft in another site.

veins of the vertebral column   A plexiform venous network that drains the blood from the vertebral column, the adjacent muscles, and the meninges of the spinal cord.

velocity   The rate of movement of a body; distance traveled per unit of time.

velopharyngeal closure   The blocking of the escape of air from the nose by raising the soft palate and contracting the posterior pharyngeal wall; occurs when making certain speech sounds and when swallowing.

velopharyngeal insufficiency   An anatomic or functional abnormality of the velopharyngeal sphincter; results in incomplete closure of the oral cavity beneath the nasal passages, as seen in cleft palate.

Velpeau's bandage   A bandage that immobilizes the elbow and shoulder by holding the brachium against the side and the flexed forearm on the chest. The palm of the hand rests on the clavicle of the opposite side.

vena cava, *pl.* venae cavae   One of the two large venous trunks that return blood from the peripheral circulation and drain into the right atrium; the inferior vena cava receives blood from the lower extremities, and from the pelvic and abdominal viscera; the superior vena cava, from the head, neck, upper extremities, and chest.

vena comitans, *pl.* venae comitantes   Companion veins; one of the paired veins that closely accompany the smaller arteries; the arterial pulsations aid venous return.

vena cordis   The veins of the heart, including the coronary veins; also called *cardiac veins.*

venereal   Pertaining to, related to, or caused by sexual contact.

venereal disease (VD)   Any contagious disorder that's sexually transmitted, including chancroid, gonorrhea, granuloma inguinale, herpes genitalis, lymphogranuloma venereum, and syphilis.

venipuncture   Puncture of a vein to withdraw a specimen of blood, perform a phlebotomy, instill a medication, start an I.V. infusion, or inject a radiopaque substance for radiologic examination.

venogram   Radiographic examination of a vein filled with contrast medium; performed before catheter insertion to check the status of blood vessels, especially if the catheter is intended for long-term use.

venom   A poison; the toxic fluid secreted by some snakes, arthropods, and other animals and transmitted by sting or bite.

venous blood gas   The concentration of oxygen and carbon dioxide in venous blood; measured to assess the adequacy of oxygenation and ventilation and to determine the acid-base status.

venous insufficiency   Abnormal circulation characterized by inadequate drainage of venous blood from a body part, usually the legs.

venous pressure   The stress exerted by blood on the walls of veins, normally 60 to 120 mm Hg in peripheral veins but elevated in conditions such as heart failure and acute or chronic constrictive pericarditis, or by venous obstruction.

venous pulse   The pulsation of a vein; can be palpated over the internal jugular vein.

venous thrombosis   Phlebothrombosis; the presence of a clot in a vein in which the vessel wall isn't inflamed.

ventilate   1. To provide with air. 2. To oxygenate blood in the pulmonary capillaries.

ventilation   The process by which air is exchanged between the lungs and the atmosphere.

ventilator   A device used in respiratory therapy to provide assisted pulmonary ventilation and positive-pressure breathing; may be used continuously or intermittently.

ventral   Denoting a position toward the belly of the body; in the anterior plane.

ventricle   A small cavity, such as those in the brain, or the lower chambers of the heart.

ventricular   Pertaining to or relating to a ventricle.

ventricular aneurysm   A localized thinning, stretching, and bulging of the wall of the left ventricle, occurring most often after myocardial infarction.

ventricular fibrillation   A cardiac arrhythmia characterized by rapid small contractions of the ventricular muscle as a result of rapid, disorganized depolarizations of the myocardial fibers.

ventricular gallop   An abnormal cardiac rhythm in which a low-pitched extra heart

sound is heard early in diastole on auscultation of the heart.

ventricular gradient   The net electrical
difference between ventricular activity of
varying durations; determined by computing
the algebraic sum of the areas within the QRS
complex and within the T wave in the electrocardiogram.

ventricular septal defect (VSD)   An
abnormal opening in the septum separating
the ventricles, usually resulting from failure
of the fetal interventricular foramen to close;
results in blood flow from the left ventricle to
the right ventricle and recirculation of blood
through the pulmonary artery and lungs.

ventriculoatrial shunt   A surgically created passageway implanted between a cerebral ventricle and the right atrium to drain
excess cerebrospinal fluid from the brain in
hydrocephalus.

ventriculocisternostomy   Surgery performed to treat hydrocephalus by creating an
opening from the third cerebral ventricle to
the cisterna magna; allows cerebrospinal fluid to drain through the shunt.

ventriculography   1. An X-ray examination of the head, after removal of the cerebrospinal fluid from the cerebral ventricles
and its replacement by air or another contrast
medium. 2. An X-ray examination of one of
the ventricles of the heart after injection of a
radiopaque contrast medium.

ventriculoperitoneal shunt   A surgically created passageway implanted between
a cerebral ventricle and the peritoneum to
drain excess cerebrospinal fluid from the
brain in hydrocephalus.

ventriculoperitoneostomy   A surgical
procedure for temporarily diverting cerebrospinal fluid in hydrocephalus, usually in
the newborn.

ventriculopleural shunt   A surgical
procedure used to correct obstructive and
communicating hydrocephalus; diverts cerebrospinal fluid from the lateral ventricle into
the pleural cavity.

ventriculoureterostomy   A surgical
procedure for directing cerebrospinal fluid
into the general circulation performed in the
treatment of hydrocephalus, usually in the
newborn.

venule   Any of the small blood vessels
that gather blood from the capillaries and
anastomose to form veins.

VEP   *abbr* visual evoked potential

vermiform appendix   The wormlike diverticulum extending from the cecum and
ending in a blind extremity.

vermis, *pl.* vermes   A worm or wormlike structure, such as the median lobe of the
cerebellum.

vernal conjunctivitis   A chronic, bilateral form of conjunctival inflammation,
thought to be allergic in origin, that recurs
during the spring and summer; marked by
photophobia and intense itching.

vernix caseosa   A cheeselike substance
that's made up of sebaceous gland secretions,
lanugo, and desquamated epithelial cells and
covers the skin of the fetus and newborn;
protects the skin agent during intrauterine
life.

verruca   1. A hyperplastic, warty skin lesion with a rough surface; caused by human
papillomavirus; may be transmitted by contact and usually appears on fingers and
hands. 2. A wartlike epidermal growth not
caused by a virus.

verruca plana   A small, smooth, tan or
flesh-colored wart seen most commonly in
children; may occur in large numbers on the
face, neck, back of the hands, wrists, and
knees.

verrucous carcinoma   A squamous cell
neoplasm of the oral cavity, larynx, or genitalia; slow-growing tumor and papillary in
appearance; usually doesn't metastasize.

verrucous dermatitis   Chromomycosis;
a chronic fungal skin condition characterized
by rough, cauliflower-like lesions.

vertebra, *pl.* vertebrae   Any one of the
33 bones of the spinal column, comprising
the 7 cervical, 12 thoracic, 5 lumbar, 5 sacral,
and 4 coccygeal vertebrae; composed of a
body, an arch, a spinous process for muscle
attachment, and pairs of pedicles and
processes.

vertebral artery   One of a pair of arteries
that branch from the subclavian arteries and
supply the muscles of the neck, the vertebrae
and spinal cord, the cerebellum, and the interior of the cerebrum.

vertebral body   The weight-supporting
central portion of a vertebra.

vertebral column   The backbone; the
flexible structure made up of 33 vertebrae
that extends from the base of the skull to the
coccyx; forms a bony case for the spinal cord
and the longitudinal axis of the skeleton.

vertex presentation   Any position of
the fetus as it enters the maternal pelvic inlet
in which the head of the fetus is the presenting part and the chin rests on the chest; a
form of cephalic presentation and the one
most favorable for delivery.

vertical transmission   Transfer of a disease or trait from one generation to the next,
either genetically or through the placenta.

vertigo   A sensation of movement in
which the patient feels himself revolving in
space (subjective vertigo) or his surroundings
revolving about him (objective vertigo); may

Vertebral column

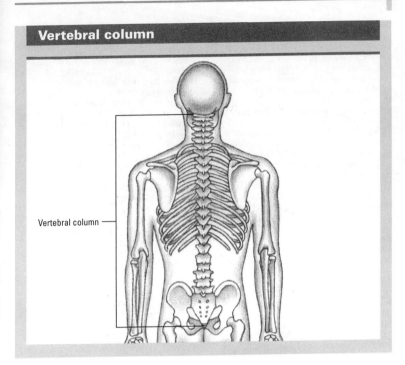

Vertebral column

result from diseases of the inner ear or from disturbances of the vestibular pathways in the central nervous system.

 TIME LINE Ear infection is a common cause of vertigo in children. Vestibular neuritis may also cause this symptom.

very-low–density lipoprotein (VLDL) A plasma protein with a density less than 1.006 g/ml; composed chiefly of triglycerides with small amounts of cholesteryl esters.

vesical fistula An abnormal passage from the urinary bladder to the body surface or to the vagina, uterus, or rectum.

vesical reflex The desire to urinate produced when the bladder is moderately distended.

vesicant An agent that causes or forms blisters.

vesicle 1. Any small anatomic sac containing liquid. 2. A small blister that contains clear fluid.

vesicoureteral reflux Abnormal backflow of urine from the bladder to the ureter; results from a congenital defect, obstruction of the bladder outlet, or lower urinary tract infection.

vesicouterine Pertaining to the bladder and the uterus.

vesicular appendix A small, fluid-filled cyst attached by a stalk to the fimbriated end of the fallopian tube; a vestige of the embryonic mesonephric duct.

vesicular breath sound A normal rustling sound heard on auscultation over the lung, characteristically higher pitched during inspiration.

vesiculitis Inflammation of a vesicle, particularly of the seminal vesicles.

vessel Any one of the channels throughout the body that convey fluids, such as blood and lymph; primarily refers to the arteries, veins, and lymphatic vessels.

vestibular Of or pertaining to a vestibule, the space at the entrance to a canal, as the vestibule of the mouth, the area between the cheeks and the teeth.

vestibular gland 1. One of a pair of small secretory glands located on each side of the vaginal orifice; also called *Bartholin's gland, greater vestibular gland.* 2. Any of the small mucous glands located between the urethral and vaginal orifices; also called *lesser vestibular gland.*

vestibule A space that serves as the entrance to a passageway.

vestige A relatively useless remnant of an organ or other body structure that had a vital function at an earlier stage of individual development or in a more primitive form of the species.

viable   Capable of sustaining life, as a normal human fetus at 28 weeks' gestation.

vibration   A form of massage administered by quick tapping with the fingertips or by a mechanical device.

vibrio   Any bacterium belonging to the genus *Vibrio*.

Vibrio cholerae   The genus and species of anaerobic, rod-shaped, motile bacteria that's the cause of cholera; found in normal and diseased human intestinal tracts and in water.

vibrio gastroenteritis   An infectious disease endemic in Asia and the Pacific islands acquired from contaminated seafood; characterized by nausea, vomiting, abdominal pain, and diarrhea; caused by *Vibrio parahaemolyticus*.

Vibrio parahaemolyticus   A species of the genus *Vibrio* that causes gastroenteritis associated with eating uncooked or undercooked shellfish, especially crabs and shrimp.

villoma, *pl.* villomas, villomata   Papilloma; a villous neoplasm that's found primarily in the bladder and large intestine.

villous adenoma   A slow-growing, soft, potentially malignant papillary polyp of the intestinal mucosa.

villous carcinoma   An epithelial tumor with many long, closely packed, fingerlike papillary outgrowths.

villous papilloma   A benign tumor with long, slender processes, usually occurring in the bladder, breast, intestine, or a cerebral ventricle.

villus, *pl.* villi   A tiny projection clustered over the surface of a mucous membrane, as in the arachnoid villi, chorionic villi, and intestinal villi; diffuses and transports fluids and nutrients.

viral hepatitis   A viral inflammation of the liver, caused by one of the hepatitis viruses.

viral infection   Any of the diseases caused by an invasion of the body or a body part by a virus pathogenic to humans.

viremia   The presence of a virus in the bloodstream.

virilization   The development of male secondary sexual characteristics in a female, including enlarged clitoris, deepened voice, and growth of facial and body hair; occurs as the result of adrenal dysfunction or hormonal medication.

virion   A complete viral particle with a central nucleoid surrounded by a protein sheath or capsid.

virologist   A microbiologist who studies viruses and viral diseases.

virology   The branch of microbiology that deals with the study of viruses and viral diseases.

virulence   The degree of pathogenicity of a microorganism, its power to produce disease as indicated by disease severity and by the organism's ability to invade host tissues.

virulent   Characterized by a high degree of pathogenicity.

virus   A minute microorganism that has no independent metabolic activity and therefore replicates only within a cell of a living host.

visceral afferent fibers   Nerve fibers that receive stimuli from smooth muscle and glandular tissue and carry impulses toward the central nervous system.

visceral lymph node   A small oval gland that drains lymph circulating in the lymphatic vessels of the abdominal and pelvic viscera.

visceral nervous system   The autonomic nervous system; the portion of the nervous system that comprises the whole complex of nerves, fibers, ganglia, and plexuses by which smooth muscle, cardiac muscle, and glandular tissue are innervated.

visceral pain   Pain caused by distention or forceful contraction of a hollow organ; characteristically severe, diffuse, and difficult to localize.

visceral peritoneum   The largest serous membrane in the body, which covers the viscera and holds it in position.

visceral pleura   The serous membrane that surrounds the lungs and lines the fissure between each lobe, separating them.

viscid, viscous   Adhesive; glutinous.

viscous fermentation   The formation of gelatinous material in milk, urine, and wine by the action of various bacilli.

viscus, *pl.* viscera   Any of the large internal organs contained in the abdominal, thoracic, or pelvic cavities.

vision   The act of seeing; sight.

visual accommodation   The process by which the eye adjusts the thickness and convexity of the lens to focus an external visual object on the retina.

visual evoked potential (VEP)   Measure of the electrical activity in the brain elicited by stimulating the retina with a repeatedly flashing light.

visual field defect   Changes in the vision that result from lesions within the visual pathway.

visual pathway   The route over which a visual sensation is transmitted from the retina to the brain; consists of an optic nerve, the optic nerve fibers traveling along the optic chiasm to the lateral geniculate body of the thalamus, and an optic tract terminating in an occipital lobe.

vital capacity (VC)   A measurement of the volume of air that can be expelled from the lungs after a maximum inspiration, representing the greatest possible breathing capacity.

vital signs   The measurements of pulse, respiratory rate, blood pressure, and body temperature.

vital statistics   Data collected by the government relating to births, deaths, marriages, health, and disease.

vitamin   Any of the group of organic substances present in foods that are essential in trace amounts for normal physiologic and metabolic function.

vitamin A   A fat-soluble substance (retinol) found in fish liver oils, dairy products, eggs, liver, and vegetables with carotene; deficiency results in night blindness and disturbances of the epithelium.

vitamin deficiency   A state or condition resulting from inadequate intake of or inability to utilize one or more vitamins.

vitamin D–resistant rickets   An inherited disease clinically similar to rickets; caused by defective renal tubular absorption of phosphate and below-normal absorption of calcium from the diet; resistant to therapeutic doses of vitamin D.

vitamin E   Any of the tocopherols, fat-soluble vitamins present in wheat germ, egg yolks, cereals, and liver; essential for normal reproduction, muscle development, and red blood cell resistance to hemolysis.

vitamin K   A group of fat-soluble vitamins present in alfalfa and other green vegetables, liver, and eggs; essential for the synthesis of prothrombin in the liver; used to treat obstructive jaundice, hemorrhagic disorders, and hypoprothrombinemia of the newborn.

vitamin K_1   Phytonadione; a viscous, oil-soluble vitamin, occurring naturally in green plants or produced synthetically; used as a prothrombinogenic agent.

vitamin K_2   Menaquinone; a fat-soluble crystalline compound that has vitamin K activity but is more unsaturated than vitamin K_1 and slightly less active biologically.

vitaminology   The study of vitamins, including their structures, actions, and function.

vitelliform   Resembling an egg yolk.

vitellin   A protein containing lecithin and found in egg yolks.

vitelline artery   Any of the embryonic arteries that circulate blood to the yolk sac from the primitive aorta.

vitelline circulation   The circulation of blood and nutrients between the developing embryo and the yolk sac through the vitelline blood vessels.

vitelline membrane   The delicate cytoplasmic membrane surrounding the yolk.

vitiligo   Absence of pigmentation.

vitreous hemorrhage   Extravasation of blood into the vitreous humor of the eye; caused by diabetic retinopathy, hypertension, retinal neovascularization, or trauma.

vitreous humor   The semigelatinous substance contained in the interstices of the stroma in the vitreous body, filling the cavity behind the lens of the eye.

vitreous membrane   Not a true membrane, but a condensation of collagen fibers in the posterior vitreous body.

viviparous   Bearing live young rather than eggs, as with most mammals and some fish and reptiles.

VLDL   *abbr* very-low–density lipoprotein.

VMA   *abbr* vanillylmandelic acid.

Vo$_2$ Symbol for oxygen uptake.

vocal cord   Either of two strong bands of elastic mucous membrane covering muscle in the larynx, attached to the angle of the thyroid cartilage.

vocal cord nodule   A small, beadlike growth that develops on the vocal cords from overuse of the voice.

vocal fremitus   The vibration of the chest wall as a person speaks; felt during auscultation of the chest.

void   To evacuate as waste matter, as in urine from the bladder.

volar   Denoting the palm of the hand or the sole of the foot.

volatile   The tendency of a liquid to evaporate rapidly.

Volkmann's canal   Any one of the small vascular canals in bone tissue connecting Haversian canals.

Volkmann's contracture   1. A serious, persistent flexion contraction of the fingers and wrist; caused by ischemia; develops after injury to the elbow region. 2. Any contracture brought about by tissue degeneration related to ischemia.

Volkmann's splint   An apparatus used in fractures of the lower leg; has a footpiece and extends from foot to knee, allowing ambulation.

volsella forceps   An instrument used to grip tissues and apply traction that has small teeth at the end of each blade.

volt   The unit of electric potential or electromotive force, the force required to send one ampere of current through one ohm of resistance.

volume The space occupied by a body, expressed in cubic units.

volvulus A knotting or twisting of the bowel on itself, causing intestinal obstruction.

vomer The flat bone forming the posterior and inferior part of the nasal septum.

vomit To forcibly expel the contents of the stomach through the mouth.

TIME LINE In a newborn, pyloric obstruction may cause projectile vomiting, while Hirschsprung's disease may cause fecal vomiting. In an infant or toddler, intussusception may lead to vomiting of bile and fecal matter. Because an infant may aspirate vomitus, as a result of his immature cough and gag reflex, position him on his side or abdomen and clear any vomitus immediately.

von Gierke's disease A form of glycogen storage disease in which a defect in glucose-6-phosphatase results in abnormally large amounts of glycogen in the liver and kidneys, causing hepatomegaly, hypoglycemia, hyperuricemia, and bleeding.

von Willebrand's disease An inherited hemorrhagic disorder characterized by prolonged bleeding time, spontaneous epistaxis and gingival bleeding, and menorrhagia; caused by a deficiency of factor VIII.

vortex, *pl.* **vortexes, vortices** 1. A whirlpool. 2. A whorled pattern, as of muscle fibers or of hairs; any structure with a whorled appearance.

VS *abbr* vital signs.

VSD *abbr* ventricular septal defect.

vulvar Pertaining to or related to the vulva.

vulvectomy The surgical excision of part or all of the vulva, performed most frequently in the treatment of neoplastic disease.

vulvocrural Of or relating to the vulva and the thigh.

vulvovaginal Of or relating to the vulva and the vagina.

VZV *abbr* varicella-zoster virus.

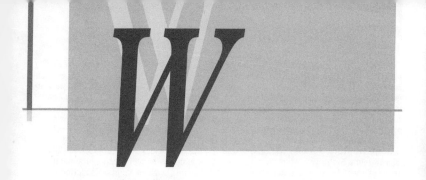

W   Symbol for tungsten.

Wagner's corpuscle   A small sensory end organ that has a connective tissue capsule and tiny stacked plates. These special organs are found in the dermis of the hand and foot, forearm, lips, tongue, palpebral conjunctiva, and mammary papilla.

Wagstaffe's fracture   A fracture in which there's separation of the internal malleolus.

walker   A light, mobile framework, about waist high, with four widely placed, sturdy legs. Made of metal tubing, walkers are used to help patients who need more support for walking than that given by a cane or crutch.

wall   A limiting structure of a space within the body — for example, the abdomen, thorax, or pelvic cavity, or of a cell.

wall eye   Deviation of the eye in which the eye turns outward; also called *exotropia*.

Wangensteen apparatus   A nasogastroduodenal catheter and suction system for treatment of a stomach or intestinal blockage.

Wangensteen tube   The catheter of a Wangensteen drainage apparatus.

warfarin poisoning   A condition resulting from an overdose of the drug warfarin or the accidental ingestion of a rodenticide that contains warfarin.

warm-blooded   Any mammal, including humans, that maintains its own warm body temperature despite changes in environmental temperatures.

washout   The administration of a gas to remove another a gas or volatile anesthetic agent.

Wassermann test   A blood test developed in 1906 and given to detect syphilis. The test is based on a complement-fixation reaction.

wasting   A gradual loss of weight accompanied by a decrease in appetite, mental activity, and vigor.

water (H_2O)   A tasteless, odorless, colorless liquid. The chemical compound has one molecule that contains one atom of oxygen and two atoms of hydrogen. It freezes at 32° F (0° C), boils at 212° F (100° C) and is found in all organic tissues.

waterborne   Carried by water; for example, typhoid fever is a waterborne disease.

Waterhouse-Friderichsen syndrome Cerebrospinal meningitis marked by cyanosis, collapse, the sudden onset of fever, petechiae, and massive bilateral adrenal hemorrhage.

watt   The unit of electrical power of work being done, expressed as one joule per second. A watt is the power produced by one ampere of current flowing with a force of one volt.

wave   In physics: an orderly, predictable disturbance in which energy moves through a medium, such as water or air, without altering the properties of the medium. Some waves, such as electromagnetic waves and X-rays, can travel through a vacuum; other waves, such as sound, can only travel through matter.

wavelength   The distance between the top of one wave and the same spot on the next one; a given point on one wave cycle and the corresponding point on the next successive wave cycle.

WBC   *abbr* white blood cell.

W chromosome, Z chromosome   The sex chromosomes of some types of insects, birds, and fishes. Females of these species have one W and one Z chromosome and are considered to be heterogametic; males have two Z chromosomes and are homogametic.

wean   1. To encourage an infant to give up breast-feeding and to substitute other foods for breast milk. 2. To withdraw someone from a substance on which the person is dependent.

weanling   An infant who has recently switched from breast milk to other foods.

weaver's bottom   A form of bursitis characterized by excruciating pain over the center of the buttock and down the back of the leg. It affects the ischial bursae of the hips of people who sit in one position for prolonged periods of time.

web A membrane or tissue that covers a space. Examples of web include the esophageal, laryngeal, subsynaptic, and terminal.

Weber test A test for determining if hearing loss is the conductive type caused by a middle-ear problem or sensorineural from an inner ear or nerve disorder.

wedge fracture A compression fracture of a vertebra. In this type of fracture, the anterior of a vertebra becomes compressed so that the vertebra takes on a wedge shape.

wedge pressure The capillary pressure in the left atrium, determined by measuring the pressure in a cardiac catheter wedged in the most distal segment of the pulmonary artery.

wedge resection The surgical removal of a triangular section of tissue or organ.

WEE *abbr* western equine encephalitis.

weeping 1. Tearing; crying; lacrimating. 2. Oozing or dripping fluid or serum.

Wegener's granulomatosis A chronic inflammatory disease affecting mostly males. The condition is characterized by the formation of tumorlike masses in the upper and lower respiratory tracks, necrotizing vasculitis, and glomerulonephritis. The disease may be triggered by hypersensitivity to an unknown antigen.

weight Heaviness; the force, or pull of gravity, exerted on a body. On the surface of the earth, mass and weight are the same.

weismannism A theory, proposed by German biologist August Weismann, that acquired characteristics can't be inherited.

Wenckebach period An incomplete heart block that can be detected with an electrocardiogram. It's marked by a progressive beat-to-beat lengthening of the PR interval.

Werdnig-Hoffmann disease A genetic disorder with muscular atrophy that begins in infancy or young childhood. Degeneration of the cells in the anterior horn of the spinal cord and the motor nuclei in the brain stem cause the progressive wasting.

Werner's syndrome Hereditary syndrome characterized by premature senility and gray hair, spindly extremities, and cataracts.

Wernicke's encephalopathy An inflammatory, hemorrhagic, degenerative condition of the brain that's characterized by lesions in several parts of the brain including the hypothalamus, mamillary bodies, and tissues surrounding ventricles and aqueducts.

West nomogram A nomogram used in estimating the body surface area of children or adults.

wet dressing A moist covering or dressing used to treat a variety of skin conditions. As the moisture in the dressing evaporates, it provides relief by cooling and drying the skin and softening dried blood. The moisture also stimulates circulation.

wet lung An accumulation of liquid in the lungs.

 CLINICAL TIP A person with wet lung may have a persistent cough and crackles at the lung bases. The condition occurs in people exposed to pulmonary irritants, such as ammonia, chlorine, dusts, sulfur dioxide, volatile organic acids, and gases of corrosive chemicals.

W/F Symbol for white female, commonly used in the initial identifying statement in a patient record.

Wharton's jelly A soft gelatinous material found in the umbilical cord. It contains collagen fibers that increase in number as the fetus ages.

wheal A smooth, slightly raised section of skin that may be either redder or paler than the surrounding area. The wheal may itch intensely, change in size and shape, and disappear within hours. It's usually a sign of allergy. Also called *hive, welt.*

wheat weevil disease A lung inflammation caused by an allergy to weevil particles in wheat flour.

wheelchair A chair with large wheels and brakes. It's used by individuals who are unable to walk and can be personalized with special brakes, armrests, seats and other features.

wheeze A whistling sound made during inhaling and exhaling; may occur as a result of asthma, hay fever, tumors, obstructions, bronchial spasm, or tuberculosis.

ALERT If a patient is wheezing, examine their degree of respiratory distress. Be alert for confusion; abnormally fast, slow or shallow respirations; increased accessory muscle use and increased chest wall motion; use of intercostal, suprasternal, or supraclavicular retractions; and stridor or nasal flaring.

white fibrocartilage A mixture of tough, white fibrous tissue and flexible cartilaginous tissue. The white fibrous tissue dominates and is divided into circumferential fibrocartilage, connecting fibrocartilage, interarticular fibrocartilage, and stratiform fibrocartilage.

white substance A tissue consisting of myelinated and unmyelinated nerve fibers and embedded in neuroglia. It's the tissue surrounding the gray matter in the spinal cord.

white thrombus 1. A collection of blood factors that contain mostly white blood cells and few or no red blood cells. 2. A collection

Wisdom teeth

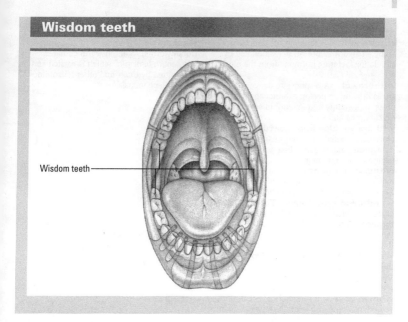

Wisdom teeth

---

of blood factors that consists primarily of blood platelets and fibrin.

whitlow An inflammation of the end of a finger or toe that may be superficial or deep and develops pus.

WHO *abbr* World Health Organization.

whole blood Blood that's unmodified, or has none of the components removed. An anticoagulant such as heparin may be added and the blood is then used for transfusion.

whorl A spiral twist. Examples of whorls include the turns of the cochlea in the inner ear, the formation of muscle fibers in the heart, and the skin swirls that create fingerprints.

WIA *abbr* waking imagined analgesia.

Widal's test A blood test to determine the presence of *Salmonella* infection.

Wilms' tumor A rapidly growing malignant kidney tumor that occurs most commonly in children under age 5, although it sometimes develops before birth. Rare cases occur later in life. Also called *adenomyosarcoma.*

Wilson's disease A rare, inherited disorder that's progressive. Symptoms include poor copper metabolism and accumulation of copper in the liver, brain, kidney, cornea, and other tissues. Also called *familial hepatitis.*

CLINICAL TIP Wilson's disease produces a characteristic rust-colored

ring around the cornea (Kayser-Fleischer ring) caused by copper deposits.

wind chill The loss of heat from a body exposed to wind. Wind chill is expressed as an "index" or as a "factor." The wind-chill index measures kilocalories per hour per square meter of skin surface. The wind-chill factor refers to the temperature felt by someone exposed to the wind; it's expressed as degrees Celsius or Fahrenheit.

winding sheet A covering used to wrap a dead body.

window An opening into a cavity or structure; it may occur naturally or be surgically created.

windowed In an orthopedic cast: an opening to relieve pressure that may inflame or irritate the skin.

winter itch Itching that occurs in people who have dry skin or atopic dermatitis, especially in the winter.

wiry pulse An abnormal pulse that's strong and intense.

wisdom tooth The last teeth on either side of the upper and lower jaw. Called the third molars, these are the last to erupt and usually appear between the ages of 17 and 21.

Wiskott-Aldrich syndrome Immunodeficiency inherited as an X-linked trait. Symptoms include eczema, inadequate T- and B-cell function, thrombocytopenia, and an increased susceptibility to infections and cancer.

witch's milk A milklike substance secreted by a newborn's breast. It's stimulated by circulating lactating hormone from the mother.

withdrawal A response to danger or stress in which a person exhibits apathy, depression, lethargy, retreat and, in severe cases, catatonia and stupor.

withdrawal bleeding Bleeding from the uterus, associated with the shedding of endometrium, that occurs when hormonal medication is discontinued.

withdrawal method A contraceptive method in which the penis is withdrawn from the vagina before ejaculation.

withdrawal symptoms The physiologic changes, which may be unpleasant, even life-threatening, that occur when alcohol, stimulants, some opiates, or other drugs are withdrawn after prolonged use.

Wolff-Parkinson-White syndrome An abnormal cardiac rhythm in which an electrocardiogram shows a short PR interval and a wide QRS complex.

woman-year In statistics: a year in the reproductive life of a sexually active woman; a unit that represents 12 months of exposure to the possibility of pregnancy.

Wood's glass Ultraviolet rays used extensively diagnose fungus infections of the scalp, such as tinea capitis, and erythrasma and to reveal porphyrins and fluorescent materials. Also called *Wood's rays, Wood's lamp.*

Wood's light An ultraviolet light used for diagnosing scalp and skin diseases such as tinea capitis. The light causes hairs infected with a fungus to glow.

woolsorter's disease An occupational disease affecting people who process sheep's wool; the lung form of anthrax.

worm A soft-bodied, elongated invertebrate of the phyla Annelida, Acanthocephala, Nemathelminthes, or Platyhelminthes. Parasitic worms infecting humans include the hookworm, pinworm, roundworm, and tapeworm.

wormian bone A tiny, smooth, segmented bone that's moist, soft, and lukewarm, and located along the serrated borders of the sutures between cranial bones.

wound An injury in which there's a break in the skin or another body structure and that has been caused by physical means.

wound irrigation Flushing a wound cavity with saline or a medicated solution.

Wright's stain A mixture of methylene blue and eosin that's used to stain blood samples for examining corpuscles and for detecting malarial parasites.

Wuchereria A genus of filarial worms (roundworms) found in warm climates. *Wuchereria bancrofti,* which is carried and transmitted by *Culex* and other mosquitoes, causes elephantiasis.

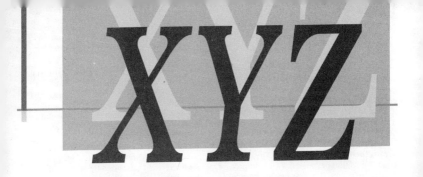

X Symbol for Kienbock unit of X-ray exposure.

xanthelasmatosis A condition in which xanthomas (tumors with excess fat or lipids) are found in tissues.

xanthine A nitrogenous compound, a by-product metabolism found in the tissues of muscles, liver, spleen, pancreas, and other organs and in urine.

xanthine derivative The methylated xanthine compounds caffeine, theomine, and theophylline that are used for their bronchodilator effects. The compounds are found naturally in plants and are routinely consumed in the form of cocoa, coffee, cola, and tea.

xanthinuria **1.** A hereditary disorder of purine metabolism in which xanthine oxidase, an enzyme, is missing. The disorder causes excessive secretion of xanthine in the urine. **2.** General term for excessive xanthine excretion.

xanthochromic, xanthochromatic A yellowish discoloration of the skin or cerebrospinal fluid.

xanthogranuloma, *pl.* xanthogranulomas, xanthogranulomata A tumor that contains granulation tissue as well as lipid or fatty deposits.

xanthoma, *pl.* xanthomas, xanthomata A fatty, yellow plaque or nodule found in the subcutaneous layer of skin, commonly around tendons; also located on the eyelids. The condition usually occurs in older women.

xanthoma disseminatum A benign condition in which small orange or brown nodules develop on the face and the mucous membranes. When the condition involves the pituitary gland, it commonly results in diabetes insipidus.

xanthoma palpebrarum A soft, yellow spot found on the eyelids.

xanthomasarcoma A giant cell sarcoma of the tendon sheaths and aponeuroses that contains xanthoma cells.

xanthoma striatum palmare A yellow plaque or nodule found in groups on the palms of the hands.

xanthoma tendinosum A movable yellow, elevated or flat, round papule or nodule found on tendons, ligaments and fascia of the hands, fingers, elbows, knees, and heels of persons with hereditary lipid storage disease.

xanthomatosis An condition marked by deposits of yellow fatty nodules in the internal organs, skin, and reticuloendothelial system.

xanthoma tuberosum A yellow or orange, large flat or elevated, round nodule found in groups on the elbows, knees, and other areas subject to injury of people with a hereditary lipid storage disease such as hyperlipoproteinemia.

xanthopsia An visual disorder where by objects appear yellowish. It can be associated with jaundice or digoxin toxicity.

xanthosis A yellowish discoloration that can be seen in degenerating tissues.

xanthurenic acid An aromatic compound, which is a metabolite of tryptophan, present in elevated amounts in the urine of patients with vitamin B_6 deficiency.

X chromosome A sex chromosome present in both sexes. Normal males have one X chromosome and normal females have two X chromosomes in their cells.

Xe Symbol for xenon.

xenogenesis **1.** Skipping generations; heterogenesis. **2.** The theoretical production of offspring who have none of the characteristics of the parents.

xenon (Xe) An inert, gaseous element. Its atomic number is 54; atomic weight, 131.30.

xeroderma A skin disorder marked by dryness, roughness, and discoloration.

xeroderma pigmentosum A rare, inherited skin disease that affects all races and begins in childhood. Symptoms include extreme sensitivity to light and development of excessive freckling, telangiectases, keratoses, papillomas, carcinoma and, possibly, melanoma in exposed skin.

CLINICAL TIP Severe ophthalmologic abnormalities may also be present: photophobia, lacrimation, keratitis, and tumors of the lid and cornea.

xerophthalmus Abnormally dry cornea and conjunctiva caused by vitamin A deficiency.

xeroradiography A diagnostic X-ray technique that produces an image photoelectrically instead of chemically. The process permits shorter exposure times and a lower radiation level than that of standard X-rays.

xiphisternal articulation The cartilaginous connection between the xiphoid process and the sternum. The joint usually hardens at puberty.

xiphoid process The smallest of three parts of the sternum, articulating caudally with the body of the sternum and laterally with the seventh rib.

X-linked Relating to traits carried on the X chromosome. Whether dominant or recessive, X-linked traits are always expressed in males because they have only one X chromosome.

X-linked dominant inheritance An inheritance sequence in which a dominant gene on the X chromosome is always expressed.

X-linked inheritance An inheritance sequence in which a trait varies according to sex because genes on the X chromosome have no counterparts on the Y chromosome.

X-linked recessive inheritance An inheritance sequence in which an abnormal recessive trait on the X chromosome is carried by females and expressed in males.

XO In genetics: the lack of either the X or Y chromosome, making each cell monosomic. In such circumstances, each cell contains a total of 45 chromosomes.

X-ray High-energy electromagnetic waves that can penetrate most substances and interact with photographic film. X-rays are used to examine structures, to destroy diseased tissue, and to make images for diagnostic purposes, such as in fluoroscopy and radiography.

X-ray microscope A microscope that can produce X-ray images on film. The images can be magnified many times with a light microscope.

X-ray pelvimetry A radiographic determination of the dimensions of the female pelvis and the diameter of the fetal head; used to determine whether the fetal head can safely pass through the pelvis during labor.

XX In genetics: the normal sex chromosome pattern in the human female.

XY In genetics: the normal sex chromosome complement pattern in the human male.

xylitol A five-carbon sugar alcohol obtained by the reduction of xylose. Xylitol is as sweet as sucrose and is used as an artificial sweetener in diabetic diets.

XYY syndrome A condition in which the human male has an extra Y chromosome, usually resulting in an increase in height but poor mental and psychological development.

Y Symbol for yttrium.

yaws An endemic, infectious, tropical disease caused by the spirochete *Treponema pertenue* and transmitted by direct contact with skin lesions of an infected person. It's characterized by chronic, ulcerating lesions anywhere on the body with eventual tissue and bone deformation and destruction if left untreated.

Yb Symbol for ytterbium.

Y chromosome The male sex chromosome in humans and many other species, appearing singly in the normal male and carried by half the male gametes and none of the female gametes.

yeast A single-celled, usually rounded, nucleated fungus that reproduces by budding. Some species are pathogenic in humans, as *Candida albicans,* which can cause athlete's foot, candidiasis, vaginitis, and thrush.

yellow cartilage The most elastic of the three main kinds of cartilage, consisting of a network of elastic fibers in a flexible, fibrous matrix. It's found in the external ear, the auditory tube, the epiglottis, and the larynx.

yellow fever An acute arbovirus infection endemic in tropical regions of the Americas and Africa. It's characterized by fever, headache, hemorrhage, jaundice, and renal damage. It's caused by a flavivirus transmitted by mosquitoes.

yellow fever vaccine A live, attenuated yellow fever virus vaccine cultured in chick embryos and used for immunization against yellow fever. It's recommended for people traveling or living in endemic areas, but shouldn't be given to persons who are immunosuppressed, pregnant, or have a known hypersensitivity to chicken or egg protein.

Yersinia pestis A small, gram-negative bacillus that causes bubonic and pneumonic plague. The primary host is the rat, but other small rodents may also carry it. It's transmitted from rat to human by the rat flea and between humans by the human body louse.

Y fracture A Y-shaped intercondylar fracture.

yin and yang In traditional Chinese medicine, the concept that describes various opposing physical forces in nature and the body, such as hot and cold, wet and dry, and active and passive. Each organ is associated with either *yin* or *yang* characteristics; and good health is believed to require a balance of *yin* and *yang* throughout the body.

Y-linked Relating to characteristics or conditions transmitted by genes carried on the Y chromosome.

yoga An ancient Hindu exercise and health maintenance program that aims to promote relaxation, and produce other health benefits, through the practice of specific positions combined with deep breathing and meditation.

yolk The nutritional material, rich in fats and proteins, stored in the ovum to supply nourishment to the developing embryo.

yolk sac An extraembryonic membrane that expands into a pear-shaped vesicle, part of which becomes the primitive gut. It's connected to the body of the embryo by the yolk stalk.

yolk stalk The long, narrow tube connecting the yolk sac with the midgut of the embryo in the early stages of prenatal development.

Young's rule A formula for calculating the approximate dose of a drug for a child age 2 or more. Divide the child's age by the sum of the child's age plus 12 to obtain the fraction of the adult dosage to give.

Y-set A device composed of plastic components, used for delivering I.V. fluids through a primary I.V. line connected to a combination drip chamber-filter section from which two separate plastic tubes lead to fluid sources.

ytterbium (Yb) A rare metallic element with an atomic number of 70 and an atomic weight of 173.04.

yttrium (Y) A scaly, gray rare metallic element with an atomic number of 39 and an atomic weight of 88.905. Radioactive isotopes of yttrium have been implanted as seeds in the body for cancer therapy.

yuppie flu Chronic infection caused by the Epstein-Barr virus; also called *chronic fatigue syndrome.*

Z chromosome A sex chromosome present in certain insects, fishes, and birds. Normal females of the species have a single Z chromosome and a W chromosome, and normal males of the species have only Z chromosomes.

Zenker's diverticulum A circumscribed herniation of the mucous membrane at the junction of the pharynx and the esophagus.

TIME LINE Hoarseness, asthma, and pneumonitis may be the only signs of esophageal diverticula in elderly patients.

zero The point on a thermometer scale at which the gradations begin. On the Celsius (centigrade) and Réaumur's temperature scales, the zero point is the freezing point of water. On the Fahrenheit scale, the zero point is set at 32° below the freezing point of water.

Ziehl-Neelsen method A stain used to detect acid-fast organisms, which appear red against a blue background. It's commonly used in the microscopic examination of sputum suspected of containing *Mycobacterium tuberculosis.*

ZIG *abbr* zoster immune globulin.

zinc (Zn) A blue-white crystalline metal with an atomic number of 30 and an atomic weight of 65.37. Zinc is an essential part of many enzymes and is needed in trace amounts in the body.

zinc deficiency A condition caused by a lack of an adequate amount of zinc in the diet, characterized by anemia, retarded growth, delayed sexual maturity, prolonged healing of wounds, and the habit of eating clay or dirt.

zinc gelatin A topical protectant prepared from zinc oxide, gelatin, glycerin, and purified water.

zinc oxide A white powder used as a topical astringent, antiseptic, and protectant and prescribed for a wide range of minor skin irritations.

zinc salt poisoning A toxic condition caused by the ingestion or inhalation of a zinc salt and characterized by colic, painful diarrhea, vomiting, and fever.

ZIP *abbr* zoster immune plasma.

zirconium (Zr) A rare metallic element with an atomic number of 40 and an atomic weight of 91.22. It's chiefly obtained from the mineral zircon.

Zn Symbol for zinc.

Zollinger-Ellison syndrome A condition characterized by severe, intractable peptic ulcers, gastric hyperacidity, elevated serum gastrin levels, and gastrinoma of the pancreas or the duodenum, which may be either benign or malignant.

zona, *pl.* **zonae** A zone or girdle encircling a region or area; an area with a specific boundary or characteristics. Examples of zona are zona arcuata, zona orbicularis, zona pellucida.

zona arcuata An inner tunnel.

zona fasciculata Middle section of the cortex of the adrenal gland.

zona glumerulosa Outer section of the cortex of the adrenal gland.

zona orbicularis The orbicular zone of the hip joint in which circular fibers of the articular capsule form a ring around the neck of the femur.

zona pellucida A transparent, noncellular layer of uniform thickness that surrounds a mammalian ovum. It's secreted by the ovum while it develops in the ovary and is retained until near the time of implantation.

zona radiata A zona pellucida that has a striated appearance caused by radiating within the membrane.

zona reticularis Inner section of the cortex of the adrenal gland.

zoogenous Derived or acquired from animals.

zoology The biology of animal life.

zoonosis A disease of animals that may be transmitted to humans. Some examples are equine encephalitis, leptospirosis, rabies, and yellow fever.

zooparasite A parasitic animal species or organism including, for example, many protozoa, worms, and arthropods.

zoopsia An hallucination in which the patient visualizes animals or insects, commonly occurring in delirium tremens.

zootoxin A poisonous substance of animal origin, such as the venom of snakes, spiders, or scorpions.

zosteriform Resembling the herpes zoster infection.

zoster immune globulin (ZIG) A passive immunizing agent currently in limited use for preventing or attenuating herpes zoster virus infection in immunosuppressed individuals who are at great risk for severe herpes zoster virus infection.

Z-plasty A plastic surgery technique in which a Z-shaped incision is made to reduce contractures of the skin around a scar or wound closure.

Zr Symbol for zirconium.

Z-track An intramuscular injection technique in which the patient's skin is pulled in such a way that the needle track is sealed off after the injection. The technique is done to minimize subcutaneous irritation and discoloration.

zygogenesis Reproduction by the union of male and female gametes and nuclei; the formation of a zygote.

zygoma 1. The long zygomatic process of the temporal bone. 2. The zygomatic arch. 3. A term sometimes applied to the zygomatic bone.

zygomatic arch The arch formed by the joint of the temporal process of the zygomatic bone and the zygomatic process of the temporal bone.

zygomatic bone One of the pair of quadrangular bones that forms the prominence of the cheek and the lower part of the eye socket. It joins with the frontal bone, the maxilla, the zygomatic process of the temporal bone, and the sphenoid bone.

zygomatic nerve Sensory branch of the maxillary division of the trigeminal nerve that supplies the skin over the cheekbone and the temple.

zygomatic process Any of several strong, bony processes that form part of the zygomatic arch.

zygomaticus major One of the muscles of the mouth arising from the zygomatic bone in front of the temporal process and inserting into the corner of the mouth. It acts to draw the angle of the mouth up and back to smile or laugh. It's innervated by the facial nerve.

zygomaticus minor One of the muscles of the mouth arising from the malar surface of the zygomatic bone and inserting into the upper lip. It acts to draw the upper lip up and out in a sad facial expression. It's innervated by the facial nerve.

zygomycosis An acute, commonly sudden and severe fungal infection caused by a class of water mold. In humans, it's usually seen in patients with chronic debilitating diseases, particularly uncontrolled diabetes mellitus, or in immunosuppressed individuals.

zygote In embryology: the fertilized ovum, or the cell, resulting from the union of the male and female gamete, that exists until the first cleavage.

zygotene The synaptic stage in the first meiotic prophase of gametogenesis in which longitudinal pairing of homologous chromosomes occurs.

Appendices

Appendix A: Medical roots, prefixes, and suffixes

In any health care setting, medical terms are in constant use. As an integral member of the health care team, you must be able to understand the medical terms used by your colleagues.

Most medical terms are derived either from ancient languages, such as Latin and Greek, or from the names of doctors or mythologic figures. Learning medical terminology is akin to learning a new language; it can be easier if you know how to analyze a term's key elements and identify word associations. Most medical terms are a combination of two or more parts. If you can successfully interpret each part separately and then combine them, you can usually grasp the essential meaning of the term. Thus, interpreting the meaning of a medical term requires knowledge of common medical roots, prefixes, and suffixes.

A *root* is the essential component, or basic meaning, of a word. Many medical roots, for example, signify a disease, procedure, or body part. Some roots appear after a prefix, before a suffix, or between a prefix or suffix. In addition, two or more roots may be combined to form a medical term, commonly with the letter "o" (for example, cardi-*o*-pulmonary and cardi-*o*-vascular).

A *prefix* is one or more letters attached to the beginning of a word or base. To determine the meaning of a prefix in a medical term, consider a familiar word that begins with the same prefix. For example, the prefix *anti-* has the same meaning (against) in both *antislavery* and *antibiotic*.

A *suffix* is one or more letters attached to the end of a word or base. When a suffix begins with a consonant, a combining vowel, such as "o," precedes the suffix. Adding a "y" to a word denotes a procedure (for example, gastroscopy). Adding -*ly* to a word denotes an act or process (for example, splenomegaly).

With a bit of practice, you'll quickly discover how easy it can be to interpret the parts of a medical term and then combine them to identify the term's meaning. For example, in *acrocyanosis*, the root *acr-* (extremities) and the vowel "o" are combined with the prefix *cyan-* (blue) and the suffix -*osis* (condition) to form a term meaning "a condition characterized by blue extremities." In *osteopathology*, the root *osteo-* refers to "bone." It's a derivative of a second root, *patho-*, meaning "disease." The suffix -*logy* is a derivative of the Latin word *logos*, meaning "the study of." Putting these identifiable parts together yields the definition of *osteopathology*: "the study of bone diseases."

Here's an extensive list of medical roots, prefixes, and suffixes, along with their meanings.

Root, prefix, or suffix	Meaning	Root, prefix, or suffix	Meaning
a(n)-	absence, without	cervic(i)(o)-	neck
ab-	away from	cheil(o)-	lip
abdomin(o)-	abdomen	chem(i)(o)-	chemical
acou-	hearing	chlor(o)-	green
acr(o)-	extremity, peak	chol(e)(o)-	bile
ad-	toward	chondr(o)-	cartilage
aden(o)-	gland	cili-	eyelid, eyelash
adip(o)-	fat	circum-	around
alb-	white	col(i)(o)-	colon
-algia	pain	colp(o)-	vagina
all(o)-	different, other	con-	with
alve-	channel, cavity	contra-	opposite
ambi-	on both sides	corpor-	body
andr(o)-	male	cost(o)-	rib
angi(o)-	vessel	crani(o)-	skull
anis(o)-	unequal	cry(o)-	cold
ankyl(o)-	crooked	cut-	skin
ante-	before, forward	cyan(o)-	blue
anti-	against	cyst(i)(o)-	bladder
apo-	away from, separate	cyt(o)-	cell
arteri(o)-	artery	dacry(o)-	tears
arthr(o)-	joint	dactyl(o)-	finger, toe
articul-	joint	deca-	ten
astro-	star	dendr(o)-	treelike
atri(o)-	atrium of heart	dent(i)(o)-	tooth
auri-	ear	derm-, -derm	skin
aut(o)-	self	dextr(o)-	right
bi-	two	di-	twice
bili-	bile	dia-	across, through
bio-	pertaining to life	digit(i)-	finger, toe
-biosis	life	dipl(o)-	double
blast-, -blast	embryonic state	disc(i)(o)-	disk-shaped
belphar(o)-	eyelid	dors(o)-	back
brachi(o)-	arm	-dorsal	back
brady-	slow	dys-	difficult, painful
brom(o)-	stench	ect(o)-	outside
bronch(o)-	bronchus	-ectomy	surgical removal
bucc(o)-	cheek	end(o)-	inward
calc-	heel	enter(o)-	intestine
capit-	head	ep(i)-	on, upon
carcin(o)-	cancer	erg(o)-	work
cardi(o)-	heart	erythr(o)-	red
caud-	tail	eso-	within
-cele	hernia, tumor	esthe-	perception, feeling
centi-	hundred	ex(o)-	outside
cephal(o)-	head	extra-	outside of, beyond
cerebr(o)-	cerebrum	fasci-	bundle

Root, prefix, or suffix	Meaning	Root, prefix, or suffix	Meaning
febri-	fever	latero-	side
fet(i)(o)-	fetus	leuk(o)-	white
fibr(o)-	fiber	lip(o)-	fat
fil-	threadlike	lith(o)-	stone
fiss-	cleft, split	lymph(o)-	lymph
galact(o)-	milk	lyo-	dissolved
gastr(o)-	stomach	-lys(i)(o)	decomposition
ger(o)-, geront(o)-	aging	macr(o)-	large, long
gest-	carry	mal-	bad, abnormal
gli(o)-	gluelike	mamm(o)-	breast
gloss(o)-	tongue	mast(o)-	breast
gluc(o)-, glyc(o)-	sweet	medi(o)-	middle
gon(o)-	semen, seed	mega-	great, large
-gram	letter, drawing	melan(o)-	black
gran-	grain, particle	meno-	menses
-graph	write, record	ment-	mind
grav(i)-	heavy	meta-	beyond, change
hem(a)(o)-	blood	-metr	measure
hepat(o)-	liver	metr(o)-	uterus
hetero-	other, different	micr(o)-	small, one-millionth
histi(o)-, hist(o)-	tissue	milli-	one-thousandth
home(o)-, hom(o)-	same	mio-	less
hyal(o)-	glasslike	mito-	threadlike
hydr(o)-	water, hydrogen	mono-	one
hyp(o)-	below, under	morph(o)-	shape
hyper-	above, beyond	multi-	many
hyster(o)-	uterus	my(o)-	muscle
idi(o)-	self, separate	myc(o)-, mycet(o)-	fungus
ile(o)-	ileum	myel(o)-	marrow, spinal cord
ili(o)-	ilium, flank	myx(o)-	mucus
infra-	beneath	narco-	stupor
inter-	between, among	nas(o)-	nose
intra-	within, into	ne(o)-	new
is(o)-	equal, identical	nephr(o)-	kidney
ischi(o)-	hip	neur(o)-	nerves
-itis	inflammation or disease	nos(o)-	disease
jejun(o)-	jejunum	nucle(o)-	nucleus
juxta-	near	ocul(o)-	eye
kerat(o)-	horny tissue, cornea	olig(o)-	few, little
kilo-	thousand	-oma	tumor
kinet(o)-	movement	omphal(o)-	navel
labio-	lips	onych(o)-	nail
lact(i)(o)-	milk	ophthalm(o)-	eye
laryng(o)-	larynx	orchi(o)-	testes
		oro-	mouth
		-osis	condition

Root, prefix, or suffix	Meaning	Root, prefix, or suffix	Meaning
-osm(o)-	sell	re-	back, contrary
oss-, oste(o)-	bone	ren(o)-	kidney
ot(o)-	ear	reticul(o)-	netlike
ov(i)(o)-	egg, ova	retr(o)-	backward
ox(y)-	oxygenation	rhin(o)-	nose
par(a)-	beside	-rrhea	fluid discharge
path(o)-	disease	rub(r)-	red
ped(o)-	child	sangui-	blood
pell-	skin	sarc(o)-	flesh
pent(a)-	five	scler(o)-	hard
peri-	around	scolio-	crooked
phako-	lens	-scope	observe
pharmaco-	drug	scot(o)-	darkness
pharyng(o)-	pharynx	semi-	half
pheo-	dusky	sens-	perception, feeling
phleb(o)-	vein	sep-	decay
-phob	abnormal fear	sept(o)-	septum
phon(o)-	sound	sider(o)-	iron
phot(o)-	light	somat(o)-	body
pico-	one-trillionth	spectro-	image
pil(i)(o)-	hair	squam(o)-	scale
-plasia	growth	sten(o)-	narrow
plasm(o)-	liquid part of blood	-stol	send
-plegia	paralysis	-stormy	opening
pleur(o)-	pleura, rib, side	sub-	under
-plasty	surgical repair	super-	above, over
plic-	fold, ridge	supra-	above, upon
-pnea	breathing	sym-	union
pneum(o)-	lung	syn-	union
pod(o)-	foot	tachy-	swift, rapid
-poiesis	production	-taxis	movement
poly-	much, many	test-	testicle
-por(o)	passageway	tetra-	four
post-	behind, after	therm(o)-	heat
-praxia	movement	thorac(o)-	chest
pre-	before, in front	thromb(o)-	clot
pro-	before, in front	-tomy	incision
proct(o)-	rectum	toxic(o)-	poisonous
prote(o)-	protein	trache(o)-	trachea
proto-	first	trans-	across, through
pseudo-	false	tri-	three
psych(o)-	mind	trich(o)-	hair
puber-	adult	-tripsy	crushing
pulmo(n)-	lung	-trophy	growth, nutrition
pyel(o)-	pelvis (kidney)	-tropic	influential
pyr(o)-	heat	ultra-	beyond
quadr(i)(u)-	four	uni-	one

Root, prefix, or suffix	Meaning	Root, prefix, or suffix	Meaning
ur(o)-	urine, urinary	vesic(o)-	bladder
-uria	urine	xanth(o)-	yellow
vas(o)-	vessel	xen(o)-	strange, foreign
ven(i)(o)-	vein	xer(o)-	dry
ventr(o)-	belly, front	xiph(o)-	sword
ventriculo-	ventricle	zyg(o)-	yoke, union
vertebr(o)-	vertebra		

Appendix B: English-Spanish translator

If you can't easily obtain the services of a translator to help you communicate with a Spanish-speaking patient, refer to the table below. It's alphabetically arranged to quickly translate medical words and phrases from English to Spanish.

English	Spanish	English	Spanish
Abdomen	Abdomen *or* vientre	Bladder	Vejiga
		Bleeding	Sangramiento
Abortion	Aborto	Blindness	Ceguera
Abscess	Absceso	Bloody stools	Sangre en las heces
Acne	Acné		
Acquired immu-nodeficiency syn-drome (AIDS)	Síndrome de im-munodeficiencia adquirida (SIDA)	Bluish skin discoloration	Descolorimiento azulado de la piel
		Bone	Hueso
Activities of daily living	Actividades nor-males de la vida cotidiana	Brain tumor	Tumor cerebral
		Breast cancer	Cáncer de la mama
		Bronchitis	Bronquitis
Addiction	Adicción	Bruises	Contusiones
Adenoids	Adenoides	Burn (first, second, or third degree)	Quemadura (de primer, segundo o tercer grado)
Adenoma	Adenoma		
Allergic reaction to a medication	Reacción alérgica a un medicamento		
		Burning on urination	Ardor al orinar
Allergy	Alergia		
Anemia	Anemia	Burning sensation	Sensación de ardor
Angina	Angina	Bursitis	Bursitis
Ankle	Tobillo	Buttocks	Nalgas
Ankle swelling	Hinchazón de tobillo	Calf	Pantorrilla
		Cancer	Cáncer
Appendicitis	Apendicitis	Cartilage	Cartílago
Arm	Brazo	Cataracts	Cataratas
Armpit	Axila	Cerebral palsy	Parálisis cerebral
Arteriosclerosis	Arteriosclerosis	Change in bowel habits	Cambio de los hábitos de evac-uación intestinal
Arthritis	Artritis		
Asthma	Asma		
Back	Espalda	Chest	Pecho
Backache	Dolor de espalda	Chest pain	Dolor del tórax (pecho)
Black, tarry stools	Heces negras, alquitranadas		
		Chickenpox	Varicela

English	Spanish	English	Spanish
Chills	Escalofríos	Encephalitis	Encefalitis
Chlamydia	Clamidia	Endocrine problem	Problema endocrinológico
Chorea	Corea		
Cold	Resfriado	Epilepsy	Epilepsia
Cold sores	Úlceras de la boca	Erection difficulties	Dificultades de erección
Colitis	Colitis		
Colon cancer	Cáncer del colon	Eye	Ojo
Confusion	Confusión, desorientación	Face	Rostro
		Facial swelling	Inflamación facial
Constipation	Estreñimiento	Faintness	Debilidad, desfallecimiento
Convulsion	Convulsión		
Coronary artery disease	Enfermedad de la arteria coronaria	Farsightedness	Hiperopía
		Fatigue	Fatiga
Cough	Tos	Fever	Fiebre
Cramp	Espasmos, calambres	Finger	Dedo de la mano
		Fistula	Fistula
Cramps	Calambres	Flatulence	Flatulencia
Crohn's disease	Enfermedad de Crohn	Floaters	Flotadores
		Flu	Influenza, gripe
Deafness	Sordera	Fluid retention	Retención de fluido
Degenerative disease	Enfermedad degenerativa	Food allergies	Alergias a alimentos
Diabetes mellitus	Diabetes melitus	Food poisoning	Intoxicación alimentaria
Diarrhea	Diarrea		
Difficulty breathing	Dificultad para respirar	Foot	Pie
		Fracture	Fractura
Difficulty speaking	Dificultad para hablar	Frostbite	Congelación
		Gallbladder attack	Ataque de la vesícular biliar
Difficulty swallowing	Dificultad para tragar		
		Gallstone	Calculo biliar
Difficulty walking	Dificultad para caminar	Gangrene	Gangrena
		Gastric ulcer	Úlcera gástrica
Diphtheria	Difteria	Gastrointestinal disorders	Trastornos gastrointestinales
Discharge	Flujo, secreción		
Dizziness	Vértigo, mareo	Genetic disorders	Trastornos genéticos
Dizzy spells	Episodios de vértigo		
		Genital sores	Llagas genitals
Double vision	Visión doble	Gestational diabetes	Diabetes gestacional
Down syndrome	Síndrome de Down		
Ear	Oreja	Glaucoma	Glaucoma
Ear Injury	Herida en el oído	Gonorrhea	Gonorrea
Eczema	Eccema	Gout	Gota
Ejaculation	Eyaculación	Groin	Ingle
Elevated blood fats	Alto contenido en lípidos sanguíneos	Gums	Encías
		Hair	Cabello *or* pelo
Elbow	Codo	Hallucination	Alucinación
Embolism	Embolismo	Halos around lights	Halos alrededor de las luces
Emphysema	Enfisema		

English	Spanish	English	Spanish
Hand	Mano	Impaired movement	Deterioro de movimiento
Handicap	Impedimento, deficiencia	Indigestion	Indigestión
Harelip	Labio leporino	Infantile paralysis	Parálisis infantil
Hay fever	Fiebro de heno	Infarct	Infarto
Head	Cabeza	Infection	Infeccíon
Headache	Dolor de cabeza	Inflammation	Inflamación
Head injury	Herida en la cabeza	Influenza	Influenza
		Injury	Herida
Hearing	Oído	Itch	Picazón, comezón
Hearing problem	Problema auditivo	Jaundice	Piel amarilla, ictericia
Heart attack	Ataque al corazón		
Heartbeat	Latido	Jaw	Mandíbula
Irregular	Irregular	Joint	Articulación
Rhythmical	Rítmico	Joint pain	Dolor de las articulaciones
Slow	Lento		
Fast (tachycardia)	Taquicardia	Kidney	Riñón
Heartburn	Acedía, acidez estomacal	Kidney stones	Cálculos en el riñón
Heart disease	Enfermedad del corazón	Knee	Rodilla
		Laceration	Laceración
Heart failure	Deficiencia cardiáca	Laryngitis	Laringitis
		Leg	Pierna
Heart murmur	Soplo del corazón	Lesion	Lesión
Heart problem	Problema del corazón	Leukemia	Leucemia
		Lice	Piojos
Heel	Talón	Ligament	Ligamento
Hemorrhage	Hemorragia	Lip	Labio
Hemorrhoids	Almorranas, hemorroides	Loss of appetite	Pérdida de apetito
		Loss of balance	Pérdida de equilibrio
Hepatitis	Hepatitis	Loss of sensation	Pérdida de sensación
Hernia	Hernia		
Herpes	Herpes	Lump	Pella, bulto
High blood pressure	Presión sanguínea alta	Lung problems	Problemas de los pulmones
High cholesterol	Colesterol alto	Malaise	Malestar
Hip	Cadera	Malaria	Malaria
Hit (on face)	Bofetada	Malignancy	Malignidad
Hives	Urticaria	Malignant	Maligno(a)
Hoarseness	Ronquera, afonía	Malnutrition	Desnutrición
Hot flashes	Acceso repentino de calor	Manic-depressive	Maníaco-depresivo(a)
Human immuno-deficiency virus (HIV)	Virus de inmunode-ficiencia humana	Measles	Sarampión
		Medications	Medicamentos
		Memory changes	Cambios en la memoria
Ill	Enfermo(a)		
Illness	Enfermedad	Meningitis	Meningitis
Immunization	Immunizacíon	Menopause	Menopausia

English	Spanish	English	Spanish
Menstrual difficulties	Dificultades con la menstruación	Overdose	Sobredosis
Metastasis	Metástasis	Overweight	Sobrepeso
Migraine	Migraña, jaqueca	Pain	Dolor
Mite	Ácaro	Growing pain	Dolor creciente
Moles	Lunares	Labor pain	Dolor de parto
Mood swings	Cambios de humor	Phantom limb pain	Dolor de miembro fantasma
Mononucleosis	Mononucleosis infecciosa	Referred pain	Dolor referido
Mouth	Boca	Sharp pain	Dolor agudo
Multiple sclerosis	Esclerosis multiple	Shooting pain	Dolor punzante
Mumps	Paperas	Burning pain	Dolor que arde
Muscle	Músculo	Intense pain	Dolor intenso
Muscle aches	Dolor de músculos	Severe pain	Dolor severo
Muscle incoordination	Falta de coordinación muscular	Intermittent pain	Dolor intermitente
Muscle spasms	Espasmos musculares	Throbbing pain	Dolor palpitante
Muscle twitching	Crispamiento muscular	Painful	Doloroso, dolorosa
Muscular dystrophy	Distrofia muscular	Painful intercourse	Dolor al tener relaciones sexuales
Mute	Mudo(a)	Palpitations	Palpitaciones
Myocardial infarct	Infarto cardíaco	Palsy	Parálisis
Myopia	Miopía	Palsy, Bell's	Parálisis facial
Nails	Uñas	Palsy, cerebral	Parálisis cerebral
Nasal discharge	Secreción nasal	Paralysis	Parálisis
Nausea	Nausea	Parkinson's disease	Enfermedad de Parkinson
Near-sightedness	Miopía	Pellagra	Pelagra
Neck	Cuello	Penile discharge	Secreción del pene
Nephritis	Nefritis	Penis	Pene
Nervousness	Nerviosidad	Pernicious anemia	Anemia perniciosa
Neuralgia	Neuralgia	Pertussis	Tos convulsiva
Neurologic disease	Enfermedad neurológica	Pimple	Grano
		Pneumonia	Pulmonía, neumonía
Night sweats	Sudor nocturno	Poison ivy	Hiedra venenosa
Nipple discharge	Secreción del pezón	Poison oak	Zumaque venenoso
Nocturia	Nocturia	Polio	Poliomielitis
Nose	Nariz	Polyps	Pólipos
Nosebleed	Hemorragia nasal	Pregnant	Embarazada
Numbness	Adormecimiento	Premature ejaculation	Eyaculación prematura
Nutrition	Nutrición	Pressure	Presión
Obesity	Obesidad	Psoriasis	Psoriasis
Osteoporosis	Osteoporosis	Pus	Pus
Obstruction	Obstrucción	Pyorrhea	Piorrea
Ophthalmia	Oftalmia	Rabies	Rabia
Osteomyelitis	Osteomielitis	Rash	Erupción
		Rectal cancer	Cáncer del recto

English	Spanish	English	Spanish
Redness	Rojez	Spotted fever	Fiebre púrpura
Relapse	Recaída	Sprain	Torcedura
Renal	Renal	Sputum	Esputo
Rheumatic fever	Fiebre reumática	Staggering gait	Andar tambaleante
Ringing in the ears	Zumbido en los oídos	Stiff neck	Tiesura del cuello, cuello rígido
Roseola	Roséola	Stiffness	Rigidez
Rubella	Rubéola	Stomach ache	Dolor del estómago
Rupture	Ruptura	Stomach ulcer	Úlcera del estómago
Scab	Costra		
Scabies	Sarna	Stress	Tensión
Scar	Cicatriz	Stroke	Ataque cerebral
Scarlet fever	Escarlatina	Suicide	Suicidio
Scratch	Rasguño	Sunburn	Quemadura del sol
Scrotal swelling	Hinchazón del escroto	Sunstroke	Insolación
		Swelling	Hinchazón
Scrotum	Escroto	Syphilis	Sífilis
Seizure	Convulsión	Systemic illness	Enfermedad sistémica
Senility	Sensoriales		
Sensory changes	Cambios sensoriales	Tachycardia	Taquicardia
		Tapeworm	Lombriz solitaria
Sexually transmit-ted disease	Enfermedad transmitida sexualmente	Tenderness	Sensibilidad
		Tendon	Tendón
		Tetanus	Tétano
Shin	Espinilla de la pierna, estrés tibial medial	Thigh	Muslo
		Throat	Garganta
		Thrombosis	Trombosis
Shock	Choque	Thrush	Afta
Shortness of breath	Falta de aire	Thyroid disease	Enfermedad de la tiroides
Shoulder	Hombro	Tingling	Hormigueo
Shuffling gait	Arrastramiento de pies al caminar	Toe	Dedo del pie
		Tongue	Lengua
Sickle cell anemia	Anemia falciforme	Tonsillitis	Amigdalitis
Sinus congestion	Congestión nasal	Tooth	Diente
Sinus infections	Infecciones de los senos paranasales	Toothache	Dolor de muela
		Toxemia	Toxemia
Skin	Piel	Trauma	Trauma
Skin ulcerations	Ulceraciones de la piel	Tuberculosis	Tuberculosis
		Tumor	Tumor
Skull	Cráneo	Typhoid fever	Fiebre tifoidea
Slipped disc	Disco desplazado	Typhus	Tifus, tifo
Smallpox	Viruela	Ulcers	Úlceras
Snakebite	Mordedura de culebra	Unconsciousness	Pérdida del conocimiento
Sore	Llaga	Undulant fever	Fiebre ondulante
Spasms	Espasmos	Unusual bleeding	Sangramiento anormal
Spider bite	Picadura de araña		

English	Spanish	English	Spanish
Urethral discharge	Secreción de la uretra	Worms	Lombriz (las lombrices)
Uremia	Uremia	Wound	Herida
Urinary frequency	Frecuencia urinaria	Wrist	Muñeca
Urinary tract	Vías urinarias	Yellow fever	Fiebre amarilla
Urinary urgency	Urgencia de orinar		
Urine	Orina		
Urine leakage	Pérdida de orina		
Uterus, prolapsed	Prolapso de la matriz		
Vaginal bleeding after intercourse	Sangramiento vaginal después de tener relaciones sexuales		
Vaginal discharge	Secreción vaginal		
Varicose veins	Várices		
Venereal disease (STD)	Enfermedad venérea		
Canker sore	Chancro		
Chancre	Chancro		
Chlamydia	Clamidia		
Cold sore	Úlceras en la boca		
Condyloma	Condiloma		
Genital wart	Verruga genital		
Gonorrhea	Gonorrea		
Herpes genitalis	Herpes genital		
Moniliasis	Moniliasis		
Syphilis	Sífilis		
Trichomonas	Tricomonas		
Vertigo	Vértigo		
Virus	Virus		
Vision	Vista		
Vision changes	Cambios en la vista		
Vomiting	Vómito		
Warmth	Tibieza		
Wart	Verruga		
Weakness	Debilidad		
Weal	Verdugón, moretón		
Weight gain	Aumento de peso		
Weight loss	Pérdida de peso		
Wheeze	Jadeo, silba		
Wheezing	Respiración jadeante		
Whiplash	Concusión de la espina cervical, lesión de latigazo		
Whooping cough	Tos ferina		

Appendix C: Table of equivalents

Metric system equivalents

Metric weight		Household	Metric
1 kilogram (kg or Kg)	= 1,000 grams (g or gm)	1 teaspoon (tsp)	= 5 ml
1 gram	= 1,000 milligrams (mg)	1 tablespoon (T or tbs)	= 15 ml
1 milligram	= 1,000 micrograms (μg or mcg)	2 tablespoons	= 30 ml
0.6 g	= 600 mg	8 ounces	= 236 ml
0.3 g	= 300 mg	1 pint (pt)	= 473 ml
0.1 g	= 100 mg	1 quart (qt)	= 946 ml
0.06 g	= 60 mg	1 gallon (gal)	= 3,785 ml
0.03 g	= 30 mg		
0.015 g	= 15 mg		
0.001 g	= 1 mg		

Metric volume

1 liter (l or L)	= 1,000 milliliters (ml)*
1 milliliter	= 1,000 microliters (μl)

Temperature conversions

Fahrenheit	Celsius	Fahrenheit	Celsius	Fahrenheit	Celsius
106.0	41.1	103.0	39.4	100.0	37.8
105.8	41.0	102.8	39.3	99.8	37.7
105.6	40.9	102.6	39.2	99.6	37.6
105.4	40.8	102.4	39.1	99.4	37.4
105.2	40.7	102.2	39.0	99.2	37.3
105.0	40.6	102.0	38.9	99.0	37.2
104.8	40.4	101.8	38.8	98.8	37.1
104.6	40.3	101.6	38.7	98.6	37.0
104.4	40.2	101.4	38.6	98.4	36.9
104.2	40.1	101.2	38.4	98.2	36.8
104.0	40.0	101.0	38.3	98.0	36.7
103.8	39.9	100.8	38.2	97.8	36.6
103.6	39.8	100.6	38.1	97.6	36.4
103.4	39.7	100.4	38.0	97.4	36.3
103.2	39.6	100.2	37.9	97.2	36.2

Temperature conversions *(continued)*

Fahrenheit	Celsius	Fahrenheit	Celsius	Fahrenheit	Celsius
97.0	36.1	94.6	34.8	92.2	33.4
96.8	36.0	94.4	34.7	92.0	33.3
96.6	35.9	94.2	34.6	91.8	33.2
96.4	35.8	94.0	34.4	91.6	33.1
96.2	35.7	93.8	34.3	91.4	33.0
96.0	35.6	93.6	34.2	91.2	32.9
95.8	35.4	93.4	34.1	91.0	32.8
95.6	35.3	93.2	34.0	90.8	32.7
95.4	35.2	93.0	33.9	90.6	32.6
95.2	35.1	92.8	33.8	90.4	32.4
95.0	35.0	92.6	33.7	90.2	32.3
94.8	34.9	92.4	33.6	90.0	32.2

Weight conversions

1 oz = 30 g   1 lb = 453.6 g   2.2 lb = 1 kg

* 1 ml = 1 cubic centimeter (cc); however, ml is the preferred measurement term used today.